TETRODOTOXIN, SAXITOXIN, AND THE MOLECULAR BIOLOGY OF THE SODIUM CHANNEL

ANNALS OF THE NEW YORK ACADEMY OF SCIENCES
Volume 479

TETRODOTOXIN, SAXITOXIN, AND THE MOLECULAR BIOLOGY OF THE SODIUM CHANNEL

Edited by C. Y. Kao and S.R. Levinson

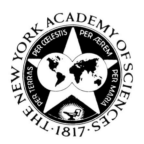

The New York Academy of Sciences
New York, New York
1986

Cover: The front cover of the paperbound edition depicts the chemical structures of saxitoxin (*top*) and tetrodotoxin (*bottom*). The background illustration on the back cover shows the amino acid sequences of the cloned sodium channels of rat brain and electric eel. Superimposed on top of this are current traces from squid giant axon. Traces were taken before (*1*) and during (*2*) action of tetrodotoxin.

Library of Congress Cataloging-in-Publication Data

Tetrodotoxin, saxitoxin, and the molecular biology of
the sodium channel.

(Annals of the New York Academy of Sciences, ISSN
0077-8923, v. 479)
Papers presented at a conference sponsored by the
New York Academy of Sciences held on Dec. 11–13, 1985 in
New York, N.Y.
Includes bibliographies and index.
1. Tetrodotoxin—Physiological effect—Congresses.
2. Saxitoxin—Physiological effect—Congresses.
3. Sodium channels—Congresses.   4. Neurotoxic agents—
Physiological effect—Congresses.   I. Kao, C. Y.
II. Levinson, S. R.   III. New York Academy of Sciences.
IV. Series.   [DNLM: 1. Ion Channels—congresses.
2. Saxitoxin—metabolism—congresses.   3. Tetrodotoxin—
metabolism—congresses.   W1 AN626YL v.479 /
QW 630 T348 1985]
Q11.N5 vol. 479   500 s   86-31231
[QP632.T46]   [591.1'88]
ISBN 0-89766-353-5
ISBN 0-89766-354-3 (pbk.)

SP
Printed in the United States of America
ISBN 0-89766-353-5 (cloth)
ISBN 0-89766-354-3 (paper)
ISSN 0077-8923

ANNALS OF THE NEW YORK ACADEMY OF SCIENCES

Volume 479
December 9, 1986

TETRODOTOXIN, SAXITOXIN, AND THE MOLECULAR BIOLOGY OF THE SODIUM CHANNEL[a]

Editors
C. Y. KAO and S. R. LEVINSON

CONTENTS

---

[a]The papers in this volume were presented at a conference entitled Tetrodotoxin, Saxitoxin, and the Molecular Biology of the Sodium Channel that was sponsored by the New York Academy of Sciences and was held on December 11–13, 1985 in New York, N. Y.

Part VI. Cellular Aspects of Sodium Channels

Part VII. Panel Discussion

Financial assistance was received from:
- AMERICAN CYANAMID COMPANY/MEDICAL RESEARCH DIVISION
- ASTRA
- NATIONAL INSTITUTE OF ENVIRONMENTAL SAFETY AND
  HEALTH—NATIONAL INSTITUTES OF HEALTH
- NATIONAL INSTITUTE OF NEUROLOGICAL AND COMMUNICATIVE
  DISORDERS AND STROKE—NATIONAL INSTITUTES OF HEALTH
- NATIONAL SCIENCE FOUNDATION
- OFFICE OF NAVAL RESEARCH (N00014-85-G-0137)
- A. H. ROBINS COMPANY
- SANDOZ, LTD.
- SCHERING PLOUGH CORPORATION
- STUART PHARMACEUTICALS
- U. S. ARMY MEDICAL RESEARCH AND DEVELOPMENT COMMAND

Preface

C. Y. KAO

Department of Pharmacology
Downstate Medical Center
State University of New York
Brooklyn, New York 11203

S. R. LEVINSON

Department of Physiology
University of Colorado
School of Medicine
Denver, Colorado 80262

Of the various ionic channels now identified, the voltage-gated sodium channel remains the most widely studied, and the one about which most is known. The voltage-gated sodium channel is significant historically as the core of the classical and influential Hodgkin-Huxley formulation of the ionic theory of bioelectric activity. Until recent years, the focus of research on the sodium channel has been biophysical, and studies were confined to the living membrane.

The toxins tetrodotoxin and saxitoxin, which have some uniquely selective actions on this channel, became generally available in the mid-1960s. In addition to becoming important tools for physiological research, they were also the first specific chemical markers by which the sodium channel could be located and isolated. As a result, great strides have been made in the last decade in biochemical studies of this channel, culminating in the recent elucidation of the primary structures of three subtypes of the channel. From now on, studies on the molecular mechanism of the functions of the sodium channel will have to be based on and constrained by knowledge of its structure.

Progress in biochemical studies of the sodium channel has been accompanied by significant new developments in the understanding of the chemistry of both tetrodotoxin and saxitoxin. Not only will these developments help studies on the sodium channel, but an improved understanding of these toxins themselves will undoubtedly lead to more and wiser uses.

At this conference we gathered together bioorganic chemists, electrophysiologists, biochemists, and molecular biologists to summarize their areas of study, our focus being the common theme of the voltage-gated sodium channel. Although tetrodotoxin and saxitoxin were our starting points, some other toxins were also included for discussion because they have added materially to our understanding of the functional aspects of the sodium channel. We have taken a broad view of the molecular biological aspect of the problem that goes beyond molecular genetics. We also feel that the voltage-gated sodium channel is especially relevant when it is reinserted into the framework of cellular function. Finally, we feel that a summary assessment of the current state of knowledge should be coupled with a peek into the near future. These points of view will become readily evident in the organization of this volume, which contains the proceedings of the conference.

It may be appropriate to recall here that we thought the conference went extremely well, and on this point the participants and the audience would undoubtedly concur. For that outcome, we owe everything to the organizational and preparatory work of

Ms. Ellen Marks and her staff, especially Ms. Barbara Parker. For those who have attended previous conferences of the New York Academy of Sciences at the Barbizon-Plaza Hotel, this conference also unintendedly marked a turning point. At the end of the conference the hotel was closed, to be razed and replaced by a luxury condominium apartment building. The voltage-gated sodium channel is a rapidly developing topic, and the timely publication of the proceedings is important. We are indebted to Mr. Bill Boland and Mr. Tom Cohn of the Editorial Department of the New York Academy of Sciences for sparing no effort to achieve that goal.

Tetrodotoxin, Tarichatoxin, and Chiriquitoxin: Historical Perspectives[a]

FREDERICK A. FUHRMAN

Stanford University School of Medicine
Stanford, California 94305

Tetrodotoxin is one of the most poisonous nonprotein substances known. It has a highly unusual chemical structure, and it acts in a specific manner on one of the most fundamental of all physiological processes: the generation of bioelectricity. If one were to seek, through isolation from natural sources or by synthesis, a compound with such pharmacological properties the search would almost certainly have failed. The discovery of tetrodotoxin (and of saxitoxin) was largely a matter of chance. Important achievements in purification and pharmacology occurred after the development of appropriate new methods and tools such as chromatography, microelectrodes, and the voltage clamp.

The first experimental work on the toxin that was eventually identified as tetrodotoxin occurred just about 100 years ago, so this volume is actually a centennial to commemorate the event. Comprehensive accounts of early poisonings in man and of the isolation of tetrodotoxin are available elsewhere.[1-5] Rather than repeat that history, I should like to give a personal account of the development of our knowledge of tetrodotoxin. I am well aware of the pitfalls of such reminiscences. As George F. Kennan wrote recently: "Historical perceptions, like *affaires de coeur,* are a matter of a particular stage in one's life; attempts at repetition are unlikely to be successful."[6] I do not expect to provide anything significant in the way of new data, but I do believe the following historical account of how knowledge about tetrodotoxin developed may have some interest of a kind that is not readily discernable from the scientific literature.

TETRODOTOXIN IN SALAMANDERS: TARICHATOXIN

In the summer of 1941, while still a graduate student, I came to Stanford University for what I thought was to be a summer's research on the metabolism of excised mammalian tissues. I was in fact to remain there for the rest of my professional career. During the course of the summer I was given two vials of pale tan powder with the suggestion that I might like to examine their effects on the metabolism of mammalian brain. One vial was labeled "Paralytic Shellfish Poison" and was a gift of Hermann Sommer and Karl Meyer at the University of California in San Francisco. It contained a very crude preparation of what we now know as saxitoxin. The other vial was labeled "Triturus Toxin" and contained the best preparation that E. L. Tatum and W. J. Van Wagtendonk had been able to prepare from the egg clusters of the local newt, *Taricha* (then *Triturus*) *torosa.*[7] We now know that it consisted of somewhat less

[a]The preparation of this paper was aided by a grant from the Ford Foundation to Stanford University.

1

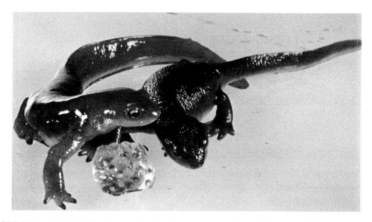

FIGURE 1. Adult California newts, *Taricha torosa,* male and female, with an egg cluster.

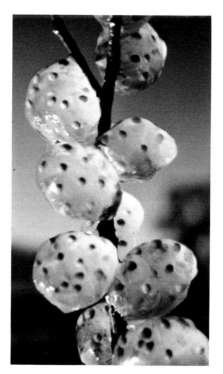

FIGURE 2. Egg clusters of the newt, *Taricha torosa,* attached to a twig. The eggs are laid under water. Each cluster is about 2 cm in diameter and contains about 20 embryos.

than 1% tetrodotoxin. I shall now refer to this toxin as tarichatoxin, although the genus remained *Triturus* for several more years.

At the time, we knew that both these toxins produced paralysis in mammals and there were suggestions that they affected the central nervous system as well as peripheral neurons.[8] There was no hint that they were related chemically or pharmacologically. Much of our thinking at that time about the mechanism of action of anesthetics and other central nervous system depressants was dominated by Quastel's hypothesis[9] that such compounds selectively inhibited the metabolism of glucose by brain tissue. Therefore, I tested the effect of both these crude preparations on the oxygen consumption and glycolysis of brain slices.[7,10] Not surprisingly, they had no effect whatsoever, a result confirmed by Quastel himself 25 years later. He then showed, however, that tetrodotoxin did inhibit the extra oxygen consumption of brain slices produced by electrical stimulation,[11] a phenomenon linked to the influx of sodium ions[12] but requiring a technique unknown in 1941. Little more was accomplished in 1941 because, during the war, most of us became involved in research on problems of more immediate importance. Work on tarichatoxin was postponed but not forgotten.

The story of tetrodotoxin in newts began in a wholly unexpected and fortuitous way. In 1932 Victor Twitty, an experimental embryologist, joined the Stanford faculty soon after completing his doctoral research at Yale University under Ross G. Harrison. At that time a popular and productive research procedure consisted of transplanting rudimentary organs between different species of amphibian embryos. At Yale, Twitty had used *Ambystoma tigrinum* and *A. punctatum* for this purpose. At Stanford he soon found that after winter rains the ponds behind the Stanford campus abounded in *Taricha torosa* (FIG. 1). These newts lay their eggs in clusters (FIG. 2) in ponds and streams. Twitty soon transplanted eye and limb rudiments from *Taricha* into *Ambystoma*, and much to his surprise found the hosts became paralyzed, but eventually recovered.[13] Injection of simple extracts of *Taricha* egg clusters into various other amphibians and mammals confirmed that the eggs did indeed contain a highly toxic substance.[14] Twitty also showed by grafting experiments that this or a similar toxin was present in other species of California newt as well as in the Japanese newt *Cynops (Triturus) pyrrhogaster* and the Eastern American newt *Notophthalmus (Triturus) viridescens.*[15]

Obviously, the next step was chemical purification of the toxin and Twitty was fortunate that a talented biochemist, E. L. Tatum (later Nobel laureate with George Beadle), was working in an adjoining laboratory. Horsburgh, Tatum, and Hall used a preparation from *Taricha* egg clusters purified mainly by precipitating impurities with ethanol, to show that in cats the toxin produced hypotension, respiratory paralysis, and unresponsiveness of the tibialis anticus muscle stimulated via the sciatic nerve.[8] Shortly thereafter Tatum and Van Wagtendonk tried various methods of further purification (adsorption, precipitation with alkaloidal reagents, high vacuum molecular distillation) without marked success.[7] They did establish that the toxic component of the mixture had a molecular weight of 200–400. Their best preparation had a lethal dose of about 64 mouse units per milligram, equivalent to about 1% tetrodotoxin. It was this preparation that I encountered in 1941.

It was thus clear 45 years ago that embryos of *Taricha torosa* contained a potent, low molecular weight neurotoxin that certainly was not a general metabolic poison. The evidence did not permit us to decide whether the toxin acted on nerve axons, the neuromuscular junction, or muscle fibers. The next logical step was to test the toxin on nerve axons, but in 1941 neither the necessary equipment nor anyone who could operate it existed at Stanford. It was not until 1946 that Robert Turner, my colleague in the anatomy department, and I were able to test tarichatoxin on the action potentials of frog nerve axons.[16] The results showed clearly that the toxin reduced the action potential and that the effect was completely reversible (FIG. 3).

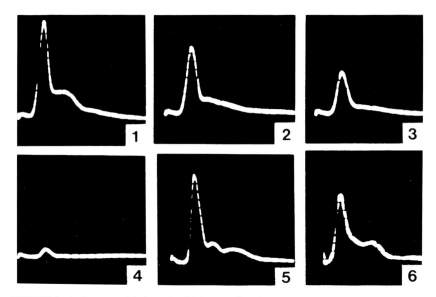

FIGURE 3. Action potentials from the tibial nerve of the frog, *Rana pipiens. 1,* normal control. *2, 3,* and *4,* 15, 30, and 60 seconds after application of crude tarichatoxin. *5,* Same nerve 2 minutes after washing. *6,* Same nerve after three cycles of toxin and washing.[16]

In 1960 I returned to the question of the chemical nature of tarichatoxin. With the development of chromatography, I thought that it might be possible to isolate the active compound, and began some experiments of this kind. Soon after, I happened to talk with the organic chemist Harry Mosher, my campus neighbor, who told me that Victor Twitty had discussed with him the feasibility of a chemical approach to a quite different problem connected with *Taricha.* Twitty had found that *Taricha* in streams of coastal California disappear after breeding, but return precisely to their "home" segment of stream the next year to lay their eggs. Twitty wondered whether a chemical cue was involved. Obviously, the problems of chemical research in this area were formidable. I immediately suggested that it might be more productive to investigate the chemical nature of tarichatoxin. I also offered to provide some partially purified material to start with. Fortunately, Harry Mosher liked my idea. A talented graduate student was available to assist him, and in a year and a half Brown and Mosher[17] obtained a crystalline compound with a lethal dose of about 10 μg/kg.

The next problem was collecting sufficient quantities of egg clusters to isolate enough pure compound for study of the chemical structure. The toxin is located in the eggs and embryos which are embedded in the gelatinous mass. Over the course of three years we were able to collect almost 1000 kg of egg clusters. It is fortunate that *Taricha torosa* lays its eggs in clusters rather than singly, as does *Taricha granulosa.* The collection of a ton of single eggs would have been an almost impossible task.

With crystalline tarichatoxin in our hands, it was obvious that such a toxic compound required definitive pharmacological investigation, and for this C. Y. Kao joined us for a summer at Stanford in 1962. We were able to establish that the major systemic effects of tarichatoxin were attributable to a block of preganglionic cholinergic and somatic motor nerves.[18] The block occurred without depolarization. Thus the pharmacological properties of the newt toxin resembled those of both saxitoxin and of tetrodotoxin from puffer fish. A search of the literature showed that no nonprotein substance with toxicity equal to or greater than these three compounds had ever been described. Unlikely as it seemed, we considered the possibility that tarichatoxin was identical with either saxitoxin or tetrodotoxin. There were sound chemical reasons for eliminating saxitoxin from consideration. However, as data accumulated, the resemblance to tetrodotoxin became even stronger. Through the kind cooperation of Professor K. Tsuda of the University of Tokyo we obtained a generous supply of authentic tetrodotoxin from puffer fish. This permitted us to make direct comparisons of the pharmacological and chemical properties of tetrodotoxin and tarichatoxin. For example, a dose of 1000 μg/kg of either compound injected into *Taricha torosa* had no effect. This resistance of animals to their own toxin is well documented for tetrodotoxin as well as for other unrelated toxins. Actually, Ishihara[19] found in 1918 that newts as well as puffer fish were resistant to tetrodotoxin, but we were unaware of this finding at the time. The nerves of *Taricha* and puffer fish are also resistant to tetrodotoxin.[20,21] Meanwhile, Harry Mosher and his group of chemists demonstrated that the IR spectra of tarichatoxin and tetrodotoxin (from fugu) were identical and that the physical properties of three acetates of the two toxins were identical. We thus came to the inevitable conclusion that tarichatoxin was tetrodotoxin even though it existed in newts.[22] All species of Salamandridae so far studied contain a toxin, but crystalline tetrodotoxin has been obtained from only two species (TABLE 1).

TETRODOTOXIN IN TETRAODONTID FISHES

Many fish belonging to the order Tetraodontiformes (Plectognathi) have been known to be poisonous since the beginning of recorded history. This is probably because many of them, in contrast to newts, are valued as food. Charles Rémy, who visited Japan in 1882 and whose research I shall soon mention, put it this way: *"la chair de ces redoubtable poissons est exquise"* ("the flesh of these redoubtable fishes is exquisite"). These fish are referred to as *fugu* or pufferfish, globefish, and swellfish, because of their ability to blow themselves up (FIG. 4). One of them, identified as *Tetraodon lineatus,* is shown on an Egyptian tomb of the Fifth Dynasty (ca. 2500 B.C.),[24] and there is evidence that the early Egyptians knew this fish to be poisonous.

TABLE 1. Tetrodotoxin in Newts of the Family Salamandridae

Species	Relative Toxicity	Habitat	Refs.
Taricha torosa[a]	high	California	59, 64
Taricha rivularis[a]	high	northern California	59, 64
Taricha granulosa[a]	high	northwestern United States	59, 64
Notophthalmus viridescens[a]	medium	eastern United States	59, 64, 65
Cynops pyrrhogaster	low	Japan	59,64
Cynops ensicauda	low	Ryukyu Islands	64
Paramesotriton hongkongensis	low	China	59
Triturus vulgaris	slight	Europe and Western Asia	64
Triturus cristatus	slight	Europe	64
Triturus alpestris	slight	Europe	64
Triturus marmoratus	slight	Europe	64

[a]Toxin tentatively or definitely identified as tetrodotoxin.

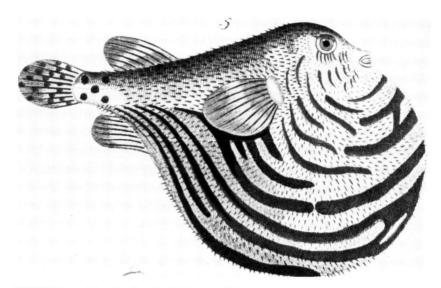

FIGURE 4. An inflated puffer fish, *Globe rayé*. (Nineteenth-century colored lithograph from the author's collection.)

The earliest Chinese materia medica, the *Pen-T'so Chin* (*The Herbal*), usually attributed to the legendary Emperor Shun Nung (2838–2698 B.C.), lists the eggs of tetraodon fishes among its drugs.[3] However, we may doubt the authenticity of the authorship, since a dragon was implicated in the birth of Shun Nung.[25] *The Herbal* was probably written in the first or second century B.C.[3] Puffer fish are clearly described and included among the drugs in the *Pen-T'so Kang Mu* (*Great Herbal*) of Li Shih-Chen in 1596. None of this, however, was known to Europeans of that era. They first learned of poisonous tetraodon fishes, and many other aspects of Japanese life, from Engelbert Kaempfer's *History of Japan*, published in London in 1727.[26] The author was physician to the Dutch embassy in Nagasaki from 1690 to 1693, at a time when Japan was closed to Europeans except for the Dutch in Nagasaki. Kaempfer obtained much of his information from translators and others by "liberally assisting them... with my advice and medicines, with what information I was able to give them in Astronomy and Mathematicks, and with a cordial and plentiful supply of European liquors." This fascinating work is illustrated with many engravings derived from Japanese sources. Kaempfer described a puffer fish thus: "Furube is another Fish, not very large. The Dutch call him Blazer, which signifys Blower, because he can blow and swell himself up into the form of a round Ball. He is rank'd among the poisonous Fish, and if eat whole, is said unavoidably to occasion death." (See FIG. 5.)

During the two centuries after Kaempfer's sojourn in Japan a number of European naturalists and physicians described poisonings by puffer fish in China, India, Malaya, Cambodia, the Philippines, Baja California, and the South Pacific. Many of these reports are listed by Halstead.[4] The best known and most vivid description of poisoning by tetraodon fish occurs in the journals of Captain James Cook[27] from the voyage of HMS *Resolution* on 8 September 1774: "About three to four o'clock in the morning (after eating some liver and roe for dinner) we were seized with most extraordinary weakness in all our limbs attended with numbness of sensation like to that caused by exposing ones hands and feet to a fire after having been pinched much by frost. I had almost lost the sense of feeling nor could I distinguish between light and heavy objects, a quart pot full of water and a feather was the same in my hand." In spite of many such case reports, no experimental work seems to have been published. A Dr. Eldridge of Yokohama[28] appended the following footnote to his brief report in 1879: "Since the above was written the writer has been engaged in experimental researches upon the *fugu* poison, his results being of so positive a nature that he hopes at no distant day to present an account of the subject more complete than any yet published." But the report seems never to have been printed.

On 14 April 1883 Charles Rémy reported to the Societé de Biologie (in Paris) the results of the first experimental work on poisonous "fougou" carried out in Japan during a visit the preceding year.[29] In an extensive article[23] he listed the five most poisonous species, from a list provided by a Dr. Geerts, and reviewed the earlier observations of others. He described the symptoms and established that the toxin was mainly in the gonads. At about this time many young Japanese traveled to Europe, principally to Germany, for further education. Upon returning to Japan they established modern experimental medical science in that country. Among them was D. Takahashi, who became the first professor of pharmacology at the University of Tokyo. In 1889 he published (with Y. Inoko) the first comprehensive study of the pharmacology of tetrodotoxin.[30] They described the hypotension and respiratory depression and noted that the heart continued to beat after the respiration had stopped.

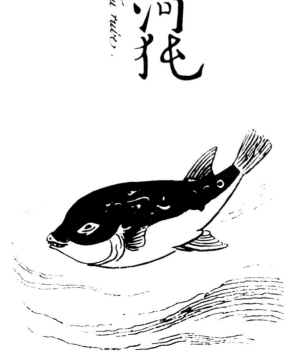

FIGURE 5. Fugu, or puffer fish, from Kaempfer's *History of Japan.*[26] (From a late seventeenth-century Japanese original.)

They attempted, without success, to purify the toxin. They also observed that tetraodon fish were resistant to their own toxin.[31] This volume commemorates the centennial of these two first series of experiments.

Renewed efforts to isolate the active principle of fugu ovaries began in Tokyo late in the 19th century and were published in detail in 1911 by Tahara (also "Tawara").[32] His best preparation, which he named "tetrodotoxin," had a toxicity of 4 mg/kg and was thus about 4% pure. It was used in many pharmacological studies for a decade or more and was awarded a United States patent in 1913.[33]

Isolation of crystalline tetrodotoxin was not achieved until 1950 by Yokoo,[34] who called the product "spheroidine." When it was later shown to be identical to a toxin isolated in 1952 by Tsuda and Kawamura[35] named tetrodotoxin, the latter name prevailed. Isolation of tetrodotoxin occurred well after that of many plant alkaloids (morphine, atropine, strychnine, etc.) and of most vitamins (*e.g.,* biotin and pantothenic acid). When the methods used for purification of these compounds were applied to puffer fish ovaries or newt eggs, they failed completely. This is now understandable because of the unique chemical properties of tetrodotoxin.

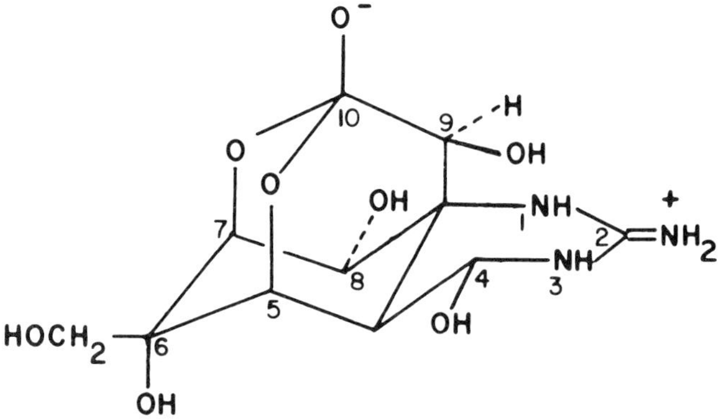

FIGURE 6. Tetrodotoxin.

Once crystalline tetrodotoxin was available, it was possible to conduct meaningful studies of chemical structure. An exciting race ensued to solve the structure of this unusual toxin. This culminated in April 1964 in Kyoto at the Natural Products Symposium of the International Union of Pure and Applied Chemistry, when the same structure (FIG. 6) was reported by chemists from four different groups headed by K. Tsuda, T. Goto, R. B. Woodward, and H. S. Mosher.

Most investigators have presumed that the toxin in all species of *Tetraodon* fish is tetrodotoxin. However, crystalline tetrodotoxin has been obtained from only about a half dozen of some 40 species of these fish. Kao[3] gives a comprehensive list of toxic Tetraodontiformes. It is now becoming evident that substances with pharmacological properties closely similar to tetrodotoxin itself occur in these fish as well as in other animals. Nakamura and Yasumoto[36] identified tetrodonic acid, 4-*epi*tetrodotoxin and anhydrotetrodotoxin in *Takifugu (Fugu) pardalis* and in *T. poecilonotus.* These compounds are far less toxic than tetrodotoxin and are easily overlooked in a search based only on toxicity. Shiomi *et al.*[37] found evidence of the presence of toxins other than tetrodotoxin in *Lagocephalus lunaris* and *Fugu niphobles.* Even the dinoflagellate toxin, saxitoxin, has been found in puffer fish.[38,39] Toxicity alone is thus not sufficient proof of the presence of tetrodotoxin even in closely related species. Identification must be based on definitive chemical evidence of the nature of the toxin.

The basic pharmacology of tetrodotoxin that eventually led to the demonstration of its highly specific action on sodium channels has a long history. Almost a century ago Takahashi and Inoko[30] found that stimulation of motor nerves in frogs poisoned with tetrodotoxin failed to elicit a response, although the muscle itself responded to direct stimulation. Ishihara,[19] in 1918, showed that sensory nerves were also blocked, and that the block was confined to the segment of a nerve that had been exposed to the toxin. A few years later, Iwakawa and Kimura[40] compared the local anesthetic action of tetrodotoxin with that of cocaine. Modern research on effects of tetrodotoxin on cellular processes began in 1960 with experiments of Narahashi and associates that made use of intracellular microelectrodes.[41] Their experiments indicated that tetrodotoxin blocked the action potential of muscle fibers by inhibiting the transient increase in conductance associated with movement of sodium ions across the membrane. This was confirmed by studies on voltage-clamped lobster axons by Narahashi et al.[42] at Duke University.[42] Shortly thereafter we provided the Duke group with a sample of tarichatoxin which they (Takata et al.[43]) found to have an identical effect. Before the paper could be published, we identified tarichatoxin as tetrodotoxin. Fortunately the results of both series of experiments were identical.

TETRODOTOXIN AND CHIRIQUITOXIN IN FROGS

In 1964 we thought that tetrodotoxin occurred only in tetraodon fishes and in newts. Although the occurrence in these two unrelated groups of animals seemed odd, it was only another among several such peculiar distributions of chemical substances. We saw no reason to look for tetrodotoxin in other animals, so we sought other toxins from amphibia. It has been suggested that brilliant colors serve as a warning to predators that the animal is poisonous. Certain vividly colored frogs of the families Dendrobatidae and Atelopidae from Central and South America have been known for centuries to be poisonous. Poisons for arrows and darts were prepared from the skins of some of them.[44] We began work on the Atelopidae because Witkop and Daly[45] had already begun investigation of toxins from the Dendrobatidae. We soon found that the skin of the brilliant orange and black *Atelopus zeteki* frog from Panama (FIG. 7) yielded a nonprotein toxin with an LD_{50} of 16 µg/kg in mice that we termed atelopidtoxin (later, zetekitoxin).[46] It produced hypotension and a variety of cardiac arrhythmias in dogs.[47] In amphibian and fish hearts it produced the rarely observed phenomenon of circus contraction. Before investigation of the chemical nature of zetekitoxin could be completed,[48] the frogs from which it was obtained were declared an endangered species, and we reluctantly sought a source from other species of Atelopidae.

Among 12 species, subspecies, and distinct populations of frogs that we studied, all were toxic. In addition to *A. zeteki,* three of these yielded enough material for chemical identification of the toxin[49] (TABLE 2). The close taxonomic relationship of these frogs is apparent from a recent systematic revision of the genus from Costa Rica and Panama that recognizes only three species: *A. varius, A. chiriquiensis,* and *A. senex.* Much to our surprise, Mosher and his associates identified the major toxin in *A. varius* from San José Province, Costa Rica (FIG. 7) as tetrodotoxin. Tetrodotoxin also occurred in a green and black frog from Costa Rica identified as *A. varius ambulatorius.* The skins and eggs of a fourth atelopid, *A. chiriquiensis* (FIGURE 8),

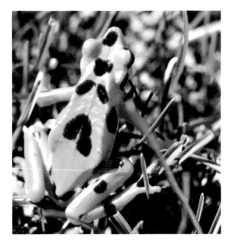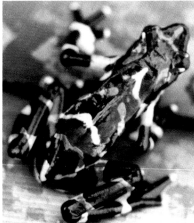

FIGURE 7. Left: *Atelopus varius* (*A. v. zeteki*) from El Vallé de Anton, Panama. Right: *Atelopus varius* (*A. v. varius*) from San Antonio de Patarra, San José Province, Costa Rica. (Photograph by H. S. Mosher.)

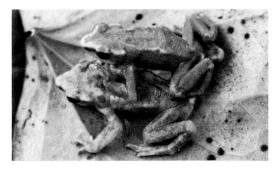

FIGURE 8. *Atelopus chiriquiensis* from Cerro de la Muerte, Costa Rica. (Photograph by H. S. Mosher.)

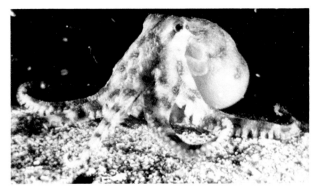

FIGURE 9. The Australian blue-ringed octopus, *Hapalochlaena maculosa*. (Photograph by K. Gillett, courtesy of M. E. H. Howden.)

yielded not only tetrodotoxin, but a new toxin designated chiriquitoxin. This analogue of tetrodotoxin differs only at C-6, where the -CH$_2$OH group is replaced by an unidentified group with a mass of 104 (FIG. 5). The LD$_{50}$ in mice was 13 μg/kg rather than the 10 μg/kg found for tetrodotoxin. Effects in anesthetized mammals were similar to those of tetrodotoxin. Kao and his associates[50] found that chiriquitoxin blocked not only the sodium channels but also interfered with movement of potassium ions. Chiriquitoxin appears to be less stable than tetrodotoxin and isolation of additional amounts has proved elusive.

TETRODOTOXIN IN OTHER ANIMALS

While investigation of the toxins in atelopid frogs was in progress, we were surprised by the announcement that tetrodotoxin occurred in a goby, *Gobius criniger,* a fish unrelated to the Tetraodontidae. This goby has been known to be poisonous for over a century.[51] In 1971 Hashimoto and Noguchi[52] reported the presence of a

TABLE 2. Tetrodotoxin in Frogs of the Family Atelopidae

Species	Color	Habitat	Organ	Toxin % Tetrodotoxin	Refs.
Atelopus varius (A. v. zeteki)	black and orange	El Vallé de Anton, Panama	skin	<5	49
Atelopus varius (A. v. varius)	black and red on yellow	San Antonio de Patarra, San José Province, Costa Rica	skin	100	49
Atelopus varius (A. v. ambulatorius)	mottled black on green	Vallé de Parrazu, Costa Rica	skin	100	49
Atelopus chiriquiensis	yellow, yellow-green, gray, rust-gray	Cerro de la Muerte, San José Province, Costa Rica	skin eggs	30	49, 66

tetrodotoxin-like substance in specimens from Amami-Oshima Island, and in 1973 they[53] isolated crystalline tetrodotoxin from them. We[54] have evidence that a toxin resembling tetrodotoxin is present in three species of California goby, but we have been unable to isolate the toxin in sufficient quantity to determine its identity.

Several cephalopod mollusks (octopuses and squid) secrete a variety of pharmacologically active substances from their posterior salivary glands. These serve to immobilize their prey. The Australian blue-ringed octopus (*Hapalochlaena maculosa*) is particularly poisonous (FIG. 9). Although only about 10 cm long, its bite can be fatal to an adult human being. The toxin from its posterior salivary glands, maculotoxin, has been known to resemble tetrodotoxin since 1970,[55] but there were conflicting reports about its identity. This was resolved in 1978 by the isolation of crystalline tetrodotoxin from this octopus.[56] The same toxin appears to be present in the eggs.[57] The occurrence of tetrodotoxin only in the posterior salivary glands of the adult octopus is quite different from the distribution in fish, newts, and frogs. In these animals the toxin is usually found in the gonads and skin.

Recently tetrodotoxin has been identified in a variety of gastropod mollusks from certain regions of the coast of Japan, as well as in a crab and a starfish (for references see ref. 58). Some of these animals also contain other toxins, and it will be of interest to learn whether analogues of tetrodotoxin can be identified in any of them.

CONCLUSION

I have mentioned that the poisonous nature of tetraodon fish has been known for several thousand years. Many fatalities have occurred, and still occur, from eating these fish. Strange as it may seem, there are two recorded cases, one fatal, of human poisoning from swallowing a newt, *Taricha granulosa*.[59,60] There are two other major types of poisoning from eating marine animals. One is, of course, paralytic shellfish poisoning. The other is ciguatera. This has been recognized as a distinct type of food poisoning since 1771.[61] The sources of the toxins causing ciguatera and paralytic

TABLE 3. Occurrence of Tetrodotoxin

Phylum	Class	Family	Common Name
Chordata	Amphibia	Salamandridae	newts
		Atelopidae	Atelopid frogs
	Osteichthys (Pisces)	Tetraodontidae	puffer fish
		Lagocephalus	
		Diodontidae	porcupine fish
		Canthigasteridae	sharp-backed puffers
		Chilomycterus	
		Gobidae	gobies
Mollusca	Gastropoda	Buccinidae, Bursidae, Terebridae, etc.	marine snails
	Cephalopoda	Octopodidae	octopuses
Echinodermata	Asteroidea	Astropectinidae	starfish
Arthropoda	Crustacea	Xanthidae	crabs

shellfish poisoning remained unknown for many years, but are now identified as dinoflagellates. Conversely, the source of tetrodotoxin, which seemed to be firmly established, is now uncertain. As long as tetrodotoxin was thought to be confined to fish of the order Tetraodontiformes, it seemed reasonable that it originated as a metabolic product, perhaps evolved for protection against predators. The discovery of tetrodotoxin in newts made this idea less certain, but perhaps still tenable. Now that tetrodotoxin has been identified in animals from six different classes in four different phyla (TABLE 3), its endogenous production becomes quite unlikely. As Mothes[62] wrote in 1981: "It is difficult to imagine that such a substance has been invented several times during evolution." Mosher and I have presented elsewhere evidence for the possible origin of tetrodotoxin.[63] This may be through a food chain or from a symbiotic organism. More evidence is presented in this volume by Yasumoto.[67] Whatever the source, tetrodotoxin has proved to be an important tool in research. Much of the knowledge about sodium channels that is presented in this volume was made possible by this fascinating compound.

ACKNOWLEDGMENTS

I thank M. E. H. Howden of Macquarie University for the fine photograph of the Australian blue-ringed octopus.

REFERENCES

1. MOSHER, H. S., F. A. FUHRMAN, H. D. BUCHWALD & H. G. FISCHER. 1964. Science 144: 1100–1110.
2. TSUDA, K. 1966. Naturwissenschaften 53: 171–176.
3. KAO, C. Y. 1966. Pharmacol. Rev. 18: 997–1049.
4. HALSTEAD, B. W. 1967. Poisonous and Venomous Marine Animals of the World, vol. 2. U. S. Government Printing Office. Washington, D. C.
5. EVANS, M. H. 1972. Int. Rev. Neurobiol. 15: 83–166.
6. KENNAN, G. F. 1985. The New Yorker. Feb. 25, 52.
7. VAN WAGTENDONK, W. J., F. A. FUHRMAN, E. L. TATUM & J. FIELD II. 1942. Biol. Bull. 83: 137–144.
8. HORSBURGH, D. B., E. L. TATUM & V. E. HALL. 1940 J. Pharmacol. Exp. Ther. 68: 284–291.
9. QUASTEL, J. H. 1939. Physiol. Rev. 19: 135–183.
10. FUHRMAN, F. A. & J. FIELD II. 1941. Proc. Soc. Exp. Biol. Med. 48: 423–425.
11. CHAN, S. L. & J. H. QUASTEL. 1956. Science 156: 1752–1753.
12. OKAMOTO, K. & J. H. QUASTEL. 1970. Biochem. J. 120: 37–47.
13. TWITTY, V. C. & H. A. ELLIOTT. 1934. J. Exp. Zool. 68: 247–291.
14. TWITTY, V. C. & H. H. JOHNSON. 1934. Science 80: 78–79.
15. TWITTY, V. C. 1937. J. Exp. Zool. 76: 67–104.
16. TURNER, R. S. & F. A. FUHRMAN. 1947. Am. J. Physiol. 105: 325–328.
17. BROWN, M. S. & H. S. MOSHER. 1963. Science 140: 295–296.
18. KAO, C. Y. & F. A. FUHRMAN. 1963. J. Pharmacol. Exp. Ther. 140: 31–40.
19. ISHIHARA, F. 1918. Mitt. Med. Fac. Tokyo Univ. 20: 375–426.
20. KAO, C. Y. & F. A. FUHRMAN. 1967. Toxicon 5: 25–34.
21. KIDOKORO, Y., A. D. GRINNELL & D. C. EATON. 1974. J. Comp. Physiol. 89: 59–72.
22. BUCHWALD, H. D., L. DURHAM, H. G. FISCHER, R. HARADA, H. S. MOSHER, C. Y. KAO & F. A. FUHRMAN. 1964. Science 143: 474–475.
23. RÉMY, C. 1883. Mem. Soc. Biol. (Paris) 35: 1–28.
24. GAILLARD, C. 1923. Mem. Inst. Francais Arch. Orient. 51: 97–100.
25. WONG, K. C. & L. T. WU. 1936. History of Chinese Medicine. 2d ed. National Quarantine Service. Shanghai.
26. KAEMPFER, E. 1727. The History of Japan. Giving an Account of the Ancient and Present State and Government of That Empire; of Its Temples, Palaces, Castles, and Other Buildings; of Its Metals, Minerals, Trees, Plants, Animals, Birds, and Fishes; etc. J. G. Scheuchzer, Trans. London.
27. BEAGLEHOLE, J. C., Ed. 1961. The Journals of Captain Cook, vol 2. Voyages of the *Resolution* and *Adventure* 1772–1775. Cambridge University Press. London. pp. 534–535.
28. ELDRIDGE, S. 1879. Med. Times Gaz. 2: 377–378.
29. RÉMY, C. 1883. C. Rend. Soc. Biol. 35: 263–265.
30. TAKAHASHI, D. & Y. INOKO. 1889. Arch. Exp. Pathol. Pharmakol. 26: 401–418.
31. TAKAHASHI, D. & Y. INOKO. 1889. Arch Exp. Pathol. Pharmakol. 26: 453–458.
32. TAHARA, Y. 1911. Biochem. Z. 10: 255–275.
33. TAHARA, Y. 1913. U. S. Patent 1 058 643.

34. YOKOO, A. 1950. J. Chem. Soc. Jpn **71:** 590–592.
35. TSUDA, K. & M. KAWAMURA. 1952. J. Pharm. Soc. Jpn **72:** 771–773.
36. NAKAMURA, M. & T. YASUMOTO. 1985. Toxicon **23:** 271–276.
37. SHIOMI, K., H. INAOKA, H. YAMANAKA & T. KIKUCHI. 1985. Toxicon **23:** 331–336.
38. KODAMA, M., T. OGATA, T. NOGUCHI, J. MARUYAMA & K. HASHIMOTO. 1983. Toxicon **21:** 897–900.
39. NAKAMURA, M., Y. OSHIMA & T. YASUMOTO. 1984. Toxicon **22:** 381–385.
40. IWAKAWA, K. & S. KIMURA. 1922. Arch. Exp. Pathol. Pharmacol. **93:** 305–331.
41. NARAHASHI, T., T. DEGUCHI, N. URAKAWA & Y. OHKUBO. 1960. Am. J. Physiol. **198:** 934–938.
42. NARAHASHI, T., J. W. MOORE & W. R. SCOTT. 1964. J. Gen. Physiol. **47:** 965–974.
43. TAKATA, M., J. W. MOORE, C. Y. KAO & F. A. FUHRMAN. 1966. J. Gen. Physiol. **49:** 977–988.
44. LEWIN, L. 1923. Die Pfeilgifte. Barth. Leipzig.
45. DALY, J. W., B. WITKOP, P. BOMMER & K. BIEMANN. 1965. J. Am. Chem. Soc. **87:** 124–126.
46. FUHRMAN, F. A., G. J. FUHRMAN & H. S. MOSHER. 1969. Science **165:** 1376–1377.
47. RANNEY, B. K., G. J. FUHRMAN & F. A. FUHRMAN. 1970. J. Pharmacol. Exp. Ther. **175:** 368–376.
48. BROWN, G. B., Y. H. KIM, H. KÜNTZEL, H. S. MOSHER, G. J. FUHRMAN & F. A. FUHRMAN. 1977. Toxicon **15:** 115–128.
49. KIM, Y. H., G. B. BROWN, H. S. MOSHER & F. A. FUHRMAN. 1975. Science **189:** 151–152.
50. KAO, C. Y., P. N. YEOH, M. D. GOLDFINGER, F. A. FUHRMAN & H. S. MOSHER. 1981. J. Pharmacol. Exp. Ther. **217:** 416–429.
51. FONSSAGRIVES, J.-B. 1877. Traité d'Hygiene Navale. 2d ed. J. B. Baillière. Paris.
52. HASHIMOTO, Y. & T. NOGUCHI. 1971. Toxicon **9:** 79–84.
53. NOGUCHI, T. & Y. HASHIMOTO. 1973. Toxicon **11:** 305–307.
54. ELAM, K. S., F. A. FUHRMAN, Y. H. KIM & H. S. MOSHER. 1977. Toxicon **14:** 45–49.
55. FREEMAN, S. E. & R. J. TURNER. 1970. Toxicol. Appl. Pharmacol. **16:** 681–690.
56. SHEUMACK, D. D., M. E. H. HOWDEN, I. SPENCE & R. J. QUINN. 1978. Science **199:** 188–189.
57. SHEUMACK, D. D., M. E. H. HOWDEN & I. SPENCE. 1984. Toxicon **22:** 811–812.
58. MARUYAMA, J. & T. NOGUCHI. 1984. Mer (Tokyo) (Bull. Soc. Fr.-Jpn Oceanogr.) **22:** 299–304.
59. BRODIE, E. D., JR., J. L. HEUSEL, JR. & J. A. JOHNSON. 1974. Copeia (no. 2). pp. 506–511.
60. BRADLEY, S. G. & L. J. KLIKA. 1981. J. Am. Med. Assoc. **246:** 247.
61. POEY, F. 1866. Repert. Fisico-Natural Isla Cuba (Havana) **2:** 1–39.(Cited in Halstead, B. W. 1978. Poisonous and Venomous Marine Animals of the World. Rev. ed. Darwin Press. Princeton, N. J.)
62. MOTHES, K. 1981. The Problem of Chemical Convergence in Secondary Metabolism. *In* Science and Scientists. M. Kageyama *et al.,* Eds.: 323–326. Jpn Scientific Soc. Press. Tokyo.
63. MOSHER, H. S. & F. A. FUHRMAN. 1984. Occurrence and Origin of Tetrodotoxin. *In* Seafood Toxins. E. P. Ragelis, Ed. Am. Chem. Soc. Symposium Series no. 262. pp. 333–344.
64. WAKELY, J. F., G. J. FUHRMAN, F. A. FUHRMAN, H. G. FISCHER & H. S. MOSHER. 1966. Toxicon **3:** 195–203.
65. LEVENSON, C. H. & A. M. WOODHULL. 1979. Toxicon **17:** 184–187.
66. PAVELKA, L. A., Y. H. KIM & H. S. MOSHER. 1977. Toxicon **15:** 135–139.
67. YASUMOTO, T., H. NAGAI, D, YASUMURA, T. MICHISHITA, A. ENDO, M. YOTSU & Y. KOTAKI. 1986. Interspecies distribution and possible origin of tetrodotoxin. This volume.

Chemistry and Biology of Saxitoxin and Related Toxins

EDWARD J. SCHANTZ

Department of Food Microbiology and Toxicology
University of Wisconsin
Madison, Wisconsin 53706

Our present knowledge of the highly lethal neurotoxin known as paralytic shellfish poison or mussel poison, and now called saxitoxin, has had a long and interesting development. This paper is a summary of some work on the paralytic shellfish poisons (PSP) that I have carried out during the past 40 years in collaboration with many of my colleagues. Its purposes are (1) to review briefly the clinical history and aspects of human paralytic shellfish poisoning, and (2) to review in some detail the development of the chemical and physical aspects of saxitoxin that may be related to its biological function of reducing the permeability at the sodium channel of nerve and muscle membranes. A thorough knowledge of the structural aspects of saxitoxin and its derivatives is essential in this respect.

CLINICAL HISTORY AND ORIGIN OF SAXITOXIN[1]

Medical records for several centuries have described cases of food poisoning from eating mussels and clams at certain times with symptoms that indicate saxitoxin or one of its derivatives was involved. The diagnosis of the paralytic form of shellfish poisoning is not difficult, particularly if symptoms occur shortly after the misfortune of eating a meal containing toxic shellfish. The symptoms in man apparently are of nervous origin and may set in immediately after the meal. A prickly feeling in the lips, tongue, and fingertips followed by numbness are the first signs of intoxication. An ataxic gait and muscular incoordination followed by ascending paralysis mark the progress of the intoxication, with death from respiratory failure in from 2 to 24 hours depending on how much of the poison was consumed. If one survives 24 hours the prognosis is good and no lasting effects of the ordeal are apparent.

One of the most puzzling phenomena associated with mussel poisoning was the unpredictable and sporadic occurrence of the poison in the mussels. The only clue to its presence was when human cases of poisoning began to appear after eating the toxic mussels. Toxicity of the mussels usually appeared quite suddenly, and often within a week or two after fatal cases of poisoning the mussels from the same location could be eaten again without harm.

Although many theories were proposed for the occurrence of poisonous shellfish throughout the eighteenth and nineteenth centuries, particularly in European countries around the North Sea, the actual cause was not known until about 1927 when outbreaks of mussel poison occurred along the central California coast. At that time Dr. Herman Sommer and colleagues at the University of California observed a particular dinoflagellate blooming around the California sea mussels at the time when many people became sick and died after eating the mussels. These investigators suspected that the dinoflagellates upon which the mussels were feeding might be poisonous. Acidic water extracts of the dinoflagellates and the mussels killed mice in

15

exactly the same manner. The dinoflagellate was identified as *Gonyaulax catenella*.[2,3] To verify this observation, Dr. Sommer placed nonpoisonous mussels in laboratory jars containing seawater cultures of *G. catenella* and found that the mussels soon become poisonous. When these mussels were placed in water containing nonpoisonous organisms, the mussels excreted or destroyed the poison within a week or two, thus establishing conclusively the relationship of *G. catenella* to the poisonous mussels. This discovery by Sommer and colleagues led Canadian investigators Needler,[4] Prakash,[5] and others to the discovery that *Gonyaulax tamarensis* (var. *excavata*) caused clams and scallops along the Northeast coast of North America and the Northeast coast of England to become poisonous. Mussels bind 90% or more of the poison in the dark gland or hepatopancreas and show no physical signs of harm that would distinguish toxic ones from nontoxic ones.

In connection with my work at the Biological Laboratories at Fort Detrick, Maryland in 1945 I had the opportunity to work with Dr. Sommer at the University of California and Dr. Byron Riegel of Northwestern University on the mussel poison problem in California. This work along with that of my colleagues led to much of the knowledge of the chemistry of saxitoxin and its derivatives that we have today.

ASSAYS FOR SAXITOXIN AND RELATED TOXINS

The early work of Sommer and associates established a good mouse assay for the poison in mussels which made quantitative work with the poison practical. A mouse unit (MU) was defined as the minimum amount of poison that would kill a 20-gram white mouse in 15 minutes when one ml of an acidified extract of mussel tissues was injected intraperitoneally. Higher amounts than the minimum kill in shorter time, that is, death times of 3, 4, 6, and 8 minutes are equivalent to 3.7, 2.5, 1.6, and 1.3 MU respectively, as illustrated in FIGURE 1.[6] When we obtained saxitoxin in the purified state we found that one MU was equivalent to 0.18 μg of saxitoxin dihydrochloride (mol wt saxitoxin = 299; saxitoxin dihydrochloride = 372). We used the mouse assay to quantitate the *in vivo* response in practically all of our work on the isolation, purification, and chemical and physical characterization of the various paralytic poisons in mussels, clams, scallops, and cultures of Gonyaulax species.

Some chemical tests[7,8] have been worked out for saxitoxin in shellfish products, but these methods require partial purification and the use of special spectral equipment, and often have been subject to considerable error. They were used only to a limited extent in our studies.

CHEMICAL AND BIOLOGICAL CHARACTERIZATION

Our work on the isolation and characterization of the poison from California sea mussels (*Mytilus californianus*) was undertaken at the suggestion of the National Academy of Sciences in 1944 when outbreaks of mussel poisoning again occurred along the central California coast. In order to obtain sufficient poison for chemical studies it was necessary (1) to collect large quantities of poisonous mussels, and (2) to work out efficient procedures for the purification of the poison. Collection of the poison from mussels was somewhat limited because of the sporadic manner in which the poisonous dinoflagellate occurred and the relatively short time we had to collect the poisonous mussels. Because mussels bind most of the poison found in their bodies in the dark gland or hepatopancreas, this gland was removed from the mussel and stored in aqueous ethanol for purification. Significant amounts of mussel poison were obtained from the sea mussels, but additional and much larger amounts were obtained by the collection of poisonous Alaska butter clams (*Saxidomas giganteus*). Through arrangements with the United States Department of the Interior and the Alaska Experimental Commission, in 1948 to 1954 I made large collections of poison from the Alaska butter clam siphons which were preserved in acidic aqueous ethanol similar to the hepatopancreas of the mussels.

Small amounts were also obtained by culturing the poisonous dinoflagellate in our laboratories at Hooper Foundation, University of California, the Biological Laborato-

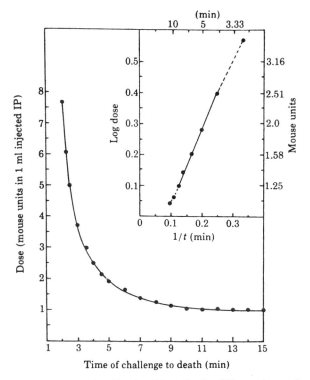

FIGURE 1. Time to death relationships in white mice for different doses of saxitoxin. The equation for the straight line relationship is log dose = $(145/t) - 0.2$, where t is in seconds.

ries, Fort Detrick, Maryland, and at the University of Wisconsin. The culturing at the Biological Laboratories was carried out with axenic cultures of *G. catenella* and *G. tamarensis* with help from Luigi Provasoli, Haskins Laboratories, who provided the axenic cultures of these organisms. The original culture of *G. catenella* was collected in 1944 from a bloom in Monterey Bay, California by Lucile Foster at the Hooper Foundation, University of California. The culture of *G. tamarensis* was collected by Provasoli from the Bay of Fundy. The poisons from California mussels, Alaska butter clams, and cultures of *G. catenella* appeared the same, but were kept separate throughout the work. They all produced the same signs of poisoning in mice and all had similar molecular weights of 300 to 400 as measured in crude extracts by the diffusion rate of the poison in a Northrop diffusion cell. Their action on cation exchange resins was also similar. The source from the Alaska butter clam siphons proved to be the best supply because, unlike the mussels, 60–70% of the poison in the whole body of the clam was contained in the siphon and remained there for periods of a year or more, which made collection possible at low tide anytime the weather permitted.

Another source of the poison was made available to me shortly after World War II in 1947 through the courtesy of the Canadian Defense Research Board and the Canadian Department of Human Services. This source was the entrails of commercial scallops collected in the Bay of Fundy. The entrails were from deep sea scallops, which are usually poisonous at all times. The poison in the scallops, however, had different properties and did not function well on cation exchange resins. As a result I stored them in acid solution (about pH 2) for later studies. Poison produced in cultures of *G. tamarensis* had properties similar to the poison from the scallops and was stored for further studies.

Early work by Riegel and Sommers in 1944 established that the poison from California mussels was a basic substance easily extracted with acidic water (pH 2), and some purification was accomplished on Decalso and activated carbon. These substances were not very efficient for purification. The new Amberlite cation exchange resins (Amberlite XE-64) developed by Rohm and Haas Company at about this time, however, proved to be ideal for the quantitative removal of the poison from crude acid extracts of poisonous shellfish containing as little as 1 MU per mg of solids. Extracts of the hepatopancreas of poisonous mussels usually contained 2 to 8 MU per mg of solids, whereas extracts of the siphons of poisonous butter clams varied considerably but usually contained around 2 MU per mg of solids. Research on purification methods at the Biological Laboratories and with Riegel's group at Northwestern University resulted in partial purification of the poison on the resin to about 3000 MU per mg of solids. Further chromatography on acid-washed and activated alumina brought the specific toxicity to 5500 MU per milligram. Chromatography repeated in various ways did not increase the specific toxicity and the poison was considered in a highly purified state in 1954. Subsequently over 20 grams of highly purified saxitoxin were prepared at the Biological Laboratories, mainly from butter clam siphons.

The poison was found to be a white hygroscopic solid very soluble in water, partly soluble in methanol and ethanol, but insoluble in most nonpolar solvents such as ethyl and petroleum ethers. It showed no absorption in the ultraviolet. Titration showed two pK_a values at 8.2 and 11.5. The optical rotation was about +130. The molecular formula was found to be $C_{10}H_{17}N_7O_4$ as the free base with a molecular weight of 299 and as the dihydrochloride salt 372. The poison can be reduced with hydrogen at room temperature and pressure in the presence of platinum black to produce a nearly nontoxic derivative with only 1–2% activity remaining. One mole of hydrogen was taken up per mole of poison in this reaction. It also reacted with certain aromatic nitro compounds to form a colored complex in much the same way as creatinine reacts with dinitrophenol in the Jaffe test and with dinitrobenzoic acid in the Benedict-Behre test. The reduced poison did not react with these reagents. The good correlation of these tests with the poison suggested to us their possible use as a quantitative chemical test to replace the mouse test where mice are hard to get and keep for assay purposes. However, certain impurities contained in clam and mussel extracts interfered sufficiently with the test for its practical use as an assay, but it was valuable for our research work with the purified poison.

Publication of our work[9,10] on the purification and characterization of the poisons from mussels, clams, and the cultured *G. catenella* generated much interest in these toxic substances and small amounts were donated to physiologists, pharmacologists, and chemists throughout the world for various studies. As a result Dr. C. Y. Kao[11] of the State University of New York and Dr. M. H. Evans[12] of the Sherrington School of Physiology, London discovered in 1964 that the poison caused death by blocking specifically the inward sodium current in nerve and muscle cell membranes, an action similar to that of tetrodotoxin from the puffer fish.

CHEMICAL STRUCTURE OF THE PARALYTIC POISONS

Our early studies on the chemical structure of saxitoxin were hampered by the fact that the highly polar nature of the molecule presented poor conditions for crystallization. Although we had crystallized saxitoxin as the helianthate in 1957, the molecule was too large to be usable for structure determination by crystallographers in X-ray diffraction studies. In July 1972, I moved to the Department of Food Microbiology and Toxicology at the University of Wisconsin, and continued the research on saxitoxin with Professors Frank Strong and Heinrich Schnoes in the Department of Biochemistry. In 1971 Wong et al.,[13] working on the structure by degradation of the molecule at the University of California, reported a proposed structure for saxitoxin. Although later shown to be incorrect, it did establish that saxitoxin essentially is a tetrahydropurine derivative. During the years that followed questions were raised by some investigators regarding the properties of the reported structure that did not seem in accord with the properties of saxitoxin. As a result we felt that more effort should be exerted on obtaining a good crystalline derivative so that crystallographic studies could be used for structure determination. Work with Strong, Schnoes and Vartan Ghazarossian at the University of Wisconsin laboratory resulted in a crystalline derivative of saxitoxin with p-bromobenzene sulfonic acid which was very suitable for crystallographic studies. Jon Clardy and colleagues, then at Iowa State University, carried out the crystallographic studies and determined the structure as presented in FIGURE 2 and TABLE 1. This structure for saxitoxin was presented at the first Conference on Poisonous Dinoflagellates in Boston, Massachusetts, in November 1974, and published in the Journal of the American Chemical Society, in March 1975.[14] On the basis of this structure, Tanino et al.[15] and Kishi, at Harvard University, synthesized D,L-saxitoxin. It was found active in blocking sodium channels in the same manner as natural saxitoxin. Later Bordner et al.[16] confirmed our structure for saxitoxin with an X-ray analysis of saxitoxin ethyl hemiketal.

Although these studies solved the structure for saxitoxin, the neutral or weakly basic poison from scallops, and that produced in cultures of G. tamarensis, was still a mystery. Its poisonous action appeared identical to saxitoxin,[17] but because of its weakly basic action on cation exchange resins (Amberlite CG-50) and electrophoresis it was assumed to be of different structure. Approximately 85% of the poison from east coast scallops and G. tamarensis cultures was eluted from the cation exchange resin above pH 4 and the remainder of 15% was removed below pH 3. On the other hand 90–95% of the poison from the west coast mussels, butter clams, and axenic G. catenella culture was eluted only below pH 3. The extracts of poisonous scallop viscera obtained from the Canadians back in 1947 were stored in acid solution and moved to the University of Wisconsin in 1972 along with extracts of cultured G. tamarensis cells. After standing in acid solution for over 20 years, we found that the poison now chromatographed on the cation exchange resins similarly to saxitoxin. The major poison in extracts of freshly collected scallop entrails obtained from the Canadian

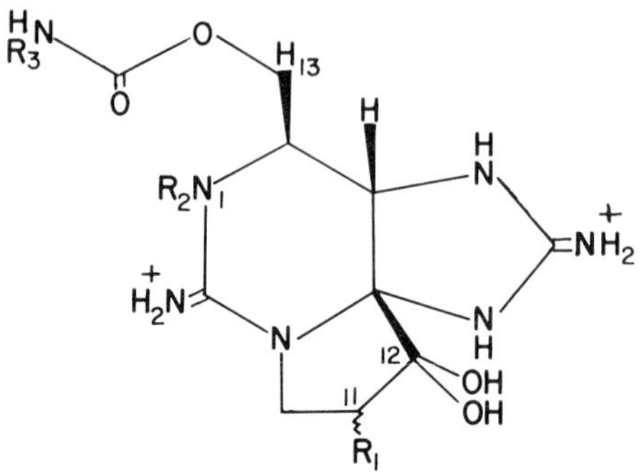

FIGURE 2. Structure of saxitoxin and some analogues (see explanation and data for TABLE 1).

Department of Human Services in 1978, however, was eluted from the cation exchange resins above pH 4, in line with the original observations. It was therefore assumed that some conversion took place in the molecule that led to a more basic structure.

Shortly after we were successful in obtaining the structure of saxitoxin, Shimizu and colleagues[18] at the University of Rhode Island purified the poison from east coast scallops and reported that the structure of the major poison from scallops and *G. tamarensis,* based on NMR studies, was 11-hydroxy saxitoxin, which he called gonyautoxin II and its epimer gonyautoxin III. This work established the similarity of *G. tamarensis* poison to saxitoxin, but in our minds it was questionable whether the proposed structure could be correct because it would not be weakly basic in character,

TABLE 1. Relation of Structure of Saxitoxin (FIGURE 2) and Some Derivatives to Biological Activity in Mice

Structure	R_1	R_2	R_3	Mouse Units per mg[a]	nMoles per Mouse Unit[b]
Saxitoxin	H	H	H	5500	0.6
Neosaxitoxin	H	OH	H	5000	0.64
α-11-Hydroxysaxitoxin sulfate	OSO_3	H	H	2500	1.06
β-11-Hydroxysaxitoxin sulfate	OSO_3	H	H	2000	1.27
Carbamoyl-*N*-sulfo-α-11-hydroxy saxitoxin sulfate	OSO_3	H	SO_3	60	35
Carbamoyl-*N*-sulfo-β-11-hydroxy saxitoxin sulfate	OSO_3	H	SO_3	600	3.5
α-Saxitoxinol	reduction to alcohol at C-12			150	24
β-Saxitoxinol	same			20	175
Decarbamoyl	acid treatment removal of C—NH₂ at C-13 ‖ O			3300	1.18

[a]Based on the dry weight of the toxin as the hydrochloride salt.
[b]Based, for comparison, on the mol wt of the toxin as a free base.

as is *G. tamarensis* poison. In our laboratory at the University of Wisconsin, Gregory Boyer had also purified the poison from freshly collected scallops on Bio-gel P-2 and acidic Al_2O_3 columns. Upon elemental analyses he found, in addition to the elements in saxitoxin, one mole of sulfur per mole of poison in the form of sulfate. Nuclear magnetic resonance studies showed this group in the 11-position making the correct structure for the major poison from scallops, and also for the poison from *G. tamarensis,* the sulfonic acid ester of 11-hydroxy saxitoxin (FIG. 2, TABLE 1). This structure was in line with the properties of *G. tamarensis* poison and was published in 1978 in the *Journal of the Chemical Society: Chemical Communications.*[19] The substitution on C-11 exists as an α- or β-epimer, and the specific toxicity of the sulfate in that position reduced the specific toxicity by about half (2500 MU/mg).

In 1978 Shimizu published the structure of an interesting saxitoxin derivative, 1-*N*-hydroxysaxitoxin,[20] which he isolated from scallops and called neosaxitoxin (FIG. 2, TABLE 1). Subsequently Boyer[21] in 1980 published the structure of both epimers (α and β) of neo-11-hydroxysaxitoxin sulfate.

Some very interesting derivatives of saxitoxin have recently been isolated by Hall and colleagues of the University of Alaska from dinoflagellates of the genus *Protogonyaulax* found along the coast of Alaska. The spectroscopic studies performed in collaboration with H. K. Schnoes and his associates at the University of Wisconsin suggested that two of these were carbamoyl-*N*-sulfo-11α-hydroxysaxitoxin sulfate and its 11β-epimer (FIG. 2, TABLE 1). X-ray analysis carried out by S. D. Darling at the University of Akron confirmed the latter structure.[22] These compounds are neutral in character.

The attenuation of toxicity associated with sulfonation of the carbamoyl group introduces a new aspect of structure-activity relationships in this group of neurotoxins. Saxitoxin has the highest specific toxicity of any of these poisons isolated thus far (see TABLE 1). In our laboratory, Ghazarossian *et al.*[23] found that removal of the carbamoyl group at C-13 by treatment of saxitoxin with 7 N HCl at 100°C reduced the toxicity to about 60%. As stated previously in our earlier work and that of Koehn *et al.,*[24] reduction of the hydrated ketone at the 12-position to a monohydroxy group reduced the toxicity to about 1–2% of the original.

It is apparent that any substitution or change in the saxitoxin molecule lowers the specific toxicity and also increases the number of molecules that cause death in a mouse. As indicated by the behavior of the various toxins on the cation exchange resins and in electrophoresis, the total net charge on the molecule is reduced to different degrees by substitution on the saxitoxin molecule. Saxitoxin and neosaxitoxin have approximately the same charge and approximately the same toxicity. The sulfate on C-11 reduces the total net charge about one-half and the toxicity about one-half. The carbamoyl-*N*-sulfo-11-hydroxysaxitoxin sulfate toxins have little or no net charge and very little toxicity. The greatest change in toxicity, however, takes place upon the reduction of saxitoxin with sodium borohydride or catalytically with hydrogen over platinum yielding the corresponding alcohol at C-12 without a loss in net charge. Schnoes and colleagues[24] have purified the individual α- and β-epimers of the alcohol and determined the specific toxicity of each at about 150 MU per mg for the α-epimer and about 20 for the β-epimer. In terms of nanomoles (nM) of toxin per mouse unit, about 23 nM of the α-epimer and about 175 nM of the β-epimer are required to produce death in a 20-gram mouse. In contrast, only 0.6 nM saxitoxin and 0.64 nM of neosaxitoxin are required to cause death.

Hall[25] has pointed out that substitution of the sulfo-radical on the carbamoyl nitrogen also caused a marked decrease in toxicity to about 60 MU per mg when the sulfate at C-11 was in the α-position and about 600 when the sulfate was in the

β-position. It is difficult to state definite figures for the toxicity in many cases because the sulfo-radical on the carbamoyl nitrogen is easily hydrolyzed and may occur also for the sulfate at C-11. It appears, however, that the sulfo-radical on the carbamoyl reduces the toxicity to a much greater extent than removal of the carbamoyl group completely. In general the presence of the sulfo-radical on the carbamoyl nitrogen in addition to the sulfate on C-11 lowers the specific toxicity to 1% to 10% (60 to 600 MU/mg) and the reduction at C-12 lowers the specific toxicity to 1% or 2% (50 to 100 MU per mg). Since binding of the toxin at the sodium channel is concentration dependent, higher concentrations of substituted or altered toxins are required around the channel than is required for saxitoxin.

Earlier in our work, we had found that purified saxitoxin was not a single component in the Craig countercount distribution.[10] We used a butanol-water system buffered at pH 8 to separate saxitoxin into a large component accounting for about 85% of the total mouse toxicity and a smaller component accounting for the remaining toxicity. When either component was acidified, the result was an equilibrium mixture of the same proportions. Elucidation of the structure of saxitoxin showed that this tautomerism was between the ketone and the dihydroxy or hydrated ketone on C-12. The hydrated or dihydroxy form is believed to be biologically active, but no definite proof can be offered. It is also the form in which saxitoxin crystallizes. Reduction eliminates the toxicity and the tautomerism. The function of the ketone form, if it is involved in toxicity, is not clear.

PUBLIC HEALTH CONSIDERATIONS

Paralytic shellfish poisoning due to saxitoxin and its derivatives is not a serious public health problem at the present time. Although the human consumption of shellfish as a source of dietary protein is increasing, the danger of food poisoning has been held down because of surveillance and control exercised by the food and drug officials in charge of food safety. The World Health Organization recognizes these paralytic poisons as an international problem and has issued protocols for the protection of the public health. The shellfish industry loses much financially from outbreaks of poisoning. Studies on the control of poisonous dinoflagellates in commercial shellfish areas are in order and should be encouraged. In order to maintain a safe food supply, the United States Food and Drug Administration, in cooperation with Canadian officials, has set up a reference standard for the mouse assay using purified saxitoxin dihydrochloride which I have prepared for them. Shellfish for sale must contain less than 80 μg of poison as saxitoxin dihydrochloride per 100 g of edible shellfish meats. This amount is well below the amount, estimated from accidental cases of poisoning, that causes symptoms of poisoning in people.

Another problem is the search for an antidote for the paralytic poisons. At present no antidote is known, and research on its development should be encouraged. The most satisfactory treatment is artificial respiration, which has saved many lives (particularly in borderline cases of poisoning). Larger doses of poison resulted in death despite this treatment.

REFERENCES

1. SCHANTZ, E. J. 1960. Biochemical studies on paralytic shellfish poisons. Ann. N. Y. Acad. Sci. **90:** 843.
2. SOMMER, H. & K. F. MEYER. 1937. Paralytic shellfish poisoning. AMA Arch. Pathol. **24:** 560.

3. SOMMER, H., W. F. WHEDON, C. A. KOFOID & R. STOHLER. 1937. Relation of paralytic shellfish poison to certain plankton organisms of the genus *Gonyaulax*. AMA Arch. Pathol. **24:** 537.
4. NEEDLER, A. B. 1949. Paralytic shellfish poisoning and *Gonyaulax tamarensis*. J. Fish. Res. Bd. Can. **7:** 490.
5. PRAKASH, A. 1963. Source of paralytic shellfish toxin in the Bay of Fundy. J. Fish. Res. Board Can. **20:** 983.
6. SCHANTZ, E. J., E. F. MCFARREN, M. L. SCHAFER & K. H. LEWIS. 1958. Purified shellfish poison for bioassay standardization. J. Assoc. Official Agric. Chem. **41:** 160.
7. BATES, H. A. & H. RAPOPORT. 1975. J. Agric. Food Chem. **23:** 237.
8. SHOPTAUGH, N. H., M. IKAWA, T. L. FOXALL & J. J. SASSNER. 1981. A fluorometric technique for the detection and determination of paralytic shellfish poisons. *In* The Water Environment. W. W. Carmichael, Ed.: 427. Plenum. New York.
9. SCHANTZ, E. J., J. D. MOLD, D. W. STANGER, J. SHAVEL, F. J. RIEL, J. P. BOWDEN, J. M. LYNCH, R. W. WYLER, B. RIEGEL & H. SOMMER. 1957. Paralytic shellfish poison. VI. A procedure for the isolation and purification of the poison from toxic clam and mussel tissues. J. Am. Chem. Soc. **79:** 5230.
10. MOLD, J. D., J. P. BOWDEN, D. W. STANGER, J. E. MAURER, J. M. LYNCH, R. S. WYLER, E. J. SCHANTZ & B. RIEGEL. 1957. Paralytic shellfish poison. VII. Evidence for the purity of the poison isolated from toxic clams and mussels. J. Am. Chem. Soc. **79:** 5235.
11. KAO, C. Y. & A. NISHIYAMA. 1965. J. Physiol. (London) **180:** 50.
12. EVANS, M. H. 1964. Brit. J. Pharmacol. **22:** 478.
13. WONG, J. L., R. OESTERLIN & H. RAPOPORT. 1971. Structure of saxitoxin. J. Am. Chem. Soc. **93:** 7344.
14. SCHANTZ, E. J., V. E. GHAZAROSSIAN, H. K. SCHNOES, F. M. STRONG, J. P. SPRINGER, J. O. PEZZANITE & J. CLARDY. 1975. The structure of saxitoxin. J. Am. Chem. Soc. **97:** 1238.
15. TANINO, H., T. NAKATA & Y. KISHI. 1977. J. Am. Chem. Soc. **99:** 2818.
16. BORDNER, J., W. E. THIESSEN, H. A. BATES & H. RAPOPORT. 1975. J. Am. Chem. Soc. **97:** 6008.
17. NARAHSHI, T., M. S. BRODWICK & E. J. SCHANTZ. 1975. Environ. Lett. **9:** 239.
18. SHIMIZU, Y., L. J. BUCKLEY, M. ALAM, Y. OSHIMA, W. E. FALLON, H. KASAI, I. MIURA, V. P. GULLO & K. NAKANISHI. 1976. J. Am. Chem. Soc. **98:** 5414.
19. BOYER, G. L., E. J. SCHANTZ & H. K. SCHNOES. 1978. Characterization of 11-hydroxysaxitoxin sulfate. J. Chem. Soc. Chem. Comm. **20:** 889.
20. SHIMIZU, Y., C. HSU, W. E. FALLON, Y. OSHIMA, I. MIURA & K. NAKANISHI. 1978. J. Am. Chem. Soc. **100:** 6791.
21. BOYER, G. L. 1980. Ph.D. thesis. University of Wisconsin. Madison.
22. WICHMANN, C. F., W. P. NIEMCZURA, H. K. SCHNOES, S. HALL, P. B. REICHARDT & S. D. DARLING. 1981. J. Am. Chem. Soc. **103:** 6977.
23. GHAZAROSSIAN, V. E., E. J. SCHANTZ, H. K. SCHNOES & F. M. STRONG. 1976. Biochem. Biophys. Res. Comm. **68:** 776.
24. KOEHN, F. E., V. E. GHAZAROSSIAN, E. J. SCHANTZ, H. K. SCHNOES & F. M. STRONG. 1981. Derivatives of saxitoxin. Bioorg. Chem. **10:** 412.
25. HALL, S. 1981. Ph.D. thesis. University of Alaska. Fairbanks, Alaska.

Chemistry and Biochemistry of Saxitoxin Analogues and Tetrodotoxin[a]

YUZURU SHIMIZU

Department of Pharmacognosy and Environmental Health Sciences
College of Pharmacy
University of Rhode Island
Kingston, Rhode Island 02881

PHYSICOCHEMICAL PROPERTIES OF SAXITOXIN ANALOGUES

The importance of saxitoxin and its analogues in neurophysiological experiments involving sodium channels cannot be overstated. In 1976, we first reported the isolation of new saxitoxin analogues, gonyautoxin-I, II, III,[1] and subsequently neosaxitoxin, gonyautoxin-IV, V, VI.[2] Since then a total of more than a dozen toxins have been isolated from various sources by the author's group and others (FIG. 1; see refs. 3 and 4 and references therein). The addition of those new toxins to the inventory of pharmacological probes has provided new insights into the mechanism of action of saxitoxin and tetrodotoxin in excitable membranes. Kao and co-workers, for example, suggested that the arrangement of two oxygen groups and guanidinium moiety in both saxitoxin and tetrodotoxin derivatives is the critical structural feature for the toxin binding.[5,6] Shimizu also pointed out structural problems associated with the classical "plug" model[7] by comparing the spatial arrangements of functional groups in the newly isolated toxin with those of saxitoxin and tetrodotoxin, and proposed a "lid" model with a simple three-point attachment to the proximity of sodium channels (FIG. 2).[3,8] Stricharz, on the other hand, interpreted experimental data for the new derivatives to show the formation of hemiketal or hemiaminoketal between the hydrated ketone at C-12 of saxitoxin and a nucleophilic group at the receptor site.[9] The possibility of such covalent bonding to the receptor has been a subject of discussion since the structure of saxitoxin was shown to possess a hydrated ketone structure.[10] A difficulty associated with such a model seems to be the absence of a comparable ketal formation site in tetrodotoxin derivatives. It is true that either hemiaminoacetal at C-4 or orthoester at C-10 could form a similar bond, but their locations relative to the essential guanidinium at C-2 are considerably different from that in saxitoxin derivatives, unless a different nucleophilic group at the site is involved in tetrodotoxin binding. The covalent binding model also may present a difficulty in explaining the activity observed with 12(OH)-dihydrosaxitoxin,[11] for which the ketal formation is prohibited.[3,8,9] At any rate discussion on this subject will continue. Some physicochemical properties of the toxins that may serve for the interpretation of the neurophysiological experimental data are discussed below.

The pK_a and Charge Distribution in Saxitoxin

The origin of the unusually low pK_a (8.4) of saxitoxin was determined, by carbon NMR[12] and proton NMR[1] studies, to be the imidazoline guanidinium group. In both

[a]The author gratefully acknowledges grants from the NIH (GM–24425 and GM–28754) which supported this work.

24

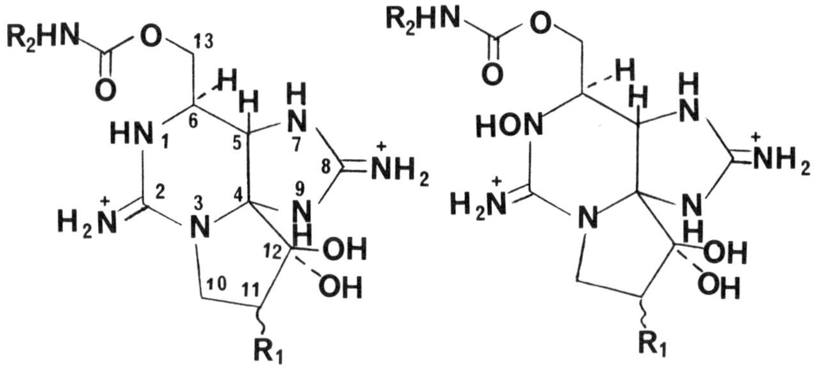

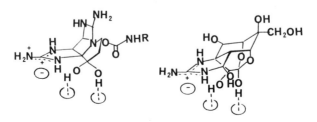

FIGURE 1. Structures of natural saxitoxin analogues.

Saxitoxin: R_1, R_2 = H
Gonyautoxin-II: R_1 = α-OSO_3^-, R_2 = H
Gonyautoxin-III: R_1 = β-OSO_3^-, R_2 = H
Gonyautoxin-V: R_1 = H, R_2 = SO_3^-
Gonyautoxin-VIII: R_1 =
(= C-2 toxin) β-OSO_3^-, R_2, = SO_3^-
Epigonyautoxin-VIII:
(= C-1 toxin) R_1 = α-OSO_3^-, R_2 = SO_3^-

Neosaxitoxin: R_1, R_2 = H
Gonyautoxin-I: R_1 = α-OSO_3^-, R_2 = H
Gonyautoxin-IV: R_1 = β-OSO_3^-, R_2 = H
Gonyautoxin-VI: R_1 = H, R_2 = SO_3^-
C-3 toxin: R_1 = β-OSO_3^-, R_2 = SO_3^-
C-4 toxin: R_1 = α-OSO_3^-, R_2 = SO_3^-

studies it was pointed out that C-12 can take the keto form at a pH range higher than 8.0. Thus saxitoxin exists in an equilibrium of three species around the physiological pH (FIG. 3). The keto form is only possible when the imidazoline guanidinium moiety is deprotonated. It was also suggested that the positive charge in the imidazoline group is not fully delocalized, and the guanidine group should be considered as an amidine, with a pK_a that was considerably lowered by substitution with an electron-withdrawing group. In fact, the X-ray crystallography data show all three nitrogen atoms, N-7, N-8, and N-9, on a plane, but the bond distance between C-8 and N-9 is longer than the others.[10] The N-9 atom does not have full SP^2 character.

The pK_a and Charge Distribution in Neosaxitoxin

Microtitration and NMR studies of neosaxitoxin indicate that the imidazoline group of neosaxitoxin also has an unusually low pK_a value of 8.65 for the imidazoline guanidinium group. In addition, there is another directly observable pK_a of 6.75, which

FIGURE 2. Three-point attachment model of saxitoxin and tetrodotoxin.[3]

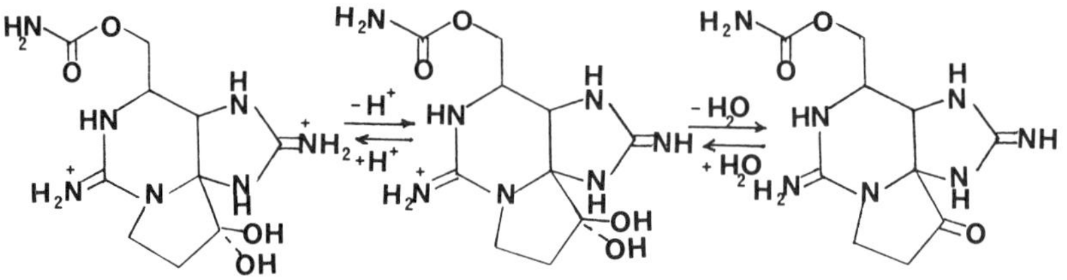

FIGURE 3. Three chemical species of saxitoxin around the physiological pH; $pK_a = 8.24$.

was previously assigned to the proton dissociation from hydroxyimmonium group at N-1 to the N-oxide type structure, on the basis of the pH dependent chemical shift study of the NMR.[13] It is analogous to the dissociation of hydroxamic acid. A recent pK_a study of oxyguanidine derivatives suggests that the pK_a can also be due to the deprotonation of the guanidinium group itself.[4] The titration of δ-N-hydroxyarginine gave pK_a values of 2.1, 7.5, and 9.2.[14] The pK_a of 7.5 seems to be the one that corresponds to the pK_a of 6.75 of neosaxitoxin. In another experiment, the pK_a of canavanine, an alkoxyguanidine derivative, was examined. The microtitration of the compound under nitrogen atmosphere gave pK_a values 2.1, 7.2, and 9.4, which are very

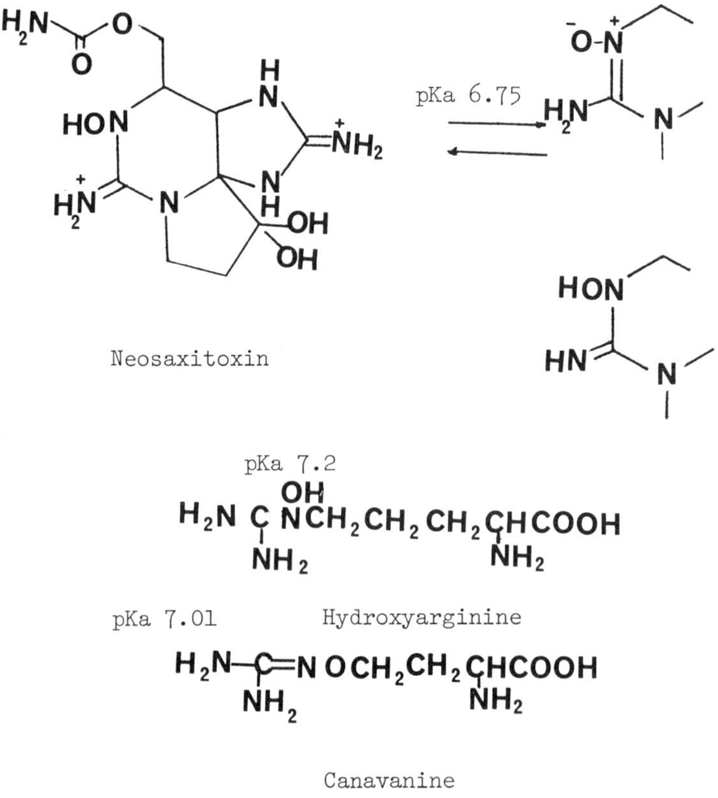

FIGURE 4. The pK_as of neosaxitoxin and oxyguanidine derivatives.

close to the reported values of 2.35, 7.01, and 2.35.[15] Because canavanine lacks a dissociable OH other than that of carboxyl group, the pK_a 7.01 must be due to the guanidinium moiety.

It is conceivable that electron-withdrawing substituents, such as oxygen or halogen, enhance the acidity of the guanidinium group, and considerably lower the pK_a. Results are thus still inconclusive as to whether the deprotonation is from the nitrogen or oxygen. In either case, however, the net charge of the substituted guanidinium moiety in the pyrimidine ring of neosaxitoxin and its derivatives becomes only slightly positive or zero around the physiological pH (FIG. 4).

The Conformation of the Toxin Molecule in Solution

The X-ray structure of saxitoxin p-bromobenzenesulfonate shows that the carbamoyl side chain is extended outward from the skeleton.[10] The comformational analysis based on the spin-spin coupling constants between H-6 and H-13 in NMR indicated that the side chain takes a similar conformation in solutions.[1] There is no evidence for the presence of a hydrogen bonding between the carbamoyl carbonyl and 12-OH or 7-NH, as might be speculated. Another important aspect of the molecular

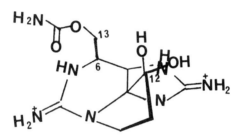

FIGURE 5. Conformation of saxitoxin and dihydrosaxitoxin in solutions.

shape is the packered conformation of the five-membered ring, which places 12-OH and 12-OH in *quassi* axial and *quassi* equatorial configuration, respectively (FIG. 5).[1] Removal of one of the hydroxyl groups at C-12 does not seem to change the ring conformation. Thus saxitoxin and dihydrosaxitoxins take the same conformation. The exact spatial arrangement of 12 and 12-hydroxyl groups or C-12 relative to C-8 guanidinium group may be critical for the toxin-receptor interactions in both models discussed earlier.

BIOGENESIS OF SAXITOXIN ANALOGUES

Now saxitoxin analogues are known to be in a number of organisms in different genera and different phyla.[4] Moreover, even in the same species, the toxigenicity drastically varies from strain to strain.[16,17] This capricious occurrence of the compounds is rather astonishing, in view of their unique structural features. The mystery was further deepened when saxitoxin and gonyautoxins were found in the macroalgae, *Jania* ssp.,[18] and the blue-green alga, *Aphanizomenon flos-aquae.*[19] One way to explain such irregular occurrences of highly peculiar structures is to consider the presence of a genetic factor common to the organisms. In an attempt to approach the problem from the molecular side, the biosynthesis of saxitoxin was first investigated.

Several speculative biosynthetic pathways had been considered for the biosynthesis of the tricyclic perhydropurine derivative. After numerous feeding experiments, the normal purine metabolic pathway was ruled out as the origin of the purine moiety. Instead the involvement of arginine or its precursor, α-ketoglutarate, was first confirmed in the formation of the toxin skeleton.[20] Subsequently it was established that ornithine, the direct precursor of arginine, can be incorporated into the toxin with a loss of the carboxyl group.[21] The feeding of [2-^{13}C, 2-^{15}N]-double-labeled ornithine to the culture of *Aphnizomenon flos-aquae* resulted in the intact incorporation of the ^{13}C-^{15}N combination into C-4 and N-9 of neosaxitoxin as shown by a ^{15}N-^{13}C spin-spin coupling in the NMR spectrum.[21]

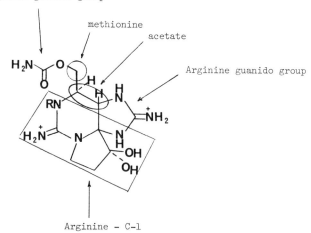

FIGURE 6. The biosynthetic origins of saxitoxin molecules.

With regard to the origin of C-5, C-6, and C-13, malonate or 3-hydroxypropionate derived from malonate was first considered to condense with arginine as a three-carbon unit.[22] Indeed [^{13}C$_2$]acetate was efficiently incorporated into C-5 and C-6 of neosaxitoxin,[21] but repeated attempts to pulse-feed ^{13}CO$_2$ and labeled 3-hydroxypropionic acid resulted in no specific incorporation of the isotopes into the toxin molecule. Another plausible pathway was the condensation of L-serine with arginine. The resulting intermediate would possess a perfect functional and stereochemical arrangement to form the toxin ring system. In fact the feeding of [3-^{13}C]serine to the culture of *A. flos-aquae* has resulted in the enrichment of C-13 of neosaxitoxin. This incorporation has proved to be very deceptive however. When [1,2-^{13}C$_2$]glycine was fed to the culture of *A. flos-aquae*, the enrichment of only C-13 carbon was observed. Since glycine is the direct precursor of serine, the experiment was expected to result in the enrichment of C-5 and C-6 carbon in neosaxitoxin. This enrichment of a single carbon, C-13, by the doubly labeled precursor can be explained by a C$_1$ transfer via tetrahydrofolate. The enrichment of C-13 by [3-^{13}C]serine can be explained likewise, because serine is also

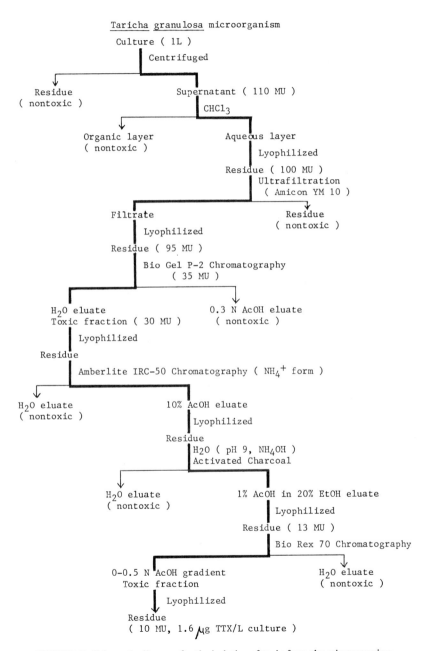

FIGURE 7. Schematic diagram for the isolation of toxin from the microorganism.

known to be a good C_1 donor to tetrahydrofolate. The feeding of [methyl-^{13}C]methionine resulted in excellent enrichment of C-13 of neosaxitoxin. Since methyltetrahydrofolate is a methyl donor in the biosynthesis of methionine and the process is considered to be rather irreversible, methionine in the form of S-adenosylmethionine (SAM) should be the direct precursor of C-13 of the toxin.

The above feeding experiments establish the origins of all carbons and nitrogens in the toxin skeleton (FIG. 6). The remaining questions are how these fragments are combined together and how this relates to the toxigenicity of the organisms.

BIOGENESIS OF TETRODOTOXIN

In parallel with the biosynthetic studies of saxitoxin, we have been investigating the biogenesis of another important sodium channel blocker, tetrodotoxin in the newts *Taricha torosa* and *T. granulosa*. In earlier studies we observed the apparent absence of the *in situ* biosynthesis of tetrodotoxin in these animals.[22] Repeated feeding experiments using sodium acetate with a high level of radioactivity confirmed the previous findings; guanidinium compounds such as creatinine and carnosine in the newt were substantially labeled, while tetrodotoxin remained unlabeled.

The possible involvement of the intestinal microflora of the newt was also investigated. The oral feeding of ^{14}C-acetate to *T. granulosa* did not result in the labeling of tetrodotoxin, and no appreciable amount of toxin was detected in the culture specimen from the intestine of the newt.

Recently we reinvestigated the toxin production by an isolate from the intestinal flora, on a suspicion that the toxin production might be very minute under artificial conditions.

New isolates were made from the washings of the newt's gut on agar plates. Independent colonies were then transferred to the liquid medium. After two days at ambient temperature, the culture (3% tryptic soy broth) was centrifuged, and the supernatant was fractionated following the mouse toxicity as shown in FIGURE 7.[23] The elution pattern and retention time of the toxic component matched exactly those of tetrodotoxin, and the toxic symptoms in mice were also indistinguishable from those of tetrodotoxin. Further chemical and neurophysiological studies of the toxin are currently in progress.

REFERENCES

1. SHIMIZU, Y., M. ALAM, Y. OSHIMA & W. E. FALLON. 1975. Biochem. Biophys. Res. Comm. **66:** 731.
2. OSHIMA, Y., L. J. BUCKLEY, M. ALAM & Y. SHIMIZU. 1977. Comp. Biochem. Physiol. **57C:** 31.
3. SHIMIZU, Y. 1982. Pure Appl. Chem. **54:** 1973.
4. SHIMIZU, Y. 1984. Paralytic shellfish poisons. *In* Progress in the Chemistry of Organic Natural Products, vol. 45. W. Herz, H. Grisebach & G. W. Kirby, Eds.: 235. Springer-Verlag, Vienna.
5. KAO, C. Y. & S. E. WALKER. 1982. J. Physiol. **323:** 619.
6. KAO, C. Y. 1983. Toxicon Suppl. **3:** 211.
7. HILLE, B. 1975. Biophys. J. **15:** 615.
8. SHIMIZU, Y., M. KOBAYASHI, A. GENENAH & Y. OSHIMA, 1984. Tetrahedron **40:** 539.
9. STRICHARTZ, G. 1984. J. Gen. Physiol. **84:** 281.
10. SCHANTZ, E. J., V. E. GHAZAROSSIAN, H. K. SCHNOES, F. M. STRONG, J. P. SPRINGER, J. O. PEZZANITE & J. CLARDY. 1975. J. Am. Chem. Soc. **97:** 6008.

11. SHIMIZU, Y., C. P. HSU & A. GENENAH. 1981. J. Am. Chem. Soc. **103:** 605.
12. ROGERS, R. S. & H. RAPOPORT. 1980. J. Am. Chem. Soc. **102:** 7335.
13. SHIMIZU, Y., C. P. HSU, W. E. FALLON, Y. OSHIMA, I. MIURA & K. NAKANISHI. 1978. J. Am. Chem. Soc. **100:** 6791.
14. SHIMIZU, Y., A. HORI & M. GHAZALA. Unpublished data.
15. BOYAR, A. & R. E. MARSH. 1982. J. Am. Chem. Soc. **104:** 1995.
16. MARANDA, L., D. M. ANDERSON & Y. SHIMIZU. 1985. Estuarine Coastal and Shelf Science. **21:** 401.
17. HALL, S. 1982. Toxins and Toxicity of *Protogonyaulax* from the Northeast Pacific. Ph.D. thesis. University of Alaska. pp. 1–196.
18. KOTASKI, Y., M. TAJIRI, Y. OSHIMA & T. YASUMOTO. 1983. Bull. Jpn Soc. Sci. Fish. **49:** 283.
19. ALAM, M., Y. SHIMIZU, M. IKAWA & J. J. SASNER, JR. 1978. J. Environ. Sci. Health **A13:** 493.
20. SHIMIZU, Y., M. KOBAYASHI, A. GENENAH & N. ICHIHARA. 1984. Biosynthesis of paralytic shellfish toxins. *In* Seafood Toxins. E. P. Ragelis, Ed. American Chemistry Society. Washington, D. C.
21. SHIMIZU, Y., M. NORTE, A. HORI & A. GENENAH. 1984. J. Am. Chem. Soc. **106:** 6433.
22. SHIMIZU, Y. & M. KOBAYASHI. 1983. Chem. Pharm. Bull. **31:** 3625.
23. GUPTA, S., K. YOUNG & Y. SHIMIZU. Unpublished.

The Chemistry of Tetrodotoxin[a]

HARRY S. MOSHER

Department of Chemistry
Stanford University
Stanford, California 94305

INTRODUCTION

The structure of tetrodotoxin (TTX, **1**) was determined over twenty years ago[1-4] and the synthesis of racemic TTX was accomplished over fifteen years ago.[5,6] These aspects of the chemistry of TTX are history, and we are now studying other facets of its chemistry.

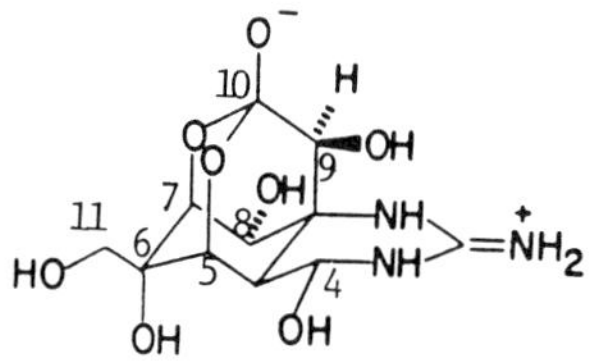

1 a   **1 b**

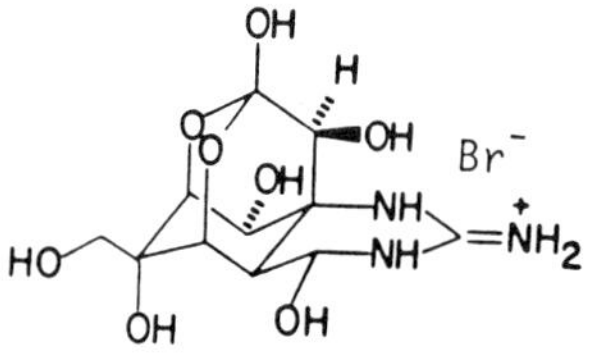

Recent tetrodotoxin chemical research has focused on modifications of the molecule that may increase its usefulness in the study of the mechanism of action of sodium channels and their role in the transmission of nerve impulses. The aims of such chemical modifications are to reveal structure activity relationships, to develop better radioactive-labeled, spin-labeled, fluorescent-labeled, or photoaffinity-labeled TTX derivatives, and to develop neuron blocking agents that can be localized and therefore used as local anesthetics. It is evident that useful molecular modifications must retain the sodium channel blocking ability of the parent TTX molecule.

The structure of crystalline TTX, including its absolute configuration, has been unequivocally established as the unique zwitterion (**la**). This and related structures rest not only on extensive chemical and spectroscopic evidence,[1-4] but also on a total of five X-ray chromatographic determinations[3,7-10] done on TTX derivatives. The last of these was on tetrodotoxin hydrobromide (**lb**). In the crystalline state TTX is stable indefinitely; in solution it is reasonably stable in dilute acid, but it very rapidly decomposes at pHs above 8. The pK_a of the guanidine group in TTX cannot be determined accurately because of decomposition in basic solution, but that of the C-10 acidic hemilactal anion is observed at 8.7. Although crystalline TTX is entirely in the

[a]The author gratefully acknowledges research support from the National Institutes of Health (grant NS14345).

32

zwitterion form **la**, in acid solution it is in the protonated hemilactal form **lb**. In both **la** and **lb** under physiological conditions the guanidine moiety is in the protonated, resonance stabilized, guanidinium form as shown below (**lc** ↔ **ld** ↔ **le**). For convenience, however, the structures will be represented with the positive charge localized on

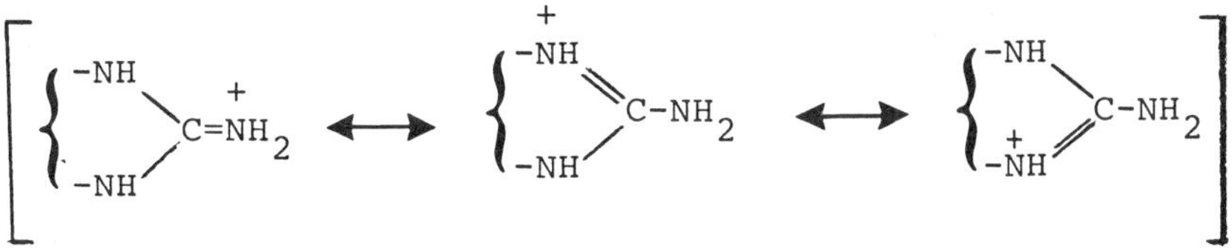

1c   **1d**   **1e**

the $=NH_2^+$ group. In solution the hemilactal and hydroxy lactone forms **lb** and **lf** are in equilibrium. The lactone appears to involve the C-8 hydroxy almost exclusively, leaving the C-5 hydroxy free. The lactone can undergo hydrolysis to the dihydroxy acid (**lg**), which has not been isolated but is known in solution as tetrotoxinic acid.[2] Strong base gives the carboxylate anion (**lh**), which has only a transitory existence. This unstable anion **lh** decomposes ultimately to quinazoline derivatives that are fluorescent and are used for the detection and analysis[4,11,12] of TTX.

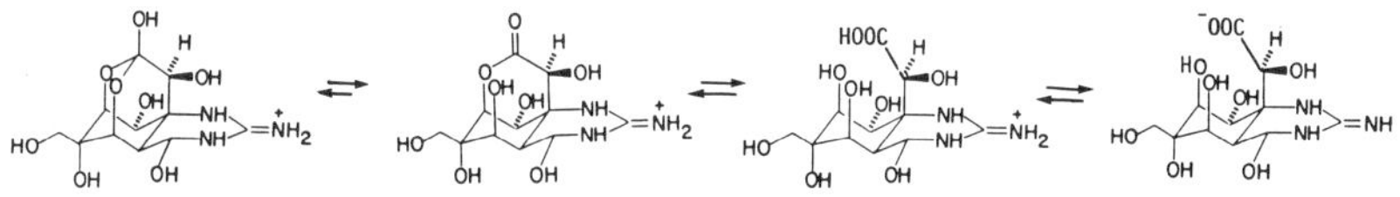

Hemilactal (**1b**)   Hydroxy-lactone (**1f**) Tetrotoxinic Acid (**1g**) Carboxylate Anion (**1h**)

Another vulnerable site of the TTX molecule is the hydroxy group at C-4. As shown in the following equilibrium, this is a potential amino-aldehyde (aminal); however, the ring form must be overwhelmingly favored. Ring closure can take place in two ways to give either the TTX configuration or the C-4 epimer[12] of TTX. This may also be the mechanism for the formation of the C-4–C-9 anhydro series of compounds of which 4,9-anhydrotetrodotoxin (**2**, anhydro-TTX) is the parent.

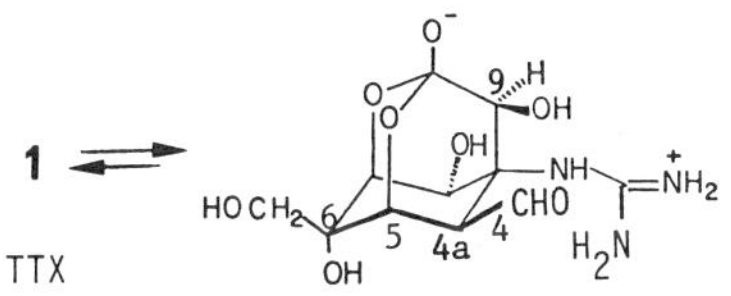

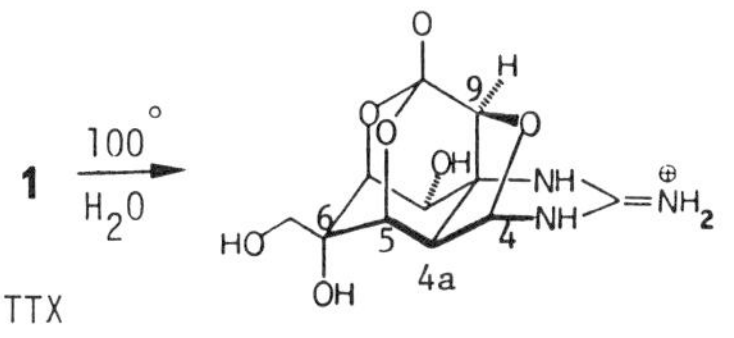

Amino-aldehyde   Anhydro-TTX

Another important chemical charactertistic of TTX is its solubility. Crystalline TTX is not soluble in water but is very soluble in dilute acid, from which it crystallizes slowly when the solution is brought back to neutrality. Crystalline TTX does not dissolve to any appreciable extent in any neutral organic solvent (*i.e.,* Et_2O, MeOH, EtOH, acetone, DMF, DMSO, or CH_3CN) and therefore it cannot be extracted from aqueous solution. Amorphous TTX, obtained by dissolving crystalline TTX in dilute acetic acid followed by lyophilization, dissolves to some extent in DMSO. Since TTX is a low molecular weight compound, it cannot be separated from salts by dialysis. If buffer solutions are used, it is preferable to employ ammonium carbonate or pyridine acetate, which can be removed by high vacuum lyophilization. These solubility characteristics, and sensitivity to base and strong acid, put severe limitations on organic chemical methods that may be used in modifying the molecule and in isolating reaction products.

A final generalization is that modifications of the TTX structure at the guanidinium end of the molecule, that is, to the right as we have written these formulas, lead to products that are inactive or, at least, have greatly reduced toxicity and sodium channel blocking ability. On the other hand, the TTX structure can be modified at the C-6 and/or C-11 portions of the molecule and still retain substantial activity.

MODIFICATIONS OF THE TTX MOLECULE

Tritiated TTX

The availability of a suitably labeled form of the agent is crucial to studies of the action of many physiologically active substances. Most such studies with TTX itself have made use of material tritiated by the Welzbach[13] method (exposing TTX to tritium gas). There is extensive degradation of TTX in this process and its purification has required exacting methods,[14,15] accompanied by large losses. The ultimate recovery of pure [³H]TTX is low (ca. 1%), and its radioactivity not particularly high (ca. 100–400 Ci/mol). A process involving hydrolysis of anhydro TTX (**2**) with tritium oxide in order to obtain tritiated TTX (0.7% chemical yield, 18,000 Ci/mole) has been reported recently.[16] The product is claimed to have 60% of the radioactivity expected for the incorporation of one ³H atom per molecule of TTX. It was proposed that the reaction involves epimerization at the anhydro bridge of **2** with ³H incorporation at C-4; however, specific evidence for this was not presented. In spite of this proposal, the chemical rationale for tritium incorporation is unclear; it would be valuable to obtain direct evidence for the nature of this reaction. An alternate approach to the tritiation problem is the incorporation of radioactivity into a reagent, which is then attached to the TTX structure. Such TTX derivatives that involve attachment of a radioactive moiety to the molecule are additional aspects of the labeling problem that are to be considered.

4,9-Anhydro Derivatives

Central to the chemistry of TTX derivatives is 4,9-anhydro-TTX (**2**, anhydro-TTX[1] or anhydro-*epi*-TTX[2]). This derivative is formed with inversion of configuration at C-4 when the oxygen bridge between C-4 and C-9 is established. The anhydro form is easily identified by virtue of the small coupling constant ($J_{4a-4} = < 1 Hz$) of the upfield C-4a proton at about 3.0 ppm with the downfield C-4 proton at about 5.5 ppm. This indicates an equatorial C-4 proton coupled to an axial C-4a proton at a dihedral angle of about 90°. In TTX itself (and those 4-substituted TTX derivatives without a 4,9-anhydro bridge) the coupling constant J_{4-4a} is about 10 Hz, corresponding to a dihedral angle between these protons of approximately 180°. The anhydro derivatives are also characterized as essentially nontoxic (at least 100 times less toxic than TTX itself). Although TTX is unstable to base, anhydro-TTX is relatively stable in dilute alkali at 20° because the C-4 aminal function is now protected. Anhydro-TTX exhibits two pK_as, one at 7.95 (C-11 hemilactal zwitterion) and another at 11.5 (guanidine group). In contrast to TTX, the more strained anhydro structure is not in measurable equilibrium with the lactone form in solution.

Anhydro-TTX is prepared in moderate-to-poor yields by selective hydrolysis (dil. HCl, 20°) of any of the acetylanhydro-TTX derivatives (3a–3d, see below) or from 11-formylanhydro-TTX (3e). Anhydro-TTX has been reported to occur in fugu.[12]

	3	**4**
Diacetate	$R^6, R^{11} = Ac; R^1, R^2, R^3, R^8, R^{10} = H$	(3a)
Tetraacetate	$R^6, R^{11}, R^8, R^{10} = Ac; R^1, R^2, R^3 = H$	(3b)
Pentaacetate	$R^6, R^{11}, R^8, R^{10}, R^3 = Ac; R^1, R^2 = H$	(3c)
Heptaacetate	all Rs = Ac.	(3d)
11-Formyl	$R^{11} = HCO; R^1, R^2, R^3, R^8, R^{10} = H$	(3e)

Goto et al.[2] reported that TTX was in equilibrium with anhydro-TTX during isolation. It was removed during purification via its crystalline picrate.

Acetylation of TTX[1-4] (Ac₂O, pyridine) gives a series of acetates (di-, tetra-, penta-, hepta-) having the basic anhydro-TTX skeleton shown in 3. Apparently the 4,9-anhydro bridge is first formed, followed by acetylation of the OH groups at C-11, C-6, C-8, and C-10 in that order. The unsubstituted NH_2 of the guanidine is the first nitrogen to be acetylated, followed by the N-1 and N-3 positions. Under forcing conditions, an octaacetate (4) is formed[3] that has a double bond between C-4 and C-4a.

Hydrolysis apparently takes place in the reverse order; first the acetyl groups on nitrogens are removed in accord with the observation that acyl guanidines are very easily hydrolyzed. The acetyls on C-10 and C-8 are removed next, leaving 6,11-diacetyl-anhydro-TTX (3a). Either 3a or 3b can be converted to anhydro-TTX (2), using hydrolysis catalyzed with NH_4OH or NEt_3. Finally, anhydro-TTX (2) can be converted back to TTX (1). Most of these transformations are not good yield processes. There is no report, to our knowledge, of a TTX derivative that has the guanidinium group selectively protected while one or more of the hydroxy groups are free.

Treatment of TTX with formic acid (99.8%, 82°C, 2 h) gives 11-formyl-4, 9-anhydro-TTX (3e, 75% yield).[1] The formyl group is readily removed by hydrolysis (dil. aqueous base) to give anhydro-TTX (2, 67% yield).[1] This probably is the method of choice for the preparation of 2.

Since the only primary alcohol group in TTX is at C-11, esterification should occur preferentially at this position. Strong and Keana[18] have studied the reaction of succinic anhydride in aqueous solution at pH 5–6 at room temperature with TTX and found that even under these mild conditions the succinylation product (ca. 5% yield) had the anhydro structure and only about 0.4% of the toxicity of TTX. This product was readily hydrolyzed back to TTX ($t_{1/2}$, 6 h; pH 7.2), presumably via anhydro-TTX.[19] A similar result was observed in the case of formylation of **1** to give **3e** and its hydrolysis back to anhydro-TTX.

Modifications at C-4

Treatment of TTX or anhydro-TTX at room temperature with methanolic or ethanolic HCl gives the 4-methoxy (**5a**) or ethoxy (**5b**) derivative.[1,2] The 4-amino derivative (**5c**) is obtained by treatment of TTX with ammonia; 4-deoxy-TTX (**5d**) is obtained by platinum-catalyzed hydrogenation of TTX in 5% HCl solution. These compounds all have the TTX stereochemistry at C-4 and not the epimeric structure which is required in the anhydro series. The toxicities (iv, mouse) of these derivatives in comparison with TTX were published by Deguchi,[20] and are given in TABLE 1, opposite

TABLE 1. Reported Toxicities of C-4 Tetrodotoxin Derivatives[20,21]

R		LD_{50} (iv) $\mu g/kg$[20,21]
OH	(**1**)	9
OCH_3	(**5a**)	341
OC_2H_5	(**5b**)	692
NH_2	(**5c**)	528
H	(**5d**)	42

formulas **5a–5d**. The same samples were restudied by Narahashi et al.[21] in the frog sciatic nerve and lobster nerve preparations with comparable results. All had sodium-channel blocking action indistinguishable from that of tetrodotoxin. The most active sample was **5d**, which was later shown[21] to be contaminated with enough of the parent TTX (**1**) to account for most of its toxicity. It would require only 0.1% to 0.3% contamination of TTX in samples **5a–5c** to give the activities shown. The analytical techniques were not sensitive enough to show these possible low orders of contamination, so it seems that at best these derivatives are on the order of 100 to 500 times less active than TTX itself.

Modifications at C-9

Refluxing TTX in water (or heating in a sealed tube at 120°C to 130°C) causes it to lose its toxicity; tetrodonic acid[1] (tetradoic acid[2]) is isolated from the solution. If the H_2O is replaced with D_2O, deuterium is incorporated at C-9. An X-ray determination of tetrodonic acid hydrobromide[1] reveals structure **6**, which differs from TTX in

Tetrodonic Acid[1] (Tetrodoic Acid[2]) (**6**)

having the 4,9-anhydro bridge and being epimeric at both C-4 and C-9. These structural features direct the carboxyl group away from the position above the carbocyclic ring, thus precluding the possibility of hemilactal or lactone forms. Tetrodonic acid, which is reported to be nontoxic, has recently been identified as a natural product accompanying TTX in fugu.[12] Tetrodonic acid has not been converted back to TTX or to *epi*-C-9-TTX. No simple C-9 derivative such as the ketone, a monoester, or an ether has been reported.

6,11-Isopropylidine, C-4 Modified Derivatives

Key compounds in Woodward's[3] structural studies were the crystalline 6,11-isopropylidine derivatives 7 and 8 (designated Gougoutas hydrochloride and Rajappa hydrochloride). The first of these was formed at room temperature on storing TTX in anhydrous methanol/acetone/HCl. The X-ray crystallographic analysis of compound

Gougoutas Hydrochloride (7)   Rajappa Hydrochloride (8)

7 revealed every atom in the tetrodotoxin structure without rearrangement. As might be expected, because of the methoxy substituent at C-4, this compound is essentially nontoxic.[22] Hydrolysis of 7 (DCl in D_2O, 20°C, 7 h) gives a 3:1 mixture[22] of TTX (1) and anhydro-TTX (2). Presumably the reaction to give 7 proceeds by first methylating the 4-hydroxy group, followed by 6,11-isopropylidination, because treatment with anhydrous acetone and HCl (25°C, 2 h) without methanol gives the anhydro derivative 8. Methylation of 8 (Me_2SO_4/MeI, 100°C, 10 h) gives the C-10 *O*-methyl derivative,[3] which cannot exist as a zwitterion and shows the classical properties of the strongly basic guanidine group.[2] From these results it is evident that modifications of TTX at C-4 and C-9, on the guanidinium end of the molecule, greatly reduce or destroy the activity of TTX.

Derivatives Modified only at C-6 and/or C-11

The TTX modifications discussed to this point were generated during the early studies conducted in connection with the proof of structure of TTX (before 1965). More recently (1975–79) several developments have given new impetus to the study of TTX derivatives. These include: (1) the report by Tsein *et al.*[23] that 11-nor-TTX (9) gave an *O*-methyloxime derivative (formulated as 10) that showed substantial, although capricious, TTX-type activity; (2) the discovery of chiriquitoxin,[24,25] isolated along with TTX from the skin of a Costa Rican frog, which had toxicity comparable to TTX and the same structure, with the exception of a different substituent in place of the C-11 CH_2OH group, as shown in 11; (3) the publication by Guillory *et al.*[26] concerning the synthesis of a photoaffinity-labeled derivative of TTX that was active and that presumably had structure 12; (4) the revelation by Lazdunsky and co-

R, R^1 =   O= or (HO)$_2$ (9)

CH$_3$ON= or [CH$_3$ONH-, HO-]   (10)

? [121 mass units]   (11)

2-(NO$_2$)-4-N$_3$-C$_6$H$_3$-NHCH$_2$CH$_2$COOCH$_2$-, HO- (12)

2-(NO$_2$)-4-N$_3$-C$_6$H$_3$-NHCH$_2$CH$_2$NH-, H-   (13)

workers[27] of their systematic and successful attack on the problem of making TTX derivatives such as 13 that were sodium-channel blocking agents.

The derivatives modified only at C-6 and/or C-11 can be divided into the following three groups: (1) those that are derived directly from the primary alcohol at C-11, *i.e.*, ROCH$_2$C^6(OH)-; (2) those that are derived from the C-11 aldehyde, OCHC^6(OH)-; and (3) those that are derived from the C-6 ketone, nor-TTX (9, O=C^6). We shall discuss the derivatives in this order.

Direct Esterification of C-11 Primary Alcohol

The one example reported to be a derivative involving only the primary alcohol at C-11 is that by Guillory *et al.*,[26] who described the esterification of TTX with *N*-(4-azido-2-nitrophenyl)-β-alanine (14), using carbonyldiimidazole (15) as coupling agent (aqueous DMF, r.t., 12 h, in the dark). The presumption is that esterification took place only at the primary alcohol group on C-11 to give 12 and that the 4,9-anhydro bridge was not formed. The nonisolated product was studied in photoaf-

finity labeling experiments. From the results, it is clear that a sodium-channel blocking substance was present in the reaction mixture. The description of the chemistry is insufficient to evaluate the chemical yield, stability, and identity of the active component. No subsequent report verifying this simple reaction has appeared. We have been unsuccessful in trying to use carbonyldiimidazole for preparing the unknown C-11 monoacetate.[22] It certainly would be very valuable if a practical, reproducible procedure for this direct esterification could be developed.

Derivatives Made via the C-11 Aldehyde

The major pathway to highly active (and radiolabeled) derivatives of TTX was pioneered by Lazdunsky and co-workers.[28,29] This method involves conversion of TTX to the C-11 aldehyde (17), followed by coupling with a substituted amine to give a Schiff's base (18), which is then reduced (NaBH$_4$ or NaCNBH$_3$) to the saturated

$$R = \quad H_2N\text{-}CH_2CH_2\text{-} \qquad\qquad\qquad (a)$$
$$HOOC\text{-}CH_2\text{-} \qquad\qquad\qquad\quad (b)$$
$$HOOC\text{-}CH_2CH_2\text{-} \qquad\qquad\quad (c)$$
$$HOOCCH(NH_2)CH_2CH_2CH_2CH_2\text{-} \quad (d)$$
$$2,4\text{-}(NO_2)\text{-}C_6H_3\text{-}NH\text{-} \qquad\qquad (e)$$
$$2\text{-}(NO_2)\text{-}4\text{-}N_3\text{-}C_6H_3\text{-}NHCH_2\overset{\overset{\displaystyle O}{\|}}{\text{-}C}NH\text{-} \quad (f)$$

derivative (**19**). Either the starting TTX or the substituted amine (or both) can be radiolabeled. The derivative **19f** with the *p*-azido grouping was shown to bind irreversibly to excitable neuron tissue upon UV irradiation. The same photoaffinity labeling ability was demonstrated by **24f** (see below). The Pfitzner-Moffatt oxidation with dimethylsulfoxide (DMSO), phosphoric acid (H_3PO_4), and dicyclohexylcarbo-diimide (DCC) was done under anhydrous conditions ($40°C$, 3–4 h) using amorphous TTX (obtained by dissolving it in dilute trifluoroacetic acid, followed by lyophiliza-tion). The yield on this oxidation (**1** → **17**) after purification was 5% to 10%. The yield of the subsequent coupling and reduction was about 20%. These yields were measured by following the coelution of biological activity and radioactivity through several purification steps (Bio Rex 70 cation exchange resin and Biogel P-2 chromatography). Thus the overall yield of purified derivatives **19a–19f** was on the order of 1% to 2%.

Bontemps *et al.*[17] have published an improved procedure for synthesis of aldehyde **17** by the same reaction but adhering to more scrupulously anhydrous conditions. In the coupling reaction with tritium-labeled ethylenediamine, a 12-fold excess of the aldehyde **17** was used so that TTX was joined at both ends of the ethylenediamine chain. This product was reduced ($NaCNBH_3$) to give [^3H]ethylenediamine ditetrodo-toxin (**20**). Even with the improved procedure, the yield after purification was low, based on TTX. Product **20** was reported to show specific binding to an excitable membrane preparation from the electric organ of the electric eel. Although this derivative contains two TTX moieties per molecule, it appears that each molecule blocks only one sodium channel.

$$TTX\text{—}NHCH_2CH_2NH\text{—}TTX$$

20

It is important to reemphasize that the TTX molecule has several chemically reactive sites. Products must be rigorously purified to homogeneity to avoid contamina-tion by radioactive artifacts. There have been no reports of chemical or NMR characterization of the products of derivatives **12** through **20**.

Derivatives of "Nortetrodotoxin"

By virtue of the $C(OH)CH_2OH$ (α-glycol) structure of TTX, periodate oxidation gives formaldehyde and nortetrodotoxin (**9**) in good yield. This compound was prepared

1   **9**

by both Tsuda[1] and Goto[2] during their structural studies that proved the presence of the HOCH$_2$C(OH) unit in TTX. Nor-TTX (**9**) was reported by Goto et al.[2] and by Tsein et al.[23] to be essentially nontoxic, whereas Tsuda and co-workers[1] did not report that it had been tested for toxicity. We have reinvestigated[30] the synthesis of nor-TTX and found it to be approximately 20% to 50% as lethal (ip in mouse) as TTX and about 20% as active as a sodium-channel blocker.[31] Nor-TTX (**9**) would appear to be an ideal compound for the preparation of active TTX derivatives; however, the problems associated with the attempted preparation of the O-methyloxime[23,30] are indicative of

9a   **9b**   **9c**

the complications with this compound as a synthon for further modifications. Although the yield of nor-TTX is excellent,[1,2,30] the NMR of the product indicates that it exists in a facile equilibrium with several forms, as indicated in **9a–9c**. It has not been obtained in crystalline form. The small carbonyl signal at 1745 cm^{-1} in the IR is that of a lactone[2,3,30,32]; the 6-keto function is hydrated even after being dried in a vacuum desiccator. There must be a complex equilibrium between lactone (**9c**), hemilactal (**9b**), zwitterionic forms and a trace of the 6-keto (**9a**) structures. This is especially apparent in the difficulties we experienced in getting reproducible NMR spectra of presumably pure samples of nor-TTX. Certainly pH was an important variable, but there appeared to be other unidentified conditions which affected the NMR spectrum.

The report by Tsein et al. on the reaction of **9** with O-methyl hydroxylamine was

9   **21a**   **21b**   **22**

based on one experiment using 1 mg of TTX. The interpretation of results was clouded by their determination that nor-TTX itself was inactive. We have repeated this experiment and conclude that the product is an equilibrium mixture **9 ⇄ 21a ⇄ 21b,** probably containing only traces of the oxime form. We were unable to isolate oxime

TABLE 2.

No.	R, R¹	Refs.
9	$0= \rightleftarrows (HO)_2$	1,2,13,30
23	H-, HO-	30
24a	H-, H_2N-	33
24b	H-, MeHN-	33
24c	H_2NCH$_2$-, HO-	34
21	MeON= $\rightleftarrows$ MeONH-, HO-	23
24d	2-(NO$_2$)-4-N$_3$-C$_6$H$_3$-NHCH$_2$C-NHN-	27
24e	2-(NO$_2$)-4-N$_3$-C$_6$H$_3$-NHCH$_2$C-NHNH-	27
24f	2-(NO$_2$)-4-N$_3$-C$_6$H$_3$-NHCH$_2$CH$_2$NH-	27
24	2-R″-C-NHCH$_2$C-NHNH- R″ = -NH$_2$	33
24g	-NHMe	33
	-N$_3$	33
24h	4-OH-3-I-C$_6$H$_3$-CH$_2$CH$_2$C-O-	33

24

21b. It is likely[30] that the hydrated form (**21a**) predominates in the presence of excess methoxyamine and it is in equilibrium with substantial amounts of nor-TTX (**9**) when the reactants are present in equivalent amounts. Attempts to reduce this mixture to a stabilized 6-methoxyamino-nor-TTX (**22**) were unsuccessful.[30] However, reduction of nor-TTX itself with $NaCNBH_3$ gave an amorphous 11-nor-TTX-6-OH (**23**) in 60% yield that had about 90% of the activity of nor-TTX and about 18% of the activity of TTX itself.[30] The C-6 configuration was assigned based on NMR spectra.[30]

In spite of these complications, nor-TTX has been used as a synthon for the preparation of a number of useful TTX derivatives. These reactions have proceeded in low yield; but by using radioactive tracer techniques, it has been possible to obtain chromatographically homogeneous, active preparations (**24e–24g**) in some cases (see TABLE 2).

Anhydro-TTX, like TTX, is oxidized by periodate in excellent yield to 11-nor-4, 9-anhydro-TTX-6,6-diol[35] (nor-anhydro-TTX, **25**) that is relatively nontoxic (as expected for an anhydro derivative). The NMR spectrum of nor-anhydro-TTX (**25**), in

noranhydro-TTX

1   **2**   **25**   **9**

contrast to that of nor-TTX (**9**), is completely reproducible and shows no sign of the lactone-hemilactal equilibrium.[35] It is also entirely in the 6,6-diol hydrated-keto form. Like nor-TTX, conditions for clean, good yield reactions with carbonyl reagents have not yet been worked out. It has been hydrolyzed to the active nor-TTX (**25 → 9**); thus it can be viewed as a protected form of nor-TTX, and its chemistry should be explored further.

FUTURE CHEMICAL RESEARCH

It is instructive to consider where future chemical research on TTX may take us. Perhaps the first priority is the improvement of procedures for making the types of molecules such as **19a–19f, 24a–24h**, and related compounds in well-characterized forms and in good yields. A closely related goal is the synthesis of specifically radioactively labeled TTX molecules for use in various studies, including the determination of the metabolic fate of TTX. Further studies should be conducted on the synthesis of chemical derivatives, including ones which can be used for selectively protecting this reactive molecule while designed transformations are performed. This work is required before we can obtain derivatives to study further structure-activity relationships. Activity studies might also lead to the synthesis of simpler active analogues that possess the sodium-channel blocking activity of TTX. There is also the challenge of preparing active derivatives with substituents that reduce the transport of TTX in the animal system and thus might be developed into local anesthetics based on the sodium-channel blocking ability. Finally, there is the goal of achieving a practical total synthesis of TTX, thus eliminating dependence upon the pufferfish as our source of TTX.

REFERENCES

1. TSUDA, K., S. IKUMA, M. KAWAMURA, R. TACHIKAWA, K. SAKAI, C. TAMURA & O. AMAKASU. 1964. Chem. Pharm. Bull, Jpn 12: 1357–1374.
2. GOTO, T., Y. KISHI, S. TAKAHASHI & Y. HIRATA. 1965. Tetrahedron 21: 2059–2088.
3. WOODWARD, R. B. 1964. Pure Appl. Chem. 9: 49–74.
4. MOSHER, H. S., F. A. FUHRMAN, H. D. BUCHWALD & H. G. FISCHER. 1964. Science 144: 1100–1110.
5. KISHI, Y., M. ARATANI, T. FUKUYAMA, F. NAKATSUBO, T. GOTO, S. INOUE, H. TANINO, S. SUGIURA & H. KAKOI. 1972. J. Am. Chem. Soc. 94: 9217–9219.
6. KISHI, Y., T. FUKUYAMA, M. ARATANI, F. NAKATSUBO, T. GOTO, S. INOUE, H. TANINO, S. SUGIURA & H. KAKOI. 1972. J. Am. Chem. Soc. 94: 9219–9222.
7. TOMIIE, Y., A. FURUSAKI, K. KASAMI, N. YASUOKA, K. MIYAKE, M. HAISA & I. NITTA. 1963. Tetrahedron Lett. 2101–2104.
8. TSUDA, K., C. TAMURA, R. TACHIKAWA, K. SAKAI, O. AMAKASU, M. KAWAMURA & S. IKUMA. 1963. Chem. Pharm. Bull. Jpn 11: 1473–1475.
9. TSUDA, K., C. TAMURA, R. TACHIKAWA, K. SAKAI, O. AMAKASU, M. KAWAMURA & S. IKUMA. 1964. Chem. Pharm. Bull. Jpn 12: 643–645.
10. FURUSAKI, A., Y. TOMIIE & I. NITTA. 1970. Bull. Chem. Soc. Jpn 43: 3332–3341.
11. YASUMOTO, T., M. NAKAMURA, Y. OSHIMA & J. TAKAHATA. 1982. Bull. Jap. Soc. Sci. Fish. 48: 1431–1437.
12. NAKAMURA, M. & T. YASUMOTO. 1985. Toxicon 23: 271–276.
13. WILZBACH, K. E. 1957. J. Am. Chem. Soc. 79: 1013–1015.
14. LEVINSON, S. R. 1975. Philos. Trans. R. Soc. London 270: 337–348.
15. BALERNA, M., M. FOSSET, R. CHICHEPORTICHE, G. ROMEY & M. LAZDUNSKY. 1975. Biochemistry 14: 5500–5511.
16. GRÜNHAGEN, H. H., M. RACK, R. STÄMPFLI, H. FASOLD & P. REITER. 1981. Arch. Biochem. Biophys. 206: 198–204.
17. BONTEMPS, J., R. CANTINEAU, C. GRANDFILS, P. LEPRINCE, G. DANDRIFOSSE & E. SHOFFENIELS. 1984. Anal. Biochem. 139: 149–157.
18. STRONG, P. N. & J. F. W. KEANA. 1976. Bioorg. Chem. 5: 255–262.
19. STRONG, P. N. 1974. Ph.D. thesis. University of Oregon. Eugene, Ore.
20. DEGUCHI, T. 1967. Jpn J. Pharmacol. 17: 267–278.
21. NARAHASHI, T., J. W. MOORE & R. N. POSTON. 1967. Science 156: 976–978.
22. NACHMAN, R. J. 1981. Ph.D. thesis Stanford University. Stanford, Calif.
23. TSIEN, R. Y., D. P. L. GREEN, S. R. LEVINSON, B. RUDY & J. K. M. SANDERS. 1975. Proc. R. Soc. Lond. Ser. B. 191: 555–559.
24. KIM, Y. H., G. B. BROWN, H. S. MOSHER, & F. A. FUHRMAN. 1975. Science 189: 151–152.
25. PAVELKA, L. A., Y. H. KIM & H. S. MOSHER. 1977. Toxicon 15: 135–139.
26. GUILLORY, R. J., M. D. RAYNER & J. S. D'ARRIGO. 1977. Science 196: 883–885.
27. CHICHEPORTICHE, R., M. BALERNA, A. LOMBET, G. ROMEY & M. LAZDUNSKY. 1979. J. Biol. Chem. 254: 1552–1557.
28. CHICHEPORTICHE, R., M. BALERNA, A. LOMBET, G. ROMEY & M. LAZDUNSKY. 1980. Eur. J. Biochem. 104: 617–625.
29. JAIMOVICH, E., R. CHICHEPORTICHE, A. LOMBET, G. ROMEY & M. LAZDUNSKY. 1980. Pflügers Arch./Eur. J. Physiol. 397: 1–5.
30. PAVELKA, L. A., F. A. FUHRMAN & H. S. MOSHER. 1982. Heterocycles 17: 225–230.
31. KAO, C. Y. 1982. Toxicon 20: 1043–1050.
32. GOTO, T., Y. KISHI, S. TAKAHASHI & Y. HIRATA. 1964. Tetrahedron Lett. 1779–1783.
33. ANGELIDES, K. J. 1981. Biochem. 20: 4107–4118.
34. KOVALENKO, V. A., V. N. PASHKOV, E. V. GRISHIN, Y. A. OVCHINNIKOV, V. P. SCHEVCHENKO & N. F. MYASOEDOV. 1982. Bioorg. Kim. 8: 710–712.
35. NACHMAN, R. J. & H. S. MOSHER. 1985. Heterocycles 21: 3055.

Interspecies Distribution and Possible Origin of Tetrodotoxin

T. YASUMOTO,[a] H. NAGAI,[a] D. YASUMURA,[a]
T. MICHISHITA,[a] A. ENDO,[a] M. YOTSU,[a] AND
Y. KOTAKI[b]

[a]Faculty of Agriculture
Tohoku University
Sendai 980, Japan

[b]Shokei Women's Junior College
Sendai 980, Japan

Tetrodotoxin (TTX) is one of the best-known marine toxins because of its frequent involvement in fatal food poisoning, its unique chemical structure, and its specific action of blocking sodium channels of excitable membranes. The toxin derives its name from the pufferfish family (tetraodontidae), but past studies have revealed its wide distribution in both terrestrial and marine animal kingdoms.[1,2] In many of the TTX-containing animals, toxin content fluctuates according to individual, region, and season. Moreover, Shimizu et al.[3] have recently confirmed that cultured pufferfish lacked the toxin but accumulated it when fed the toxic pufferfish livers. The observation strongly suggests a food chain origin of the toxin.

In pursuit of the alleged toxin elaborator, we tested herbivorous fish and crabs, their food algae, planktivorous annelids, and epiphytic bacteria for the presence of TTX. Detection of low levels of TTX was facilitated by two types of high-performance liquid chromatographic (HPLC) analyzer. Anhydrotetrodotoxin (anhydTTX) and 4-epitetrodotoxin (epiTTX) coexisting with TTX were also determined. Some specimens were also tested for the presence of paralytic shellfish toxins (PST) because these toxins often existed in pufferfish,[4] crabs,[5,6] and in an alga.[7]

This paper deals with detection of TTX and its derivatives in the viscera of herbivorous fish, xanthid crabs, an annelid, an alga, and in bacterial culture broth. Coexistence of TTX and PST in some specimens is also described.

MATERIALS AND METHODS

Specimens

The specimens used for toxin analyses and the places from which they were obtained are listed as follows. Xanthid crabs (*Zosimus aeneus*) were obtained from Negros Island, the Philippines, from Viti Levu Island, Fiji, and from Okinawa, Japan; other species (*Atergatis floridus* and *A. integerrimus*) were from Negros Island. Parrotfish (*Ypsiscarus ovifrons*) were from Wakayama and Hyogo Prefectures; another species (*Scarus gibbus*) was from Okinawa. Angelfish (*Pomacanthus semicirculatus*) were from Okinawa. Annelids (*Pseudopotamia occelata*) were from Miyagi Prefecture. Red calcareous algae (*Jania* sp.) were from Okinawa and from the Gambier Islands, French Polynesia. Bacteria (*Alteromonas* sp.) were isolated from the Okinawan *Jania* sp. (in a previous paper it was described as *Pseudomonas* sp.).[8]

Reference Compounds

TTX, *epi*TTX, and anhydTTX isolated from pufferfish in a previous study[4] were used as references. An authentic sample of 2-amino-6-hydroxymethyl-8-hydroxy-quinazoline (C-9 base) was prepared from TTX following the method of Tsuda *et al.*[10] Reference PST were prepared by Oshima *et al.* from cultured cells of *Protogonyaulax tamarensis.*[11]

Toxin Analyses

Homogenized specimens were extracted with hot 0.02 N acetic acid and filtered. The filtrate was adjusted to pH 5.0 with dil. sodium hydroxide solution and passed through a charcoal column. The column was washed with water and the toxins were eluted with an aqueous solution containing 20% ethanol and 1% acetic acid. After evaporation of the solvent, the residue was dissolved in water and passed through a column packed with Amberlite CG-50 (NH_4^+). The column was washed with water and the toxins were eluted with 0.5 N acetic acid. The eluate was used for HPLC analyses.

Two types of fluorometric HPLC analyzer (analyzer-I and analyzer-II) were used to analyze TTX analogues. Analyzer-I separates toxins on a reversed phase column (Develosil ODS, 0.8 × 25 cm) by paired-ion chromatography and measures fluorescence intensities of alkaline degradation products of the toxins.[12] Analyzer-II uses a cation exchange gel column (Hitachi gel 3011C, 0.5 × 40 cm) with a citrate buffer solution for separation and detects toxins on the same principle.[13]

Analyses of saxitoxin analogues were performed by a fluorometric HPLC analyzer, which separates toxins on a cation exchange gel column (Hitachi gel 3011C, 0.4 × 100 cm) with a citrate buffer and measures fluorescence intensities of alkaline oxidation products of the toxins.[14]

Thin-layer chromatography (TLC) of toxins was performed on precoated silica gel 60 plates (Merck) using the following solvents: (a) pyridine-ethyl acetate-acetic acid-water (75:35:15:30), (b) *tert*-butanol-acetic acid-water (2:1:1), (c) phenol-water-28% ammonium hydroxide (13:2:18), and (d) 1-butanol-acetic acid-water (2:1:1). TTX analogues were detected as fluorescent spots with 10% potassium hydroxide in methanol and saxitoxin analogues with 1% hydrogen peroxide.

A mouse assay method proposed by Kawabata[15] was used for TTX, and the official mouse assay method[16] for saxitoxin analogues.

Extraction of Bacterial Toxins

The *Alteromonas* sp. was cultured in a medium (3% sodium chloride and 1% Polypeptone of Daigoeiyo Kagaku Co.) at 25°C for 12 days without aeration. The culture broth (12 liters) was centrifuged at 800 rpm. The precipitated cells were extracted with 50 ml of 0.02 N acetic acid for 10 min on a boiling water bath. After cooling to the room temperature, the solution was centrifuged and 50 μl of the supernatant was injected to the HPLC analyzer-I.

The culture broth after the removal of cells was acidified to pH 3.0 with acetic acid, boiled for 20 min, and evaporated to dryness. The residue was extracted with 500 ml of methanol containing 1% acetic acid to remove sodium chloride. The extract was evaporated and reextracted in a similar manner. After removal of the solvent by evaporation, the residue was dissolved in water. The solution was adjusted to pH 5.5

with dilute sodium hydroxide and passed through a charcoal column (4 × 4 cm). The column was washed and the toxins were eluted with 20% ethanol containing 1% of acetic acid. The toxic residue after evaporation of the solvent was used for HPLC analyses and for further purification.

Purification of Toxins

Purification of TTX analogues was carried out as described previously by successive treatments of extracts on columns of charcoal, Amberlite CG-50 (NH$_4$$^+$), Bio-Rex 70 (COO$^-$), Bio-Gel P-2, and Hitachi gel 3011C.[9] Similar procedures were also employed for purification of PST.[11]

Preparation of C-9 Base

Samples presumed to contain TTX analogues were heated in 2 N sodium hydroxide solution or in a 60% methanol solution containing 10% sodium hydroxide for 45 min. The solution was adjusted to pH 3.5 with hydrochloric acid and extracted with butanol. After evaporation of the butanol solution, the residue was chromatographed on a Develosil ODS column using an aqueous solution containing 5% acetonitrile and 0.02 N trifluoroacetic acid as the mobile phase. The eluate was monitored by the absorbance at 260 nm and fractions having the same retention volumes as the reference C-9 base were collected. The chromatographic purification was repeated and the samples thus obtained were subjected to spectral measurements.

Spectral Measurements

Mass spectra were measured with a Hitachi M-80 spectrometer or with a JMX DX303 spectrometer, ^{1}H NMR spectra with a Nicolet NT-300 (300 MHz) spectrometer, and UV spectra with a Hitachi 124 spectrometer.

RESULTS

Crabs

The occurrence of TTX, epiTTX, and anhydTTX was indicated by HPLC analyses in Z. aeneus from Philippines, Fiji, and Okinawa. This species had been confirmed to accumulate PST in previous studies.[5,6] However, the relative ratios of TTX analogues to PST varied markedly in individual specimens. In a single specimen one toxin family was overwhelmingly dominant over the other, as shown in TABLE 1.

Only one specimen of A. integerrimus was lethal to mice (2.2 MU/g) and TTX; epiTTX and anhydTTX were the major toxins in this specimen. On the other hand, PST constituted over 99% of the mouse lethality in a highly toxic specimen (730 MU/g) of a related species (A. floridus).

Z. aeneus specimens shown to contain TTX were combined and used for toxin extraction. The purified toxin proved to be identical with TTX by spectral measurements. The ^{1}H NMR spectrum taken in D$_2$O solution exhibited proton signals assignable to H-4 and H-4a of TTX at δ 2.21 ppm (doublet, J = 10.0 Hz) and at δ 5.36 ppm (d, J = 10.0 Hz), respectively. Other proton signals between δ 3.6 and 4.7 ppm also matched those of TTX. The secondary ion mass spectrum taken on a Hitachi M-80 spectrometer using glycerol as the matrix exhibited ions assignable to $(M + H)^+$ and $(M + Na)^+$ of TTX, respectively, at m/z 320 and 342.

Fish

The occurrence of a water soluble toxin in the viscera of *Y. ovifrons, S. gibbus,* and *P. semicirculatus* was indicated by the mouse assay, though at very low levels (below 0.2 ppm). Toxic signs induced in mice resembled those caused by TTX. High-pressure liquid chromatography analyses indicated the presence of TTX, *epi*TTX, and anhydTTX. The toxin was extracted from 8 kg of *S. gibbus* livers and purified by successive chromatography on columns of charcoal, Amberlite CG-50 (NH_4^+), Bio-Rex 70, and Bio-Gel P-2. As the amount of the toxin was too small for further purification to proceed, a semipure sample (118 mg, 100 MU) was subjected to alkaline degradation. Subsequent purification of the degradation products on a Develosil ODS column yielded a compound chromatographically indistinguishable

TABLE 1. Relative Proportions of Tetrodotoxin (TTX) and Paralytic Shellfish Toxins (PST) in Xanthid Crabs (*Zosimus aeneus*) Collected at Negros Island, the Philippines

Specimen No.	Body Weight (g)	Lethal Potency $(MU/g)^a$	TTX (%)	PST (%)
1	106	28	99	1
2	83	36	6	94
3	104	15	99	1
4	60	259	2	98
5	51	48	99	1
6	47	47	99	1
7	64	84	99	1
8	81	215	2	98

*The lethal potency is expressed in a saxitoxin mouse unit.

from the authentic C-9 base. The mass spectrum of the isolated compound was identical with that of C-9 base in showing ions at m/z 191 $(M)^+$, 174 $(M-OH)^+$, and 162 $(M-HCO)^+$. Thus the parrotfish toxin was shown to yield C-9 base, as does TTX.

Annelids

Occasional rises of mouse lethality of *P. occelatus* were observed in a year-round monitoring. In July 1982 the lethal potency rose to 24 MU/g. Analyses with HPLC analyzer-II suggested the presence of TTX, *epi*TTX, and anhydTTX. The major toxin (3.9 mg, 820 MU) purified from 50 g of the annelid proved to be indistinguishable from TTX by TLC (R_f 0.64 by solvent a, 0.46 by solvent b, and 0.34 by solvent c).

Specimens collected in July 1984 did not contain TTX or its derivatives. Instead, gonyautoxin-2 and gonyautoxin-3 were detected by the HPLC analyzer. Two toxic components were purified and proved to be identical with reference gonyautoxin-2 and gonyautoxin-3, respectively, by TLC (R_f 0.71 and 0.76 with solvent b, and 0.49 and 0.66 with solvent d).

Algae

The occurrence of TTX, epiTTX, and anhydTTX in algal samples from the Gambier islands and Okinawa was indicated by HPLC analyses. The chromatograms showed anhydTTX to be the major component in Okinawan sample and TTX in the Gambier sample. Purification of the extracts from 300 g of Okinawan algal sample afforded a compound indistinguishable from the reference anhydTTX by TLC (R_f 0.69 by the solvent b). The anhydTTX concentration in the algae showed remarkable fluctuations, both regionally and seasonally. The highest concentration observed was 44 ppb.

Alteromonas sp.

Fluorometric HPLC analyses indicated that the amounts of TTX and derivatives in the bacterial cells were less than 10 μg, respectively, if there were any. Two compounds (A, 200 μg and B, 55 μg) indistinguishable by HPLC from TTX and anhydTTX, respectively, were obtained from the culture broth (FIG. 1). TLC comparison using solvent b confirmed that compounds A and B give spots (R_f 0.64 and 0.71) comparable with those of reference TTX and anhydTTX (R_f 0.64 and 0.70), respectively.

Compound A killed mice by intraperitoneal injection of a dose of 770 ng with typical signs of TTX intoxication, such as dyspnea and spasmodic movements. The median death time (4 min 20 sec) of two mice (ddY, male, 15.0 g each) was close to the

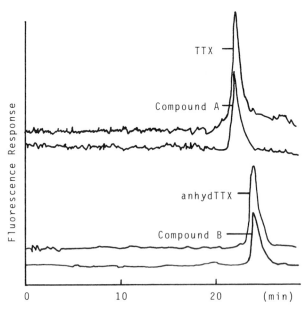

FIGURE 1. Comparison of compounds A and B isolated from the culture broth of *Alteromonas* sp. with tetrodotoxin (TTX) and anhydrotetrodotoxin (anhydTTX) by fluorometric HPLC analyzer-I.

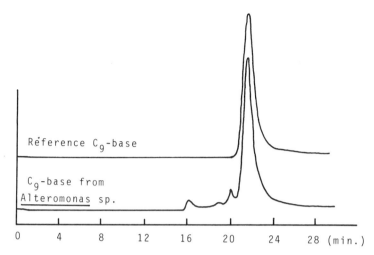

FIGURE 2. Chromatographic comparison between the degradation product of bacterial toxin and the reference C-9 base. Column, Develosil ODS (2 × 25 cm); mobile phase, 0.5 N acetic acid containing 5% acetonitrile; flow rate, 3.0 ml/min; monitoring, 260 nm.

expected death time (4 min 25 sec) given by Kawabata[15] for the same dose of TTX. A mouse (15.0 g) administered with a partially purified sample containing 12 μg of B died 4 minutes and 30 seconds after injection, but two mice given half the dose survived.

A partially purified sample containing A and B was subjected to alkaline degradation. Subsequent purification of the degradation products afforded a compound chromatographically indistinguishable from the reference C-9 base (FIG. 2). The mass spectrum of this compound agreed with that of C-9 base in showing ions at m/z 191 (M)$^+$, 174 (M-OH)$^+$, and 162 (M-HCO)$^+$. Thus the bacterial sample was confirmed to yield C-9 base upon alkaline treatment, as do TTX and its derivatives. FAB mass spectra of A and B taken on a JMX DX303 using glycerol as the matrix exhibited ions at m/z 320 and 302, which were assignable to (M + H)$^+$ ions of TTX and anhydTTX, respectively (FIG. 3). Thus all the chromatographic and spectral data show that A and B isolated from the culture of a *Alteromonas* sp. are identical with TTX and anhydTTX, respectively.

DISCUSSION

This study indicates that TTX is first produced by bacteria and transmitted to other animals through the food chain, at least in coral reef environments. Interestingly, fish species found to contain TTX were taxonomically close to pufferfish. Remote species, such as surgeonfish, unicornfish, and rabbitfish, did not contain TTX, even though they had been collected from the same area. *Y. ovifrons* is known to cause occasional poisoning when the liver is ingested but the toxin was suggested to be different from TTX.[17] *S. gibbus* is frequently involved in ciguatera, but contribution of TTX to manifestation of human symptoms may be negligible, as judged from its low concentration.

Xanthid crabs have been known to accumulate PST and thus cause fatal poisoning when ingested.[5,6] The occurrence of TTX was first noticed in *A. floridus*.[18,19] However, there seems to be no previous report on TTX in *Z. aeneus*, the most frequently implicated species in poisoning. It is noteworthy to point out that in individual *Z. aeneus* specimens the ratio between TTX and PST was heavily tilted to one toxin family and that crabs collected at the same area differed in the toxic principle.[20] It may be interesting to add that two other xanthid crabs, *Lophozozymus pictor* and *Demania alcalai*, from the same area of Negros Island, were also highly toxic but contained palytoxin, a highly lethal toxin of zoanthids belonging to the genus *Palythoa*.[21]

The occurrence of PST in the planktivorous annelid is explainable by the occasional proliferation of the toxic dinoflagellate, *Protogonyaulax tamarensis*, in the

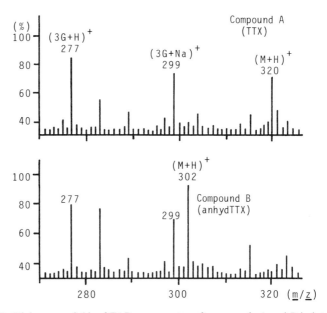

FIGURE 3. Higher mass fields of FAB mass spectra of compounds A and B isolated from the culture broth of *Alteromonas* sp. Spectra were taken with a JMX DX303 spectrometer using glycerol as the matrix.

sampling area. The origin of TTX in the annelid is not known at present. However, bacterial flocks in the sea may be suggested as the primary source.

The detection of TTX and anhydTTX in *Jania* sp. adds to the previous finding of PST in this alga[7] and points to its importance in the food chain. Interestingly, *Alteromonas* sp. (previously assigned to *Pseudomonas* sp.) converts gonyautoxins to saxitoxin and neosaxitoxin by reductively eliminating the 11-hydroxysulfate group.[8]

The discovery of *Alteromonas* sp. explains the food chain transmission of TTX, at least in coral reef environments. However, the occurrence of other TTX-producing bacteria is predictable, judging from the diversity of TTX-containing species and the many different environments in which they are found. Another point worth mentioning is the coexistence of TTX and PST in several species. In addition to our discovery of saxitoxin in pufferfish, both toxin families were newly found to occur in the crabs, the annelid, and the alga.

REFERENCES

1. MOSHER, H. S. & F. A. FUHRMAN. 1984. Occurrence and origin of tetrodotoxin. *In* Seafood Toxins. E. P. Ragelis, Ed. A.C.S. Symposium Series **262**: 332–344. American Chemical Society. Washington, D.C.
2. ONOUE, Y., T. NOGUCHI & K. HASHIMOTO. 1984. Tetrodotoxin determination methods. *In* Seafood Toxins. E. P. Ragelis, Ed. A.C.S. Symposium Series **262**: 345–355. American Chemical Society. Washington, D. C.
3. SHIMIZU, C., T. MATSUI, H. SATO & K. YAMAMORI. 1984. Pufferfish toxin. Mar. Sci. Mon. (Tokyo) **16**(10): 560–565.
4. NAKAMURA, M., Y. OSHIMA & T. YASUMOTO. 1984. Occurrence of saxitoxin in puffer fish. Toxicon **22**(3): 381–385.
5. HASHIMOTO, Y. 1979. Marine Toxins and Other Bioactive Metabolites. Japan Scientific Society Press. Tokyo.
6. YASUMOTO, T., Y. OSHIMA & Y. KOTAKI. 1983. Analyses of paralytic shellfish toxins in coral reef crabs and gastropods with the identification of the primary source of toxins. 1983. Toxicon (Suppl. 3):513–516.
7. KOTAKI, Y., M. TAJIRI, Y. OSHIMA & T. YASUMOTO. 1983. Identification of a calcareous red alga as the primary source of paralytic shellfish toxins in coral reef crabs and gastropods. Bull. Jpn. Soc. Fish. **49**(2): 283–286.
8. KOTAKI, Y., Y. OSHIMA & T. YASUMOTO. 1985. Bacterial transformation of paralytic shellfish toxins in coral reef crabs and a marine snail. Bull. Jpn. Soc. Sci. Fish. **51**(6): 1009–1013.
9. NAKAMURA, M. & T. YASUMOTO. 1985. Tetrodotoxin derivatives in puffer fish. Toxicon **23**(2): 271–276.
10. TSUDA, K., S. IKUMA, M. KAWAMURA, R. TACHIKAWA, K. SAKAI, C. TAMURA & O. AMAKASU. 1964. Tetrodotoxin. VII. On the structures of tetrodotoxin and its derivatives. Chem. Pharm. Bull. **12**(11): 1357–1374.
11. OSHIMA, Y., T. HAYAKAWA, M. HASHIMOTO, Y. KOTAKI & T. YASUMOTO. 1982. Classification of *Protogonyaulax tamarensis* from Northern Japan into three strains by toxin composition. Bull. Jpn. Soc. Sci. Fish. **48**(6): 851–854.
12. YASUMOTO, T. & T. MICHISHITA. 1985. Fluorometric determination of tetrodotoxin by high performance liquid chromatography. Agric. Biol. Chem. **49**(10): 3077–3080.
13. YASUMOTO, T., M. NAKAMURA, Y. OSHIMA & J. TAKAHATA. 1982. Construction of a continuous tetrodotoxin analyzer. Bull. Jpn. Soc. Sci. Fish. **48**(10): 1481–1483.
14. OSHIMA, Y., M. MACHIDA, K. SASAKI, Y. TAMAOKI & T. YASUMOTO. 1984. Liquid chromatographic-fluorometric analysis of paralytic shellfish toxins. Agric. Biol. Chem. **48**(7): 1707–1711.
15. KAWABATA, T. 1978. Pufferfish toxin. *In* The Manual for the Methods of Food Sanitation Tests, vol. II. Bureau of Environmental Health. Ministry of Health and Welfare, Japan. Japan Food Hygenic Association. Tokyo. pp. 232–240.
16. A.O.A.C. 1980. Paralytic shellfish poison. *In* Official Methods of Analysis of the Association of Officials. 13th ed. W. Horwitz, Ed.: 298. Assoc. Official Anal. Chem. Washington, D. C.
17. FUSETANI, N., S. SATO & K. HASHIMOTO. 1985. Occurrence of a water soluble toxin in a parrotfish (*Ypsiscarus ovifrons*) which is probably responsible for parrotfish liver poisoning. Toxicon **22**(1): 105–112.
18. ENDEAN, R., R. LEWIS, P. GYR & J. WILLIAMSON. 1983. Toxic material from the crab *Atergatis floridus*. Toxicon (Suppl. 3): 111–113.
19. NOGUCHI, T., A. UZU, K. KOYAMA, J. MARUYAMA, Y. NAGASHIMA and K. HASHIMOTO. 1983. Occurrence of tetrodotoxin as the major toxin in a xanthid crab *Atergatis floridus*. Bull. Jpn. Soc. Fish. **49**(12): 1887–1892.
20. YASUMURA, D., Y. OSHIMA, T. YASUMOTO, A. C. ALCALA & L. C. ALCALA. 1986. Tetrodotoxin and paralytic shellfish toxins in Philippine crabs. Agric. Biol. Chem. **50**(3): 593–598.
21. YASUMOTO, T., D. YASUMURA, Y. OHIZUMI, M. TAKAHASHI, A. C. ALCALA & L. C. ALCALA. 1986. Palytoxin in two species of xanthid crab from the Philippines. Agric. Biol. Chem. **50**(1): 163–167.

Structure-Activity Relations of Tetrodotoxin, Saxitoxin, and Analogues[a,b]

C. Y. KAO

Department of Pharmacology
Downstate Medical Center
State University of New York
Brooklyn, New York 11203

INTRODUCTION

Tetrodotoxin (TTX) and saxitoxin (STX) are important neurobiological tools because of their selective and high-affinity blockade of the voltage-gated sodium channel of many excitable membranes.[1] As such they have not only aided in the isolation of the sodium channel macromolecule, but are also potentially useful in further structural clarification of the channel protein. Although their sources and chemical structures are quite different, their biological actions are virtually identical in that they share the unique channel specificity and a channel affinity measured in equilibrium dissociation constants of nanomolar concentrations. The similarities of their actions imply the presence of similarities in chemical structures, which when identified can help in the understanding of their interactions with the sodium channel. More specifically, a better understanding of their interactions with the channel protein could lead to the recognition of the binding site which in turn could serve as a landmark for orientation in additional structural clarification.

Until recently, few studies of the structure-activity relations of either toxin have been successful. In the case of tetrodotoxin, most derivatives made during chemical studies of its structure in the early 1960s were too extensively modified to be of much revelatory value.[2,3] In the case of saxitoxin, questions about its structure were not resolved until it was successfully crystallized in 1975.[4,5] The separatory and detection technologies of the day for both toxins were such that contamination with minute amounts of the highly potent toxins themselves could not be excluded with certainty, rendering suspect some observations on the weaker analogues.[6]

For lack of specific information, explanations of how tetrodotoxin and saxitoxin blocked the sodium channel were based largely on unproven assumptions. A widely adopted working hypothesis depicted the blockade as resulting from the entrance of the guanidinium end of the toxin molecules into the sodium channel and the toxin acting somewhat like a plug.[7] Further elaborations suggested that the guanidinium group was lodged against the selectivity filter of the channel, and some covalent bond was formed between the receptor and identified groups in each toxin molecule.[8]

Since the mid-1970s, a number of natural and synthetic analogues of both tetrodotoxin and saxitoxin have been discovered and made. Many of these compounds have only limited and discrete alterations from the parent compound, making it easier

[a]This work was supported in part by a grant from the National Institute of Neurological and Communicative Disorders and Stroke (NS 14551).
[b]This paper is dedicated to Steven E. Walker.

to relate a change in biological effects with a modification of chemical structure. Equally important are advances in the technologies of separation, detection, and characterization that have vastly improved confidence in the purity of the newer analogues. From experiments with some of the analogues, and other simpler manipulations of the chemical states of certain groups in tetrodotoxin, saxitoxin and neosaxitoxin, my colleagues and I have been able to identify the active groups in each toxin, and also to recognize some stereospecially similar functionalities in the two toxin molecules.[9] These results have led us to believe that the binding site for tetrodotoxin and saxitoxin is most probably located on the external surface of the membrane and not inside the sodium channel.

MATERIAL AND METHODS

The details of the material and methods used can be found in the primary publications.[9-11] Briefly, the work was done on either the isolated, and often internally perfused, squid giant axon, or on the isolated skeletal muscle fiber of the frog. The electrophysiological criteria used for assaying the activities of the various compounds were either changes in the maximum rate of rise of the action potential ($\dot{V}_{max}$), or the residual sodium current (I_{Na}) in the voltage-clamped preparation. With either method, the end point was compared with that in the same preparation before treatment with the toxin. Moreover, the effects of an analogue were always compared with those of the parent toxin itself. Therefore, the emphasis is on relative potencies rather than absolute specific potencies, an important point when one considers that quantitative determinations of the contents of the various toxin compounds still depend primarily on bioassays, rather than on specific chemical methods. It should be recognized that owing to the complex and nonlinear relation between the sodium conductance and the total membrane current, as expressed in the maximum rate of rise of the action potential, the ED_{50} based on that criteria is about 2.5 to 3 times higher than the ED_{50} obtained on residual sodium current in voltage-clamped preparations. The use of relative potencies with respect to the parent toxins also unifies observations from the different methods.

The various toxin compounds used were supplied by our chemist colleagues. Tetrodotoxin analogues were supplied by Profs. H. S. Mosher and T. Yasumoto, and saxitoxin analogues by Prof. H. K. Schnoes and Dr. F. E. Koehn. The identity and purity of each compound has been checked by various physical means, and the toxicity had been determined by a mouse-lethality bioassay method. For our use, all the compounds were in lyophilized form, accurately weighed and in sealed ampoules. We prepared the initial stock solutions in slightly acidified deionized water. Subsequently, working solutions were prepared by dilutions into the appropriate physiological saline solution.

RESULTS AND DISCUSSION

Before entering into a comparison of the relative potencies of the various analogues, I should first make the clarification that all the compounds share the specificity of the parent toxin in blocking only the sodium channel. All the compounds tested also occupy the same receptor as the parent toxin.[9]

Tetrodotoxin Analogues

The Guanidinium Group

FIGURE 1 shows a list of tetrodotoxin analogues that we have examined for relative potencies. In tetrodotoxin, there is only one guanidinium group that has a pK_a of over

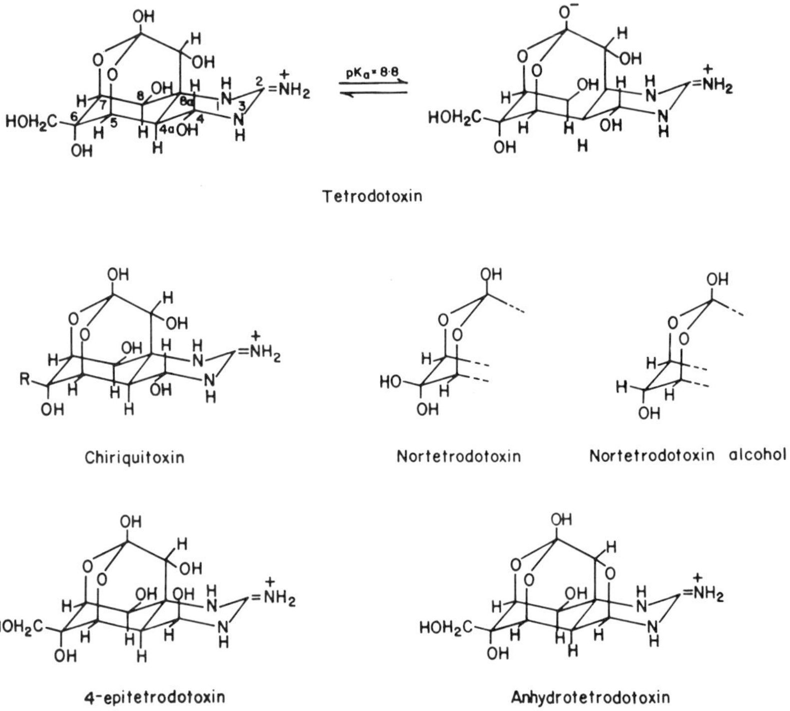

FIGURE 1. Structure of tetrodotoxin and some analogues studied. The *top row* shows protonation-deprotonation relation of C-10 -OH group. The role of this group was tested by manipulating pH of solution. The *middle row* shows three analogues modified on the C-6 position. Chiriquitoxin, a natural analogue in skin and eggs of Costa Rican frog *Atelopus chiriquensis,* has unidentified modification (R) of 104 mass units.[14-18] Nortetrodotoxin is shown as ketone hydrate on C-6, which exists in complex equilibrium with ketone form and lactone form (see Mosher[22]). The molecule to right of the broken line is identical to tetrodotoxin. Nortetrodotoxin alcohol has alcohol on C-6 (see Pavelka *et al.*[19] and Mosher[22]). In the *bottom row,* positions of -H and -OH on C-4 in 4-*epi*tetrodotoxin are reversed from those in tetrodotoxin. Anhydrotetrodotoxin is formed by dehydration between C-4 and C-9. See Nakamura and Yasumoto[21] and Kao and Yasumoto.[11] (Reprinted with permission from Toxicon **23**, Kao and Yasumoto, copyright 1985, Pergamon Press.)

11.[2,12,13] At physiological pHs it is always protonated and positively charged. There is no easy way to test the role of the guanidinium group in channel blockade, except perhaps by some drastic chemical modification that might also introduce other complex changes in the rest of the molecule. All our opinions about the role of this guanidinium group are therefore dependent on comparisons with the active guanidinium group in saxitoxin.

The C-6 Groups

The C-6 end of the molecule is almost directly across from the quanidinium end. In early chemical studies on TTX, most modifications were made around the guanidinium end, and most products were inactive.[2] However, periodate oxidation did lead to nortetrodotoxin which was either not tested for toxicity[2] or believed to be inactive.[13] When chiriquitoxin was discovered,[14-16] it was soon established that it only differed structurally from tetrodotoxin in an unidentified modification on the C-6 end, and that it was equally lethal to mice[17] and equally potent in blocking the sodium channel in frog muscle fiber[18] (FIG. 2).

Although the equipotency with tetrodotoxin escaped general appreciation, it was an important stimulus, leading to a reexamination of modifications on the C-6 end. As is now recognized, nortetrodotoxin is not a simple substance, but probably exists in solution as an equilibrium between several states.[19] It can be anywhere from 0.08 to 0.25 as potent as tetrodotoxin[20] (FIG. 2). The potency of nortetrodotoxin alcohol is within the same general range.[20] All these observations on the C-6 modified compounds show that the C-6 end is not important for blocking the sodium channel.

The C-4 and C-9 Groups

A number of C-4 analogues were made by Tsuda et al.,[2] and tested by Deguchi[3] and Narahashi et al.[6] The most potent among them was deoxytetrodotoxin, which was found to be 0.15 as active as tetrodotoxin on the lobster giant axon.[6] Unfortunately, that sample was found to contain 15% tetrodotoxin,[6] casting some doubts on the validity of those studies.

Normally, in tetrodotoxin the -OH group on C-4 points away from the C-9 and C-10 groups. In tracing the natural metabolism of tetrodotoxin in puffer fish, Nakamura and Yasumoto[21] discovered a new compound, 4-epitetrodotoxin, in which the positions of the -H and -OH were just reversed from those in tetrodotoxin. This compound, with such a minute change in structure, turns out to be 0.4 as potent as tetrodotoxin[11] (FIG. 3a).

In anhydrotetrodotoxin, the C-4 and C-9 groups are joined by an oxygen bridge. Goto et al.[13] had explained the formation of this compound by postulating the existence of a 4-epi compound, and the loss of one mole of water from C-4 and C-9. On the residual sodium current of internally perfused squid axon, anhydrotetrodotoxin was found to be about 0.02 as potent as tetrodotoxin[11] (FIG. 3a). Therefore, the -OH groups on C-4 and C-9 are both important for the channel-blockade property of tetrodotoxin.

The C-10 Group

This group in tetrodotoxin has some unusual chemical properties.[22] In solution, there is an equilibrium between the protonated and uncharged form and the deprotonated negative form with a pK_a of 8.8.[2,12,13] In the latter form, the whole molecule becomes a zwitterion because the guanidinium group is already positively charged. In several earlier studies on the effects of pH on the potency of tetrodotoxin, the cationic form of tetrodotoxin was found to be more potent than the zwitterionic form,[23-27] with

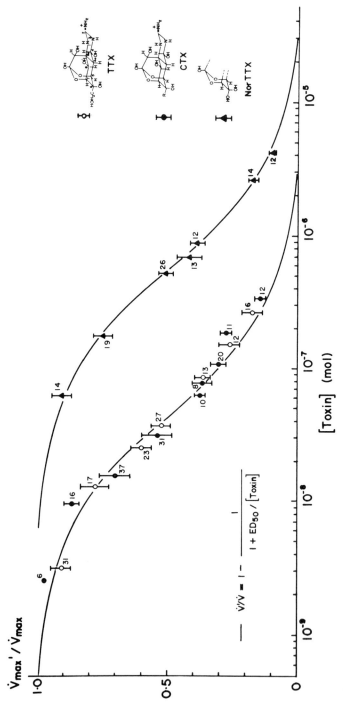

FIGURE 2. Dose-dependent relations of modified tetrodotoxin analogues at C-6. *Ordinate,* Response measured as maximum rate of rise of action potential of frog muscle fiber in toxin ($\dot{V}_{max}'$) normalized to that without toxin ($\dot{V}_{max}$). *Abscissa,* Concentration of toxin on logarithmic scale. *Symbols* represent means ±1 S.E.M.; *numbers* indicate number of fibers tested. *Solid line* is based on biomolecular reaction. Chiriquitoxin is equipotent with tetrodotoxin, whereas nortetrodotoxin is 0.08 as potent.

the relative potencies agreeing well with that expected from the abundance of the protonated C-10 group. Camougis *et al.*[23] suggested that the deprotonated O^- group on C-10 could represent a loss of a potential hydrogen-bonding site, or be repelled by some fixed anionic charge in the receptor.

In all these studies, only single doses of tetrodotoxin at different pHs were used. In a recent reexamination of this problem, we used several doses to construct dose-

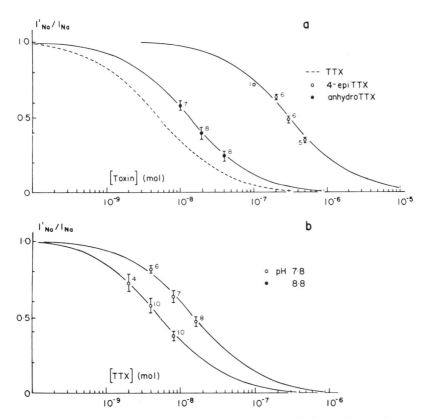

FIGURE 3. (a) Dose-response relations of 4-*epi*tetrodotoxin and anhydrotetrodotoxin. Response (*ordinate*) is based on residual sodium current in squid axon; 4-*epi*tetrodotoxin is 0.4 as potent as tetrodotoxin, and anhydrotetrodotoxin is 0.02 as potent. (b) Influence of state of C-10 -OH group on potency of tetrodotoxin. At pH 8.8, 50% of C-10 group is deprotonated; at pH 7.8, 10% is in this state. Tetrodotoxin is 2.7 times more potent at pH 7.8 than at pH 8.8, indicating that protonated C-10 is important for channel blockade. See Hu and Kao.[10]

response curves at pHs 7.8 and 8.8, and found that the relative potencies (ratio of 2.7) far exceeded what one might expect (ratio of 1.8) from changes in the relative abundance of the C-10 protonated form[10] (FIG. 3b). However, in a low ionic strength medium, not only was the potency of tetrodotoxin significantly reduced, but the relative potencies at pH 7.8 and 8.8 came close to that expected from the protonation relation (ratio of 1.7). Our interpretation is that the C-10 -OH participates in some hydrogen bonding to the receptor site. In the low ionic strength medium, the influence of the surface charge on the membrane extends farther into the surrounding solution, and displaces the toxin molecule out of range of effective hydrogen bonding. In support of this idea is the observation of Nachman[28] that a C-10 methoxy derivative of tetrodotoxin has no significant lethality.

In summary, the relative potencies of tetrodotoxin and the analogues studied are: tetrodotoxin at pH 7.8 (1), chiriquitoxin (1), nortetrodotoxin (0.08–0.25), nortetrodotoxin alcohol (*ca* 0.1), 4-*epi*tetrodotoxin (0.4), anhydrotetrodotoxin (0.02), and tetrodotoxin at pH 8.8 (0.37).

Saxitoxin and Analogues

The Active Guanidinium Group

FIGURES 4 and 5 show the structures of the saxitoxin analogues that we have studied. The first questions to be asked about the two guanidinium functions in these compounds (in spite of widely accepted assumptions) are whether the guanidinium group is involved in blocking the sodium channel, and if it is, which one of the two might be the active group. These questions were answered by the same set of experiments which took advantage of the rather different pK_a of the two guanidinium groups.[29] The pK_a of the 1,2,3 guanidinium is 11.6, and that of the 7,8,9 group is

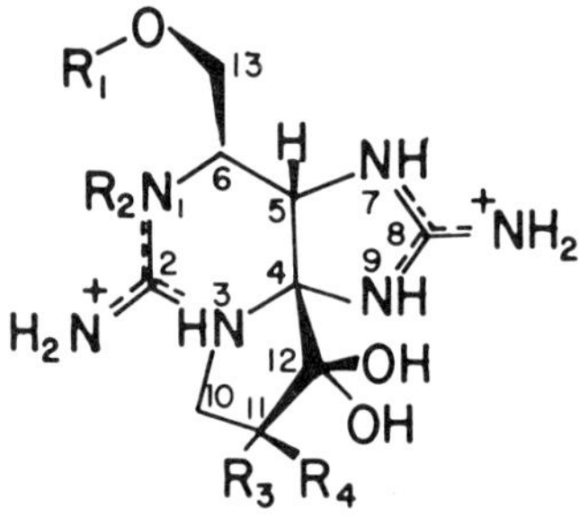

	R₁	R₂	R₃	R₄
Saxitoxin	$CONH_2$	H	H	H
Neosaxitoxin	$CONH_2$	OH	H	H
Decarbamylsaxitoxin	H	H	H	H
11α(-OSO₃)STX, Gonyautoxin II	$CONH_2$	H	OSO_3	H
11β(-OSO₃)STX, Gonyautoxin III	$CONH_2$	H	H	OSO_3
11α(-OH)STX	$CONH_2$	H	OH	H

FIGURE 4. Saxitoxin analogues modified on N-1 (neosaxitoxin), C-11, and C-13 (decarbamylsaxitoxin). Except for decarbamylsaxitoxin and 11α-(-OH) saxitoxin, the compounds are natural analogues.

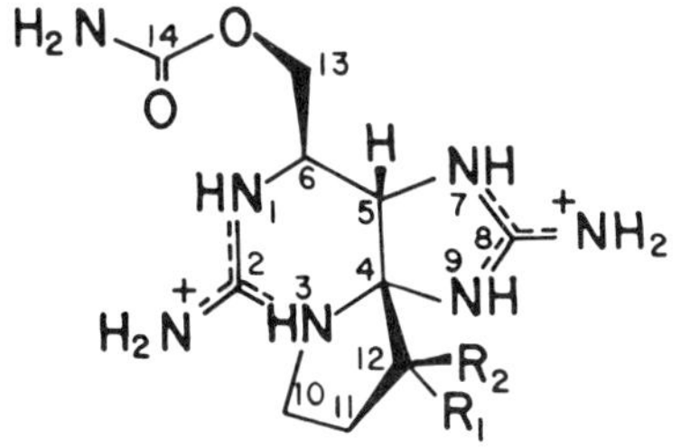

	R_1	R_2
Saxitoxin	OH	OH
α Saxitoxinol	OH	H
β Saxitoxinol	H	OH
Saxitoxin ethylene thioketal		
Saxitoxin oxime	=N-OH	
Saxitoxin methyloxime	=N-OCH₃	
Saxitoxin carboxymethyloxime	=N-OCH₂COOH	

FIGURE 5. C-12 modified analogues of saxitoxin, all of which are synthetic.

8.25.[30,31] Within the physiological range of pHs the 1,2,3 group is almost entirely protonated, whereas the 7,8,9 group can be either protonated or deprotonated depending on the pH.

An examination of the relative potencies of saxitoxin at pHs 7.25 and 8.25 shows that STX is 1.77 to 1.79 times more potent at pH 7.25 than at 8.25, a ratio that corresponds closely with the relative abundance (1.8) of the protonated form of the 7,8,9 group (TABLES 1A and 1B). The relative abundance of the protonated form of the 1,2,3 group at the same pHs would remain essentially 1.0. These observations indicate that the 7,8,9 group is the guanidinium group directly involved in blocking the sodium channel, and that the protonated cationic form is the active form.[29] Although these observations suggested that the 1,2,3 group was probably not directly involved in channel blockade, newer information suggests that it is involved in binding.[32]

The Carbamoyl Group

Ghazarossian et al.[33] first discovered that hydrolytic decarbamylation of saxitoxin led to a product which retained 60% of the toxicity of saxitoxin in mouse-lethality bioassay. This observation has been confirmed and extended by Koehn et al.,[34] and the same product when tested on the isolated frog muscle fiber was found to be 20% as potent as STX in blocking the sodium channel,[9] the difference probably attributable to the different assay systems used. Moreover, natural STX was decarbamylated, and the product then recarbamylated by reacting with chlorosulfonylisocyanate.[35] The three compounds were physically characterized and also tested on the squid axon. Whereas the natural and recarbamylated STXs were equally potent in blocking the sodium channel, the decarbamylated STX was one-fifth as potent (FIG 6).[36] Therefore it can be safely concluded that the carbamoyl group contributes to, but is not essential for, channel blockade.

The C-11 Groups

Several analogues were sulfated on the C-11 position (also known as gonyautoxins), of which we have studied the α and β epimers of 11-(OSO_3)-STX and 11-α-(OH) STX. Modifications on the C-11 group are of interest because of their proximity to the C-12 group, which are of critical importance for channel blockade (see below). The sulfate substituents are not only sterically large but also strongly negative at physiological pHs.[37] Yet their influence on blocking the sodium channel appears to be relatively small, because the relative potencies as compared with saxitoxin are STX

TABLE 1. Comparison of Relative Abundance of Protonated Guanidinium Groups with Relative Potencies of Saxitoxin at pHs 7.25 and 8.25

A.	Protonated Guanidium Group	pK_a	Relative Abundance
	1, 2, 3	11.6	1.0
	7, 8, 9	8.25	1.8
B.	Relative Potencies		
	Squid axon[a]		1.79
	Frog muscle[b]		1.77

[a] From Kao et al.,[29] potency at pH 7.25.
[b] From Hu and Kao,[32] potency at pH 8.25.

(1) : 11β-(OSO_3)-STX (0.42) : 11α-(OSO_3)-STX (0.2) : 11α-(OH)-STX (0.1) (FIG. 7).[38] These observations suggest that the C-11 groups are not critical for channel blockade.

The C-12 Groups

The ketone function on C-12 normally exists in a hydrated state.[4,5,30,34] Although in solution an equilibrium exists between the hydrated and unhydrated forms, significant amounts of the carbonyl form appear only when the 7,8,9 guanidinium is deprotonated at pHs above 8.5.[31] The two hydroxyl groups in the hydrated ketone can be reduced selectively to produce either the α or the β epimer of saxitoxinol.[34] Nonselective reduction leads to a mixture of the two epimers in a ratio of 2.7α to 1β. Historically a reduction product of saxitoxin, known as dihydrosaxitoxin, was found to be only 1% or 2% as toxic as saxitoxin. However, the product was not fully characterized, and there was some uncertainty about the possible contamination with unreduced saxitoxin.[39]

We have assayed the saxitoxinols produced by Koehn et al.[34] on both the squid axon and the frog muscle,[9,38] and found both individual epimers to be not more than 1% to

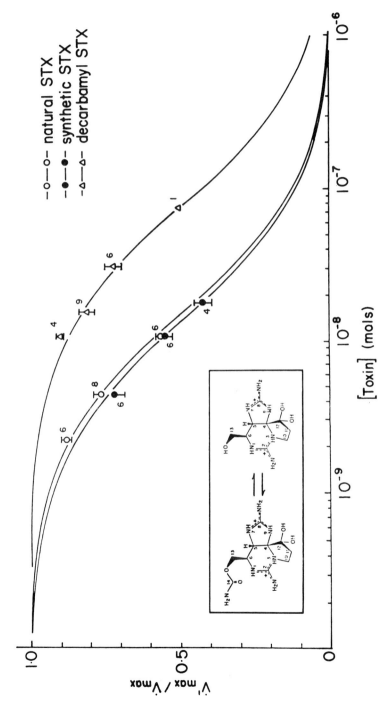

FIGURE 6. Dose-response relations of decarbamylsaxitoxin on squid axon. *Inset:* Carbamoyl group of saxitoxin can be hydrolyzed off in strong HCl,[33,34] and product can be recarbamylated by reacting with chlorosulfonylisocyanate.[35] Natural and recarbamylated saxitoxin are equally potent in reducing $\dot{V}_{max}$ in squid axon, whereas decarbamylsaxitoxin is 20% as potent. Curve for decarbamylsaxitoxin was shifted to the right by increasing the ED_{50} five times (based on data from frog muscle fiber, Kao and Walker[9]). The resultant curve fit the experimental data well. See Koehn *et al.*[36]

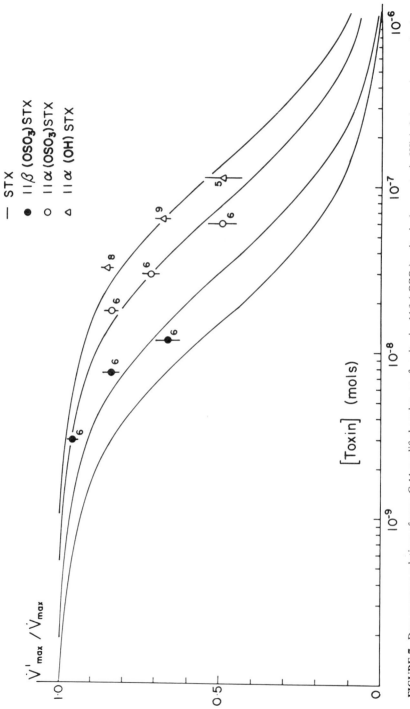

FIGURE 7. Dose-response relations of some C-11 modified analogues of saxitoxin. 11β-(-OSO$_3$)saxitoxin (gonyautoxin III) is 0.4 as active as saxitoxin, 11α-(-OSO$_3$)saxitoxin (gonyautoxin II) is 0.2 as potent, and 11α-(-OH) saxitoxin is 0.1 as potent.

2% as active as saxitoxin. At that level of weak activity, the question of possible contamination by saxitoxin is just as valid as it was historically. It is satisfactorily answered in part by the use of improved chemical technology, but more effectively by an insightful experiment by Koehn. Assuming that the limit of his detection of saxitoxin was at the 1% level of contamination, he reduced the product again sequentially. The second reduction product should then have no more than 0.01% contaminating saxitoxin. The two reduction products were equally potent at about 1% of saxitoxin, the second being 100 times more potent than can be attributed to any contaminating saxitoxin. There were some differences in the responsiveness of the squid axon and the frog muscle to the saxitoxinols, the squid axon being about 10 times less sensitive. However, the α epimer is about four times more potent than the β epimer. Three oximes[40] and a thioketal[38] modified on C-12 are all either very weak or inactive.

These observations not only show the critical role of the C-12 hydroxyl groups in the channel blockade of saxitoxin, they also show that any covalent bonding mechanism involving these groups, as first proposed by Hille,[8] is rather unlikely because the alcohol functions in saxitoxinols cannot form covalent bonds. In spite of these findings, there has been a revival recently of the theory of a covalent bonding mechanism at this site.[41] The new proposal involves a two-step mechanism in which the 7,8,9 guanidinium group is first deprotonated upon adsorption to the receptor. Then the C-12 hydrated ketone shifts to the carbonyl form which undergoes the postulated covalent reaction with some amino group in the receptor. One important basis for the proposal is an observation that neosaxitoxin was four to eight times more potent than saxitoxin at about neutral pH. This observation was associated with a separate chemical observation that the methylene hydrogens on C-11 in neosaxitoxin apparently exchanged much faster with deuterium than the corresponding hydrogens in saxitoxin.[42] Since the H-D exchange requires a carbonyl at C-12,[42] it was reasoned that the higher potency of neosaxitoxin must reflect the more abundant presence of the carbonyl form than in saxitoxin.

At least two significant difficulties are associated with this entire proposal. First, there is no information available at this time on the hydrated ketone-carbonyl equilibrium in neosaxitoxin. Second, when neosaxitoxin is reduced to neosaxitoxinol, the lethality of the product is markedly reduced, but some intrinsic activity remains.[37] The situation is similar to that of saxitoxinol where the C-12 groups are in an alcohol centrifugation, which cannot form covalent bonds because of prohibitive energetics. As will be made clear below, the enhanced potency of neosaxitoxin probably has a different explanation.

The 1,2,3 Guanidinium Group

By relating the abundance of the protonated form of the guanidinium groups and the potency of saxitoxin at different pHs, we have identified the 7,8,9 group and excluded the 1,2,3 group as being directly involved in channel blockade.[29] Recent detailed studies[32] on the effect of pH on the actions of neosaxitoxin show that the potency of channel blockade is strongly influenced by the protonation-deprotonation of the N-1 -OH group. Because the pK_a of this group is 6.75,[42] it is mostly deprotonated and negatively charged at neutral and alkaline pHs, and mostly protonated and uncharged at pHs below 6.5. At pH 7.8, neosaxitoxin and saxitoxin are equally potent. At pH 7.25 and 6.5, neosaxitoxin is about 1.8 and 3.5 times more potent than saxitoxin, but at pH 8.25, neosaxitoxin is only half as potent as saxitoxin (even though one would have expected a slightly greater potency from a more alkaline pK_a of the 7,8,9 guanidinium than in STX).

When the interactions of the two toxins are tested in constant-ratio mixtures,[9] they obviously compete for the same receptor site. The results of the interactions at pH 6.5 agree with the theoretical expectation to within 2%, with both saxitoxin and neosaxitoxin acting at full efficacy. However, the results at pH 8.25 can only fit the theoretical expectation if the efficacy of neosaxitoxin were 0.75 and that of saxitoxin remained at 1.0. This outcome suggests that the 1,2,3 group has an influence on the binding of the whole molecule to the channel protein. An efficacy factor of 0.75 suggests that when the N-1 group is mostly negatively charged, 25% of the successful collisions of the neosaxitoxin molecules with the receptor site failed to result in an effective blockage of the sodium channel. Therefore, we visualize the N-OH group as interacting with some distinct receptor group. In the protonated form it could form a hydrogen bond, in the deprotonated form it could be repelled by the anionic receptor group.

The relative potencies of saxitoxin and the analogues studied are: saxitoxin (1), tetrodotoxin (1), neosaxitoxin (1.0–1.8), saxitoxin at pH 8.25 (0.6), decarbamylsaxitoxin (0.2), 11β-(-OSO$_3$)-saxitoxin (gonyautoxin III) (0.4), 11α-(-OSO$_3$) saxitoxin (gonyautoxin II) (0.2), 11α-(-OH) saxitoxin (0.1), 12α-saxitoxinol (0.002–0.01), 12β-saxitoxinol (0.003), saxitoxin ethylene thioketal, ($\ll 0.01$), saxitoxin oxime

TABLE 2. Active Groups of Tetrodotoxin and Saxitoxin[a]

Tetrodotoxin	Saxitoxin
(1,2,3 guanidinium)	7,8,9 guanidinium
C-9 -OH	C-12 -OH
C-10 -OH	C-12 -OH
C-4 -OH	—
(C-8 -OH)	carbamoyl

[a]Groups in parentheses cannot be verified by direct experimental data.

(0.0005), saxitoxin methyloxime (0.0006), and saxitoxin carboxymethyloxime (0.007).

Surface Receptor as a Possible Toxin-binding Site

Similarities of the Active Groups in Tetrodotoxin and Saxitoxin

From the experimental data with each toxin and its analogues, the groups that are essential for blocking the sodium channel can be identified as shown in TABLE 2. An inspection of molecular models of the toxins shows remarkable stereospecific similarities in these identified active groups, even though the molecules themselves are chemically different (see color plate of models in Kao and Walker[9]). The 7,8,9 guanidinium group in saxitoxin corresponds to the only guanidinium in tetrodotoxin. The C-12 hydroxyl groups of saxitoxin correspond to the C-9 and C-10 hydroxyl groups in tetrodotoxin. The carbamoyl function in saxitoxin corresponds to the C-8 hydroxyl in tetrodotoxin. The C-4 hydroxyl group in tetrodotoxin has no counterpart in saxitoxin. With the exception of the guanidinium and C-8 functions in tetrodotoxin, the role of every group listed is supported by experimental evidence.

A Surface Receptor as the Binding Site

If two molecules as different as tetrodotoxin and saxitoxin have virtually identical biological actions of a unique nature, it must mean that they react with their receptors in a common way. The active groups as identified above could not fit into a single common site inside the sodium channel in a plugging model. There is also other discordant evidence against such a plugging conformation.[43,44] The toxin molecules can be accommodated in a single common receptor site only if that receptor were located on the external surface of the membrane near the orifice of the sodium channel. Previously, I had suggested that the C-12 hydroxyls of saxitoxin and the C-9 and C-10 counterparts in tetrodotoxin might nestle in some sort of a crypt in the receptor while the guanidinium group projects partly across the orifice of the sodium channel.[45] In this simplest of possible schemes, it is thought that the guanidinium group is electrostatically attracted to ionized carboxylate groups in the receptor, and that the various hydroxyl groups hydrogen-bond with them. In this scheme, the impression is that over the dimensions of the toxin molecules, the surroundings of the sodium channel are more-or-less planar. Such a scheme would remain plausible if it were not for our recent finding that the N-1 hydroxyl of neosaxitoxin might be involved rather significantly in binding.[32] Possibly the cationic 1,2,3 guanidinium of saxitoxin is also involved in some electrostatic interaction with the same group, but its contribution could not be easily detected by any channel-blocking activity. If these interpretations were plausible, then the tetrodotoxin and saxitoxin binding site and the surroundings of the external orifice of the sodium channel cannot be simply planar, but are more likely to be in a crevice or a fold in the large protein molecule,[46] where both the C-12 -OHs and the 1,2,3 guanidinium of saxitoxin and the N-1 -OH of neosaxitoxin can interact with different carboxylate groups. The same carboxylate groups can interact with the sterospecifically similar groups in tetrodotoxin.

ACKNOWLEDGMENT

The performance of this work has depended first and foremost on the generous and sustained help of my chemist colleagues, especially H. S. Mosher, T. Yasumoto, S. K. Schnoes, and F. E. Koehn. I am also indebted to P. N. Kao and S. L. Hu for their devoted and stimulating collaboration.

REFERENCES

1. KAO, C. Y. 1966. Tetrodotoxin, saxitoxin and their significance in the study of excitation phenomenon. Pharm. Rev. **18**: 997–1049.
2. TSUDA, K., S. IKUMA, M. KAWAMURA, R. TACHIKAWA, K. SAKAI, C. TAMURA & O. AMAKASU. 1964. Tetrodotoxin VII. On the structure of tetrodotoxin and its derivatives. Chem. Pharm. Bull. **12**: 1357–1374.
3. DEGUCHI, T. 1967. Structure and activity in tetrodotoxin derivatives. Jap. J. Pharm. **17**: 267–278.
4. SCHANTZ, E. J., V. E. GHAZAROSSIAN, H. K. SCHNOES, F. M. STRONG, J. P. SPRINGER, J. O. PEZZANITE & J. CLARDY. 1975. The structure of saxitoxin. J. Am. Chem. Soc. **97**: 1238–1239.
5. BORDNER, J., W. E. THIESSEN, H. A. BATES & H. RAPOPORT. 1975. The structure of a crystalline derivative of saxitoxin: The structure of saxitoxin. J. Am. Chem. Soc. **97**: 6008–6112.

6. NARAHASHI, T., J. W. MOORE & R. N. POSTEN. 1967. Tetrodotoxin derivatives: Chemical structure and blockage of nerve membrane conductance. Science **156:** 976–979.
7. KAO, C. Y. & A. NISHIYAMA. 1965. Actions of saxitoxin or peripheral neuromuscular systems. J. Physiol. (London) **180:** 50–66.
8. HILLE, B. 1975. The receptor for tetrodotoxin and saxitoxin, a structural hypothesis. Biophys. J. **15:** 615–619.
9. KAO, C. Y. & S. E. WALKER. 1969. Active groups of saxitoxin and tetrodotoxin as deduced from actions of saxitoxin analogues on frog muscle and squid axon. J. Physiol. (London) **323:** 619–637.
10. HU, S. L. & C. Y. KAO. 1985. The pH dependence of the tetrodotoxin-blockade of the sodium channel and implications for toxin binding. Toxicon **24:** 25–31.
11. KAO, C. Y. & T. YASUMOTO. 1985. Actions of 4-epitetrodotoxin and anhydrotetrodotoxin. Toxicon **23:** 725–729.
12. MOSHER, H. S., F. A. FUHRMAN, H. D. BUCHWALD & H. G. FISCHER. 1964. Tarichatoxin-tetrodotoxin, a potent neurotoxin. Science **144:** 1100–1110.
13. GOTO, T., Y. KISHI, S. TAKAHASHI & Y. HIRATA. 1965. Tetrodotoxin. Tetrahedron **21:** 2059–2088.
14. KIM, Y. H., G. B. BROWN, H. S. MOSHER & F. A. FUHRMAN. 1975. Tetrodotoxin: Occurrence in Atelopid frogs of Costa Rica. Science **189:** 151–152.
15. PAVELKA, L. A., Y. H. KIM & H. S. MOSHER. 1977. Tetrodotoxin-like compounds from the eggs of the Costa Rican frog, *Atelopus chiriquensis*. Toxicon **15:** 135–139.
16. FUHRMAN, F. A. 1986. Tetrodotoxin, tarichatoxin, and chiriquitoxin: Historical perspectives. This volume.
17. FUHRMAN, F. A., G. L. FUHRMAN, Y. H. KIM & H. S. MOSHER. 1976. Pharmacology and chemistry of chiriquitoxin—a new tetrodotoxin-like substance from the Costa Rican frog *Atelopus chiriquensis*. Proc. West. Pharmacol. Soc. **19:** 381–384.
18. KAO, C. Y., P. N. YEOH, M. D. GOLDFINGER, F. A. FURHMAN & H. S. MOSHER. 1981. Chiriquitoxin, a new tool for mapping ionic channels. J. Pharm. Exp. Ther. **217:** 416–429.
19. PAVELKA, L. A., F. A. FUHRMAN & H. S. MOSHER. 1982. 11-nortetrodotoxin-6,6-diol and 11-nortetrodotoxin-6-ol. Heterocycles **17:** 225–230.
20. KAO, C. Y. 1982. Actions of nortetrodotoxin on frog muscle and squid axon. Toxicon **20:** 1043–1050.
21. NAKAMURA, M. & T. YASUMOTO. 1985. Tetrodotoxin derivative in puffer fish. Toxicon **23:** 271–276.
22. MOSHER, H. S. 1986. The chemistry of tetrodotoxin. This volume.
23. CAMOUGIS, G., B. H. TAKMAN & J. R. P. TASSE. 1967. Potency difference between the zwitterion form and the cation forms of tetrodotoxin. Science **156:** 1625–1627.
24. HILLE, B. 1968. Pharmacological modifications of the sodium channels of frog nerve. J. Gen. Physiol. **51:** 199–219.
25. OGURA, Y. & Y. MORI. 1968. Mechanism of local anaesthetic action of crystalline tetrodotoxin and its derivatives. Eur. J. Pharm. **3:** 58–67.
26. NARAHASHI, T., J. W. MOORE & D. T. FRAZIER. 1969. Dependence of tetrodotoxin blockage of nerve membrane conductance on external pH. J. Pharm. Exp. Ther. **169:** 224–228.
27. ULBRICHT, W. & H. H. WAGNER. 1975. The influence of pH on equilibrium effects of tetrodotoxin on myelinated nerve fibers of *Rana esculenta*. J. Physiol. (London) **252:** 159–184.
28. NACHMAN, R. J. 1981. Synthetic approaches to tetrodotoxin analogs. PhD. thesis. Stanford University, Palo Alto, Ca.
29. KAO, P. N., M. R. JAMES-KRACKE & C. Y. KAO. 1983. The active guanidinium group of saxitoxin and neosaxitoxin identified by the effects of pH on their activities on squid axon. Pfluegers Arch. **398:** 199–203.
30. ROGERS, R. S. & H. RAPOPORT. 1980. The pK$_a$'s of saxitoxin. J. Am. Chem. Soc. **102:** 7335–7339.
31. SHIMIZU, Y., C. P. HSU & A. GENENAH. 1981. Structure of saxitoxin in solution and stereochemistry of dihydrosaxitoxins. J. Am. Chem. Soc. **103:** 605–609.

32. HU, S. L. & C. Y. KAO. 1986. Comparison of saxitoxin and neosaxitoxin binding to the sodium channel of frog muscle. Biophys. J. **49:** 41a.
33. GHAZAROSSIAN, V. E., E. J. SCHANTZ, H. K. SCHNOES & F. M. STRONG. 1976. A biologically active acid hydrolysis product of saxitoxin. Biochem. Biophys. Res. Comm. **68:** 776–780.
34. KOEHN, F. E., V. E. GHAZAROSSIAN, E. J. SCHANTZ, H. K. SCHNOES & F. M. STRONG. 1981. Derivatives of saxitoxin. Bioorg. Chem. **10:** 412–428.
35. TANINO, H., T. NAKATA, T. KANEKO & Y. KISHI. 1977. A stereospecific total synthesis of d,1-saxitoxin. J. Am. Chem. Soc. **99:** 2818–2819.
36. KOEHN, F. E., H. K. SCHNOES & C. Y. KAO. 1983. On the structure and biological properties of decarbamylsaxitoxin. Biochim. Biophys. Acta **734:** 129–132.
37. WICHMANN, C. F. 1981. Characterization of dinoflagellate neurotoxins. PhD. thesis. University of Wisconsin. Madison, Wis.
38. KAO, C. Y., P. N. KAO, M. R. JAMES-KRACKE, F. E. KOEHN, C. F. WICHMANN & H. K. SCHNOES. 1985. Actions of epimers of 12-(OH)-reduced saxitoxin and of 11-(OSO₃)-saxitoxin on squid axon. Toxicon **233:** 647–655.
39. SCHANTZ, E. J. 1960. Biochemical studies on paralytic shellfish poison. Ann. N. Y. Acad. Sci. **90:** 8433–855.
40. HU, S. L., C. Y. KAO, F. E. KOEHN & H. K. SCHNOES. 1985. Actions of saxitoxin oximes on frog skeletal muscle fibers. J. Gen. Physiol. **86:** 13a.
41. STRICHARTZ, G. S. 1984. Structural determinants of the affinity of saxitoxin for neuronal sodium channel. J. Gen. Physiol. **84:** 281–305.
42. SHIMIZU, Y., C. F. HSU, W. E. FALLON, Y. OSHIMA, I. MIURA & K. NAKANISHI. 1978. Structure of neosaxitoxin. J. Am. Chem. Soc. **100:** 6791–6793.
43. SPALDING, B. 1980. Properties of toxin-resistant sodium channels produced by chemical modification in frog skeletal muscle. J. Physiol. (London) **305:** 485–500.
44. MOCZYDLOWSKI, E., S. HALL, S. S. GARBER, G. S. STRICHARTZ & C. MILLER. 1984. Voltage-dependent blockade of muscle Na⁺ channels by guanidinium toxins. J. Gen. Physiol. **84:** 687–704.
45. KAO, C. Y. 1983. New perspectives on the interaction of tetrodotoxin and saxitoxin with excitable membranes. Toxicon (suppl.) **3:** 211–219.
46. NODA, M., S. SHIMIZU, T. TANABE, T. TAKAI, T. KAYANO, T. IKEDA, H. TAKAHASHI, H. NAKAYAMA, Y. KANAOKA, N. MINAMINO, K. KANGAWA, H. MATSUO, M. A. RAFTERY, T. HIROS, S INAYAMA, H. HAYASHIDA, T. MIYATA & S. NUMA. 1984. Primary structure of *Electrophorus electricus* sodium channel deduced from cDNA sequence. Nature **312:** 121–127.

Kinetics of TTX-STX Block of
Sodium Channels[a]

W. ULBRICHT, H.-H. WAGNER, AND J. SCHMIDTMAYER

Physiologisches Institut
Universität Kiel
D-2300 Kiel, Federal Republic of Germany

INTRODUCTION

Tetrodotoxin (TTX) and saxitoxin (STX) have become almost indispensable tools in studying excitable membranes. When applied in large doses these toxins help to separate ionic currents, to identify, by way of selective block, current through the so-called sodium channel, and to measure gating currents in these channels. This paper is concerned with the action of lower concentrations employed to study the rate and extent of toxin block as a reflection of the toxin–binding-site reaction. Because of the high specificity of this reaction the binding site must be an integral part of the sodium channel protein. Hence determination of blocking kinetics, as modified by temperature, pH, and other parameters, may yield valuable information about the location and the molecular environment of the site.

This paper presents earlier published results as well as new unpublished data obtained from amphibian myelinated nerve fibers. This preparation is particularly well suited for kinetic measurements because the nodal membrane is readily accessible to the bath solution. Thus the continuously superfused node of Ranvier, introduced by Stämpfli in 1958,[1] permits a change of K^+ concentration at the membrane with a halftime of only 20 ms (see ref. 2). Such high rates of exchange were achieved in a chamber which was better suited for recording action potentials than for voltage clamping. Hence when a very fast exchange of solutions was desired the maximum rate of rise of the action potential was the measured signal. Most of our experiments, however, were done in a conventional voltage clamp setup[3] under continuous superfusion where the exchange was about 20 times slower but still much faster than the rates of toxin action.

ONSET AND OFFSET OF TOXIN ACTION

The first quantitative description of TTX and STX action on frog nerve fibers was given by Hille,[4] who proposed that block of Na channels was due to a one-to-one reaction of the kind

$$\text{TTX} + R \underset{k_{2T}}{\overset{k_{1T}}{\rightleftharpoons}} \text{TTX-}R,$$

where one TTX (or STX) molecule reversibly binds to one receptor, R, per channel

[a]Support for this work from the Deutsche Forschungsgemeinschaft is gratefully acknowledged.

68

with binding immediately leading to block; k_{1T} and k_{2T} are the forward and dissociation rate constants. The underlying idea of toxin-induced block being an all-or-none event for the individual channel has since been confirmed in fluctuation experiments on frog nerve,[5] or for example, in single channel experiments on neuroblastoma cells.[6] Another tacit assumption of a homogeneous population of sodium channels with respect to their toxin-binding properties, however, has recently been questioned.[7] Nevertheless the toxin-induced reduction of peak I_{Na} fits well the hypothesis of one type of channels. At equilibrium with a given TTX concentration, [TTX], the fraction p_{T^∞} of channels left unblocked (and hence contributing to I_{Na}) would be

$$p_{T^\infty} = 1/(c_T + 1), \tag{1}$$

where $c_T = [TTX]/K_T$ is a dimensionless toxin concentration and $K_T = k_{2T}/k_{1T}$ is the

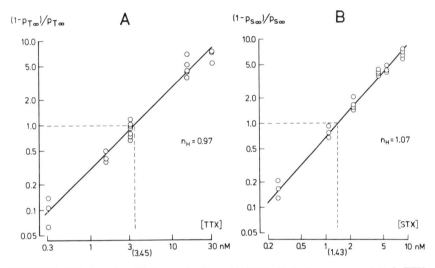

FIGURE 1. Hill plots of equilibrium toxin effects. (A) TTX effect where p_{T^∞} = peak I_{Na} in TTX, normalized to I_{Na} in control. Line of regression with slope, $n_H = 0.97$ (21 pairs of observations, $r = 0.99$, room temperature); $(1 - p_{T^\infty})/p_{T^\infty} = 1.0$ denotes mean $K_T = 3.45$ nM. Plot of data of TABLE 1 in Schwarz *et al.*[9] Reprinted by permission from the *Journal of Physiology*. (B) STX effect with p_{S^∞} defined analogous to p_{T^∞}. Line of regression with slope, $n_H = 1.07$ (26 pairs of observations, $r = 0.99$, average temperature 16°C). (From Wagner and Ulbricht.[8] Reprinted by permission from Springer-Verlag.)

equilibrium dissociation constant. For a one-to-one reaction a Hill plot of log $[(1 - p_{T^\infty})/p_{T^\infty}]$ vs. log [TTX] should yield a straight line of slope 1.0. This was indeed observed as shown for TTX in FIGURE 1A and also for STX in FIGURE 1B, where p_{S^∞} is the unblocked fraction of channels in the presence of STX. From FIGURE 1A one calculates $K_T = 3.45$ nM; in later experiments using a different batch of TTX, K_T was about 2 nM.[8]

If the reaction scheme is valid, the time course of site occupation on sudden application of toxin should be exponential with a time constant, τ, where

$$1/\tau = k_{1T} [TTX] + k_{2T} = k_{2T}(c_T + 1) = k_{2T}/p_{T^\infty}. \tag{2}$$

On washout, when $[TTX] = 0$, $1/\tau = k_{2T}$, that is, independent of the previously applied concentration.

As outlined before, the membrane of a Ranvier node is readily accessible so that the toxin concentration can be raised or decreased so fast it approaches a step change compared with the rates of blocking or unblocking. These rates were studied by recording the peak sodium current, I_{Na}, during trains of depolarizing impulses in the voltage clamp on changing solutions in a continuous-perfusion chamber. FIGURE 2 shows that onset of block by 3.1 and 15.5 nM TTX was indeed exponential, with time constants of 45.0 and 17.4 s, respectively, at room temperature. Offset on washing following either treatment was also exponential with a common mean time constant of 77 s. Equation 2 accounts for these results with $k_{1T} = 2.9 \times 10^6$ M^{-1}s^{-1} and $k_{2T} = 1.3 \times 10^{-2}$s^{-1}. Note that $k_{2T}/k_{1T} = K_T = 4.5$ nM, whereas from equilibrium results in this experiment, $p_{T^*} = 0.49$ and 0.15 in 3.1 and 15.5 nM TTX, one calculates $K_T = 3.0$ and 2.4 nM (see axon k in ref. 9). This difference is also borne out by the mean values from this series of experiments where k_{1T} was 2.96×10^6 M^{-1}s^{-1} and $k_{2T} = 1.42 \times 10^{-2}$s^{-1} so that $k_{2T}/k_{1T} = 5.10$ nM vs. $K_T = 3.45$ nM as determined from p_{T^*} (see FIGURE 1A). The discrepancy was smaller if k_{1T} was determined solely from the onset time constant at two toxin concentrations in each preparation which yielded a somewhat larger average k_{1T} (3.25×10^6 M^{-1}s^{-1}) and hence a smaller ratio k_{2T}/k_{1T} (4.37 nM).[9] Comparable results were obtained with STX, where at 16°C the analogous ratio of mean rate constants, k_{2S}/k_{1S}, was 1.76×10^{-2} s$^{-1}/1.01 \times 10^7$ M^{-1}s^{-1} (1.74 nM vs. 1.38 nM from p_{S^*}).[8]

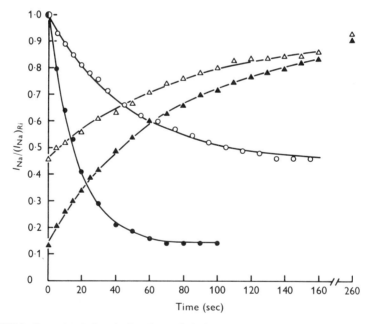

FIGURE 2. Onset (*circles*) and offset (*triangles*) of the action of 3.1 nM (*open symbols*) and 15.5 nM TTX (*filled symbols*). Ordinate, Peak I_{Na} normalized to the control value. *Abscissa*, Time after solution change. Onset time constants, $\tau_{on} = 45$ and 17 s; offset time constants, $\tau_{off} = 77$ and 78 s, respectively. (From Schwarz *et al.*[9] Reprinted by permission from the *Journal of Physiology*.)

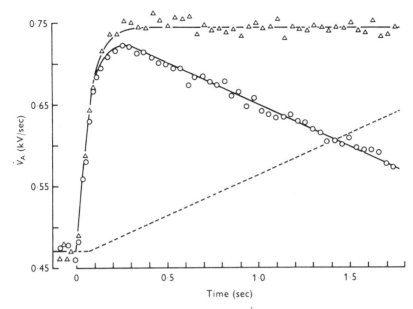

FIGURE 3. Latency of the effect of 155 nM TTX on $\dot{V}_A$, the maximum rate of rise of action potentials elicited every 20 ms. *Ordinate*, $\dot{V}_A$ in kV/s; *abscissa*, time after start of Na$^+$ effect. *Triangles* refer to a change from 59 to 118 mM Na$^+$ without toxin, *circles* to a change from 59 mM Na$^+$ to 118 mM Na$^+$ plus 155 nM TTX. The *dashed line* gives the difference between the two curves. T = 20.8°C. (From Schwarz *et al.*[9] Reprinted by permission from the *Journal of Physiology.*)

The reason for this small but consistent discrepancy between kinetic and equilibrium data is unclear and could suggest that the assumed reaction scheme is an oversimplification. This also raises the question whether we measure true rates of reaction. The answer is affirmative in the sense that we can exclude diffusional access to the binding site to limit the observed rates of block. The reasons are (1) a very short latency of action, (2) a high Q_{10} for the rate of blocking and especially unblocking, and (3) comparable results on purified Na channel preparations.

The latency was tested in current clamp experiments as illustrated by FIGURE 3, using the maximum rate of rise, $\dot{V}_A$, of periodic action potentials as a measure.[9] The triangles show the fast increase of signal on changing from 50% to 100% Na$^+$, whereas the circles refer to a change from toxin-free 50% Na$^+$ to 100% + 155 nM TTX which led to a fast increase in $\dot{V}_A$ (Na$^+$ effect) followed by a slower decrease (toxin effect). The difference between the two curves, the TTX effect proper, is given as an interrupted line starting with a delay of about 75 ms which could be accounted for by unimpeded diffusion of TTX through the thin unstirred layer surrounding the nodal membrane and the relative insensitivity of $\dot{V}_A$ to low degrees of site occupation.

The other argument against access limitation is based on the temperature dependence of onset and offset. Arrhenius plots yielded activation energies of 29.3, 85.5, and 41.0 kJ/mole for K_T, k_{2T}, and k_{1T} (57.3 kJ/mole for k_{1T} derived from onset alone). This corresponds to a Q_{10} (between 12° and 22° C) of 1.5, 3.4, and 1.8 (2.3), respectively. Interestingly the ratio of Q_{10} of k_{2T} over that of k_{1T} derived solely from onset agrees better with Q_{10} of K_T from equilibrium results. At any rate the Q_{10} values, especially those for the offset rate, seem to be too large for the access to be rate limiting.[9]

Finally, a purified sarcolemma preparation whose toxin-binding site ought to be particularly accessible and to which [³H]STX bound with a K_d = 1.43 nM (at 0°C) yielded a rate of dissociation of $1.7 \times 10^{-2} s^{-1}$ at 15°C,[10] almost identical with our frog node results k_{2S} = $1.76 \times 10^{-2} s^{-1}$ at about 16°C.[8] With the isolated sarcolemma the Q_{10} of the dissociation rate was clearly larger (2.6) than for the association rate (1.9), in agreement with our k_{2T} and k_{1T} results mentioned before. In a comparable binding study with [³H]TTX to solubilized garfish nerve a dissociation constant of $1.58 \times 10^{-2} s^{-1}$ was found at 20°C,[11] close to our mean k_{2T} of $1.42 \times 10^{-2} s^{-1}$ at room temperature.[9]

RATES OF STX-TTX INTERACTION

STX and TTX, although chemically quite different, cause such similar effects that a common binding site was soon suspected and confirmed in experiments with labeled toxin by mutual displacement (for a review see ref. 12). However, because binding studies are complicated by the presence of unspecific sites, it seemed worthwhile to test the common-site hypothesis in voltage clamp experiments on intact nodes of Ranvier. Such experiments are based on the fact that the rates of STX action are larger than those of TTX action. Thus in a series of experiments which yielded K_S = 1.4 nM (see also FIGURE 1B) and K_T = 2.0 nM, we found k_{1S} = 2.3 k_{1T} and k_{2S} = 1.7 k_{2T} (16°C).

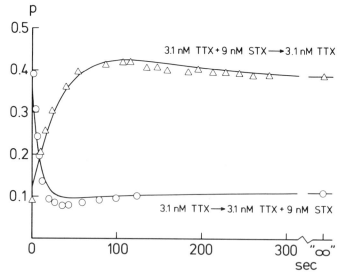

FIGURE 4. Nonmonotonic time course of block when TTX and STX compete for the same binding site. *Ordinate,* Fraction, p, of channels left unblocked. *Abscissa,* Time after solution change. *Circles* refer to adding 9 nM STX after equilibration in 3.1 nM TTX, *triangles* to a change back to 3.1 nM TTX after equilibration in the mixture. The curves were computed from the mean results of the series, k_{2S} = $1.4 \times 10^{-2} s^{-1}$, k_{2S}/k_{2T} = 1.7; c_T = 1.6, c_S = 0 or 6.3; 14.8°C. (From Wagner and Ulbricht.[8] Reprinted by permission from Springer-Verlag.)

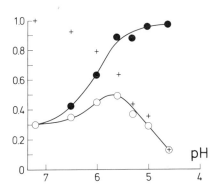

FIGURE 5. Effect of pH on the maximum rate of rise, $\dot{V}_A$ of action potentials in 15.5 nM TTX and in toxin-free solutions. *Ordinate,* $\dot{V}_A$ relative to its value in normal Ringer solution at pH 7.2; *abscissa,* pH. The points denote mean values after equilibration in 15.5 nM TTX (*open circles*), 1 s after changing back to neutral toxin-free solution (*filled circles*) and after equilibration in TTX-free solutions of the respective pH (+). The curves were drawn by eye. (From Ulbricht and Wagner.[17] Reprinted by permission from the Royal Society, London.)

Although one cannot distinguish block by STX from that by TTX, adding the faster acting STX after equilibrating a node in TTX should result in a nonmonotonic time course of additional block provided STX and TTX bind to the same site and binding limits the rates of block. Conversely, after equilibration in a STX-TTX mixture, taking out STX should lead to a nonmonotonic recovery from block since STX dissociates faster from the sites than TTX can occupy its due share of freed sites. This was indeed observed as shown in FIGURE 4. For a better understanding one should realize that at equilibrium in the mixture, I_{Na} is proportional to $p'_{S,T^*} = 1 - y'_{S^*} - y'_{T^*}$, where $y'_{S^*} = c_S/(c_S + c_T + 1)$ and $y'_{T^*} = c_T/(c_S + c_T + 1)$ are the fractions of channels occupied by STX and TTX, respectively, the prime denoting the presence of another ligand. In TTX alone, $p_{T^*} = 1 - y_{T^*}$ with $y_{T^*} = c_T/(c_T + 1)$ which is equivalent to equation 1. Hence $y'_{T^*} < y_{T^*}$ that is, the fraction of TTX-blocked channels in the presence of STX is smaller than in the same TTX concentration alone. Calculations [8] show that the overshoot during partial recovery from block is more pronounced the larger the value of k_{2S}/k_{2T}. It should be mentioned that simply adding STX to STX never results in a nonmonotonic time course of additional block. The observed transients in the STX-TTX experiments, on the other hand, are a direct indication of competition for the same site and they can be quantitatively accounted for with the separately determined rate constants of STX and TTX action.

EXTENT AND RATE OF TOXIN ACTION AT LOW pH

At alkaline pH the TTX effect was decreased, most likely due to changes in the toxin molecule whose cationic form (actually two tautomers) is converted into the zwitterion form with an apparent pK'_a of 8.8.[13,14] Our equilibrium results were fully compatible with the idea that only the cationic form is active.[15] This was also borne out by kinetic experiments which showed reduced onset rates and unchanged offset rates as if [TTX] was simply reduced in equation 2.[16]

At acid pH where TTX block was also reduced the situation was more complex and effects on the toxin molecule could be excluded. FIGURE 5 gives a summary of equilibrium results obtained in the current clamp.[17] As in FIGURE 3, $\dot{V}_A$, the maximum rate of rise of action potentials, was the measure. Open circles refer to the signal after equilibrating the node in 15.5 nM TTX at various pH values. Between pH 7.2 and 5.6 the signal increased, that is, block was relieved, although acid pH per se blocks sodium channels (as shown by the crosses). At more acid pH the signal in the toxin solution was not much different from that in the toxin-free solution of the same pH. The reason for this unexpected nonmonotonic dependence on pH was revealed on suddenly changing to neutral toxin-free Ringer solution leading to an immediate recovery of V_A (filled circles) measured after 1 s; recovery was almost 100% following pH 4.6. Obviously in acid solutions TTX binds much less and block is predominantly by protons, an effect that can be quickly reversed on going neutral. This suggests that binding to the site by TTX cations and by protons is mutually exclusive. As in the case of TTX-STX interaction, that of TTX-H$^+$ would predict I_{Na} in acid toxin solution to be proportional to $p'_{T,H^*} = 1 - y'_{T^*} - y'_{H^*}$, where $y'_{T^*} = c_T/(c_T + c_H + 1)$ is the fraction of channels blocked by TTX and $y'_{H^*} = c_H/(c_T + c_H + 1)$ is the fraction of channels blocked by protons with $c_H = [H^+]/K_H$. Since site occupation by TTX is practically unchanged after a 1-s wash, the filled circles of FIGURE 5 reflect $y'_{T^*} < y_{T^*}$ where $y_{T^*} = c_T/(c_T + 1)$ refers to neutral toxin solution ($c_H \approx 0$). However, V_A is not linearly related to I_{Na} and thus p_T, so a quantitative test has to be done in voltage clamp experiments.[9] Before results are presented it should be noted that block of sodium channels by protons depends on membrane potential and is described, according to Woodhull,[18] by

$$K_H = b_{-1}/b_1 \exp(\delta EF/RT), \qquad (3)$$

where $b_{-1}/b_1 = K_H$ for $E = 0$, δ is a dimensionless quantity, E is the observed membrane potential, F = Faraday, R = gas constant, and T = absolute temperature. Our data[15] yielded a mean $b_{-1}/b_1 = 2.04 \mu M$ and $\delta = 0.34$. With $K_H(E)$, c_H becomes voltage dependent and thus could influence the fraction of channels blocked by TTX at low pH. Hence at acid pH, p'_{T,H^*} should depend on voltage, or more precisely, on the holding potential, E_{HP}, during equilibration. This was indeed observed as illustrated by TABLE 1, in which p_T^* is the ratio of I_{Na} in acid toxin solution to I_{Na} in acid toxin-free solution. Clearly, except for pH 7.2, $p_T^* (E_{HP} = -90 \text{ mV}) > p_T^* (E_{HP} = -50 \text{ mV})$, in agreement with the idea that c_H increases (K_H decreases) at more negative E as predicted by equation 3 so that fewer channels should be blocked by TTX at constant c_T. The idea that c_T and hence K_T, are independent of E_{HP}, at least between -90 and -50 mV, is supported by the insensitivity of p_T^* at pH 7.2, where c_H is negligible (0.10 and 0.06, respectively). TABLE 1 also illustrates the enormous decrease of TTX effect in acid solutions. Thus 3.1 nM TTX at pH 7.2 causes approximately the same effect as 93.0 nM at pH 5.3 (at $E_{HP} = -90$ mV).

The quantitative fit of our results was improved by allowing for changes in local [TTX] at the outer membrane surface due to partial titration of negative surface charges at low pH. The concomitant change in surface potential, ΔE, was estimated from the observed shift along the potential axis of $P_{Na}(E)$, the sodium permeability as a function of membrane potential. The effective K_T thus became

$$K_T = \exp(-\Delta EF/RT) [TTX]/c_T. \qquad (4)$$

Since STX acts as a divalent cation, the surface potential effect should be more pronounced with this toxin. We have done only one series of pertinent experiments with 4.5 nM STX which yielded $p_{S^*} = 0.21$ at neutral pH, whereas block was considerably relieved at pH 5.6 where $p'_{S,H^*} = 0.57$ ($E_{HP} = -70$ mV in either case). This pH effect could almost exclusively be explained in terms of a proton-STX competition, but a final assessment clearly requires a wider range of pH and [STX] to be tested.[8] Surface-potential-modified TTX and STX action has been deduced from results on Ranvier nodes in Ca^{2+}-rich solutions[19] and in the presence of La^{3+} and Mg^{2+} (ref. 20). In the latter paper, NO_3^- and SCN^- were tested as well. These anions produce a shift, ΔE, in the opposite direction, *i.e.*, to more negative potentials and at the same time increase the toxin effect. Interestingly, in this and the Ca^{2+} study mentioned, only a fraction of the surface potential, deduced from ΔE, was required to account for the assumed change in local toxin concentration.

The kinetics of toxin action is also affected by low pH. In the case of simple proton-TTX competition and when H^+ binds so fast that instant equilibrium can be assumed,[18] onset should be exponential with a time constant, τ', as defined by[21]

$$1/\tau' = k_{2T}(c'_T + 1) = k_{2T}/p'_{T,H^*}, \tag{5}$$

where $c'_T = c_T/(c_H + 1)$. During offset $(c'_T = 0)$, $1/\tau' = k_{2T}$, that is, as in the absence of c_H (see equation 2). However, as shown in FIGURE 6, offset at pH 5.6 (filled triangles) was almost twice as fast as at pH 7.2 (open triangles). Onset, on the other hand, was slower at pH 5.6 (filled circles) than at neutral pH (open circles).

TABLE 1. Dependence of $p^*_{T\infty}$, the Ratio of I_{Na} in Acid TTX Solution over I_{Na} in Acid Toxin-Free Solution, on Holding Potential, E_{HP}, during Equilibration[a]

pH	[TTX] nM	$p^*_{T\infty}(E_{HP} = -50$ mV$)$	n	$p^*_{T\infty}(E_{HP} = -90$ mV$)$	n
7.2	3.1	0.52 ± 0.03	3	0.50 ± 0.01	3
5.2	15.5	0.60 ± 0.05	4	0.80 ± 0.02	4
5.3	31.0	0.53 ± 0.02	4	0.74 ± 0.02	3
5.3	93.0	0.24 ± 0.02	4	0.48 ± 0.02	3

[a] Mean values ± SEM at 15.5°–18.8°C. From Ulbricht and Wagner.[16]

The observed increased rates of dissociation at low pH forced us to assume that acid changed k_{2T} to some larger value k'_{2T}. Moreover, since k'_{2T} depended not only on pH but also on holding potential, it was better correlated with $c_H = [H^+]/K_H(E)$ than with $[H^+]$. To give an example, following treatment with 31 or 93 nM TTX at pH 5.3, washout yielded an average $k'_{2T} = 1.9 \times 10^{-2}s^{-1}$ for $E_{HP} = -50$ mV $(c_H = 4.86)$ but $k'_{2T} = 2.8 \times 10^{-2}s^{-1}$ for $E_{HP} = -90$ mV $(c_H = 8.35)$. A comparable correlation of k'_{1T} with c_H was less satisfactory especially since the determination of k'_{1T} depends on the assumed mechanism of TTX-H^+ interaction.[16] Thus without additional independent data we cannot estimate to what extent true changes in K_T, *i.e.*, in the ratio k'_{2T}/k'_{1T} and changes as defined by equation 4 are involved. There was, however, a fair agreement between the ratio of onset and offset time constants on one hand and the equilibrium effect on the other hand; at any tested pH

$$\tau'_{on}/\tau'_{off} = p'_{T,H^*}, \tag{6}$$

equivalent to the ratio at neutral pH as derived from equation 2. TABLE 2 attests to the general validity of equation 6 for a wide range of toxin concentrations, pH values, and holding potentials. It should be noted that with STX (at $E_{HP} = -70$ mV) the effect of acid pH was less marked, k'_{2S} at pH 5.6 being only $1.33 \times k_{2S}$ whereas the equivalent ratio k'_{2T}/k_{2T} was 2.7. Again, since only one [STX] was tested at one acid pH, the

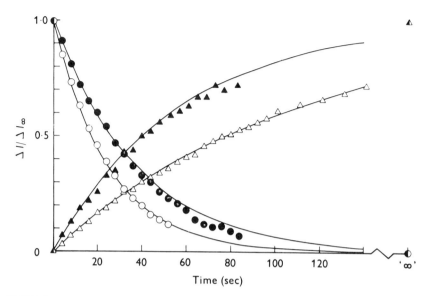

FIGURE 6. Rate of TTX action on I_{Na} at acid and neutral pH. *Ordinate*, Normalized I_{Na} increment $\Delta I/\Delta I_\infty = (I - I_T)/(I_{Ri} - I_T)$, where I is the peak I_{Na} at time t, and I_{Ri} and I_T are currents after equilibration in Ringer solution and 15.5 nM TTX. *Abscissa*, Time after solution change. *Open symbols* refer to onset (*circles*) and offset (*triangles*) at pH 7.2 with $\tau_{on} = 23.2$ s and $\tau_{off} = 111.2$ s; *filled symbols* refer to onset and offset at pH 5.6 with $\tau'_{on} = 27.6$ s and $\tau'_{off} = 57.7$ s; T = 15.5°C. (From Ulbricht and Wagner.[16] Reprinted by permission from the *Journal of Physiology*.)

TABLE 2. Comparison of Mean Ratios (± SEM) of Onset and Offset Time Constants, τ_{on}/τ_{off}, and Equilibrium Effects (± SEM) $p^*_{T\infty}$ or $p^*_{S\infty}$ from Peak I_{Na} in Toxin Solution over I_{Na} in the Respective Control for Various Combinations of Toxin Concentrations, pH Values, and Holding Potentials, E_{HP}

pH	[TTX] (nM)	E_{HP} (mV)	τ_{on}/τ_{off}	$p^*_{T\infty}$	n	Source (Ref.)
7.2	3.1	−70	0.61 ± 0.03	0.51 ± 0.01	7	9
7.2	15.5	−70	0.24 ± 0.01	0.19 ± 0.01	7	9
5.6	15.5	−70	0.69 ± 0.02	0.58 ± 0.01	3	16
5.6	31.0	−70	0.42 ± 0.03	0.41 ± 0.01	4	16
5.3	31.0	−50	0.67 ± 0.07	0.53 ± 0.02	4	16
5.3	31.0	−90	0.70	0.73	2	16
5.3	93.0	−50	0.29 ± 0.08	0.24 ± 0.02	4	16
5.3	93.0	−90	0.46 ± 0.01	0.48 ± 0.02	4	16

pH	[STX] (nM)	E_{HP} (mV)	τ_{on}/τ_{off}	$p^*_{S\infty}$	n	Source (Ref.)
7.2	1.1	−70	0.57 ± 0.06	0.56 ± 0.02	3	8
7.2	2.3	−70	0.41 ± 0.04	0.38 ± 0.02	4	8
7.2	4.5	−70	0.30 ± 0.01	0.21 ± 0.02	7	8
7.2	5.6	−70	0.21 ± 0.04	0.19 ± 0.01	4	8
7.2	9.0	−70	0.18 ± 0.03	0.13 ± 0.01	4	8
5.6	4.5	−70	0.61 ± 0.05	0.57 ± 0.02	7	8

significance of this result is limited. The reason for the pH-dependent changes in kinetics remains unclear; the relation between k'_{2T} and c_H, which on average was 10^2 $k'_{2T} = 0.89 + 0.28\ c_H$, bears signs of acid catalysis.[16]

STX AND PROCAINE DO NOT INTERACT

The preceding section has shown that the "blocking" agent H^+ interferes with TTX and STX binding. Local anesthetics, the classical blocking agents, on the other hand do not seem to bind to the TTX-STX receptor. This was studied in detail with procaine and STX in voltage clamp experiments,[22] which showed that the presence of STX did not influence rate and extent of procaine action. The results are best

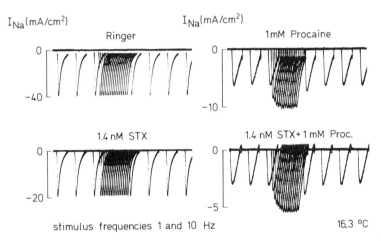

FIGURE 7. Effect of changing the pulse frequency from 1 to 10 Hz and back to 1 Hz on peak I_{Na} observed with constant depolarizing pulses of 60 mV amplitude preceded by 50-ms hyperpolarizing prepulses (by 40 mV). Standing pictures were photographed on moving film leading to overlapping records at 10 Hz. Note that the lower records were taken at twice the gain of the respective upper record to compensate for the 50% reduction by 1.4 nM STX. I_K was not eliminated; T = 16.3°C. (From Wagner and Ulbricht.[22] Reprinted by permission from Springer-Verlag.)

understood if one realizes the consequence of each sodium channel bearing two separate and independent sites, one for STX, the other for procaine. If we postulate that a channel is blocked on occupation of either site or both, the fraction, Y, of channels blocked in a STX-procaine mixture would be

$$Y = y_P + y_S - y_P y_S, \tag{7}$$

where y_S is the fraction of toxin sites occupied by STX and y_P is the fraction of local anesthetic sites occupied by procaine. For $y_S = y_{S^*} = $ const. we derive

$$dY/dt = dy_P/dt\ (1 - y_{S^*}). \tag{8}$$

Hence, after equilibration in a given [STX], a change in occupancy y_P of the procaine site should result in a linearly related change in channel block. The changes in y_P had to be achieved by provoking use-dependent procaine action since the rate of action is too fast to limit the rate of block on solution change even under optimum conditions.[23] FIGURE 7 illustrates an STX-procaine experiment in which test pulses, preceded by hyperpolarizing prepulses, were applied to the membrane at a rate of 1 Hz, then 10 Hz, and finally 1 Hz again. In Ringer solution or in 1.4 nM STX, stepping up the pulse frequency did not change I_{Na}, whereas in procaine the typical "use"-dependent recovery from block ensued. In the mixture the very same pattern was observed after doubling the amplification as predicted by equation 8 for $p_{S^*} = 1 - y_{S^*} \approx 0.5$ as obtained with 1.4 nM STX. The mean stationary results were very well fitted by equation 7 since in single-drug runs 1 mM procaine yielded $y_{P^*} = 0.81$ and 1.4 nM STX yielded $y_{S^*} = 0.49$, whereas in 1 mM procaine + 1.4 nM STX Y_∞ was 0.9, exactly as predicted. Note that in the case of STX-procaine competition, Y would have been measurably smaller. Independence of local anesthetic and toxin action was also found in binding studies (for literature see ref. 22).

The idea of separate and independent sites implies unimpeded access to the procaine site when the external toxin receptor is occupied. This seems feasible because procaine most likely acts either as a neutral molecule directly from the membrane pool or as a cation from the axon interior.[24] It should be noted, however, that in gating current measurements on squid axons 100 nM TTX was found to enhance block (*i.e.,* reduction of gating current) by the quaternary lidocaine derivative QX-314 (see ref. 25).

RATES OF TTX ACTION OF SODIUM CHANNELS WITH MODIFIED GATING

The alkaloid veratridine induces dramatic changes in sodium channel gating leading, during sustained depolarizations, to a secondary slowly increasing Na$^+$ current, I_s, followed, on repolarization, by a slowly decaying inward current tail.[26] If, after equilibration in 45 μM veratridine, the membrane is subjected to a depolarizing pulse of about 3-s duration this tail current occurs before I_s reaches a steady value. During a train of 3-s impulses elicited every 5 s the current remains inward and follows a pattern as shown in the first period in the upper panel of FIGURE 8A. Application of 31 nM TTX at the arrow leads to a progressive decrease in tail current I_t, due to the block of modified sodium channels. In the lower panel the decrease is plotted as a function of time for the onset and washout of TTX action; the results could be fitted with $k_{1T} = 3.6 \times 10^6$ M^{-1}s^{-1} and $k_{2T} = 1.14 \times 10^{-2}$s^{-1}, comparable to the results in the absence of alkaloid. The stationary reduction of I_t was to 0.07 of $(I_t)_{\text{TTX-free}}$ corresponding to $K_T = 2.4$ nM.[27]

FIGURE 8B illustrates the rate of TTX action during a depolarizing pulse lasting for 15 s. Trace 1 shows the slowly increasing inward I_s which, after about 5 s, abruptly turned outward as a Na-free TTX solution (300 nM) was applied. This outward current was most likely carried by Na$^+$ and K$^+$ through the modified sodium channels whose selectivity is decreased[28]; they nevertheless are blocked by TTX in an exponential fashion yielding τ_{on} of 1.36 s.[29] With our mean rate constants extracted from results in alkaloid-free TTX solutions, $k_{1T} = 3 \times 10^6$ M^{-1}s^{-1} and $k_{2T} = 1.4 \times 10^{-2}$s^{-1} (see ref. 9), one would expect $\tau_{on} = 1.09$ s in 300 nM TTX. The observed value was slightly larger, probably because the solution was old. With a freshly prepared 1-μM TTX solution applied to another node of Ranvier τ_{on} was 0.27 s, even slightly faster than the predicted 0.33 s. Thus the results of FIGURE 8 suggest that whatever happens to the gating mechanism in veratridine does not noticeably interfere with TTX block.

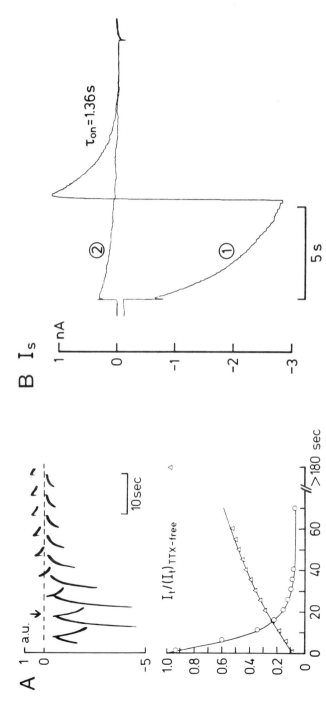

FIGURE 8. TTX effect in the presence of veratridine. (**A**) Effect of changing (at the *arrow*) to 31 nM TTX in a fiber treated with 45 μM veratridine and subjected every 4.9 s to a 2.8-s depolarizing pulse (by 40 mV). *Upper panel*, Original current record in arbitrary units (a.u.), *lower panel*, plot of tail currents, I_t, normalized to the value in TTX-free alkaloid solution. Onset (*open circles*) with τ_{on} = 8.5 s, offset (*triangles*) with τ_{off} = 87.5 s; T = 20.6°C. (From Ulbricht.[27] Reprinted by permission from Springer-Verlag.) (**B**) Effect of 300 nM TTX in the presence of 60 μM veratridine on slowly changing current, I_s, during 15-s depolarizing impulses. Trace 1, $I_s(t)$ when 5 s after the start of the impulse the solution was changed from 108 mM Na$^+$ plus 25 μM benzocaine to Na$^+$-free solution containing 300 nM TTX. Note the immediate current reversal (Na$^+$ effect) followed by an exponential decline (τ_{on} = 1.36 s) of outward current through modified sodium channels. Trace 2, 30 s later in the TTX solution. All solutions contained 10 mM TEA to block potassium channels; T = 19.3°C. (From Ulbricht and Stoye-Herzog.[29] Reprinted by permission from Springer Verlag.)

We have also tested TTX on sodium channels of nodes pretreated with chloramine-T (Cl-T; 0.6 nM for 60 s) which slows inactivation and renders it incomplete.[29-31] FIGURE 9 presents $I_{Na}(t)$ during 15-ms test pulses of constant amplitude; 10 mM TEA was in all solutions to suppress I_K. The upper traces were obtained before, the lower traces after Cl-T treatment. In each panel trace 1 refers to toxin-free solution, trace 2 to the current 16 s after changing to 10 nM TTX, and trace 3 after equilibration in this toxin solution. As one can see, the persistent I_{Na} observable after Cl-T treatment is blocked in proportion to the peak I_{Na}.

In some of the experiments each $I_{Na}(t)$ record was analyzed with a least square routine[32] to fit the formal description of inactivation[33,34]

$$I_{Na} = I_0(0) \exp(-t/\tau_0) + I_1(0) \exp(-t/\tau_1) + I_2, \qquad (9)$$

where I_0 and I_1 are the fast and slowly inactivating components ($\tau_1 \approx 5\,\tau_0$) and I_2 is the

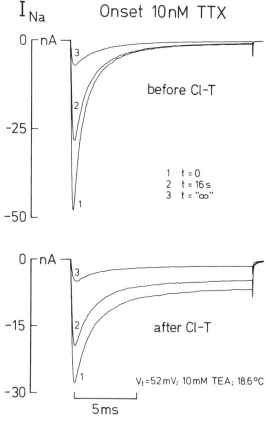

FIGURE 9. Effect of TTX on $I_{Na}(t)$ before (*upper panel*) and after a 60-s treatment with 0.6 mM chloramine-T (*lower panel*) during constant depolarizing impulses (15 ms, amplitude 52 mV). Traces 1 were obtained in toxin-free solution, traces 2 at 16 s after changing to 10 nM TTX, and traces 3 after equilibration in this toxin solution. All solutions contained 10 mM TEA to block potassium channels. T = 18.6°C.

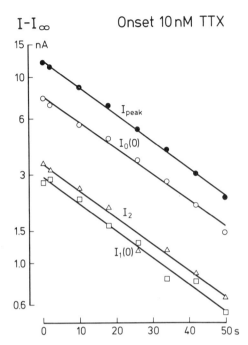

FIGURE 10. Decrease of peak I_{Na} (*filled circles*) and I_{Na} components during onset of action of 10 nM TTX. *Ordinate,* Difference between momentary current, I, and current, I_∞, after equilibration in 10 nM TTX; logarithmic scale. *Abscissa,* Time after solution change. The components as defined by equation **9** were extracted from records of the kind shown in FIGURE 9 by a nonlinear least squares routine. The lines of regression correspond to $\tau_{on} = 29.8$ s for peak I_{Na} (*filled circles*), 31.0 s for $I_0(0)$ (*open circles*), 30.0 s for $I_1(0)$ (*squares*), and 30.2 s for I_2 (*triangles*). T = 21°C.

persistent component. Extrapolation to $t = 0$ yielded $I_0(0)$ and $I_1(0)$, which in FIGURE 10 are plotted together with I_2 and peak I_{Na} as a function of time after changing to 10 nM TTX. The parallel straight lines in this semilogarithmic plot show that in Cl-T-treated fibers, as in untreated ones, peak I_{Na} decreases exponentially during onset of TTX action and that the reduction of the different components follows the same time course. This latter fact fits well the notion that these components are due to different states of a homogeneous channel population[31] rather than of two or more types of channels with supposedly different sensitivity to TTX.[7]

Thus at first sight Ranvier nodes treated with Cl-T did not react much differently to TTX than before treatment. On closer look, however, minor but consistent differences could be observed. Thus onset in 20 nM TTX was somewhat slower than before Cl-T treatment, as already suggested by traces 2 in FIGURE 9 which show that within 16 s reduction of peak I_{Na} was 48% complete before treatment but only 36% after Cl-T. The mean τ_{on} (± SEM) was 39.6 ± 1.4 s after vs. 26.4 ± 1.6 s before Cl-T treatment ($n = 6$; 17°C). Offset after Cl-T was slightly faster, τ_{off} being 82.1 ± 6.7 s vs. 89.3 ± 5.3 s; this difference, however, was not statistically different. These results point to a reduction of k_{1T} from 2.7×10^6 to 1.3×10^6 M^{-1}s^{-1} at almost unchanged k_{2T} (from 1.1×10^{-2} to 1.2×10^{-2} s^{-1}). A decrease in k_{1T} at constant k_{2T} should lead to an increase in K_T and indeed from the mean $p_{T^\infty} = 0.21 \pm 0.01$ before treatment, and

0.28 ± 0.02 after Cl-T we compute a change of K_T from 2.7 to 3.9 nM. At present we cannot explain this relatively small loss in affinity, nor do we know whether a systematic error is involved since the irreversible Cl-T action does not permit us to vary the sequence of runs. Sea anemone toxin ATX II, on the other hand, acts reversibly on Ranvier nodes[34] and produces effects similar to those of Cl-T.[31,35,36] In three experiments with 5 μM ATX II, addition of 7.5 nM TTX reduced the peak I_{Na} to $p_{T^*} = 0.30 \pm 0.003$, corresponding to $K_T = 3.2$ nM; the sodium current persisting at the end of a 15-ms test pulse was reduced to 0.26 ± 0.02 which did not significantly differ. In these early experiments we did not test TTX in the absence of ATX II nor did we determine onset or offset rates; the equilibrium results in the ATX II-TTX mixture, however, were quite comparable with our previous results[9] so that any ATX II-TTX interaction as has been suggested[36] must be rather weak.

ACKNOWLEDGMENTS

We wish to thank Ms. E. Dieter for competent help with the experiments and the figures and Ms. G. Ach for typing the manuscript.

REFERENCES

1. STÄMPFLI, R. 1958. Helv. Physiol. Acta **16**: 127–145.
2. ULBRICHT, W. 1982. Physiol. Rev. **61**: 785–828.
3. NONNER, W. 1969. Pfluegers Arch. **309**: 176–192.
4. HILLE, B. 1968. J. Gen. Physiol. **51**: 199–219.
5. SIGWORTH, F. J. 1980. J. Physiol. **307**: 131–142.
6. QUANDT, F. N. & T. NARAHASHI. 1985. Neurosci. Lett. **54**: 77–83.
7. BENOIT, E., A. CORBIER & J. M. DUBOIS. 1985. J. Physiol. **361**: 339–360.
8. WAGNER, H.-H. & W. ULBRICHT. 1975. Pfluegers Arch. **359**: 297–315.
9. SCHWARZ, J. R., W. ULBRICHT & H.-H. WAGNER. 1973. J. Physiol. **233**: 167–194.
10. BARCHI, R. L. & J. B. WEIGELE. 1979. J. Physiol. **295**: 383–396.
11. HENDERSON, R. & J. H. WANG. 1972. Biochemistry **11**: 4565–4569.
12. RITCHIE, J. M. & R. B. ROGART. 1977. Rev. Physiol. Biochem. Pharmacol. **79**: 1–50.
13. TSUDA, K., S. IKUMA, M. KAWAMURA, R. TACHIKAWA, K. SAKAI, C. TAMURA & O. AMAKASU. 1964. Chem. Pharm. Bull. **12**: 1357–1374.
14. GOTO, T., Y. KISHI, S. TAKAHASHI & A. HIRATA. 1965. Tetrahedron **21**: 2059–2088.
15. ULBRICHT, W. & H.-H. WAGNER. 1975. J. Physiol. **252**: 159–184.
16. ULBRICHT, W. & H.-H. WAGNER. 1975. J. Physiol. **252**: 185–202.
17. ULBRICHT, W. & H.-H. WAGNER. 1975. Phil. Trans. R. Soc. London B **270**: 353–363.
18. WOODHULL, A. M. 1973. J. Gen. Physiol. **61**: 687–708.
19. HILLE, B., J. M. RITCHIE & G. R. STRICHARTZ. 1975. J. Physiol. **250**: 34–35P.
20. GRISSMER, S. 1984. Pfluegers Arch. **402**: 353–359.
21. RANG, H. P. & J. M. RITTER. 1970. Mol. Pharmacol. **6**: 357–382.
22. WAGNER, H.-H. & W. ULBRICHT. 1976. Pfluegers Arch. **364**: 65–70.
23. RIMMEL, C., A. WALLE, H. KESSLER & W. ULBRICHT. 1978. Pfluegers Arch. **376**: 105–118.
24. HILLE, B. 1977. J. Gen. Physiol. **69**: 497–515.
25. CAHALAN, M. D. & W. ALMERS. 1979. Biophys. J. **27**: 39–56.
26. ULBRICHT, W. 1969. Ergeb. Physiol. **61**: 17–71.
27. ULBRICHT, W. 1974. In Biochemistry of Sensory Function. L. Jaenicke, Ed.: 351–366. Springer-Verlag. Heidelberg.
28. NAUMOV, A. P., YU. A. NEGULYAEV & E. D. NOSYREVA. 1979. Tsitologiya **21**: 692–696. In Russian.
29. ULBRICHT, W. & M. STOYE-HERZOG. 1984. Pfluegers Arch. **402**: 439–445.
30. WANG, G. K. 1984. J. Physiol. **346**: 127–141.
31. SCHMIDTMAYER, J. 1985. Pfluegers Arch. **404**: 21–28.

32. SCHMIDTMAYER, J., M. STOYE-HERZOG & W. ULBRICHT. 1983. Pfluegers Arch. **398:** 204–209.
33. CHIU, S. Y. 1977. J. Physiol. **273:** 573–596.
34. ULBRICHT, W. & J. SCHMIDTMAYER. 1981. J. Physiol. (Paris) **77:** 1103–1111.
35. BERGMAN, C., J. M. DUBOIS, E. ROJAS & W. RATHMAYER. 1976. Biochim. Biophys. Acta **455:** 173–184.
36. ROMEY, G., J. B. ABITA, H. SCHWEITZ, G. WUNDERER & M. LAZDUNSKI. 1976. Proc. Natl. Acad. Sci. U.S.A. **73:** 4055–4059.

Use- and Voltage-Dependent Block of the Sodium Channel by Saxitoxin

VINCENT L. SALGADO, JAY Z. YEH,
AND TOSHIO NARAHASHI

Department of Pharmacology
Northwestern University Medical School
Chicago, Illinois 60611

INTRODUCTION

Saxitoxin and tetrodotoxin have long fascinated electrophysiologists because of their remarkable specificity and potency of action on sodium channels in various excitable membranes.[1,2] Much effort has been made to elucidate the mechanism of sodium channel blocking action by these toxins. Kao and Nishiyama[3] first proposed that the tetrodotoxin and saxitoxin molecules, which are too large to pass through the sodium channel, physically blocked the passage of other ions by binding in the channel, acting on the channel like a cork in a bottle, with the guanidinium group of the toxin being the cork. This seemed to be a reasonable hypothesis then since free guanidinium ions can pass through the channel, and since the TTX and STX molecules are thought to be too bulky to pass through the Na channel. This notion was further elaborated by Hille.[4] By comparing the structure of TTX with STX, and by incorporating the theory of ion permeation through the channel, Hille proposed a hypothetical structural basis to account for the Na channel blocking action of these two toxins.

Hille proposed that the progress of an ion through the open sodium channel can be simulated by the passage of the ion over a series of energy barriers according to Eyring rate theory.[5] The highest energy barrier in the channel is viewed as being the basis for the channel's selectivity among different permeating ions. This barrier is viewed mechanistically as being the narrowest part of the channel, and would require ions to shed at least some of their water of hydration. Hille termed this constriction the "selectivity filter," proposing that it consists of a 3×5Å oxygen-lined constriction that allows close interaction of the partially dehydrated ion with a highly negative field strength site, presumably an ionized carboxylic acid. This selectivity filter is also the binding site for both H^+ and Ca^{2+} ions[6]. Since the site is located within the membrane field, the blocking action is expected to vary with voltage according to a Boltzmann distribution. This is indeed the case for the block in the presence of H^+ and Ca^{2+} ions.[6,7]

In Hille's model for toxin block, the guanidinium group was pictured as being bound to a carboxylic acid group in the selectivity filter, with five hydrogen bonds forming between the toxin molecule and the lining of the sodium channel. This TTX-carboxylic acid binding hypothesis was supported by experiments with trimethyloxonium tetrafluoroborate (TMO), a carboxyl group alkylating reagent. After the treatment of nerve or muscle membranes with TMO, TTX could no longer bind to the sodium channel[8] nor block the sodium currents.[9] However, the TTX-resistant channels had normal selectivity and were still sensitive to hydrogen ion block, suggesting that the carboxyl group necessary for TTX binding is distinct from that in the selectivity filter.

Two other lines of evidence further argue against STX and TTX binding to the selectivity filter. Binding to the selectivity filter should produce voltage-dependent block; for example, block becomes more pronounced with membrane hyperpolarization and with increasing positive charge on the toxin molecule. Although voltage dependence of toxin block was indeed found recently with sodium channels incorporated into bilayer membranes and activated by batrachotoxin treatment,[10–12] the voltage dependence of block caused by several STX derivatives was not influenced by a net charge ranging from 0 to +2. This is not consistent with binding to the selectivity filter. Indeed, Moczydlowski *et al.*[12] concluded that the voltage dependence of toxin binding is due to a voltage-dependent conformational equilibrium of the toxin receptor, rather than to the movement of the charged blocking molecule into an applied electric field within the channel pore. The second line of evidence comes from structure-activity studies of STX, its analogues, and TTX. Kao and Walker[13] proposed a new view for the toxin blocking action. In this view, the binding site for STX and TTX is located in the outside surface of the membrane, rather than in the selectivity filter; the active guanidinium group is electrostatically attracted by fixed anionic charges around the orifice of the sodium channel, thereby obstructing the channel more like a lid than a plug. Unlike the plugging model, in the lid model it is not obligatory for the toxin to exhibit a voltage-dependent block, since the toxin binding site is located outside the membrane field.

Voltage dependence of block as observed in bilayer membranes has not yet been demonstrated in intact membrane preparations. Ulbricht and Wagner[14] failed to detect any voltage-dependent block in the presence of TTX at pH 7.2 in the node of Ranvier. In constrast, at pH 5.2, the TTX block was less pronounced at -90 mV than at -50 mV, which is opposite to what the channel plugging model would predict. They suggested that voltage-dependent H^+ ion binding to the selectivity filter reduced TTX block at hyperpolarizing potentials. They suggested that at low pH, the voltage-dependence of block arose from the voltage-dependent binding of H^+ ions to the selectivity filter, causing a decrease in TTX block. In this model, toxin binding is assumed to be independent of membrane potential.

In addition to the possible voltage dependence, there is evidence that TTX block is use dependent. This is suggested by the work of Gage *et al.*,[15] who demonstrated that block of sodium current in squid giant axons by a crude maculotoxin was dependent upon stimulus rate. A purified maculotoxin was subsequently shown to be identical to TTX.[16] Cohen *et al.*[17] used cardiac Purkinje fiber to demonstrate that TTX blocks Na currents in a use-dependent manner. However, use dependence of the TTX block of the sodium channels in nerve membranes remains to be demonstrated.

The present study was undertaken to examine both use and voltage dependence of TTX and STX block of axonal sodium channels. STX was used in most studies, because its dissociation rate is much faster than that of TTX. We have found that STX block of axonal sodium channels is indeed voltage-dependent, and that both STX and TTX block are use-dependent.

METHODS

Giant axons (175–250 μm in diameter) isolated from the circumoesophageal connectives of the crayfish, *Procambarus clarki,* were cannulated and internally perfused as described by Lund and Narahashi.[18] Voltage clamp experiments were performed using the double sucrose-gap technique originally developed by Julian *et al.*[19,20] The chamber consisted of three compartments separated by two sucrose streams. The central pool, which was grounded, contained the experimental node; the right-hand pool, containing isotonic KCl solution to depolarize the membrane, was used to measure internal potential, and the left-hand pool, containing van Harreveld's solution, was used to apply current to voltage clamp the membrane in the central pool.

When measuring current amplitude with the sucrose-gap method, it was essential to minimize fluctuations in node width. This was done visually by keeping the image of the node fixed with respect to the eyepiece reticle of a stereomicroscope. During the course of any experiment the node area remained within ± 7% of the initial value. The node tended to remain constant, requiring only occasional adjustment, and changes occurred slowly enough that during a normal set of measurements lasting several minutes the accuracy was much better than this amount of fluctuation. Where errors were known to occur because of a change of node width, the data were discarded.

The standard solutions and their compositions (mM) were as follows: van Harreveld solution (205 NaCl, 5.4 KCl, 10 CaCl$_2$, standard internal solution (170 K-glutamate, 50 KF, 15 NaCl, and isotonic KCl solution (265 KCl, 15 NaCl). After voltage clamping the node, the internal and external solutions were changed to the test solutions. Two internal solutions of differing sodium concentration were used, both containing cesium and no potassium, to eliminate current through potassium channels. These solutions and their compositions (mM) were: 15 Na internal solution (170 CsOH, 50 CsF, 15 NaCl, and 135 glutamic acid) and 50 Na internal solution (135 CsOH, 50 CsF, 50 NaCl, and 135 glutamic acid). The external solutions (mM) were 205 Na, 10 Ca external solution (205 NaCl, 10 CaCl$_2$) and 50 Na, 10 Ca external solution (50 NaCl, 160 tetramethylammonium chloride [TMA · Cl], 10 CaCl$_2$). All internal solutions were buffered at pH 7.35 with 5 mM Hepes, and all external solutions, except sucrose and isotonic KCl, were buffered at pH 7.5 with 3 mM Hepes. In the text and figure legends, the solutions used are given in the form external Na,Ca/internal Na. The temperature for all experiments was maintained at 9°–10°C by a circulating water bath.

Voltage pulse application, data acquisition, and analysis were done with a PDP11/34 computer. In order to eliminate linear leak and capacitive currents, P-P/4 protocols were used, in conjunction with an analog signal subtractor. This protocol consisted of a pulse (P) followed by four pulses of one-forth the amplitude (P/4). The sum of the currents associated with the four P/4 pulses was subtracted from the current associated with P.

RESULTS

Use-Dependent Block of Sodium Channels by STX

FIGURE 1 shows an example of use dependence of STX block. The peak outward sodium current (I_p) evoked by 8 ms pulses to +60 mV during wash-in of 20 nM STX in the external solution is plotted against time after introducing STX. Initially, pulses were applied at a frequency of 2/min for 400 s, and a steady-state level of block was reached, with the peak current reduced to 42% of control. Beginning at 400 s, the pulse rate was increased to 12/min, and the block nearly doubled within the next 95 s, with the peak declining to only 22% of control. When pulse rate was then decreased to 0.66/min, a partial relief of block was observed, a final peak current returning to 53% of control. This experiment clearly demonstrates that the block of crayfish axon sodium channels by STX depends strongly on stimulus rate. Use-dependent block was also demonstrated with TTX, but its onset and offset rates were much slower than with STX.

Slow Onset of Use-Dependent Block

While attempting to measure recovery from use-dependent STX block, we noticed that block continued to increase for several seconds after the end of a 10-s train of depolarizing pulses. This delayed development of block was investigated further with a two-pulse protocol in which the interval between a conditioning pulse and a test pulse was varied, allowing 90 s for equilibration between pulse pairs. The amplitude of peak test pulse current relative to peak conditioning pulse current is plotted against interpulse interval for each pulse pair in FIGURE 2 for two axons under identical conditions but at two different STX concentrations. Extra block developed slowly, reaching a peak at about 5 s in 50 nM STX and 10 s in 20 nM STX. The data are

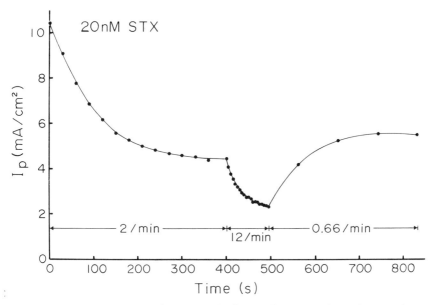

FIGURE 1. Peak sodium current during wash-in of 20 nM STX. Wash-in was begun at time 0, while a test pulse to +60 mV was applied every 30 s. An apparent steady-state level of block was attained by 400 s, but when the stimulus rate was increased to 12/min, the block increased, and when the rate was decreased to 0.66/min, the block decreased. 50 Na/50 Na, 50 Ca solutions were used, with a holding potential of −120 mV.

reasonably well fit by the sum of a falling and a rising exponential function of the form

$$I_{\Delta t}/I_0 = 1 + C(e^{-t/\tau_1} - e^{-t/\tau_2}), \qquad (1)$$

where $I_{\Delta t}$ and I_0 refer to the current amplitudes associated with the test and conditioning pulses, respectively, τ_1 and τ_2 are time constants, and C is coefficient for the exponential function.

Two types of mechanism are conceivable to explain the biphasic time course shown in FIGURE 2. In the first type, STX binds rapidly to channels during the pulse, but block does not occur simultaneously with binding. Rather, block requires a slow change

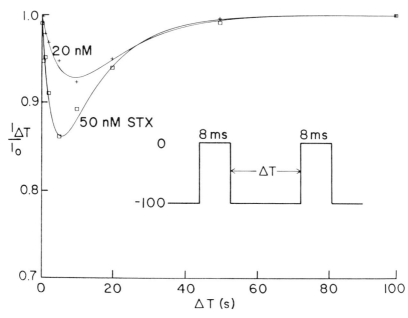

FIGURE 2. Two-pulse recovery protocol, showing delayed development of extra STX block. The protocol (*inset*) consists of an 8 ms conditioning pulse to 0 mV, followed after various intervals (ΔT) by an identical test pulse. Ninety seconds were allowed for recovery between pulse pairs. The plot of peak current during the test pulse normalized to that during the conditioning pulse shows that extra block did not develop during the conditioning pulse, but rather during the first 5–10 s after the conditioning pulse. Extra block then decayed to the resting level within 90 s. Comparing the data for 20 and 50 nM STX, we can see that the rate of onset of extra block is proportional to STX concentration. The continuous curves are plots of equation **1** with $C = 0.36$, $\tau_1 = 7.5$ s, and $\tau_2 = 13$ s for 20 nM STX, and $C = 0.28$, $\tau_1 = 3$ s and $\tau_2 = 13$ s for 50 nM STX. The holding potential was -100 mV. 15 Na/205 Na, 10 Ca solutions were used.

of the STX-bound channel that occurs during the interpulse interval. The fact that the rate of onset of extra block during the interpulse interval in FIGURE 2 is proportional to STX concentration is not compatible with this type of mechanism, because the rate of conversion of the STX-channel complex from the bound to the blocked state should not depend on STX concentration. In the second type of mechanism, binding of STX to free Na channels occurs slowly during the interpulse interval following the conditioning pulse. Experiments to verify the validity of the second hypothesis were performed as described below.

If the slow onset of use-dependent extra block seen in FIGURE 2 is due to slow binding of STX to free Na channels, the onset of use-dependent block during rapid stimulation would be limited by the rate of binding of STX. This is substantiated in FIGURE 3. Peak currents were measured during stimulation at various rates following equilibration of block at rest in 5 or 10 nM STX. In the presence of 10 nM STX, a decrease in the interstimulus interval from 10 s to 2 s enhanced and facilitated the development of use-dependent block, but further decrease in the interval below 2 s had no additional effect. The minimum time constant for development of use-dependent block was 48 s in 10 nM STX (solid curve *b*, FIG. 3). In 5 nM STX, the minimum time constant was increased to 83 s (curve *a*). These results are consistent with the idea that the rate of onset of use-dependent block is limited by the slow binding of STX to the channels.

Pulse Duration and Use-Dependent Block

From the experiments described in the preceding section it appears that use-dependent block is a two-step process, consisting of a fast step occurring during the pulse that makes more channels available for block, followed by slow binding of STX to these newly available channels during the interpulse interval. The important question now is how the channels are made available for extra block during the pulse. A first step in answering this question is to examine the dependence of extra block on pulse duration. A two-pulse protoocol similar to the one described in FIGURE 2 was used, but in this case the duration of the conditioning pulse was varied and the interval between conditioning and test pulses was kept constant at 10 s to allow extra block induced by the conditioning pulse to reach its maximum value (see FIG. 2). The peak current

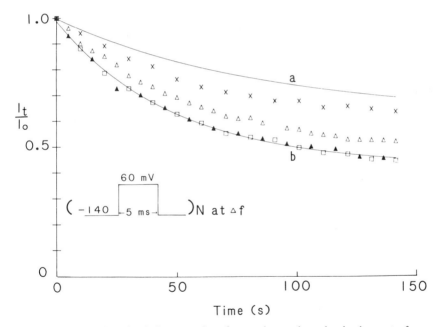

FIGURE 3. Repetitive stimulation at various frequencies to show the development of use-dependent STX block. A train of pulses (5 ms) to $+60$ mV was given at various frequencies and the peak currents normalized to that during the first pulse of the train were plotted. The symbols for pulse frequencies were *cross symbols,* 0.1 Hz; *unfilled triangles,* 0.2 Hz; *unfilled squares,* 0.5 Hz; *filled triangles,* 2 Hz. Not every current is plotted. Curve *b* shows an exponential fit to the data with a time constant of 48.6 s. The holding potential was -140 mV, and the STX concentration was 10 nM. 50 Na/50 Na, 50 Ca solutions were used. Curve *a* shows the limiting time course obtained from similar measurements in 5 nM STX (raw data not shown). The limiting time constant is 82.7 s. The limiting time constant of development of use dependence is therefore proportional to STX concentration.

evoked during the test pulse was normalized to the peak current evoked in the absence of a conditioning pulse, and plotted against conditioning pulse duration in FIGURE 4. Extra block became maximal for 1 ms pulses. The inset in FIGURE 4 shows that peak current evoked at the test pulse potential (+20 mV). Clearly, 1 ms is not even long enough for all of the channels to inactivate, and conditioning pulses longer than 1 ms, which inactivated the channels completely, did not enhance the extra block. Thus the extra block by STX does not require inactivation. Since most channels open within 1 ms, the process that makes channels available for use-dependent block by STX must occur shortly after opening.

Membrane Potential and Use-Dependent Block

Use-dependent block caused by STX was found to be a function of membrane potential. FIGURE 5 shows an example of the experiment in which the STX use-dependent block was measured at various holding potentials. The axon was equilibrated with 10 nM STX at a holding potential of −120 mV. After a 3-min rest, the axon was stimulated once every 5 s for 95 s. The peak currents in response to subsequent stimuli were normalized to the first peak current. By the end of 95 s of stimulation, the block had doubled over the resting value. The holding potential was then stepped to −160 mV, and the block was allowed to equilibrate at rest for 3 min. Another period of stimulation was then begun from the new holding potential, and the peak currents, normalized to the first peak at that holding potential, were plotted. Clearly, hyperpolarization enhanced the use dependence of STX block. The time constant for development of use-dependent block was relatively independent of potential, suggesting that the effect of hyperpolarization is to increase the number of channels that become available for extra block during a pulse, rather than to increase the rate of binding of STX during the interpulse interval.

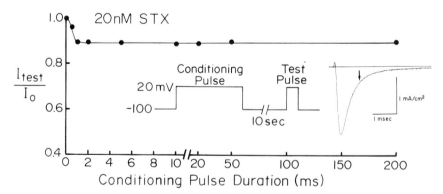

FIGURE 4. Use-dependent block by STX as affected by conditioning pulse duration. A two-pulse protocol was used (*inset*). The duration of the conditioning pulse to +20 mV was varied from 0 to 200 ms, and the test pulse was given after a delay of 10 s to allow extra block to reach a maximum. Ninety seconds were allowed for recovery between pulse pairs. The plot of peak test pulse current vs. conditioning pulse duration, normalized to the test pulse current in the absence of a conditioning pulse, shows that maximal extra block is achieved with conditioning pulses only 1 ms in duration. The inset shows the sodium current at +20 mV, with an *arrow* marking 1 ms. The holding potential was −100 mV, and the STX concentration was 20 nM. 15 Na/205 Na, 10 Ca solutions were used.

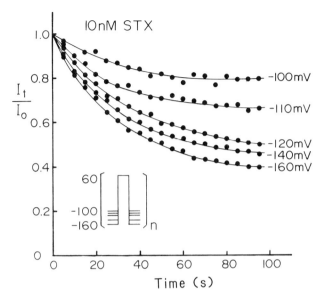

FIGURE 5. Repetitive stimulation at various holding potentials. Pulses (5 ms) to +60 mV were given at 5-s intervals, and the peak current normalized to that during the first pulse of the train was plotted. Resting block was allowed to equilibrate at each holding potential. Note that hyperpolarized holding potentials enhance use dependence. 50 Na/50 Na, 10 Ca solutions were used.

Voltage Dependence of Resting Block by STX

The degree of resting block produced by STX (and TTX) depends on the holding potential (E_H) and on the external Ca^{2+} ion concentration (FIG. 6). Concentrating first on the Ca^{2+} ion effect, we see that STX is much more potent at 10 mM Ca^{2+} than at 50 mM Ca^{2+}. Secondly, holding potential has virtually no effect on resting block at 10 mM Ca^{2+}, but at 50 mM Ca^{2+}, block is strongly voltage dependent, being minimal at −120 mV, and more intense at increasing depolarization or hyperpolarization. These results indicate that Ca^{2+} ions not only interact indirectly with the channel through their effect on the surface potential, but also interact directly with the channel.

DISCUSSION

The present results demonstrate that STX block of axonal sodium channels is both voltage and use dependent. The use-dependent block in the presence of STX differed markedly from that produced by local anesthetics in two major aspects. First, use-dependent block by STX developed after a single conditioning pulse, after a 5–10 s delay (FIG. 2). This delay is interpreted as being due to the slow rate of STX binding to newly available Na channels. Note that local anesthetics require multiple pulsing with short interpulse intervals for use-dependent block to develop, allowing the drug enough time to enter the channel. Local anesthetics, especially quaternary ones, are only able to enter the channel while it is open. STX, of course, is able to bind to the channel at any time. Secondly, even a very short depolarizing conditioning pulse (1 ms) is sufficient to allow maximal use-dependent block to occur. FIGURE 4 shows that conditioning pulses longer than 1 ms did not produce a more effective block.

The voltage- and use-dependence of STX block can be explained by a model based

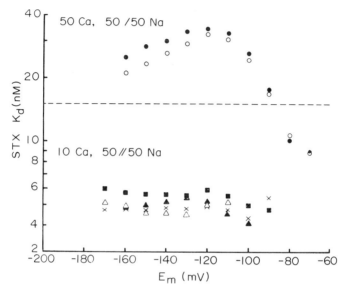

FIGURE 6. External Ca^{2+} ions affect the voltage dependence of resting block by STX. Block was measured from the ratio of peak currents evoked by test pulses before and after equilibration with STX. The peak currents from various holding potentials were measured first in control and then in the presence of STX, allowing 90 s for resting. This procedure avoids use dependence, and also corrects for slow inactivation. The data were converted into apparent K_ds, and plotted in these figures. Each symbol in each solution represents a different experiment. At all potentials where K_d was measured in both solutions, K_d in 50 mM Ca was higher than that measured in 10 mM Ca. The *dashed line* represents the predicted K_d from the change in surface potential when external Ca is increasing from 10 to 50 mM. The reduction of the negative surface potential of 13.6 mV was estimated from the degree of shift of the h_∞ curve when going from 10 to 50 mM Ca.

on ion-toxin interaction as illustrated in the following scheme:

$$C \underset{k_{-0}}{\overset{[I]}{\rightleftharpoons}} C—I$$
$$[T]k_0 \updownarrow \qquad [T]k_1 \updownarrow \quad k_{-1}$$
$$T—C \qquad\qquad T—C—I \qquad\qquad (2)$$

The following three assumptions are made. (1) Permeant cations in the external solution (*i.e.*, Na and Ca), denoted as I, can enter the closed channel, C, so that there would be two distinct closed states: C, the empty channel, and C-I, the channel containing an ion (for simplicity, we assume that the channel can contain only one ion at a time). (2) The toxin binding site is superficial, near the external mouth of the channel, and outside of the transmembrane field. (3) The toxin can bind to both of the closed states to form T-C and T-C-I, but its affinity for C-I is lower than for C, because of electrostatic repulsion between the toxin molecule outside and the ion inside the channel.

With this model, use dependence with the features we have seen could arise as follows. Because the toxin is assumed to occlude the channel at the external mouth, the transition from T-C-I to T-C cannot occur, so the ion is effectively trapped in the channel. Upon depolarization, the m gate would open and the trapped ion might escape through the inner mouth of the channel. Upon repolarization the channel would close, but it would be in state T-C rather than T-C-I as it was before the pulse. The total block, given by the sum of the amounts of T-C and T-C-I, remains unchanged immediately after the pulse. However, the equilibrium that was present before the pulse has now been perturbed, and a slow redistribution of channels among the various states is expected to occur as toxin binds to C-I and dissociates from T-C. If the initial rate of binding of toxin to C-I exceeds the rate of dissociation from T-C, the block will increase temporarily, with a time course and concentration dependence similar to that seen in FIGURE 2. This mechanism is also consistent with the result of FIGURE 4 in that use-dependent block requires channel opening, and that of FIGURE 5 in that the magnitude of use-dependent block is increased by hyperpolarization. The latter effect is expected because the magnitude of use-dependent block is dependent upon the number of channels in state T-C-I, which increases with hyperpolarization.

The ion trapping mechanism presented above to explain use-dependent block assumes that the affinity of STX for state C-I is lower than that for state C. Hyperpolarization is expected to increase occupancy of state C-I, thereby decreasing the average affinity of the channels for STX, and thus the steady-state voltage dependence predicted by this model could explain voltage dependence between -60 and -120 mV.

The decrease in K_d as the membrane potential is hyperpolarized below -120 mV in 50 Ca could be due to several effects. In our model, we would have to assume that the channels become saturated with calcium at -120 mV and the decrease in K_d must be due to an increase in the STX affinity of these Ca-blocked channels. We can propose three mechanisms: (1) Ca ions migrate deeper into the channels, increasing the distance between themselves and the toxin, and thus decreasing the repulsion, (2) the toxin itself might have some intrinsic voltage dependence because of its binding to a site within the transmembrane field, and (3) the channels undergo a conformational change that gives them a greater affinity for STX at negative potentials. Recent work with reconstituted sodium channels in the bilayer membrane provided evidence for mechanism 3[12] and against mechanism 2. Such mechanism will account for the voltage-dependent block observed at membrane potentials more negative than -120 mV. Mechanism 1 is also plausible because the voltage dependence of STX block was abolished when the external Ca was reduced to 10 mM (FIG. 6).

There is some evidence that STX and TTX have no intrinsic voltage dependence of block.[14,17] However, recent data on batrachotoxin-modified sodium channels incorporated into lipid bilayers have shown that block is indeed voltage dependent, with the K_d increasing e-fold for 30 to 40 mV depolarization.[10,11] The mechanism of this voltage dependence is not known, but Moczydlowski *et al.*[12] concluded that it was not due to binding of the toxin molecule within the membrane field, because several toxin analogues, regardless of net charge, produced the same voltage-dependent effect. It is possible, therefore, that the voltage-dependent effect they have seen is due to a voltage-dependent conformational change in the channel protein itself.

The positive voltage dependence of K_d we have seen between -180 and -120 mV, which has a slope similar to that in the bilayer experiments quoted above, may be due to the same mechanism. However, the negative voltage dependence of K_d we have observed under certain conditions, and the unique use dependence we have observed with STX suggest that STX block is even more complex than this. We have explained these additional effects as being due to antagonism of STX binding by calcium and sodium ions in the lumen of the channel. Thus, the two essential features of our model are voltage-dependent conformational change and calcium entry into the closed state of the channel. In our model, the closed channel can exist in two states for the control and in four states in describing the interaction of STX with the closed channel.

Further Applications of the Model

There are several interesting phenomena in the literature that can be explained by our model. Papers by Ulbricht and Wagner[14,22] provide interesting data that could not be satisfactorily explained at the time, but appear to be consistent with our model. The first paper[14] shows that TTX and H^+ ions appear to compete for a single binding site, and at low pH, TTX block can be relieved by large negative holding potentials, to the extent predicted if only the binding of H^+ is voltage dependent. However, these results are inconsistent with the single site model, because if TTX and H^+ bind to the same site, both should be affected equally by potential, so there would be no voltage dependence. These results are consistent with our model, however, in which voltage-dependent binding of H^+ to the selectivity filter would electrostatically inhibit TTX binding to its more superficial receptor. Voltage dependence due to Ca was probably not seen in this case because of the low Ca concentration (2 mM).

A major finding of their second paper[22] was that the dissociation rate constant of TTX was directly proportional to $[H^+]$, indicating that H^+ can catalyze the dissociation of toxin from its receptor. This effect was not understandable in terms of the single site model, but it can be readily explained by our model. If the toxin binds to a carboxyl group at the surface receptor (see INTRODUCTION), it is possible that H^+ ions can catalyze the dissociation of toxin by protonating that carboxyl group, as long as the H^+ ions have access to the carboxyl group when the toxin is bound. Thus our model accounts for both of these findings, which seemed paradoxical in terms of the single site model.

There is another effect of TTX that is relevant to this discussion. Tetrodotoxin and quaternary lidocaine (QX-314), when present together, reduce the gating current in squid giant axons.[23] By itself TTX does not affect the gating current, but QX-314 alone can reduce the gating current during repetitive stimulation, presumably by getting stuck in the inner mouth of the open channel. Cahalan and Almers[23] suggested that TTX, when bound, stabilized QX-314 in the channel because it would prevent sodium ions in the external solution from entering the channel and speeding dissociation of QX-314 from its receptor by repulsion. This is exactly the explanation of our model, except that in addition to Na, Ca would also play a role in causing dissociation of QX-314.

REFERENCES

1. NARAHASHI, T. 1974. Chemicals as tools in the study of excitable membranes. Physiol. Rev. **54:** 813.
2. CATTERALL, W. A. 1980. Neurotoxins that act on voltage-sensitive sodium channels in excitable membranes. Ann. Rev. Pharmacol. Toxicol. **20:** 15–43.
3. KAO, C. Y., & A. NISHIYAMA. 1965. Actions of saxitoxin on peripheral neuromuscular systems. J. Physiol. **180:** 50–66.
4. HILLE, B. 1975. The receptor for tetrodotoxin and saxitoxin. Biophys. J. **15:** 615–619.

5. WOODBURY, J. W. 1971. Eyring rate theory and model of the current-voltage relationship of ion channels in excitable membranes. *In* Chemical Dynamics: Papers in Honor of Henry Eyring. J. Hirschfelder, Ed.: 601–607. New York.
6. WOODHULL, A. M. 1973. Ionic blockage of sodium channels in nerve. J. Gen. Physiol. **61:** 687–708.
7. YAMAMOTO, D., J. Z. YEH & T. NARAHASHI. 1984. Voltage-dependent calcium block of normal and tetramethrin-modified simple sodium channels. Biophys. J. **45:** 337–344.
8. REED, J. K. & M. A. RAFTERY. 1976. Properties of the tetrodotoxin binding component in plasma membranes isolated from *Electrophorus electricus*. Biochemistry **15:** 944–953.
9. SPALDING, B. C. 1980. Properties of toxin-resistant sodium channels produced by chemical modification in frog skeletal muscle. J. Physiol. **305:** 485–500.
10. FRENCH, R. J., J. F. WORLEY III & B. P. BEAN. 1984. Voltage-dependent block by saxitoxin of sodium channels incorporated into planar lipid bilayers. Biophys. J. **45:** 301–310.
11. MOCZYDLOWSKI, E., S. S. GARBER & C. MILLER. 1984. Batrachotoxin activated Na^+ channels in planar lipid bilayers: Competition of tetrodotoxin block by Na^+. J. Gen. Physiol. **84:** 665–686.
12. MOCZYDLOWSKI, E., S. HALL, S. S. GARBER, G. S. STRICHARTZ & C. MILLER. 1984. Voltage-dependent blockade of muscle Na^+ channels by guanidinium toxins: Effect of toxin charge. J. Gen. Physiol. **84:** 687–704.
13. KAO, C. Y. & S. E. WALKER. 1982. Active groups of saxitoxin and tetrodotoxin as deduced from actions of saxitoxin analogues on frog muscle and squid axon. J. Physiol. **323:** 619–637.
14. ULBRICHT, W. & H. -H. WAGNER. 1975. The influence of pH on equilibrium effects of tetrodotoxin on myelinated nerve fibres of *Rana esculenta*. J. Physiol. **252:** 159–184.
15. GAGE, P. W., J. W. MOORE & M. WESTERFIELD. 1976. An octopus toxin, maculotoxin, selectively blocks sodium current in squid axons. J. Physiol. **259:** 427–443.
16. SHEUMACK, D. D., M. E. H. HOWDEN, I. Spence & R. J. QUINN. 1978. Maculotoxin: A neurotoxin from the venom glands of the octopus *Hapalochlaeua maculosa* identified as tetrodotoxin. Science *199: 188–189.*
17. COHEN, C. J., B. P. BEAN, T. J. COLATSKY & R. W. TSIEN. 1981. Tetrodotoxin block of sodium channels in rabbit Purkinje fibers. J. Gen. Physiol. **78:** 383–411.
18. LUND, A. E. & T. NARAHASHI. 1981. Modification of sodium channel kinetics by the insecticide tetramethrin in crayfish giant axons. *Neurotoxicol. 2: 213–229.*
19. JULIAN, F. J., J. W. MOORE & D. E. Goldman. 1962. Membrane potentials of the lobster giant axon obtained by use of the sucrose-gap technique. J. Gen. Physiol. **45:** 1195–1216.
20. JULIAN, F. J., J. W. MOORE & D. E. GOLDMAN. 1962. Current-voltage relations in the lobster giant axon membrane under voltage clamp conditions. J. Gen. Physiol. **45:** 1217–1238.
21. ARMSTRONG, C. M. & F. BEZANILLA. 1974. Charge movement associated with the opening and closing of the activation gate of the Na channels. J. Gen. Physiol. **63:** 533–552.
22. ULBRICHT, W., & H. -H. WAGNER. 1975. The influence of pH on the rate of tetrodotoxin action on myelinated nerve fibres. J. Physiol. **252:** 185–202.
23. CAHALAN, M. D. & W. ALMERS. 1979. Interactions between quaternary lidocaine, the sodium channel gates, and tetrodotoxin. Biophys. J. **27:** 39–56.

On the Mechanism by Which Saxitoxin Binds to and Blocks Sodium Channels[a]

GARY STRICHARTZ,[b,c] THOMAS RANDO,[b]
SHERWOOD HALL,[d] JANE GITSCHIER,[e]
LINDA HALL,[f] BARBARAJEAN MAGNANI,[b]
AND CHRISTINA HANSEN BAY

[b]*Anesthesia Research Laboratories
Brigham and Women's Hospital
Boston, Massachusetts 02115*

[c]*Department of Pharmacology
Harvard Medical School
Boston, Massachusetts 02115*

[d]*Food and Drug Administration
Washington, D.C. 20204*

[f]*Department of Genetics
Albert Einstein College of Medicine
Bronx, New York 10461*

INTRODUCTION

Saxitoxin is a highly specific inhibitor of sodium channels in excitable membranes, usually with high affinity, and showing rapid and complete reversibility. Inasmuch as saxitoxin (STX) and another agent, tetrodotoxin (TTX), bind with high affinity to most sodium channels, studies of their binding site and of their mechanism of action may reveal interesting information about the physiology of the channel itself. In this paper we report the results of four approaches to examine the action of STX: (1) studies of the binding of natural derivatives of saxitoxin, (2) studies of the potency of synthetic analogues of STX, (3) studies of the interference of STX binding by divalent metal and monovalent organic cations, and (4) studies of the interaction between saxitoxin and drugs that modify the gating of Na channels.

METHODS

The methods applied in these experiments include standard biochemical and electrophysiological techniques. Binding of tritiated STX (*STX) prepared by the method of Ritchie *et al.*[1] was studied in intact walking leg of lobster (*H. americanus*)[2] and in isolated membranes of mammalian brain[3] and of extracts of *Drosophila*

[a]Much of the research reported here was supported by grants from the USPHS (NS 12828 and NS 18467 to GS, and NS 13881 to LH). T. Rando holds a National Service Award (2T 32 GM07753–06) from NIGMS.
[e]Present address: Department of Medicine and Howard Hughes Medical Institute, University of California at San Francisco, San Francisco, Calif. 94143.

96

melanogaster heads.[4] The affinities of the unlabeled derivatives and of various cations were determined by competition with *STX in equilibrium binding experiments.[5,6] Physiological actions of the toxins were assayed in three different systems: (1) sodium currents of the frog node of Ranvier under voltage clamp,[7] (2) compound action potentials of the frog sciatic nerve in a sucrose-gap mode,[8] and (3) single Na channels in black lipid membranes activated by batrachotoxin (BTX).[9] From these various methods we have derived both equilibrium dissociation constants (K_d) and rate constants for toxin binding and dissociation. Some of the results reported here have been published previously, whereas others have appeared only in abstract form and will be published in their entirety in the future.

RESULTS AND DISCUSSION

The Potency of Naturally Occurring Derivatives of STX

The equilibrium K_d values of 12 natural derivatives of saxitoxin have been measured in brain membranes. Structures of these molecules are shown in FIGURE 1. Their R components and K_d values are listed in TABLE 1. For comparison, the affinities for blocking single BTX-activated sodium channels have been included, as have the relative potencies for blocking action potentials in frog nerve. A close agreement exists among the relative affinities measured by the three methods, showing that binding of these toxins closely underlies their channel-blocking activity and that the presence of BTX does not alter the order of their affinities, even though it modifies the details of their physiological action, as we describe below.

Several clear trends appear from examination of FIGURE 1 and TABLE 1. First, oxygenation at the N-1 position increases the potency, as does addition of a sulfate at the 11-β position. In contrast, sulfation at the 11-α position reduces potency slightly, and -SO_3 substitution at N-21 on the carbamyl "tail" reduces potency drastically. Some of these changes in K_d occur almost independently of each other, but the ones that increase potency, in general, are strongly modulated by other substituents.

Equilibrium K_d values represent the ratio of the rate constant for toxin dissociation to that for toxin binding. Investigations of the blocked and unblocked times of single channels yield these constants directly[9,10] as does analysis of the inhibition and recovery of macroscopic currents.[7,11,12] The binding rate constants are positive exponential functions of the net charge on the toxins; divalent STX binds most rapidly, monovalent B1 less rapidly, and neutral GTX4 even more slowly. The dissociation rate constants do not vary predictably with toxin charge but instead reflect the strength of the toxin:receptor complex. For example, all derivatives oxygenated at N-1 dissociate from the receptor more slowly than their nonoxygenated homologues, and all toxins sulfonated at 11-β dissociate more slowly than their sulfate-free counterparts.[9,10] The latter fact provides a telling observation about the toxin:receptor complex; the 7,8,9-guanidinium moiety of the toxin[14] probably forms an ionic bond with a negative charge on the receptor,[8,13] yet the addition of the negatively charged sulfate at the 11-β position in GTX3 still increases the energy of binding. When the added sulfate is closer to the essential guanidinium group, at the 11-α position in GTX2, the potency is lowered and dissociation is faster. Similarly, addition of the acidic hydroxyl at N-1 reduces the toxin's net charge but increases the strength of binding. Therefore, total binding must include forces other than ionic bonds.

Since it is known that another change in toxin chemistry wrought by N-1 hydroxylation is an increase in the probability of the keto form at C-12, judged on the

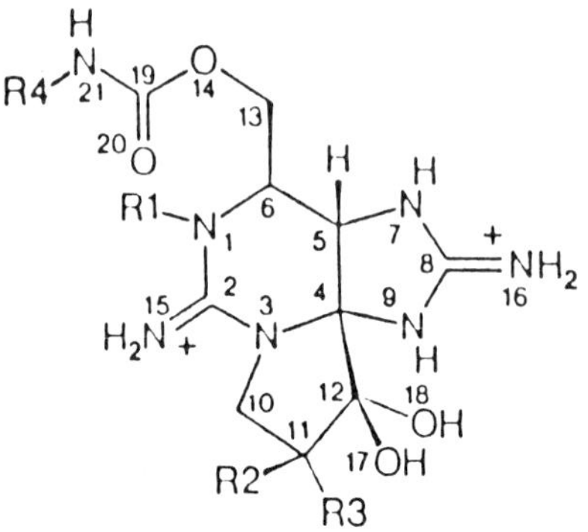

FIGURE 1. The structures of naturally occurring saxitoxin derivatives (see TABLE 1 for R components).

basis of an increased rate of exchange of C-H hydrogens,[15] an involvement of this group bears consideration. In neutral solution STX exists less than 1% in the keto form, being almost entirely consigned as a hydrated ketone, the dihydroxyl gem-diol.[16] Raising the pH promotes appearance of the ketone, via an electron shift towards C-4 concomitant with deprotonation of the 7,8,9-guanidinium. Binding of STX to ion-exchange resins

TABLE 1. Structures of Naturally Occurring Saxitoxin Derivatives (see FIG. 1) and Their Relative Dissociation Constants or Inverse Efficacies for Saturable Binding to Mammalian Brain, Inhibiting Frog Action Potentials, and Blocking Single Na Channels in Rat Muscle

Compound	R1	R2	R3	R4	Binding $(K_i/K_{STX}{}^a)$	AP Inhibition (Relative $ED_{50}{}^b$)	Channel Block $(K_d/K_{STX}{}^c)$
STX	H	H	H	H	≡1	≡1	≡1
BI	H	H	H	SO_3^-	39.5 ± 6.9	—	41.9
GTX2	H	H	OSO_3^-	H	2.92 ± 0.20	4.55 ± 0.005	6.5
C1	H	H	OSO_3^-	SO_3^-	800 ± 124	—	581
GTX3	H	OSO_3^-	H	H	0.54 ± 0.04	0.735 ± 0.043	1.04
C2	H	OSO_3^-	H	SO_3^-	10.8 ± 1.4	—	34.9
Neo	OH	H	H	H	0.23 ± 0.01	0.223 ± 0.011	0.279
B2	OH	H	H	SO_3^-	4.51 ± 5.8	—	44.2
GTX1	OH	H	OSO_3^-	H	2.48 ± 0.2	—	3.49
C3	OH	H	OSO_3^-	SO_3^-	2400	—	535
GTX4	OH	OSO_3^-	H	H	0.298 ± 0.054	—	—
C4	OH	OSO_3^-	H	SO_3^-	4.13 ± 0.3	—	—
TTX					4.91 ± 0.7	2.98^d	6.28

^{a}In rabbit brain membranes (K_{STX} = 0.96 ± 0.07 nM); 150 mM Na^+, 2 mM Ca^{2+}, pH = 7.2, 4°C.

^{b}In frog sciatic nerve ($EC50_{STX}$ = 8.0 nM); 110 mM Na^+, 2 mM Ca^{2+}, pH = 7.2, 19°–21°C (ref. 6).

^{c}In rat t-tubular channels opened by BTX (0.2 μM) (K_{STX} = 4.3 nM at 0 mV); 200 mM Na^+, 0.1 mM EDTA, pH = 7.4, 23°–25°C (refs. 7, 10).

^{d}Data from relative inhibition of Na currents in voltage-clamped frog node of Ranvier (ref. 5).

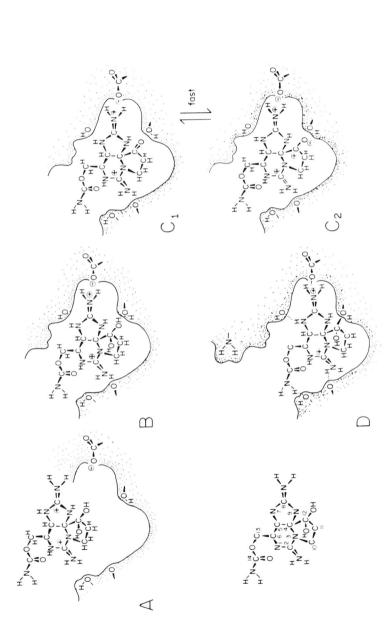

FIGURE 2. A multistep scheme for the binding of STX to high-affinity Na channels. Initial ionic binding of the 7,8,9-guanidinium to an anionic group of the receptor (*A,B*) leads to dehydration of the gem-diol at position 12, producing a ketone (*C₁*) that exists in rapid equilibrium with its carbo-cation (*C₂*). A secondary covalent bond can form between the receptor and the C-12 moiety (*D*). Dissociation is a two-stage reaction, with the rate-limiting step being the breaking of the covalent bond, a reaction which is acid catalyzed (cf. ref. 11) and slowed by deuterated solvents (ref. 7).

and to negatively charged membrane surfaces has a similar effect.[3] We believe that the ketone may also be induced by toxin dehydration following initial ionic binding to the receptor. Accordingly, we view the overall binding scheme as a two-stage process (FIGURE 2), beginning with the formation of an ionic bond between the 7,8,9-guanidinium and the receptor and the subsequent destabilization and dehydration of the gem-diol. Secondary to this dehydration, the induced ketone is able to form a covalent bond with the receptor. Selective reduction of the gem-diol to either 12α- or 12β-dihydrosaxitoxin yields molecules with differential potencies about 0.05 and 0.001 that of native STX, respectively, proving that the covalent bond is not absolutely essential for toxin action.[8,17,18] The toxin may be able to bind by the first partial reaction, dissociating rapidly but still providing some blocking action. Alternatively, the reduced saxitoxinols may form hydrogen bonds with the receptor groups that may normally bind covalently to STX ketones.

Synthetic STX Analogues

One limitation in quantifying the potencies of derivatives formed by modification of natural toxins is that trace remnants of unmodified toxins may partially account for toxic actions, especially when the apparent potencies are so low that they could arise from undetectable levels of native toxins.[17,19] This problem does not occur when synthetic analogues are used, since they are usually intermediates in multistep processes that lead to products of increasing potency. Seven such compounds, including the end product, synthetic saxitoxin, were made by Professor Y. Kishi of Harvard University and have been tested by action potential blockade and *STX competition. Their structures are shown in FIGURE 3. All of the compounds, including synthetic STX ($\pm$STX), occur as racemic mixtures and only half of the total molecules may have the correct stereochemistry for binding to sodium channels.[20]

Analogues that vary systematically at the carbamyl substituent on C-6 and at the gem-diol at C-12 were tested. The results of a typical *STX competition experiment are shown in FIGURE 4. Increasing concentrations of $\pm$STX (compound 1) reduce the amount of *STX bound saturally to brain membranes at one radioligand concentration. Parallel competition experiments were performed, with unlabeled STX and several of the synthetic analogues displacing *STX from membranes under otherwise identical conditions. The concentrations of the analogues which displaced half of the saturally bound *STX are listed in TABLE 2. The relative values agree within a factor of two with the potencies determined by impulse blockade (data not shown) when both could be tested.

The results of these experiments are somewhat surprising. Decarbamyl $\pm$ STX (compound 2) appears to be twice as potent as $\pm$STX (compound 1), but concentrations of the synthetic analogues are only known within a factor of 2, so this apparent potency difference may be insignificant. Since synthetic STX, as provided, was equipotent to native STX, whereas in principle it should have been only half as potent, we believe that the estimated $\pm$STX concentration was only half of the true value. In the same system, native decarbamyl-STX was about half as potent as native STX, in agreement with several previous reports.[17,21]

Further changes in the substituents at C-6 continued to lower the toxin potency. Compounds 3 and 5 have affinities that are 10^{-3} and 3×10^{-5}, respectively, that of native STX. These changes are far greater than that due to decarbamylation alone, and far exceed the uncertainty in the quantity of material tested. The nature of

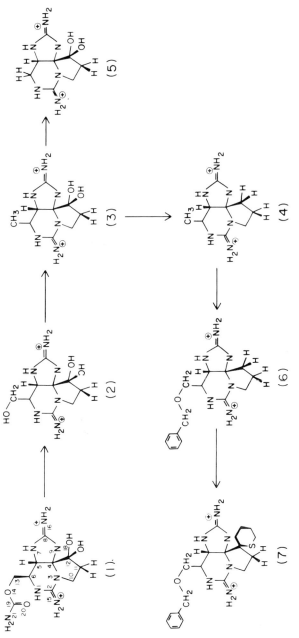

FIGURE 3. Structures of synthetic saxitoxin (*1*) and six synthetic analogues.

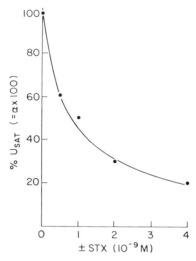

FIGURE 4. The inhibition of saturable *STX binding by increasing concentrations of synthetic saxitoxin. *STX at 0.5 nM was equilibrated with rabbit brain membranes, at 2°–4°C (cf. ref. 3).

substituents at C-6 profoundly affects binding. Examination of molecular models of STX reveals the close apposition of these groups to the 1,2,3-guanidinium moiety and to the gem-diol at C-12. Both steric and inductive factors could modify the chemistry of the 1,2,3-guanidinium, and steric interactions might also alter the reactivity of C-12 hydroxyls and ketones.

The role of the ketone at C-12 was tested directly with analogues 4, 6, and 7. Unfortunately, the limited material available prevented us from testing these compounds as completely as the others. In impulse-blocking experiments we found that compound 4, which contains a methylene at C-12 and can demonstrate neither hydroxyl nor carbonyl activities, has an EC50 value of 5–10×10^{-4} M. Although this is far greater than the EC50 for $\pm$STX (compound 1:4–8×10^{-9} M) it is only 300–500-fold greater than that of the direct precursor with a ketone at C-12, analogue 3, which has an EC50 of 1–3×10^{-6} M. We conclude that saxitoxin need not have any

TABLE 2. *STX Binding Competition by Synthetic Analogues[a]

Synthetic Analogue	$K_{0.5}(M)$[b]
1	1×10^{-9}
2	5×10^{-10}
3	1×10^{-6}
4	n.a. (2×10^{-4})[c]
5	4×10^{-5}
6	1×10^{-3}
7	2×10^{-4}
STX (native)	1×10^{-9}
decarbamyl STX	4×10^{-9}

[a]See FIGURE 3 for structures.
[b]Concentration to halve saturable binding, at 0.5 nM *STX.
[c]Insufficient material to test binding: value listed is for relative impulse blocking action.

oxygen-containing groups at C-12 to be active and that while the gem-diol form contributes significantly to the final binding energy of STX, other parts of the moleculae also bond to the receptor.

Interference with Toxin Binding by Various Cations

Since the sodium channel is highly cation selective and since STX and TTX are believed to act near the outer opening of the channel's ion pathway, it is not surprising that cations interfere with toxin binding. In an early publication Kao and Nishiyama[22] thoughtfully proposed that guanidinium moieties of TTX and STX entered the channel pore, as permeant guanidinium ions were known to, but could proceed further for only a limited distance resulting in an effective "plugging" of the pore. This hypothesis was elaborated by Hille in a speculative model[23] based largely on studies showing competition between STX and a variety of metal cations and H^+ for a common binding site.[13,24] Sodium conductance was titrated as if a single essential acidic group with pK_a 5.0–5.5 controlled the passage of ions,[25,26] and the binding of both STX and TTX varied with pH in a remarkably similar manner.[13,24,27,28] Other experiments showed that a charged guanidinium group at positions 7, 8, 9 in STX[8,14] also was essential for any blocking action, and an ionic bond between that positively charged moeity on STX (and, by analogy, on TTX) and the acidic group on the sodium channel appears to be an inevitable element in toxin binding and channel blocking.

The relationship between this cation binding site and the functional activities of the channel should provide strong evidence about the mechanism of toxin action. The original notion that the toxin was bound at the channel's selectivity filter[23] has been challenged by observations that ion selectivity is unchanged in toxin-insensitive channels, produced chemically[29] or biologically.[30,31] We have conducted a series of experiments over several years to examine the ways in which cations that are known to ineract with the channel's permeability pathway modify the binding and action of TTX and STX and its derivatives.

Cations may interfere with toxin binding through two separate mechanisms. They may bind directly to the toxin binding site, thereby inhibiting toxin occupancy by steric interference. (This is really a strong electrostatic repulsion, as is all steric hindrance at the molecular level.) Cations may also bind to a site nearby the toxin receptor and modulate toxin binding by changing the electrical potential at the receptor, where the toxin is bound, relative to the bulk solution, where the toxin is free. The effect may lower the apparent toxin affinity, but does not necessarily abolish binding. These two mechanisms may be discriminated by the dependence of the binding inhibition on the cation concentration. Specifically, for the case of direct occupancy of the toxin site the inhibition will be competitive and the potency of any particular cation will be characterized by a single inhibitory dissociation constant, K_i, which will be identical regardless of the toxin ligand used to probe the site's occupancy. For the case of electrostatic interference from a nearby site, the apparent potency of the interfering cation should increase with the charge on the ligand being tested; polyvalent toxins will be affected more than monovalent toxins, and monovalent more than neutral. Earlier studies comparing divalent STX and monovalent TTX had already demonstrated a greater effect of elevated Ca^{2+} ions on STX.[13,32] Quite recent work using other treatments to modulate the potential at the membrane surface confirmed these results.[33-35]

We have examined the changes produced by divalent metals in K_d values of a set of STX derivatives having net charges ranging from +2 to 0. The K_ds were determined in equilibrium binding experiments with brain membranes. Labeled saxitoxin (*STX)

TABLE 3. Ratio of Toxin Affinity in High and Low Calcium

Compound	Toxin Charge	$\dfrac{K_d(2 \text{ mM Ca}^{2+})^a}{K_d(42 \text{ mM Ca}^{2+})}$	n
*STX	+2	0.275 ± 0.023	14
Neo-STX	+1.25	0.402 ± 0.069	7
GTX2	+1	0.431 ± 0.065	7
GTX3	+1	0.495 ± 0.123	3
B-1	+1	0.676 ± 0.050	3
C-2	0	1.33 ± 0.089	5
TTX	+1	0.379 ± 0.070	7

^{a}Means ± SEM, with n observations.

was used to probe channel occupancy and the binding competition by the STX derivatives was measured in low (2 mM) and high (22 or 42 mM) Ca^{2+} solutions in the presence of 150 mM Na^+. The ratios of the K_d values in 42 mM calcium to those in 2 mM Ca^{2+} are collected in TABLE 3. If the elevation of the K_d values was exclusively due to a competitive inhibition by Ca^{2+}, then the relation of the K_d values would be given by

$$K_d^{app} = K_d^0(1 + [Ca^{2+}]/K_{Ca}), \tag{1}$$

where K_d^{app} is the measured K_d, K_d^0 the value with no Ca^{2+} present, and K_{Ca} the dissociation constant for Ca^{2+} at the toxin binding site. For competitive inhibition, the ratio of K_d^{app} at any two Ca^{2+} concentrations is a function of $[Ca^{2+}]$ and K_{Ca} only, and not of the tested ligand; clearly that is not the case in TABLE 2. Here the elevation of K_d^{app} depends on the net charge of the toxin, with the more positive toxins being affected more strongly.

The dependence on toxin charge of the response to elevated Ca^{2+} is qualitatively consistent with electrostatic interactions occurring between the bound toxin and charged groups fixed on the membrane at a distance from the toxin binding site. Divalent cations interact with fixed anionic charges on the membrane, rendering the local electrical potential at the binding site less negative and thereby reducing the apparent affinity for the toxin. The cation:fixed charge interaction can be described as the net effect of actual ionic bonding plus screening.[36] Screening of fixed charges follows from the diffuse accumulation of cations near the membrane and should be independent of cation species but dependent only on cation charge. In contrast, binding of cations to charged membrane groups varies with the particular cation, the order of affinity depending on the nature of the anionic group.[37] The total interaction produces a change in electrical surface potential which, if it originates sufficiently far from the binding site, is experienced equally by all toxins of the same net charge. But if the electrostatic interactions originate very close to the binding site, then toxins that have different specific charge distributions may react differently, even if they carry the same net charge. The distances between the separate charges on the toxin and the fixed charges on the membrane must be comparable to the Debye length for the given solution in order for such discrimination to occur.[38]

Our experiments showed that STX binding was depressed by divalent cations selectively; the order of effectiveness was $Ni^{2+} > Ca^{2+} \geq Mn^{2+} > Mg^{2+}$. Binding rather than screening alone explains this differential effect. The anionic groups binding the toxin appear to be close to the toxin binding site, for the effects of a particular divalent metal cation depended on the toxin tested. For example, elevated Ca^{2+} (42 mM) increased the K_d values for GTX2, GTX3 (and TTX) by the same extent (see TABLE 3), but had a significantly smaller effect on Bl, although all three toxins carry net charge $+1$. The relative results with elevated Ni^{2+} (not shown) are comparable, except that the TTX affinity is reduced only half as much as those of GTX2 and GTX3. Therefore, modulation of toxin binding by divalent metal cations appears to be due to fixed groups on the membrane very close to the toxin binding site. Direct competitive binding contributes little to the antagonism. This conclusion is supported by the anomalous response of toxin C2 to Ca^{2+}; in the presence of 40 mM Ca^{2+} C2 binds more tightly than in 2 mM Ca^{2+}. The net zero charge on CX2 results from the sum of the two positively charged guanidinium groups and two negatively charged sulfates (FIGURE 1, TABLE 1), located where those for GTX3 and Bl are each found alone. Perhaps Ca^{2+} ions form a bridge between sulfates on the toxin and anionic groups located on the receptor. Or perhaps divalent cations change the conformation of the receptor when they bind, via some allosteric mechanism, and thereby alter the juxtaposition of charged groups at the binding site to those on the receptor. This second hypothesis is difficult to test, but cannot be discounted on the basis of present evidence. We can conclude that the overall effect of divalent cations on the binding of guanidinium toxins is complex and can be described neither by direct competition nor a simple action of the diffuse double layer.

Monovalent metal cations also inhibit the binding of saxitoxin[6,13,39] and tetrodotoxin.[26,40–42] Their ability to do this parallels their ability to impede the flow of Na^+ through the channel and is consistent with a toxin binding site located at the channel pore. However, there appear to be at least two titratable anionic groups in the channel[29,43] and both may be sites for binding alkali metal cations. We attempted to probe the involvement with STX binding of these functionally defined acid groups by examining a series of organic cations. These cations had known physiological actions,[44,45] and we hoped that their larger size and less symmetrical shapes would discriminate the sites in the channel better than the small, spherically symmetrical metal ions did.

The results of such competition studies are shown in TABLE 4. Data listed include those from binding competition to lobster walking leg nerves and to membrane extracts of heads of *Drosophila*.[4,46] In addition, the equivalent dissociation constants for

TABLE 4. Effect of Organic Cations on Saturable *STX Binding

	K_i(STX Binding)(mM)[a]		$K_{block}(G_{Na})$(mM)[d]
Cation	Lobster Walking Leg Nerve[b]	*Drosophila* Brain[c]	Frog Nerve
Hydrazine	160 ± 60	—	—
Ammonium	241 ± 97	61.3 ± 11.1	368
Methyl-Hydrazine	404 ± 56	—	—
Methyl-Guanidine	660 ± 60	16.3 ± 2.5	27–40
Guanidine	670 ± 60	10.2 ± 1.4	122
Formamidine	700–800	26.5 ± 5.6	80
Acetamidine	>800	52.9 ± 0.9	80
Methylamine	>1000	—	00

[a]K_i values are from averages ($\pm$SD) of 4 determinations at each of 4 or 5 cation concentrations.

[b]Substituted cation replaces tetramethylammonium chloride to give total monovalent cation of 440 mM in artificial sea water (cf. ref. 2).

[c]Incubation medium contains 0.2 mM Ca^{2+} and choline chloride to give 200 mM total monovalent cation (cf. ref. 46).

[d]Apparent affinity for external binding site of Na channel (after ref. 45).

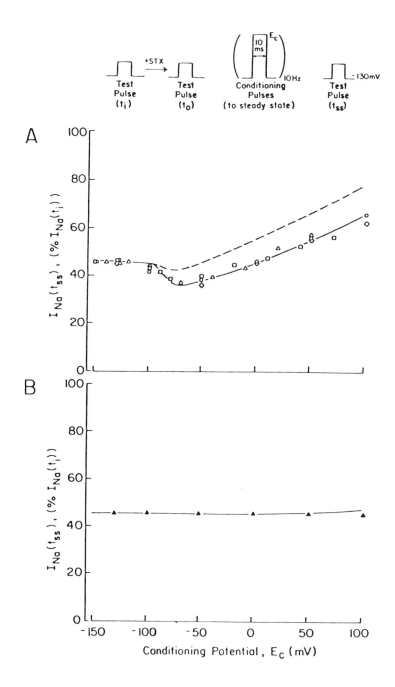

inhibition of Na^+ permeability in frog nerve are listed in the right-hand column.[45] The ionic conditions for these three procedures are quite different; binding to lobster nerve was conducted in artificial sea water containing 50 mM Mg^{2+} and 10 mM Ca^{2+} and an amount of tetramethylammonium ion sufficient to maintain the total monovalent cation at 440 mM[2], whereas fly heads were studied in 0.2 mM Ca^{2+} and enough choline chloride to maintain monovalent cations at 200 mM.[46] Frog nerves were voltage clamped in Ringer solution containing 2 mM Ca^{2+} and Na^+ balanced against the cation being tested to total 110 mM monovalent cation.

Despite a few similarities, there are many differences between the K_d values for STX binding and those for Na permeability. For example, whereas methylamine is essentially ineffective on both activities, both guanidine and methyl guanidine are about equipotent in displacing STX, yet are markedly different in their ability to block Na^{2+} current. And in fly brain, ammonium and acetamidine are nearly equal in inhibiting STX whereas they differ about four-fold in Na^+ current blocking potency. The results listed for *Drosophila* membranes are very similar to those published for rat brain synaptosomes[39] and rat skeletal muscle,[47] and appear to represent a high affinity binding site found in some invertebrates and most vertebrates. Assuming that these results also describe STX binding to Na channels of frog myelinated nerve, we conclude that it is possible for ions like guanidinium and ammonium to inhibit toxin binding while having little effect on sodium flux. The site where these cations inhibit STX binding, therefore, cannot also be the locus of their action which lowers Na^+ permeability, and must instead be located at a point more removed from the channel's pore. This conclusion is consistent with previous results showing that chemical modification of the channel by carboxyl selective acylating reagents produced insensitivity to TTX but affected ion permeation little and metal cation selectively not at all.[29,43,48]

The much higher K_i values for the lobster nerve arise to a large degree from the much higher concentrations of metal cations, particularly divalent ones, present in the sea water. The K_d values for STX in this preparation range from 10–20 nM, compared to 1–5 nM in the fly and the mammalian systems, and the inhibitory ion concentrations are also about 10 times higher.[2] Although it is difficult to evaluate the contribution of the ionic conditions to the raised K_i values, it seems unlikely that the order of inhibitory potency of cations is altered by such ionic differences. Therefore, we suggest that the lobster sodium channels are biochemically distinct from other channels having a high affinity for STX. (Others have concluded the same based on electrophysiological data.[49])

FIGURE 5. (A) Voltage-dependent block of BTX-modified channels by STX. Na channels in the frog node of Ranvier were modified by BTX (I_{Na} [t_i]) and then treated with 1.5 nM STX, which caused a reduction of the BTX-modified current to a new value (I_{Na} [t_o]). When the node was then depolarized to various conditioning potentials (E_c) at a frequency of 10 Hz, the inhibition by STX was modulated: for -100 mV < 0 mV the block was enhanced, for $E_c > 0$ mV the block was relieved, and for $E_c < -100$ mV there was no change. The symbols show the results from 4 experiments (the values are normalized such that the resulting blocks (I_{Na} [t_o]) are all identical). The *dashed line* is the voltage-dependent modulation of STX block predicted from single-channel studies (ref. 9) if the modulation were to occur only for open channels. The *solid line* is the same prediction with the voltage dependence shifted by 50 mV. **(B)** In the absence of BTX, no change of the STX inhibition was observed with this pulse protocol. However, the solid line shows the theoretical prediction based on the same model which produced the solid line in **A**. There is virtually no change predicted because in channels not modified by BTX the open state is extremely short-lived and thus does not allow for voltage-dependent modulation of STX block.

Effects of Guanidinium Toxin on Channel Gating

The concept that STX and TTX inhibit sodium channels by binding at the outer opening and preventing the permeation of sodium ions has emerged from experimental results of the past 15 years. Regardless of the details of binding, this inhibitory mechanism was assumed to exclude any involvement of channel gating, for the rates[11,12] and equilibrium levels[50,51] of toxin binding appeared to be independent of membrane potential, and the gating currents that arise from channel activation and closing were unaffected by these toxins.[52] The block by guanidinium toxins of BTX-activated channels in planar bilayers, however, shows a clear voltage dependence,[9,53,54] with rate constants for blocking and for dissociation both affected by voltage, although in the opposite direction, and to the same extent irrespective of the net charge on the toxin. At more positive depolarizations the blocking rate slows and dissociation accelerates, leading to a reduced probability of toxin occupancy. This

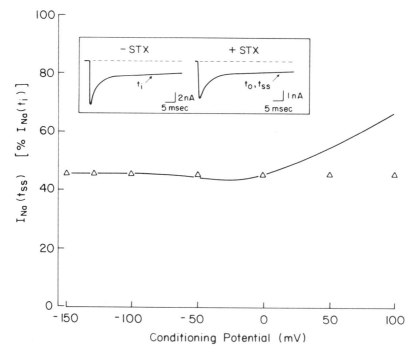

FIGURE 6. Lack of voltage-dependent block of chloramine-T-modified channels by STX. Nodal channels were modified by chloramine-T (ref. 56) and otherwise treated identically as described in FIGURE 5. The *symbols* show the results of three separate experiments, normalized to the same resting block ($I_{Na}[t_o]$). The *solid curve* is based on the same model as the solid curve in FIGURE 5, and differs from it only because BTX-modified channels begin to open at -100 mV whereas chloramine-T-modified channels begin to open at -60 mV. The model is based on the assumptions that STX binds in a voltage-dependent manner to open channels but not to closed channels, thus no modulation of block is predicted at conditioning potentials more negative than that required to open channels. *Inset* shows chloramine-T-modified currents without (*left*) and with (*right*) STX (1.5 nM). The current records with STX before (t_o) and after a train of conditioning pulses (t_{ss}) superimpose completely.

TABLE 5. STX Binding in the Presence of Gating Modifiers[a]

Modifier	% Saturable Binding[b]
Aconitine (10^{-4} M)	88.6 ± 2.3 (n = 36)[c]
Batrachotoxin (10^{-6} M)	89 ± 2.0 (n = 4)[d]
Leiurus q. venom (1–5 μg/ml)	97 ± 7.5 (n = 8)[e]
Centruroides s. venom (1–5 μg/ml)	104 ± 8.7 (n = 6)[e]

[a]Walking leg nerves of lobster, in TMA seawater, as described in ref. 2.
[b]Expressed as fraction of binding in absence of modifiers.
[c]*STX = 4–20 nM; Scatchard analysis showed K_{STX} increased from 19 nM to 28 nM by aconitine.
[d]*STX = 7 nM.
[e]*STX = 3–30 nM.

effect continues throughout the testable voltage range, well beyond potentials where the gating of BTX-activated channels reaches saturation, and appears to be due to changes in channel conformation and not to direct effects on the toxin molecules.[9,10]

We have observed the same phenomenon in frog myelinated nerve. The inhibition of BTX-modified Na currents by STX was continuously decreased over potentials from -60 to $+100$ mV, but was constant from -150 to -100 mV (FIG. 5A, ref. 55). Since BTX-modified channels in node are maximally in the open state at voltages above -60 mV but fully closed below -100 mV, we conclude that voltage-dependent block occurs in BTX-modified open but not in closed channels.

The relaxation times for STX binding, at 1–2 nM concentrations, are tens of seconds, yet the open state lifetime of normal channels is on the order of milliseconds. This may explain why no voltage dependence of STX block was observed in normal nodal currents (FIG. 5B). Kinetic restrictions notwithstanding, it is also possible that voltage-dependent block is a unique feature of BTX-opened channels. This possibility was tested in channels maintained in the open state by chloramine-T treatment, which irreversibly prevents inactivation.[56] STX inhibition of currents through these channels was not altered by membrane potential but was equal to that predicted for normal channels[7] (FIG. 6). Therefore BTX, as well as other "activator" compounds,[57] renders a form of open sodium channels that interacts with STX in a uniquely voltage-dependent mode.

Binding data also shows an effect of activators on STX.[6] Both BTX and aconitine produced significant reductions in *STX binding to lobster nerve (TABLE 4). The binding inhibition was activator-dose dependent but never exceeded 20%, and Scatchard analysis indicated a decrease in STX affinity. Since these experiments were conducted in the absence of Na^+, only modest membrane depolarizations would have resulted from the increased probability of channel opening. We believe that the activators modulate STX binding in this preparation through an allosteric mechanism, as shown previously for activators and scorpion α-toxins.[58] In the case of the α-toxins the binding is enhanced, whereas with STX it is depressed. Interestingly, the venoms from two different scorpions, both containing α-toxins, were without effect on STX binding (TABLE 5).

Even in the absence of activator drugs we observe modification of channel gating by saxitoxin. Long depolarizations convert channels to a nonconducting form from which they slowly return.[59] Recovery from such "slow inactivation" normally occurs over several hundred milliseconds. Saxitoxin increases the fraction of channels which are converted to this slowly inactivated form, and decelerates the rate of recovery (FIG. 7). (The rapid rate of recovery of channels in the "fast inactivated" state is unchanged.) Both modifications of slow inactivation may be explained by the stabilization of slowly inactivated channels by STX, present at concentrations that block half the channels before the conditioning pulse. However, the binding reaction that subserves this effect must differ from the normal inhibitory mechanism, because the time constant for normal blocking-unblocking is approximately 50 seconds,[7,12] yet the slowed recovery occurs more than 100 times faster. We offer two explanations of this discrepancy. One is that conditioning pulses convert channels to a conformation that binds STX with a higher affinity, but with a much faster dissociation rate constant, and, therefore, an even greater binding rate constant. The other is that toxin

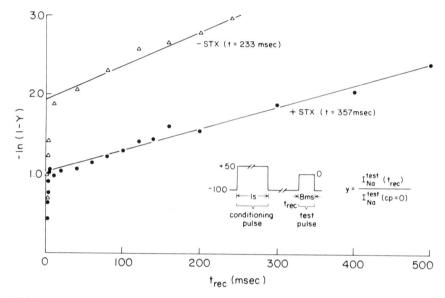

FIGURE 7. The effect of STX on slow inactivation of Na channels. Na channels in the frog node of Ranvier were driven to the slow inactivated state by a 1-s depolarization to +50 mV. The recovery from that pulse was measured by a brief test pulse at various times after the conditioning (see pulse inset). In untreated nodes, the recovery occurred in two phases—a rapid phase ($t = 0.96$ ms) and a slow phase ($t = 233$ ms). The fraction of the Na current which exhibited the slow recovery was 15%. When the node was treated with 2 nM STX and the procedure was repeated, two changes were observed. First, and more consistent, the fraction of the current which recovered slowly was increased, in this case to 50%. Second, and quite variable, the time constant of the slow phase was increased, in this case to 357 ms. The time constant of the rapid phase of recovery was unchanged by STX.

molecules may bind to channels without directly inhibiting ion passage, and that this mode of action is enhanced by long depolarizations. But whatever the correct explanation, the notion that STX and TTX action can be described by a simple, one-step binding reaction must be altered to accommodate these new results.

ACKNOWLEDGMENTS

We thank Dr. Edward Moczydlowski for his comments on the manuscript, and Mr. Richard Roscoe for assistance in programming the computer model for voltage-dependent block. The able technical assistance of Ms. Isobel Heyman and Ms. Maria Schoen is gratefully acknowledged.

REFERENCES

1. RITCHIE, J. M., R. B. ROGART & G. R. STRICHARTZ. 1976. J. Physiol. (London) **261:** 477–494.
2. STRICHARTZ, G. R. & C. M. HANSEN BAY. 1981. J. Gen. Physiol. **77:** 205–221.
3. STRICHARTZ, G. 1982. Mol. Pharmacol. **21:** 343–350.
4. GITSCHIER, J., L. T. HALL & G. R. STRICHARTZ. 1980. Biochim. Biophys. Acta **595:** 291–312.
5. STRICHARTZ, G. R., S. Hall & Y. SHIMIZU. 1984. Biophys. J. **45:** 286a.
6. HANSEN BAY, C. M. & G. R. STRICHARTZ. 1978. Biophys. J. **21:** 207a.
7. HAHIN, R. & G. R. STRICHARTZ. 1981. J. Gen. Physiol. **78:** 113–139.
8. STRICHARTZ, G. 1984. J. Gen. Physiol. **84:** 281–305.
9. MOCZYDLOWSKI, E., S. HALL, S. S. GARBER, G. S. STRICHARTZ & C. MILLER. 1984. J. Gen. Physiol. **84:** 687–704.
10. MOCZYDLOWSKI, E., A. UEHARA & S. HALL. 1986. *In* Ion Channel Reconstitution. C. Miller, Ed. Plenum. New York.
11. ULBRICHT, W. & H. H. WAGNER. 1975. J. Physiol. **252:** 185–202.
12. WAGNER, H. H. & W. ULBRICHT. 1975. Pfluegers Arch. **359:** 297–315.
13. HENDERSON, R., J. M. RITCHIE & G. R. STRICHARTZ. 1974. Proc. Natl. Acad. Sci. U.S.A. **71:** 3936–3940.
14. KAO, P. N., M. R. JAMES-KRACKE & C. Y. KAO. 1983. Pfluegers Arch. **398:** 199–203.
15. SHIMIZU, Y., C. P. HSU, W. E. FALLON, Y. OSHIMA, I. Miura & K. NAKANISHI. 1978. J. Am. Chem. Soc. **100:** 6791–6793.
16. SHIMIZU, Y., C. P. HSU & A. GENENAH. 1981. J. Am. Chem. Soc. **103:** 605–609.
17. KAO, C. Y. & S. E. WALKER. 1982. J. Physiol. **323:** 619–637.
18. KAO, C. Y., P. N. KAO, M. R. JAMES-KRACKE, F. E. KOEHN, C. F. WICHMANN & H. K. SCHNOES. 1985. Toxicon **23:** 647–655.
19. HU, S. L., C. Y. KAO, F. E. KOEHN & H. K. SCHNOES. 1985. J. Gen. Physiol. **86:** 13a–14a.
20. TANINO, H., T. NAKATA, T. KANEKO & Y. KISHI. 1977. J. Am. Chem. Soc. **99:** 2818–2819.
21. GHAZAROSSIAN, V. E., E. J. SCHANTZ, H. K. SCHNOES & F. M. STRONG. 1976. Biochem. Biophys. Res. Comm. **68:** 776–780.
22. KAO, C. Y. & A. NISHIYAMA. 1965. J. Physiol. (London) **180:** 50–66.
23. HILLE, B. 1975. Biophys. J. **15:** 615–619.
24. HENDERSON, R., J. M. RITCHIE & G. R. STRICHARTZ. 1973. J. Physiol. (London) **235:** 783–804.
15. HILLE, B. 1975. Fed. Proc. **34:** 1318–1321.
26. WOODHULL, A. M. 1973. J. Gen. Physiol. **61:** 687–708.
27. COLQUHOUN, D., R. HENDERSON & J. M. RITCHIE. 1972. J. Physiol. (London) 95–126.
28. ULBRICHT, W. & H. H. WAGNER. 1975. J. Physiol. (London) **252:** 159–184.
29. SPALDING, B. C. 1980. J. Physiol. (London) **305:** 485–500.
30. PAPPONE, P. E. 1980. J. Physiol. (London) **306:** 377–410.
31. HUANG, M. L. Y., W. A. CATTERALL & G. EHRENSTEIN. 1979. J. Gen. Physiol. **73:** 839–854.
32. HILLE, B., J. M. Ritchie & G. R. STRICHARTZ. 1975. J. Physiol. (London) **250:** 34P–35P.
33. GRISSMER, S. 1984. Pfluegers Arch. **402:** 353–359.
34. NEUMCKE, B. & R. STAMPFLI. 1984. Pfluegers Arch. **401:** 125–131.
35. NEUMCKE, B. & R. STAMPFLI. 1986. Prog. Zool. **33:** In press.
36. MCLAUGHLIN, S. G. A., G. SZABO & G. EISENMAN. 1971. J. Gen. Physiol. **58:** 667–687.
37. MCLAUGHLIN, S., N. MULRINE, T. GRESALFI, G. VAIO & A. MCLAUGHLIN. 1981. J. Gen. Physiol. **77:** 445–473.
38. ALVAREZ, O., M. BRODWICK, R. LATORRE, A. MCLAUGHLIN, S. MCLAUGHLIN & G. SZABO. 1983. Biophys. J. **44:** 333–342.

39. WEIGELE, J. B. & R. L. BARCHI. 1978. FEBS Lett. 95: 49–53.
40. REED, J. K. & M. A. RAFTERY. 1976. Biochem. 15: 944–953.
41. REED, J. K. & W. TRZOS. 1979. Arch. Biochem. Biophys. 195: 414–422.
42. FRELIN, C., P. VIGNE & M. LAZDUNSKI. 1981. Eur. J. Biochem. 119: 437–442.
43. SIGWORTH, F. J. & B. C. SPALDING. 1980. Nature 283: 293–295.
44. HILLE, B. 1971. J. Gen. Physiol. 58: 599–619.
45. HILLE, B. 1975. J. Gen. Physiol. 66: 535–560.
46. GITSCHIER, J. M. 1981. Tritiated-saxitoxin as a probe for voltage-sensitive sodium channels in wild-type, mutant, and aneuploid *Drosophilia melanogaster.* Ph.D. thesis. Massachusetts Institute of Technology. Cambridge, Ma.
47. BARCHI, R. L. & J. B. WEIGELE. 1979. J. Physiol. (London) 295: 383–396.
48. GULDEN, K. -M. & W. VOGEL. 1985. Pfluegers Arch. 403: 13–20.
49. POOLER, J. P. & D. P. VALENZENO. 1979. Biochim. Biophys. Acta 555: 307–315.
50. ALMERS, W. & S. R. LEVINSON. 1975. J. Physiol. (London) 247: 483–509.
51. KRUEGER, B. K., R. W. RATZLAFF, G. R. Strichartz & M. P. BLAUSTEIN. 1979. J. Mem. Biol. 50: 287–310.
52. ARMSTRONG, C. M. & F. BEZANILLA. 1974. J. Gen. Physiol. 63: 533–552.
53. KRUEGER, B. K., J. F. WORLEY R. J. FRENCH. 1983. Nature 303: 172–175.
54. HARTHSHORNE, R. P., B. U. KELLER, J. A. TALVENHEIMO, W. A. CATTERALL & M. MONTAL. 1985. Proc. Natl. Acad. Sci. U.S.A. 82: 240–244.
55. RANDO, T. A. & G. R. STRICHARTZ. 1986. Biophys. J. 49: 785–794.
56. WANG, G. K. 1984. J. Physiol. (London) 346: 127–141.
57. GARBER, S. S. & C. MILLER. 1985. J. Gen. Physiol. 86: 14a–15a.
58. CATTERALL, W. 1977. J. Biol. Chem. 252: 8669–8676.
59. PEGANOV, E. M., KHODOROV, B. I. & L. SHISHKOVA. 1973. Bull. Exp. Biol. Med. 76: 1014–1017.

Interactions of Scorpion Toxins with the Sodium Channel

HANS MEVES,[a] J. MARC SIMARD,[b]
AND DEAN D. WATT[c]

[a]Physiologisches Institut
Universität des Saarlandes
D-6650 Homburg, Federal Republic of Germany

[b]Division of Neurosurgery
University of Texas Medical Branch
Galveston, Texas 77550

[c]Department of Biochemistry
Creighton University
Omaha, Nebraska 68178

INTRODUCTION

Less than two decades have passed since Koppenhöfer and Schmidt[1] described the effects of a scorpion venom on sodium (Na) currents. In the brief interval since, the isolation of numerous scorpion toxins has fostered the study of their chemical properties and physiological effects, adding measurably to our understanding of the sodium channel. Nearly 100 toxins have been isolated and their amino acid compositions analyzed. The primary structures of more than one-third of these toxins have been elucidated and models of the tertiary structure of two have been proposed (for review, see ref. 2). By comparing the findings from studies on specific binding, it has become evident that there are two classes of scorpion toxins, each of which has distinct effects on Na currents. Additional data indicate that the scorpion toxins may also be distinguished on the basis of certain determinants of binding or of effect, namely depolarization and pH.

It is important to note that the scorpion toxins interact with the sodium channel in ways that are clearly distinguishable from those of tetrodotoxin (TTX) and saxitoxin (STX). The scorpion toxins bind with high affinity to sites on the sodium channel that are different from the binding sites for TTX and STX (for review, see ref. 3). This accords with the observation that the saturation of TTX binding sites (300 nM TTX) does not prevent the reduction of charge immobilization observed with venom from *Leiurus quinquestriatus*.[4] As further described below, the effects of the scorpion toxins differ from those of TTX and STX in two important ways: (1) the effects of some scorpion toxins are enhanced at low pH whereas the effect of TTX is reduced,[5] and (2) the action of the scorpion toxins is strongly dependent on membrane potential whereas the effects of TTX and STX on nerve membranes are not (for literature, see ref. 6).

The various properties of the scorpion toxins are well exemplified by the two classes of toxins found in the venom of the American scorpion, *Centruroides sculpturatus* (for review, see ref. 7). In this communication, we review the structural and electrophysiological characteristics of these toxins, emphasizing the coherence of findings that supports the existence of two distinct classes of scorpion toxins.

CHEMICAL STRUCTURE

Venom from a single species of scorpion is a mixture of many different substances, including a large number (>20) of different, low molecular weight proteins. Many of these small proteins have neurotoxic activity in a variety of host species. The neurotoxins commonly contain 60–70 amino acids, although a few "insect" toxins contain only 30–40 amino acids. These proteins are single chains cross-linked by four disulfide bridges, which must be intact for biological activity.[8,9] The amino acid sequences of approximately 30 toxins isolated from ten different species of scorpions have been reported and tabulated.[2,10,11]

The tertiary structure of toxin var3 from *C. sculpturatus*[12] contains structural features believed to be typical of other scorpion toxins, an assumption supported by the NMR studies of Arseniev *et al.*[13] The model (FIG. 1A) shows that a molecule of toxin var3 is composed of a dense core of secondary structure, which contains two and one-half turns of α-helix (residues 23–31, inclusive), and a short stretch of β-pleated sheet composed of three antiparallel strands (residues 1–4, 37–41, and 46–50, inclusive).[12,14] Strand S_1 of the β-sheet begins at the NH_2 terminus (residues 1–4) and is connected through a polypeptide chain to the one exposed disulfide bridge (cysteines 12–65). The other elements of secondary structure are linked by short loops of polypeptide chain (FIG. 1A). Residues 32–36 connect the carboxyl end of the α-helix with strand S_3 of the β-sheet; residues 42–45 connect strand S_3 with strand S_2 of the β-sheet; residues 51–65, which form a comparatively long stretch of contorted polypeptide chain, connect strand S_2 of the β-sheet to the COOH-terminal disulfide bridge which joins Cys-65 with Cys-12. The contorted polypeptide chain leading to the COOH terminus contains the four prolines in toxin var3.

The structure of toxin var3 is stabilized by many hydrogen bonds and by the covalent linkages of four disulfide bridges.[14] The α-helix is linked to strand S_2 of the β-sheet by two disulfide bridges (Cys 25-Cys 46 and Cys 29-Cys 48). A third disulfide bridge (Cys 16-Cys 41) covalently links strand S_3 of the β-sheet with the loop that leads to the NH_2-terminal end of the α-helix. These three disulfide bridges are buried within the molecule.[12] The pattern of the disulfide bridges in toxin var3 resembles that originally reported for toxin II from *Androctonus australis* (cysteines 12–63, 16–36, 22–46, 26–48)[15] and is considered typical for all long-chain "mammal" scorpion toxins. A long-chain "insect" toxin from *A. australis* has a different bridging pattern than the "mammal" toxins.[16] The short-chained "insect" toxins also have four disulfide bridges but their locations have not yet been determined.[16,17]

The primary structure of toxin var3 from *C. sculpturatus* was compared to that of 23 other scorpion toxins by aligning their amino acid sequences so that the cysteines were in register, leaving gaps where necessary to maximize homology. (Complete tabulated comparisons are given in refs. 2, 10, and 11.) Several regions of conserved primary sequence were observed, including the sequences composing the three strands of β-sheet (TABLE 1). For example, in strand S_1, lysine-1 is substituted only by another basic amino acid (arginine), glutamate-2 is substituted only by another dicarboxylic acid (aspartate), glycine-3 is substituted only by its homologue (alanine), and tyrosine-4 is invariant.[18] FIGURE 1B (area enclosed by dashed line) illustrates an exposed region of conservative substitution in the space-filling model on the same side as the β-sheet.

An additional structural feature of note in the model of toxin var3 is the presence of an extensive hydrophobic patch on the surface of one side of the molecule (FIG. 1B, dark region). Seven of the eight aromatic side chains in the molecule are located in this region. As shown in the figure, this hydrophobic patch coincides in part with the region of conservative substitution. The region of conserved amino acids and the unique

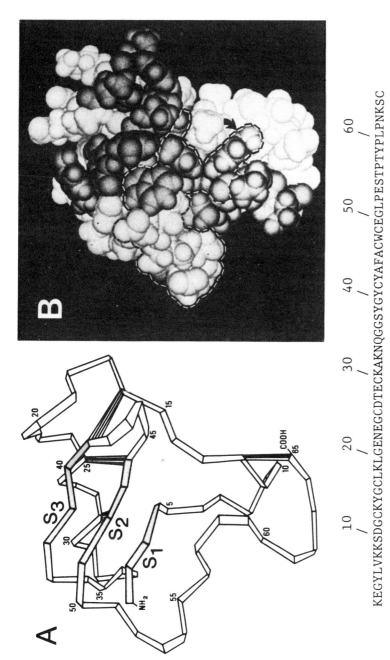

KEGYLVKKSDGCKYGCLKLGENEGCDTECKAKNQGSYGYCYAFACWCEGLPESTPTYPLPNKSC

10   20   30   40   50   60

FIGURE 1. Model of toxin var3 from *C. sculpturatus*. (**A**) The ribbon model of the polypeptide chain, kinked at each α-carbon atom, shows the three strands of antiparallel β-sheet (*gray areas*) and the positions of the disulfide bridges (*multiple lines*). The numbers correspond to the amino acids in the numbered sequence below. (**B**) The space-filling model of the same side of the molecule as in **A** shows a region of hydrophobic residues (*darkened area*) and an exposed region of conserved amino acids (*dashed lines*). Also included within the dashed line is the tyrosine at position 58 (*arrow*), which is not a conserved residue. (Adapted from Fontecilla-Camps *et al.*[18])

TABLE 1. Conserved Sequences in the β-Sheet of 24 Scorpion Toxins

	1	2	3	4		
S_1	Lys (15)	Glu (6)	Gly (19)	Tyr (24)		
	Arg (9)	Asp (18)	Ala (5)			
	37	38	39	40	41	
S_2	Ser (22)	Tyr (5)	Gly (23)	Tyr (20)	Cys (24)	
	Asp (1)	Gly (3)	Ser (1)	Ser (2)		
	Gly (1)	Lys (1)		His (1)		
		—^{a} (15)		Lys (1)		
	45^b	46	47	48	49^c	50
S_3	Ala (21)	Cys (24)	Trp (17)	Cys (24)	Glu	Gly
	Gly (2)		Tyr (7)		variable	
	Ser (1)					

Numbers above each sequence correspond to the position in the chain of toxin var3 from *C. sculpturatus,* whose residues are listed in the first line of each of the three sequences, S_1–S_3 (see FIG. 1). Listed below each sequence are amino acid substitutions; numbers in parentheses give the frequency of a given residue in 24 toxins.
^{a}The dash at position 38 of S_2 indicates a deletion in the aligned sequences.
^{b}In sequence S_3, residue 45 is not part of the β-sheet.
^{c}Residues 49–50 show high variability in amino acid substitutions in the 24 toxins. See refs. 2, 10, and 11 for references to original sequences.

hydrophobic patch suggest that this side of the molecule is associated with biological activity, an assumption consistent with the effects of modification of certain specific amino acids in other toxins (for review, see ref. 19).

EFFECTS ON SODIUM-CHANNEL CURRENTS

Although the structural features of the long-chain scorpion toxins do not permit a distinction between classes of toxins, voltage clamp studies of Na currents indicate that a distinction between two classes is warranted. One class of toxins slows inactivation and has minimal effects on activation, whereas the other class shifts the voltage dependence of activation without appreciably slowing inactivation. Toxins from both classes alter the voltage dependence of inactivation and make inactivation incomplete.

FIGURE 2A illustrates the slow turning-off of the inward current, compared to the control, in a node of Ranvier treated with 3.3 μg/ml of toxin V from *C. sculpturatus.* This effect was first reported with whole venom from *L. quinquestriatus*[1] and has since been demonstrated in the node of Ranvier by treatment with several isolated toxins, including toxin IIα from the same venom,[20] toxins M$_7$ and 2001 from *Buthus eupeus,*[21] toxins V and XII from *Buthus tamulus,*[22] and toxins V and var1–3 from *C. sculpturatus.*[23] The existence of this class of toxins in the venom of *C. sculpturatus* has been confirmed independently using a toxin (named IVα) isolated by different methods.[24] Slowing of inactivation has also been observed in neuroblastoma cells[25] and in crayfish,[26] cockroach,[27] and squid[28] axons with toxins I and II from *A. australis,* as well as in frog muscle[29] and tunicate eggs[30] with isolates from *L. quinquestriatus.* In the *Sepia* giant axon, however, one of the toxins from this class produces only a block of the Na current without slowing inactivation.[26] It is apparent from FIGURE 2A that the peak Na current and the Na activation kinetics are not substantially altered by this class of toxins. It is noteworthy, however, that venom from *L. quinquestriatus,* which slows inactivation, also produces a small negative shift of the $m_\infty(E)$ curve,[1,4] an effect more typical of the second class of toxins (see below). This last observation has not been confirmed with any isolated toxins from this class.[52]

In the node of Ranvier, toxins from this class change the voltage dependence of inactivation. The $h_\infty(E)$ curve becomes flatter and nonmonotonic, *i.e.,* inactivation is not only incomplete but increases at positive potentials. This effect was originally observed with whole venom from *L. quinquestriatus*[1] and is illustrated in FIGURE 2B (closed circles), with 3.3 μg/ml of toxin V from *C. sculpturatus*. Toxin M_7 from *B. eupeus*[21] and toxin IIα from *L. quinquestriatus*[24] produce a similar effect in the node.

The second class of toxins affects the Na current in the node of Ranvier in a very different way. These toxins decrease the Na current and shift the voltage dependence of activation to more negative potentials. In a node tested without a conditioning pulse, treatment with this class of toxins from *C. sculpturatus* decreases Na currents by half and shifts the $I_{Na}(E)$ and $P_{Na}(E)$ curves to more positive potentials than the control (see FIG. 2 of ref. 31). However, when test pulses are preceded by strong depolarizing conditioning pulses, inward currents are observed at potentials more negative than in either the control or the toxin-treated node tested without a conditioning pulse. FIGURE 3 shows inward currents during test pulses to -72 and -52 mV in a node treated with 6.1 μg/ml of toxin III from *C. sculpturatus*. In the absence of a conditioning pulse, no inward current was observed at -72 mV (**A**), and only a small current was observed at -52 mV (**B**). In comparison, larger inward currents were induced when the test pulses were preceded by depolarizing conditioning pulses (**C** and **D**). The smaller superimposed currents in panels **C** and **D** are those resulting from the conditioning pulse alone at the holding potential (-92 mV).

The larger inward currents at negative potentials that are associated with the conditioning pulse give rise to a shift of the descending branch of the $I_{Na}(E)$ curve (FIG. 4, top-left panel). The magnitude of the shift depends on several factors, including the

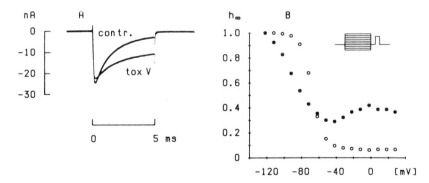

FIGURE 2. (A) Slowing of inactivation with 3.33 μg/ml of toxin V from *C. sculpturatus* (*tox V*). An inward current which inactivates normally is also shown (*contr.,* normal Ringer solution). The membrane currents in a node of Ranvier were recorded during 5-ms test pulses to -22 mV from a holding potential of -92 mV. Capacitative and leakage currents not subtracted. (B) Voltage dependence of inactivation in the control (normal Ringer solution O) and following treatment with 3.3 μg/ml of toxin V from *C. sculpturatus* (●). Prepulses of varying amplitude (40 ms) were followed after a 0.5 ms pause by a constant test pulse to -22 mV. The peak current minus the TTX-insensitive current was normalized (ordinate) and plotted against the prepulse potential (abscissa). Holding potential, -92 mV. (**A** From Hu *et al.*[31]; **B** from Meves *et al.*[23])

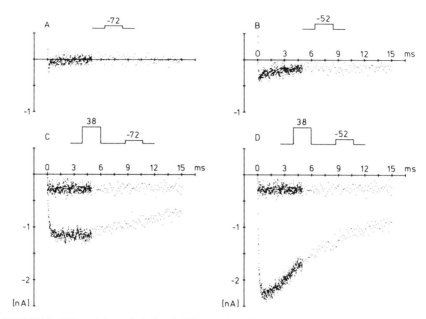

FIGURE 3. Effect of 6.1 μg/ml of toxin III from *C. sculpturatus*. The Na currents in a node of Ranvier were recorded in the presence of 6 nM TTX to reduce the effect of series resistance. Test pulses to -72 mV (**A**) and -52 mV (**B**) produced no or very little inward current. The same test pulses preceded by a depolarizing conditioning pulse (15 ms to $+38$ mV followed by a 20 ms pause) produced larger, slowly inactivating inward currents (**C** and **D**). The smaller currents in panels **C** and **D** are those recorded 20 ms after the conditioning pulse at the holding potential, -92 mV. TTX-insensitive currents were subtracted. The Ringer solution contained 110 mM NaCl, 2.5 mM KCl, 1.8 mM CaCl$_2$, 12 mM TEA, and 4 mM MOPS, pH 7.2, in addition to TTX and toxin III. The ends of the fiber were cut in 113 mM CsCl + 7 mM NaCl. Temperature, 12°C. (H. Meves, unpublished.)

interval between the conditioning and test pulses, the strength of the conditioning pulse, and the concentration of toxin.[23,32,33] These effects were first demonstrated with whole venom from *C. sculpturatus*[32] and have been observed with several isolated toxins from the same species of scorpion, including toxins I, III, IV, VI, and VII.[23,31,33] Toxins isolated by different methods from the same venom (named Iα–IIIα and IIIβ) also produce these effects in the node.[20,24] Similar observations that indicate a shift in the voltage dependence of activation have been made in the node of Ranvier with toxin II from *Centruroides suffusus suffusus*[34] and in the node[35,36] as well as in neuroblastoma cells[37] with toxin γ from *Tityus serrulatus*. In both preparations, the shift with toxin γ was observed without preceding depolarization, although in the node depolarization enhanced it.[36] In skeletal muscle, both toxin II from *C. suffusus suffusus* and toxin γ from *T. serrulatus* produce only a block of Na currents.[38,39]

Quantitative analysis indicates that the kinetics of activation are altered by treatment with toxins III and IV from *C. sculpturatus*.[31] The value of τ_m measured in the presence of toxin without a conditioning pulse is about 1.5 times larger than normal. The time-to-peak of the inward current is prolonged, an effect which is diminished at negative potentials by a depolarizing conditioning pulse (FIG 4, top-right panel). A depolarizing conditioning pulse also shifts the voltage dependence of τ_m to more negative potentials (FIG. 4, bottom). In the experiment described in FIGURE 4, a strong hyperpolarization to -142 mV was interposed between the conditioning and test pulses to allow the value of τ_m to be fitted as a third-order process (see below).

Unlike the first class, toxins in the second class do not substantially slow inactivation of sodium currents in the node of Ranvier (see FIG. 1 of ref. 31). As with the voltage dependence of activation, however, the voltage dependence of inactivation is also shifted to more negative potentials by toxin VII from *C. sculpturatus*.[33] Toxin γ from *T. serrulatus* also shifts the $h_\infty(E)$ curve in neuroblastoma cells[37] but not in the node.[35] In the node, this class of toxins from *C. sculpturatus* makes inactivation incomplete,[23,33] whereas inactivation is complete in both the node[36] and in neuroblastoma cells[37] with toxin γ from *T. serrulatus*.

The shift of the $h_\infty(E)$ curve observed with toxin VII from *C. sculpturatus* was measured with a three-pulse program (FIG. 5B, inset b). The first depolarizing pulse in

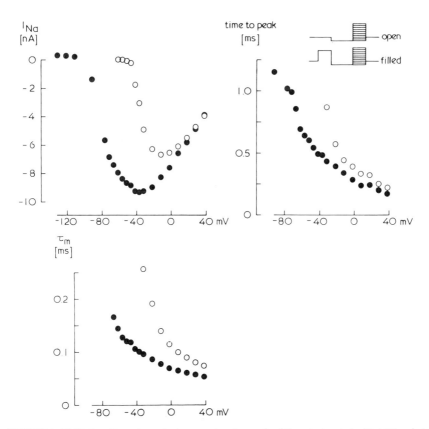

FIGURE 4. Shifts in voltage-dependent parameters in a node of Ranvier treated with 1.33 µg/ml of toxin IV from *C. sculpturatus*. Peak Na current, time-to-peak and time constant of activation (τ_m) are plotted against the potential of the test pulse. The pulse sequence consisted of a 20 ms hyperpolarizing prepulse to -142 mV, either alone (O) or preceded by a 15 ms pulse to $+38$ mV (●), followed by 1 ms test pulses to varying potentials (see inset). Holding potential, -92 mV. Leakage and capacitative currents subtracted by means of an analogue circuit. (From Hu *et al.*[31])

the sequence (+38 mV, 15 ms) induces an inward current on repolarization which reflects the characteristic shift in the voltage dependence of activation (FIG. 5Aa). The magnitude of the depolarization-induced current depends on the transiently shifted value of activation and on the steady-state value of inactivation.[32] This current turns on as inactivation is removed (going from +38 to −72 mV in the example shown) and slowly decays as the activation variable returns to its normal value at the polarized potential. As shown in FIG. 5Ab, this inward current is rapidly turned off and on by a small hyperpolarizing pulse given during its course. The magnitude of the inward current immediately following the hyperpolarizing pulse (the peak of the tail current, Fig. 5Ab) reflects the instantaneous value of the inactivation variable, that is its value at the membrane potential during the preceding pulse. The tail current decays as inactivation assumes its new value (going from −92 to −72 mV). The normalized tail currents were used to measure the voltage dependence of h_∞ following treatment with toxin VII (FIG. 5B, closed circles). The curve is shifted to more negative potentials, compared to the control (open circles), but by less than the shift in the voltage dependence of activation.[33] A shift is also observed by measuring inward currents during test pulses to −12 mV (FIG. 5B, squares). Unlike the effect with the first class of toxins (FIG. 2B), the $h_\infty(E)$ curve is not flattened and remains monotonic.

As indicated above, the kinetics that govern the turning-on of the Na current are changed by toxins III and IV from *C. sculpturatus*. In the absence of a conditioning pulse, small test pulses give rise to inward currents that turn on with a sigmoidal time course, as occurs in normal fibers (see FIG. 7A, +). Similar results are obtained in neuroblastoma cells with toxin γ from *T. serrulatus*.[37] When test pulses are preceded by a depolarizing conditioning pulse, however, inward currents at relatively negative potentials turn on with an exponential time course after treatment with venom (FIG 6) or toxins III or IV from *C. sculpturatus*.[31] Panel A of FIGURE 6 shows a noninactivat-

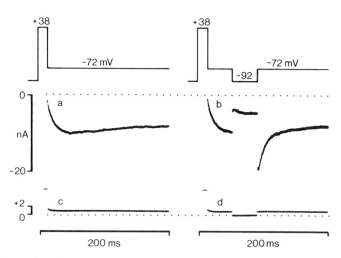

FIGURE 5A. Effect of 0.2 μg/ml of toxin VII from *C. sculpturatus* on steady-state inactivation. The node had previously been exposed to toxin at pH 5.7 for 10 min. (a) Inward current at −72 mV following a 15 ms depolarizing pulse to +38 mV. (b) Inward current produced as in a, but modulated by a 40 ms hyperpolarizing pulse to −92 mV. The tail current results from the further removal of inactivation by the hyperpolarizing pulse. Holding potential, −92 mV. (c), (d) Same as a and b, but following addition of 300 nM TTX. (From Simard *et al.*[33])

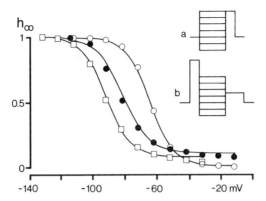

FIGURE 5B. Normalized peak inward currents plotted against the potential of an 80 ms prepulse. O = Control run prior to addition of toxin, obtained using pulse program a (test potential, -12 mV). □ = Currents obtained after treatment with toxin with the same pulse program as control run, except that the prepulse of variable amplitude was preceded by a conditioning pulse to $+38$ mV for 15 ms. ● = Normalized peak tail currents measured at -62 mV; the prepulse of variable amplitude (80 ms) was preceded by a 15 ms conditioning pulse to $+38$ mV (pulse program b). Holding potential, -92 mV. TTX-insensitive currents subtracted. (From Simard *et al.*[33])

ing inward current during a 10 mV test pulse to -82 mV following a conditioning pulse. Panels B and C of the figure show on an expanded time scale the exponential rise and decay of inward currents with test pulses to the same potential. Note that turning-on of the current is not delayed after onset of the depolarization (FIG. 6B). Interposing a strong hyperpolarizing potential ($E = -142$ mV) between the depolarizing conditioning pulse and the test pulse delays the rising phase sufficiently so that it can be fitted as a third-order process.[31] An exponential time course for the rising phase of the Na current has also been described in fibers treated with batrachotoxin,[40] although with this toxin the current rises after a small initial delay.[41]

The exponential rise of the Na current almost coincides with the exponential rise of the gating current. In FIGURE 7, the time course of the charge movement (squares) is plotted with the rising phase of the Na current ($+$) after treatment with toxin IV from *C. sculpturatus*. In the absence of a conditioning pulse, there is a pronounced delay between the rise of the charge movement and the rise of the Na current (FIG. 7A). This is similar to observations in normal fibers[42] and in fibers treated with venom from *L. quinquestriatus* (see FIG. 5 of ref. 4), a venom which slows inactivation without greatly affecting activation. However, with a depolarizing conditioning pulse, both the charge movement and the Na current begin together at the onset of depolarization and both follow a simple exponential time course (FIG. 7B). With a conditioning pulse, the rise time of the Na current ($\tau_{onNa} = 136$ μs) is somewhat slower than the rise time of the gating current ($\tau_{ongate} = 89$ μs). First-order kinetics for both the charge movement and the Na current are also observed in fibers treated with batrachotoxin, although with this toxin I_{Na} begins after an initial delay of about 70 μs, and τ_{ongate} is 1.14 times larger than τ_{onNa}.[41]

The reaction scheme

$$A \text{ (resting)} \rightleftarrows B \text{ (intermediate)} \rightleftarrows C \text{ (intermediate)} \rightleftarrows D \text{ (open)}$$

describes a model of the Na channel going from the resting state through various

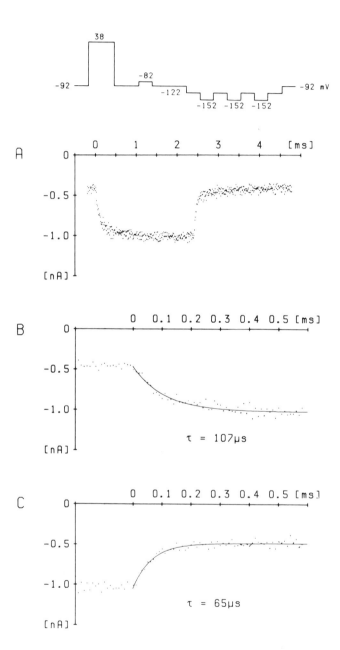

nonconducting intermediate states into the open state. This model can be used to explain several of the findings on Na currents that are observed with this class of toxins, if it is assumed that (1) binding of toxin to the Na channel increases the energy barrier for the transition $B \rightleftarrows C$ in both the forward and backward directions and (2) depolarization overcomes this barrier in the forward direction but polarization does not in the backward direction. Thus, without prior depolarization, the probability of the channel opening from the resting state would be less than normal because of the barrier. After a depolarization, the probability of the channel residing in state C, that is, in a state near the open state, would be increased, and as a consequence, the probability of its opening would be increased. For a channel in state C, the final transition to the open state would proceed without delay as a single-order rate process with exponential kinetics. Finally, relaxation in the backward direction to the resting state would be slowed because of the energy barrier, with repolarization or hyperpolarization only returning the channel to the nonconducting state C.

SPECIFIC BINDING TO EXCITABLE MEMBRANES

Studies on the specific binding of scorpion toxins to excitable membranes have demonstrated the existence of two classes of saturatable, noninteracting binding sites (TABLE 2), as first reported by Jover and colleagues.[45] They designated the two groups α and β, the α group being represented by toxin II from *A. australis,* and the β group by toxin II from *C. suffusus suffusus.* A third toxin, toxin γ from *T. serrulatus,* has also been labeled and used in binding studies.[47] A variety of preparations has been investigated, including rat brain synaptosomes, chick heart cells, electroplaque membrane, and frog muscle. Competitive inhibition of specific binding of the ^{125}I-labeled toxins by nonlabeled toxins allows their classification into two groups. Thus, the α toxins but not the β toxins inhibit the binding of ^{125}I-labeled toxin II from *A. australis* and the β toxins but not the α toxins inhibit the binding of ^{125}I-labeled toxin II from *C. suffusus suffusus* or ^{125}I-labeled toxin γ from *T. serrulatus* (TABLE 2).

Specific binding of the toxins correlates, in part, with effects on Na currents. Toxin II from *A. australis* exhibits the first class of effect on Na currents, that is, it slows inactivation. Of the toxins listed in TABLE 2 that inhibit binding of ^{125}I-labeled toxin II from *A. australis,* only toxin I from the same species has been studied in voltage clamp experiments and it too slows inactivation. Among the toxins that do not inhibit binding, all except toxins V and var1–3 from *C. sculpturatus* shift the voltage dependence of activation. It is surprising that toxins V and var1–3, which slow inactivation, do not also inhibit binding.[46] A better correlation is found for the β group of toxins. All of the toxins that inhibit the binding of ^{125}I-labeled toxin II from *C. suffusus suffusus* or of

---

FIGURE 6. Exponential rise and fall of Na current. Inward currents were recorded in Na-poor Ringer solution in a node of Ranvier treated with 5 μg/ml of venom from *C. sculpturatus.* (A) Average of three records of inward current during 2.4 ms pulses to -82 mV, 40 ms after the 15 ms conditioning pulses to $+38$ mV. Holding potential, -92 mV. The capacitative and leakage currents were estimated with -30 mV pulses, scaled appropriately and subtracted. (B) Rise time of the Na current at -82 mV, same pulse program as A except that the duration of the test pulse was reduced to 0.6 ms. (C) Decay of the Na current at -92 mV, same as B, but showing the decay of the Na current at the end of the 0.6 ms test pulse. The rise and decay of the currents were fitted with exponential functions having time constants of 107 μs (B) and 65 μs (C). The Na-poor Ringer solution had two-thirds of the usual Na replaced by tetramethylammonium and included 12 mM TEA to block K$^+$ current. The ends of the fiber were cut in 113 mM CsCl + 7 mM NaCl. Temperature, 12°C. (H. Meves, unpublished.)

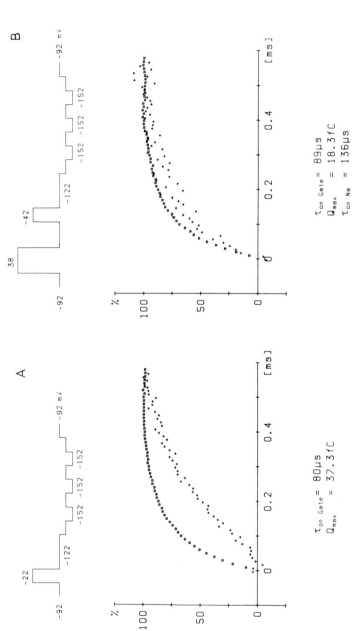

FIGURE 7. Time course of charge movement and activation of Na current in a node of Ranvier treated with 5 μg/ml of toxin IV from *C. sculpturatus*. The pulse programs for measuring the Na current and the gating current are shown at the top of each panel. The Na currents (+), recorded in Na-poor Ringer solution (two-thirds of the normal amount of the Na replaced by Tris), were divided by $\exp(-t/\tau_h)$, inverted with respect to the usual convention and normalized. The gating currents (□), recorded in the presence of 300 nM TTX, were integrated and normalized with respect to the charge value at the end of the record. **(A)** Currents during test pulses to −22 mV without a conditioning pulse. **(B)** Currents during test pulses to −42 mV, 40 ms after a 15 ms conditioning pulse to +38 mV. The gating currents in **A** and **B** and the Na current in **B** were fitted with exponential functions having the time constants indicated. Temperature, 12°C. (H. Meves, unpublished.)

[125]I-labeled toxin γ from *T. serrulatus* have been studied in voltage clamp experiments and found to shift the voltage dependence of activation. In addition, some toxins which do not inhibit their binding, notably toxins I and II from *A. australis* and toxins V and var1–3 from *C. sculpturatus*, belong to the class that slows inactivation.

EFFECTS OF DEPOLARIZATION AND pH ON BINDING AND EFFECT

Specific binding experiments have also shown that the binding affinity of some toxins is decreased by increasing $[K^+]_o$. In some studies,[47,49] increasing $[K^+]_o$ has been

TABLE 2. Summary of Literature on Competitive Binding

Inhibition	No Inhibition
α Group ^{125}I-labeled toxin II from *A. australis*	
A. australis	*C. sculpturatus*
toxin I[43-45]	toxins III, IV, V, var1–3[46]
B. occitanus	*C. suffusus suffusus*
toxin I[43–45]	toxin II[44,45]
L. quinquestriatus	*T. serrulatus*
toxins IV and V[44,45]	toxin γ[47]
T. serrulatus	
tityustoxin[47]	
β Group ^{125}I-labeled toxin II from *C. suffusus suffusus*	
C. sculpturatus	*A. australis*
toxins III and IV[46]	toxins I and II[45]
T. serrulatus	*B. occitanus*
toxin γ[48]	toxin I[45]
	C. sculpturatus
	toxins V, var1–3[46]
	L. quinquestriatus
	toxins IV and V[45]
	T. serrulatus
	tityustoxin[48]
β Group ^{125}I-labeled toxin γ from *T. serrulatus*	
C. suffusus suffusus	*A. australis*
toxin II[39,47]	toxin II[39,47]
	T. serrulatus
	tityustoxin[39,47]

correlated with depolarization by using a labeled ion distribution technique. The dependence of binding on membrane potential was first suggested by Catterall *et al*,[49] who studied the binding of an unnamed toxin from *L. quinquestriatus* on neuroblastoma cells. Similar findings have been made with ^{125}I-labeled toxin II from *A. australis* in chick heart cells[43] and in rat brain synaptosomes.[44,45] Both of these toxins exhibit the first class of effect on Na currents, that is they slow inactivation.[26,29] Conversely, the specific binding of ^{125}I-labeled toxin II from *C. suffusus suffusus* or of ^{125}I-labeled toxin γ from *T. serrulatus*, toxins which exhibit the second class of effect on Na currents, is not affected by increasing $[K^+]_o$.[45,47]

The correlate of these binding studies is the demonstration that the effect of toxin

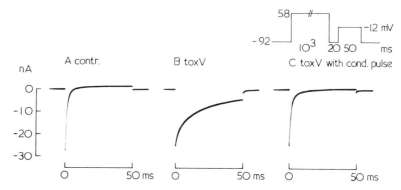

FIGURE 8. Removal of effect of toxin V from *C. sculpturatus* by a depolarizing conditioning pulse. **(A)** Na current during 50 ms test pulse to -12 mV in normal Ringer solution. Holding potential, -92 mV. **(B)** Na current during same test pulse following treatment with toxin. **(C)** Same as **B** except that the test pulse was preceded by a 1-s conditioning pulse to $+58$ mV, with a 20-ms pause before the test pulse. Leakage current not subtracted. (From Meves *et al.*[50])

on Na currents is diminished by depolarization. Such an effect has been observed with toxin M$_7$ from *B. eupeus*[21] and toxin V from *C. sculpturatus*,[50] both of which slow inactivation. FIGURE 8 illustrates that the slowing of inactivation with toxin V is essentially reversed by a one-second conditioning pulse to $+58$ mV (compare **A** and **C** in FIG. 8). In FIGURE 9, the effect of toxin V, expressed as normalized late inward

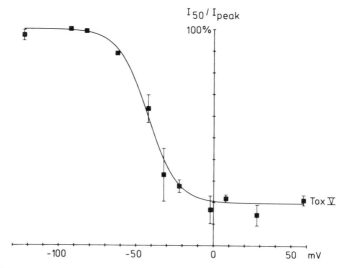

FIGURE 9. Voltage dependence for removal of effect of toxin. Average values for 9 nodes of Ranvier treated with 3.3–10 µg/ml of toxin V from *C. sculpturatus*. The effect of toxin was measured as inward current at 50 ms/peak I_{Na} during test pulses to -12 mV. The value I_{50}/I_{Na} was normalized with respect to the value without a conditioning pulse and plotted against the prepulse potential. Holding potential, -92 mV; TTX-insensitive currents subtracted. (From Meves *et al.*[50])

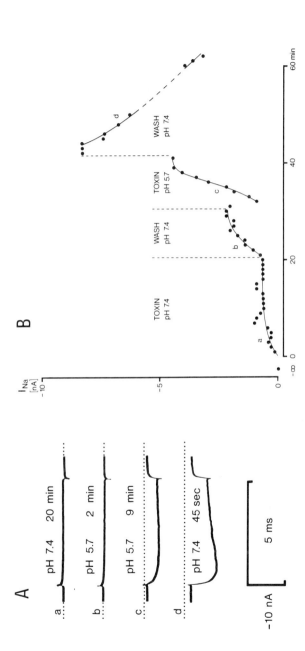

FIGURE 10. Enhanced effect of toxin VII from *C. sculpturatus* by pretreatment at pH 5.7. (**A**) Original records of currents in a node of Ranvier. (**B**) Values of I_{Na} during test pulses to -62 mV, 20 ms after a 15 ms conditioning pulse to $+38$ mV. (**Aa**) Twenty min after start of toxin VII, 0.1 µg/ml, pH 7.4 (segment **Ba**). The solution was then changed to toxin-free Ringer solution, pH 7.4, which in some fibers caused an increase in I_{Na} (segment **Bb**), but in others caused a decrease. (**Ab**) 2 min, and (**Ac**) 9 min after the start of toxin VII, 0.1 µg/ml, pH 5.7 (segment **Bc**). (**Ad**) One min after record **Ac** and 45 s after changing to toxin-free Ringer solution, pH 7.4 (segment **Bd**). Dotted lines in **A** indicate zero current. Vertical lines in **B** indicate times of solution changes. Capacitative and leakage current not subtracted in **A** but estimated from hyperpolarizing pulses and subtracted in **B**. Holding potential, -92 mV. (**A** from Simard *et al.*[33]; **B** from Simard, unpublished)

current, is plotted against the potential during a depolarizing conditioning pulse. The effect of toxin decreases with depolarization, showing a sigmoidal voltage dependence. Note that approximately 20% of the toxin effect is not removed by strong depolarization. Although the curve resembles the steady-state inactivation curve, the potential at half-maximum effect is about 20 mV more positive than the half-maximum potential of the $h_\infty(E)$ curve.[50] A reduction of toxin effect with preceding depolarization is not observed with the class of toxins that shifts the voltage dependence of activation. Indeed, as described above, the effects of these toxins on the node of Ranvier are manifested, not decreased, by a strong depolarizing conditioning pulse.

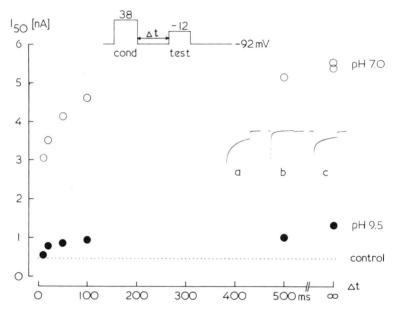

FIGURE 11. Effect of pH and of interpulse interval on the action of toxin V from *C. sculpturatus*. The Na current at the end of a 50 ms test pulse to -12 mV is plotted against the interval between a 30 ms conditioning pulse to $+38$ mV and the test pulse. Holding potential, -92 mV. The node of Ranvier was treated with 5 μg/ml of toxin V at pH 7.0 (MOPS buffer); the pH was changed to 9.5 (CHES buffer) to obtain one set of values (●), after which the pH was returned to 7.0 to obtain another set of values (○). Original current records during test pulses without conditioning pulses are shown. The three records were obtained with toxin. Record **a** at pH 7.0, record **b** at pH 9.5, and record **c** on returning to pH 7.0. TTX-insensitive current subtracted from the values plotted but not from the original records shown. (H. Meves, unpublished.)

A different determinant of binding has been described for toxins that shift the voltage dependence of activation. The specific binding of ^{125}I-labeled toxin II from *C. suffusus suffusus* depends on pH. Binding is maximum at pH 5–6 and decreases rapidly as pH 8 is approached. This effect is observed in electroplaque membrane,[48] frog skeletal muscle,[38] and in rat brain synaptosomes.[51] The correlate of these binding studies is the demonstration that the effect at pH 7.4 of toxin VII from *C. sculpturatus* is enhanced by pretreatment at pH 5.7.[33] FIGURE 10A shows original current records and FIGURE 10B the peak inward currents during test pulses to -62 mV following a depolarizing conditioning pulse in a node treated with 0.1 $\mu g/ml$ of toxin VII. At pH 7.4, 20 min of exposure to toxin resulted in a negligible effect (record Aa, segment Ba). After a brief wash, exposure to toxin at pH 5.7 resulted in a sigmoidal increase in toxin effect with time, which reached a maximum at 9 min (records Ab and Ac, segment Bc). Changing to pH 7.4 rapidly removes the blocking effect of H^+ (record Ad and segment Bd), and demonstrates the large effect of toxin at pH 7.4 following exposure to pH 5.7, compared to the initial effect of toxin at pH 7.4.

An effect of pH is not restricted to the second class of toxins. The characteristic slowing of inactivation observed with toxin V from *C. sculpturatus* is much less pronounced at pH 9.5 (FIG. 11b) than at pH 7.0 (FIGS. 11a and 11c). The inward current at 50 ms (I_{50}) at pH 9.5 is less than the value at pH 7.0, but is larger than the control value without toxin at pH 7.0 (FIG. 11, values at ∞). As discussed above, the effect of toxin V is decreased by a preceding depolarizing conditioning pulse. FIGURE 11 shows that, at both neutral pH and pH 9.5, the interval between the depolarizing conditioning pulse and the test pulse determines the extent to which the effect of toxin is removed by the conditioning pulse. Complete removal of the effect of toxin requires the combined use of an increase in pH and a depolarizing conditioning pulse applied with minimal delay before the test pulse.

SUMMARY

It is evident from the data reviewed that scorpion toxins can be distinguished on the basis of three properties: their effects on Na currents, their specific binding to excitable membranes, and the effects of depolarization and pH on binding and on effect. Additional work with other scorpion toxins is required to establish the degree of correlation between the three properties for each class of toxin. Further investigations with this family of homologous proteins will undoubtedly contribute not only to our understanding of the toxins themselves but also to our understanding of the structure and function of the Na channel.

REFERENCES

1. KOPPENHÖFER, E. & H. SCHMIDT. 1968. Die Wirkung von Skorpiongift auf die Ionen-ströme des Ranvierschen Schnürrings. I. Die Permeabilitäten P_{Na} und P_K. Pfluegers Arch. **303:** 133–149.
2. WATT, D. D. & J. M. SIMARD. 1984. Neurotoxic proteins in scorpion venom. J. Toxicol.-Toxin Rev. **3:** 181–221.
3. CATTERALL, W. A. 1984. The molecular basis of neuronal excitability. Science **223:** 653–661.
4. NONNER, W. 1979. Effects of *Leiurus* scorpion venom on the "gating" current in myelinated nerve. *In* Advances in Cytopharmacology, vol. 3. B. Ceccarelli & F. Clementi, Eds.: 345–352. Raven. New York.
5. ULBRICHT, W. & H. H. WAGNER. 1975. The influence of pH on equilibrium effects of tetrodotoxin on myelinated nerve fibres of *Rana esculenta*. J. Physiol. (London) **252:** 159–184.
6. FRENCH, R. J., J. F. WORLEY III & B. K. KRUEGER. 1984. Voltage-dependent block by saxitoxin of Na channels incorporated into planar lipid bilayers. Biophys. J. **45:** 301–310.
7. MEVES, H., J. M. SIMARD & D. D. WATT. 1984. Biochemical and electrophysiological

characteristics of toxins isolated from the venom of the scorpion *Centruroides sculpturatus*. J. Physiol. (Paris) **79**: 185–191.

8. HABERSETZER-ROCHAT, C. & F. SAMPIERI. 1976. Structure-function relationships of scorpion neurotoxins. Biochemistry **15**: 2254–2261.

9. WATT D. D. & M. E. McINTOSH. 1972. Effects on lethality of toxins in venom from the scorpion *Centruroides sculpturatus* by group specific reagents. Toxicon **10**: 173–181.

10. DUFTON, M. J. & H. ROCHAT. 1984. Classification of scorpion toxins according to amino acid composition and sequence. J. Mol. Evol. **20**: 120–127.

11. POSSANI L. D., B. M. MARTIN, I. SVENDSEN, G. S. RODE & B. W. ERICKSON. 1985. Scorpion toxins from *Centruroides noxius* and *Tityus serrulatus*. Primary structure and sequence comparison by metric analysis. Biochem. J. **229**: 739–750.

12. FONTECILLA-CAMPS, J. C., R. J. ALMASSY, F. L. SUDDATH, D. D. WATT & C. E. BUGG. 1980. Three-dimensional structure of a protein from scorpion venom: A new structural class of neurotoxins. Proc. Natl. Acad. Sci. U.S.A. **77**: 6496–6500.

13. ARSENIEV, A. S., V. I. KONDAKOV, V. N. MAIOROV & V. F. BYSTROV. 1984. NMR solution spatial structure of 'short' scorpion insectotoxin I_5A. FEBS Lett. **165**: 57–62.

14. ALMASSY, R. J., J. C. FONTECILLA-CAMPS, F. L. SUDDATH & C. E. BUGG. 1983. Structure of variant-3 scorpion neurotoxin from *Centruroides sculpturatus* Ewing, refined at 1.8Å resolution. J. Mol. Biol. **170**: 497–527.

15. KOPEYAN, C., G. MARTINEZ, S. LISSITZKY, F. MIRANDA & H. ROCHAT. 1974. Disulfide bonds of toxin II of the scorpion *Androctonus australis* Hector. Eur. J. Biochem. **47**: 483–489.

16. DARBON, H., E. ZLOTKIN, C. KOPEYAN, J. VAN RIETSCHOTEN & H. ROCHAT. 1982. Covalent structure of the insect toxin of the North African scorpion *Androctonus australis* Hector. Int. J. Pept. Protein Res. **20**: 320–330.

17. GRISHIN, E. V. 1981. Structure and function of *Buthus eupeus* scorpion neurotoxins. Int. J. Quant. Chem. **19**: 291–298.

18. FONTECILLA-CAMPS, J. C., R. J. ALMASSY, F. L. SUDDATH & C. E. BUGG. 1982. The three-dimensional structure of scorpion neurotoxins. Toxicon **20**: 1–7.

19. ROCHAT, H., H. DARBON, E. JOVER, M. F. MARTIN, J. BABLITO & F. COURAUD. 1984. Interaction of scorpion toxins with the sodium channel. J. Physiol. (Paris) **79**: 334–337.

20. WANG, G. K. & G. STRICHARTZ. 1982. Simultaneous modifications of sodium channel gating by two scorpion toxins. Biophys. J. **40**: 175–179.

21. MOZHAYEVA, G. N., A. P. NAUMOV, E. D. NOSYREVA & E. V. GRISHIN. 1980. Potential-dependent interaction of toxin from venom of the scorpion *Buthus eupeus* with sodium channels in myelinated fibre. Biochim. Biophys. Acta **597**: 587–602.

22. SIEMEN, D. & W. VOGEL. 1983. Tetrodotoxin interferes with the reaction of scorpion toxin (*Buthus tamulus*) at the sodium channel of the excitable membrane. Pfluegers Arch. **397**: 306–311.

23. MEVES, H., N. RUBLY & D. D. WATT. 1982. Effect of toxins isolated from the venom of the scorpion *Centruroides sculpturatus* on the Na currents of the node of Ranvier. Pfluegers Arch. **393**: 56–62.

24. WANG, G. K. & G. R. STRICHARTZ. 1983. Purification and physiological characterization of neurotoxins from venoms of the scorpions *Centruroides sculpturatus* and *Leiurus quinquestriatus*. Mol. Pharmacol. **23**: 519–533.

25. BAZAN, M. & P. BERNARD. 1984. Effect of α-neurotoxins from scorpion venom on sodium current in neuroblastoma cells. J. Biophys. Med. Nucl. **8**: 3-8.

26. ROMEY, G., R. CHICHEPORTICHE, M. LAZDUNSKI, H. ROCHAT, F. MIRANDA & S. LISSITZKY. 1975. Scorpion neurotoxin—a presynaptic toxin which affects both Na^+ and K^+ channels in axons. Biochem. Biophys. Res. Commun. **64**: 115–121.

27. PELHATE, M. & E. ZLOTKIN. 1982. Actions of insect toxin and other toxins derived from the venom of the scorpion *Androctonus australis* on isolated giant axons of the cockroach (*Periplaneta americana*). J. Exp. Biol. **97**: 67–77.

28. PICHON, Y. & M. PELHATE. 1984. Effect of toxin 1 from *Androctonus australis* Hector on sodium currents in giant axons of *Loligo forbesi*. J. Physiol. (Paris) **79**: 318–326.

29. CATTERALL, W. A. 1979. Binding of scorpion toxin to receptor sites associated with sodium channels in frog muscle. Correlation of voltage-dependent binding with activation. J. Gen. Physiol. **74**: 375–391.

30. OKAMOTO, H., K. TAKAHASHI & N. YAMASHITA. 1977. One-to-one binding of a purified scorpion toxin to Na channels. Nature **266:** 465–468.

31. HU, S. L., H. MEVES, N. RUBLY & D. D. WATT. 1983. A quantitative study of the action of *Centruroides sculpturatus* toxins III and IV on the Na currents of the node of Ranvier. Pfluegers Arch. **397:** 90–99.

32. CAHALAN, M. D. 1975. Modification of sodium channel gating in frog myelinated nerve fibres by *Centruroides sculpturatus* scorpion venom. J. Physiol. (London) **244:** 511–534.

33. SIMARD, J. M., H. MEVES & D. D. WATT. 1986. Effects of toxins VI and VII from the scorpion *Centruroides sculpturatus* on the Na currents of the frog node of Ranvier. Pfluegers Arch. **406:** 620–628.

34. COURAUD, F., E. JOVER, J. M. DUBOIS & H. ROCHAT. 1982. Two types of scorpion toxin receptor sites, one related to activation, the other to inactivation of the action potential sodium channel. Toxicon **20:** 9–16.

35. JONAS, P., W. VOGEL, E. C. ARANTES & J. R. GIGLIO. 1986. Toxin γ of the scorpion *Tityus serrulatus* modifies both activation and inactivation of sodium permeability of nerve membrane. Pfluegers Arch. **407:** 92–99.

36. ZABOROVSKAYA, L. D. & B. I. KHODOROV. 1985. Effect of *Tityus* γ toxin on the activation process in sodium channels of frog myelinated nerve. Gen. Physiol. Biophys. **4:** 101–104.

37. VIJVERBERG, H. P. M., D. PAURON & M. LAZDUNSKI. 1984. The effect of *Tityus serrulatus* scorpion toxin γ on Na channels in neuroblastoma cells. Pfluegers Arch. **401:** 297–303.

38. JAIMOVICH, E., M. ILDEFONSE, J. BARHANIN, O. ROUGIER & M. LAZDUNSKI. 1982. *Centruroides* toxin, a selective blocker of surface Na$^+$ channels in skeletal muscle: Voltage-clamp analysis and biochemical characterization of the receptor. Proc. Natl. Acad. Sci. U.S.A. **79:** 3896–3900.

39. BARHANIN, J., M. ILDEFONSE, O. ROUGIER, S. V. SAMPAIO, J. R. GIGLIO & M. LAZDUNSKI. 1984. Tityus γ toxin, a high affinity effector of the Na$^+$ channel in muscle, with a selectivity for channels in the surface membrane. Pfluegers Arch. **400:** 22–27.

40. KHODOROV, B. I. 1978. Chemicals as tools to study nerve fiber sodium channels. Effects of batrachotoxin and some local anesthetics. *In* Membrane Transport Processes, vol. 2. D. C. Tosteson, Y. A. Ovchinnikov & R. Latorre, Eds.: 153–174. Raven Press. New York.

41. DUBOIS, J. M. & M. F. SCHNEIDER. 1985. Kinetics of intramembrane charge movement and conductance activation of batrachotoxin-modified sodium channels in frog node of Ranvier. J. Gen. Physiol. **86:** 381–394.

42. NEUMCKE, B., W. NONNER & R. STÄMPFLI. 1976. Asymmetrical displacement current and its relation with the activation of sodium current in the membrane of frog myelinated nerve. Pfluegers Arch. **363:** 193–203.

43. COURAUD, F., H. ROCHAT & S. LISSITZKY. 1980. Binding of scorpion neurotoxins to chick embryonic heart cells in culture and relationship to calcium uptake and membrane potential. Biochemistry. **19:** 457–462.

44. JOVER, E., N. MARTIN-MOUTOT, F. COURAUD & H. ROCHAT. 1980. Binding of scorpion toxins to rat brain synaptosomal fraction. Effects of membrane potential, ions, and other neurotoxins. Biochemistry. **19:** 463–467.

45. JOVER, E., F. COURAUD & H. ROCHAT. 1980. Two types of scorpion neurotoxins characterized by their binding to two separate receptor sites on rat brain synaptosomes. Biochem. Biophys. Res. Comm. **95:** 1607–1614.

46. WHEELER, K. P., D. D. WATT & M. LAZDUNSKI. 1983. Classification of Na channel receptors specific for various scorpion toxins. Pfluegers Arch. **397:** 164–165.

47. BARHANIN, J., J. R. GIGLIO, P. LÉOPOLD, A. SCHMID, S. V. SAMPAIO & M. LAZDUNSKI. 1982. *Tityus serrulatus* venom contains two classes of toxins; *Tityus* γ toxin is a new tool with a very high affinity for studying the Na$^+$ channel. J. Biol. Chem. **257:** 12553–12558.

48. WHEELER, K. P., J. BARHANIN & M. LAZDUNSKI. 1982. Specific binding of toxin II from *Centruroides suffusus suffusus* to the sodium channel in electroplaque membranes. Biochemistry. **21:** 5628–5634.

49. CATTERALL, W. A., R. RAY & C. S. MORROW. 1976. Membrane potential dependent binding of scorpion toxin to action potential Na$^+$ ionophore. Proc. Natl. Acad. Sci. U.S.A. **73:** 2682–2686.

50. MEVES, H., N. RUBLY & D. D. WATT. 1984. Voltage-dependent effect of a scorpion toxin on sodium current inactivation. Pfluegers Arch. **402:** 24–33.
51. JOVER, E., J. BABLITO & F. COURAUD. 1984. Binding of β-scorpion toxin: A physicochemical study. Biochemistry. **23:** 1147–1152.
52. WANG, G. K. & G. STRICHARTZ. 1985. Kinetic analysis of the action of *Leiurus* scorpion α-toxin on ionic currents in myelinated nerve. J. Gen. Physiol. **86:** 739–762.

Toxins That Modulate the Sodium Channel Gating Mechanism[a]

TOSHIO NARAHASHI

Department of Pharmacology
Northwestern University Medical School
Chicago, Illinois 60611

INTRODUCTION

The discovery of the highly selective action of tetrodotoxin (TTX) on the sodium channel has led to a widespread use of the toxin as a tool for a variety of studies of ion channels.[1,2] It is equally important that the original TTX study has stimulated the use of other toxins and chemicals exhibiting specific actions for the study of excitable membranes. These studies have in turn led to the discovery of unique actions of certain other toxins. Instead of blocking the sodium channel, these toxins have been shown to alter the kinetics of the sodium channel drastically. Depending on the nature of kinetic changes, the net result in the physiological function may be exhibited by a prolongation of action potential, repetitive discharges, membrane depolarization, synaptic disturbances, or a combination of any of these changes. Since the changes in the sodium channel gating kinetics are very drastic and specific, these toxins are also becoming extremely useful tools for the analysis of channel function. Examples of such toxins include batrachotoxin (BTX), grayanotoxin (GTX), veratridine, and pyrethroids. The present paper gives highlights of our studies of some of these toxins.

BATRACHOTOXIN AND GRAYANOTOXIN

Membrane Depolarization

Batrachotoxin is one of the toxic principles contained in the skin secretion of Colombian poison arrow frog *Phyllabates aurotaenia*.[3] Our earlier studies have clearly demonstrated that BTX depolarizes the squid axon membrane by prolonged opening of sodium channels.[4,5] One of these experiments is illustrated in FIGURE 1. When applied internally to a squid giant axon BTX caused a large depolarization, eventually reversing the polarity of the membrane potential. The membrane potential was rapidly restored by lowering the external sodium concentration to a very low level (*e.g.,* 1 mM) or by applying TTX externally. These observations show that the sodium channels are opened by BTX, resulting in a large depolarization.

Grayanotoxins are contained in the leaves of plants belonging to the family Ericaceae (*Leucothoe, Rhododendron, Andromeda, Kalmia*). These toxins also cause a large depolarization of the membrane by opening the sodium channels in much the same way as BTX.[6-8]

[a]This work was supported by NIH grants NS14143 and NS14144.

Sodium Channel Gating Kinetics

Later studies by Khodorov and his associates with the nodes of Ranvier of the frog showed that BTX kept the sodium channels open for a long period of time.[9-12] The voltage dependence of the sodium channel opening was shifted drastically in the hyperpolarizing direction. These two changes in sodium channel gating function would cause a large membrane depolarization.

Grayanotoxins have also been shown to exert effects very similar to those of BTX.[13] An example of such an experiment is shown in FIGURE 2. When the squid axon membrane perfused internally with 20 mM tetraethylammonium to block the potassium channels was depolarized from a holding potential of -150 mV to -10 mV, a

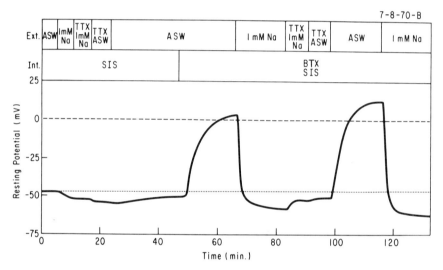

FIGURE 1. Effects of internal perfusion of 550 nM batrachotoxin (*BTX*) on the resting membrane potential of a squid giant axon. The large BTX-induced depolarization in artificial sea water (*ASW*) is reversed by lowering the sodium concentration to 1 mM, and antagonized by tetrodotoxin (*TTX*) applied externally. *SIS*, standard internal solution. From Narahashi *et al.*[4]

transient inward sodium current was followed by a small steady-state sodium current (FIG. 2B). After internal application of grayanotoxin I (GTXI) at a concentration of 5 μM, the transient current was decreased in amplitude while the steady-state current was increased slightly. These two changes became more pronounced as the concentration of GTXI was increased up to 100 μM (FIG. 2B). When the membrane was depolarized to -70 mV from -150 mV in the control axon, no sodium current was generated (FIG. 2A). After application of GTXI, however, a slow, steady-state current was produced upon step depolarization, and its amplitude increased with increasing concentration of GTXI (FIG. 2A). Thus GTXI causes the slow steady-state current to be generated at a large negative potential (-70 mV) where no transient current is produced in normal axons. FIGURE 2B also shows that with increasing concentration of GTXI, the peak amplitude of transient current decreases whereas the amplitude of

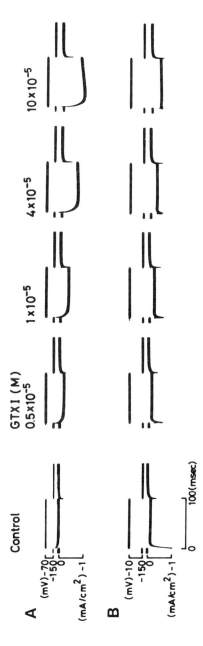

FIGURE 2. Effects of various concentrations of grayanotoxin I (*GTXI*) on membrane sodium currents associated with a step depolarization from a holding potential of (**A**) −150 mV to −70 mV or (**B**) to −10 mV. In the presence of GTXI, a slow inward sodium current appears at −70 mV where no sodium current is generated in the control. At −10 mV, the peak sodium current is decreased by GTXI whereas the slow current is increased. From Seyama and Narahashi.[13]

slow steady-state current increases. This suggests that a population of sodium channels is modified by GTXI in a concentration-dependent manner to generate the slow current.

Single Sodium Channels

Patch clamp experiments with the cultured neuroblastoma cells N1E-ll5 have revealed that the open time of single sodium channels is greatly prolonged after application of BTX[14] (FIGS. 3A and 3E). Prior to BTX application, the open time was described by a Poisson distribution with a mean of 2.2 ms (FIG. 3C). The probability of openings during a step depolarizing pulse followed a time course similar to that of the sodium current recorded from a whole cell membrane (FIG. 3D). After application of 10 μM BTX, the open time was expressed by a double exponential function with time constants of approximately 2 ms and 60 ms (FIG. 3G). The probability of openings during a depolarizing step mimicked the time course of the whole cell sodium current in the presence of BTX (FIG. 3H). The amplitude of single sodium channel current was decreased somewhat by BTX (FIGS. 3B and 3F). Whether the decrease is due to a genuine decrease in single channel conductance or high-frequency flickerings remains to be seen.

When the amplitude of individual sodium channel current was plotted against the individual open time, a unique feature of BTX modification was unveiled (FIG. 4). After exposure to BTX, the sodium channels were divided into two populations; one had the amplitude and the open time comparable to those of the normal channels, and the other had smaller amplitudes and much longer open times. The former represents the unmodified sodium channels, and the latter the BTX-modified channels. This strongly suggests that BTX modifies individual sodium channels in an all-or-none manner. It was also shown that BTX-modified sodium channels opened at large negative potentials.

Site of Action in the Sodium Channel

The results of experiments described in preceding sections indicate that BTX keeps the individual sodium channels open for a long period of time, that the channels open at large negative potentials, and that the sodium current recorded from the whole cell or a large membrane area (e.g., squid giant axon) shows no inactivation. In order to determine the site and mode of action of BTX in the sodium channel, two pharmacological probes, pronase and local anesthetic agent, were used in voltage clamp experiments with squid axons.[15,16]

Batrachotoxin removed the sodium current inactivation in squid axons in much the same way as in frog nodes of Ranvier or neuroblastoma cells. The tail current associated with a step repolarization from a depolarized level underwent no drastic change, the only detectable change being a slight slowing. These results indicate that the inactivation (h) gate is impaired by BTX. It should also be pointed out that the effect of BTX becomes apparent only after applying repetitive stimulations. This indicates that the sodium channel must be open for BTX to exert the effect.

Our earlier study showed that procaine prevented BTX from exerting the depolarizing action on squid axons.[5] In the presence of TTX, BTX had no effect on the membrane potential. When both TTX and BTX were removed, a depolarization ensued because the effect of irreversibly bound BTX was unveiled as the reversible antagonist TTX was washed out. In the presence of procaine, BTX also failed to cause

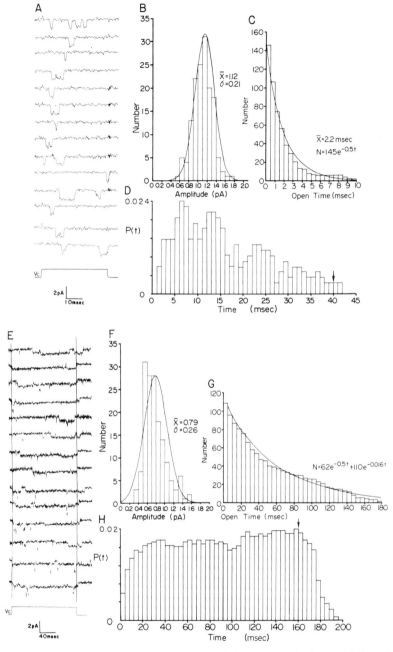

FIGURE 3. Single sodium channel currents recorded by the patch clamp technique from neuroblastoma cells in the absence and presence of 10 μM batrachotoxin (BTX). (A–D) Control. (A) Sample records of single sodium channel currents. (B) Amplitude histogram. (C) Open time distribution. (D) Probability of channel openings during a depolarizing pulse which ends at the arrow. (E–H) Corresponding figures in the presence of BTX. See text for further explanation. From Quandt and Narahashi.[14]

depolarization. However, when both procaine and BTX were removed, no depolarization was observed. This result was interpreted as indicating that procaine occupied the BTX binding site, thereby preventing the subsequently applied BTX from binding. Thus when both chemicals were washed out, procaine simply was dissociated from the site causing no depolarization.

In order to determine the site of action of BTX more precisely, pronase and N-octylguanidine were used as tools in squid axons. Pronase is known to destroy the inactivation gate, thereby causing a prolonged, noninactivating sodium current to appear. [17,18] Octyguanidine has been shown to block the open sodium channel in a manner similar to that of local anesthetics.[19] When octylguanidine was applied internally to the pronase-treated axons, the sodium current exhibited an apparent inactivation indicating that the octylguanidine blocked the sodium channel after it had

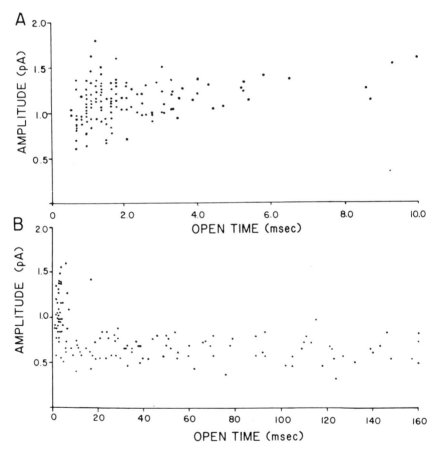

FIGURE 4. Two populations of sodium channels in the presence of 10 μM batrachotoxin (BTX). The amplitude of each sodium channel is plotted against its open time. (A) Control. (B) BTX. In BTX, sodium channels are divided into two populations, one with near normal characteristics, and the other with prolonged open times and reduced amplitudes. From Quandt and Narahashi.[14]

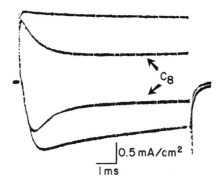

FIGURE 5. Effects of N-octylguanidine (C_8) on the sodium currents in the squid axon pretreated internally with pronase. The sodium channels are blocked by C_8 when they are open. From Kirsch et al.[19]

opened (FIG. 5). However, when the axon was pretreated with BTX resulting in removal of sodium inactivation, no effect of the subsequently applied octylguanidine was observed.[15] This suggests that BTX and octylguanidine bind to the same sodium channel site. This site is located within the sodium channel near its inner mouth.[19] Furthermore, BTX exerted its effect on the pronase-pretreated axon as evidenced by appearance of sodium currents at large negative potentials such as -70 mV. All of these observations have led to the scheme in which BTX binds to the octylguanidine site located near the inner mouth of the sodium channel and which is bound by the inactivation gate at its closed configuration.[15]

PYRETHROIDS

History, Chemistry, and Classification

Pyrethroids are the synthetic derivatives of the pyrethrins, natural toxins which are active ingredients contained in the flowers of *Chrysanthemum* species. The pyrethrum insecticides were used extensively until the end of World War II, but their uses have declined as a number of synthetic insecticides were developed after the War. Meanwhile, the environmental impact of such potent and long-lasting insecticides became a major concern, reviving interest in the pyrethrum insecticides, which are biodegradable. A large number of derivatives of pyrethrins have since been synthesized and tested for their insecticidal activities and mammalian toxicities, and some of them have been developed into very useful insecticides.

Pyrethrins and pyrethroids are esters of various alcohols and acids. Chrysanthemic acid and its analogues are common among many pyrethroids, and 3-phenoxybenzyl and 5-benzyl-3-furylmethyl groups are used in many pyrethroids. Synthetic pyrethroids may be divided into two groups: type I pyrethroids do not have a cyano group at the α position, whereas type II pyrethroids do contain an α cyano group (FIG. 6).[20] The presence of an α cyano group alters the physiological effect on the sodium channel in an interesting manner.

Resting and Action Potentials

When applied to an isolated nerve fiber such as cockroach, crayfish, and squid giant axons, the classical type I pyrethroids (*e.g.,* allethrin and tetramethrin) caused repetitive after-discharges to be induced by a single stimulus. This was due to an increase and prolongation of the depolarizing after-potential which reached the threshold membrane potential for action potential generation. The resting potential was not appreciably affected by low concentrations of pyrethroids which caused repetitive discharges. Reviews of earlier studies have been published.[21,22]

Type II pyrethroids containing an α cyano group as represented by deltamethrin, cyphenothrin, and fenvalerate depolarize the giant axon membrane without inducing repetitive discharges. The depolarization was reversed by lowering the external sodium concentration (*e.g.,* to 1mM) or by applying TTX externally.[23] Thus the sodium channels are kept open by the pyrethroids, causing a membrane depolarization.

Sodium Channel Gating Kinetics

The effects of both type I and type II pyrethroids on the resting and action potentials can be accounted for by drastic changes in the gating kinetics of sodium channels. Detailed voltage clamp analyses have been performed for the type I

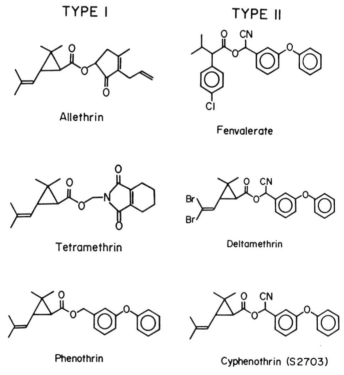

FIGURE 6. Structures of type I and type II pyrethroids. From Narahashi.[20]

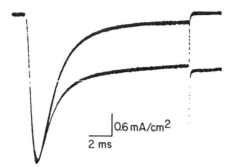

FIGURE 7. Effects of 1 μM allethrin on the sodium current of a squid axon. The record with a large steady-state current and tail current was taken after application of allethrin. From Narahashi and Lund.[28]

pyrethroids tetramethrin and allethrin, both of which have almost identical effect on the sodium channel.[24-28]

FIGURE 7 illustrates an example of a voltage clamp expereiment with a squid giant axon.[28] In order to record the sodium channel current only, the axon was perfused internally with a Cs-substituted K-free solution. Upon step depolarization, the peak transient sodium current appeared and was followed by a small steady-state sodium current. Upon step repolarizing the membrane, a very brief tail current was generated. Following internal perfusion of allethrin at a concentration of 1 μM, the steady-state sodium current was increased markedly while the peak current remained unchanged.

The tail current was also increased in amplitude and decayed very slowly. No change was found in a variety of peak current parameters after application of tetramethrin or allethrin, including the voltage dependence of the peak conductance, τ_m and τ_h.[27] The tail current associated with a step repolarization applied near the peak of sodium current decayed with a single exponential time couse in the normal axon, but exhibited a dual exponential time course after application of tetramethrin. The fast phase of tail current in tetramethrin had the same time constant and voltage dependence as those of the control axon. By contrast, the voltage dependence of the slow phase of tail current in tetramethrin was shifted in the direction of hyperpolarization by as much as 80 mV.[26] Furthermore, the time constant of the slow phase of tail current was independent of the tetramethrin concentration although the initial amplitude of the slow tail current was concentration dependent.[27] These results indicate that the peak transient current in the pyrethroid-poisoned axon represents opening of normal sodium channels, and that the large steady-state current and tail current represent opening of the pyrethroid-modified sodium channels. The concentration independent slow tail current time constant suggests an all-or-none modification of individual sodium channels.

Type II pyrethroids also modify the steady-state sodium current during a step depolarizing pulse and the tail current upon repolarization. The increases in the amplitudes of the both currents were less than that caused by type I pyrethroids. However, the time constant of tail current in type II pyrethroids was much longer than that in type I pyrethroids. For example, in crayfish giant axons the time constant of tail current in cyphenothrin, a type II pyrethroid, was estimated to be several minutes at -120 mV as against 225 ms in tetramethrin.[23]

An example of an experiment with a cyphenothrin-poisoned crayfish giant axon is shown in FIGURE 8.[23] Record A represents the control sodium current before application of cyphenothrin. Records B, C, and D, were taken at various times after internal perfusion of 1µM cyphenothrin as indicated in the chart record (E) which was taken with a higher gain but at a slower speed. It is clearly shown that although the slow tail currents were small in amplitude they accumulate as repetitive stimuli were applied even at a very low frequency. Tetrodotoxin applied toward the end of the experiment abolished the tail current, indicating that the tail currents were generated in the sodium channels. It should also be pointed out that the peak sodium current became gradually smaller with progress of time after introduction of the pyrethroid. This suggests that an increasing population of sodium channels was slowly modified by cyphenothrin. The very slow sodium current and a slight shift of the slow sodium-current–membrane potential relationship in the hyperpolarizing direction account for the observed membrane depolarization.

Rate of Channel Modification

When a depolarizing pulse is applied to a pyrethroid-poisoned axon, the modified, slow tail current develops with a characteristic time course. The time course can be measured by plotting the initial amplitudes of the slow tail currents at various moments

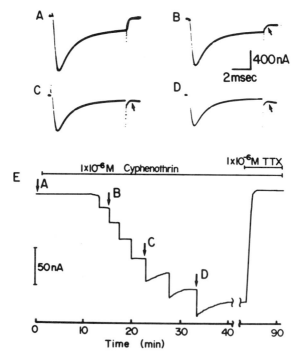

FIGURE 8. Effects of cyphenothrin on the sodium current of the crayfish giant axon. The currents were generated by an 8 ms depolarizing step to −20 mV from a holding potential of −100 mV (A) before and (**B–D**) after treatment with 1 µM cyphenothrin. The *upward arrows* in **B, C,** and **D** indicate a small increase in inward tail current. The change in holding current with time is shown in a chart record (**E**), in which each increase in inward current was elicited by the depolarizing step. The downward arrows mark the times at which records **A–D** were taken. From Lund and Narahashi.[23]

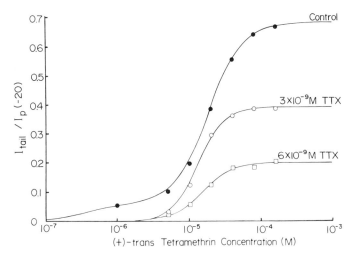

FIGURE 9. Dose-response relationships for (+)-*trans* tetramethrin before and after pretreatment with 3×10^{-9} M and 6×10^{-9} M tetrodotoxin (TTX). The slowly decaying tail current (I_{tail}) amplitude after 15 ms conditioning pulses is normalized to the peak current recorded at -20 mV, $I_p(-20)$, before application of tetramethrin. From Lund and Narahashi.[32]

during a depolarizing pulse.[27] In the tetramethrin-poisoned squid axon, the slow tail current developed with a dual exponential time course, with time constants of 1.3 ms and 24.3 ms. When the sodium channel inactivation was removed by internal perfusion of pronase or N-bromoacetamide, the slow phase disappeared. This suggests that the second phase of the time-dependent tail current growth observed in the presence of sodium inactivation results from the reopening of the unmodified sodium channels when they are changed from the inactivated state to the modified open state.

Similar experiments were performed with deltamethrin-poisoned squid axons.[29] The slow tail current developed slowly with a multiple time course, with time constants of 11 ms and 300 ms.

Stereospecificity

Because the pyrethroid molecule usually has two chiral centers, four isomers are available for each species of pyrethroid. For example, tetramethrin exists in the (+)-*trans*,(+)-*cis*, (−)-*trans* or (−)-*cis* form. Stereospecificity of the insecticidal action and mammalian toxicity has been studied extensively. The (+) isomers are usually much more potent than the (−) isomers in killing insects as well as affecting the nerve.[30,31]

Stereospecificity of pyrethroids has also been demonstrated at the sodium channel level.[32] The experiments were performed with internally perfused squid giant axons, and the initial amplitude of the slow tail current was taken as a measure of the modified open sodium channel population. When the tail current amplitute normalized to the peak sodium current amplitude is plotted against the concentration of (+)-*trans* tetramethrin, a dose-response curve can be constructed (FIG. 9). Tetrodotoxin at concentrations of 3 and 6 nM decreased the maximum amplitude of tail current without much shifting the dose-response curve, indicating a noncompetitive antagonism.

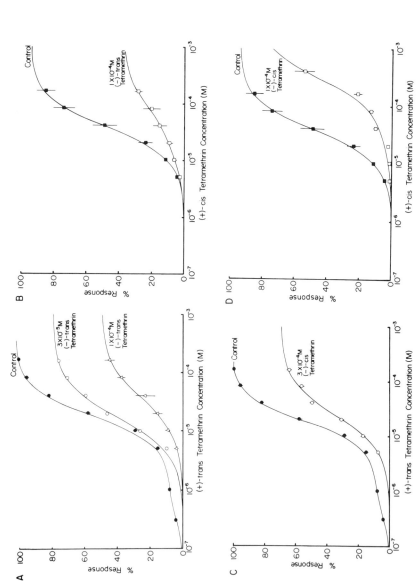

FIGURE 10. Dose-response relationships obtained as in FIGURE 9 and plotted as percent of the maximum response. **(A)** Antagonism of $(+)$-trans tetramethrin by 3×10^{-5} M and 1×10^{-4} M $(-)$-trans tetramethrin. **(B)** Antagonism of $(+)$-cis tetramethrin by 1×10^{-4} M $(-)$-trans tetramethrin. **(C)** Antagonism of $(+)$-trans tetramethrin by 3×10^{-5} M $(-)$-cis tetramethrin. **(D)** Antagonism of $(+)$-cis tetramethrin by 1×10^{-4} M $(-)$-cis tetramethrin. Values shown are mean ± SEM, $n = 3$. From Lund and Narahashi.[32]

The tail current was virtually not affected by (−)-*trans* and (−)-*cis* tetramethrin. However, when pretreated with either of these inactive isomers, the active (+)-*trans* or (+)-*cis* tetramethrin subsequently applied became less effective. As is shown in FIGURES 10A–C, noncompetitive antagonism was observed for (−)-*trans* tetramethrin against (+)-*trans* tetramethrin, (−)-*trans* against (+)-*cis,* and (−)-*cis* against (+)-*trans.* However, (−)-*cis* tetramethrin antagonized (+)-*cis,* tetramethrin in a competitive manner (FIG. 10D).

These results can be explained by a scheme illustrated in FIGURE 11 in which a *trans* site, a *cis* site, a negative allosteric site, and a TTX site are assumed to be present in the sodium channel. For example, (−)-*trans* tetramethrin binds to the negative allosteric site with a high affinity, thereby antagonizing the action of (+)-*trans* tetramethrin on the *trans* site in a noncompetitive manner. On the other hand, (−)-*cis* tetramethrin binds to the *cis* site with a high affinity, thereby antagonizing the action of (+)-*cis* tetramethrin on the same site in a competitive manner. Because of the high degree of stereospecificity, these (−) isomers can be useful tools for determining the sites of action of other channel modulators in the sodium channel.

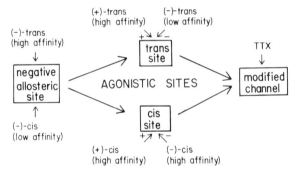

FIGURE 11. Hypothetical model for the interactions of tetramethrin with the sodium channel. See text for explanation. From Lund and Narahashi.[32]

Single Sodium Channel

Prolonged sodium current as recorded from the giant axon exposed to pyrethroids would predict that some drastic changes occur at the single channel level. Patch clamp experiments were performed with the cultured neuroblastoma cell N1E-ll5.[33] In the normal neuroblastoma cell membrane, individual sodium channels opened for about 2 ms during the early phase of a 40 ms depolarizing step (FIG. 12A). After application of tetramethrin, the sodium channels opened for a longer period of time at almost any time during a 160 ms depolarizing step (FIG. 12B). The amplitude of single sodium channel current was not affected by tetramethrin. The open times (lifetimes) of single channels followed a Poisson distribution with a time constant of 1.7 ms in the control (FIG. 12C). After application of tetramethrin, however, the open time distribution was expressed by two exponential functions, one with a time constant of 1.8 ms which is similar to that of the control and the other with a time constant of 17 ms (FIG.12D). The channels with the shorter open times represent the normal, unmodified population, whereas those with the longer open times represent the tetramethrin-modified popula-

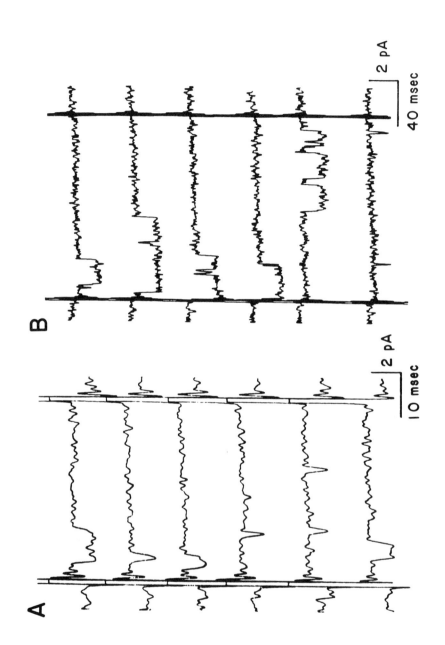

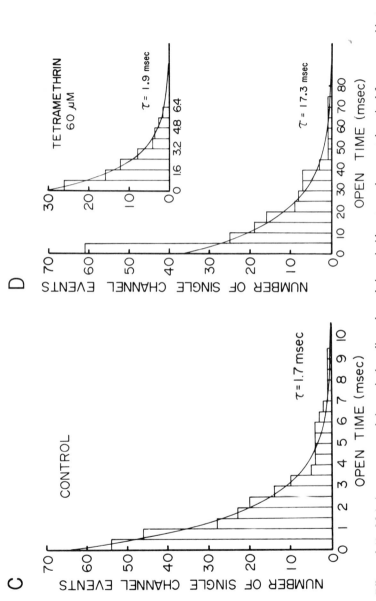

FIGURE 12. Effects of 60 μM (+)-*trans* tetramethrin on single sodium channels in an inside-out membrane patch excised from a neuroblastoma cell (N1E-ll5 line). (**A**) Sample records of sodium channel currents (inward deflections) associated with step depolarizations from −90 mV to −50 mV. (**B**) Sample records of sodium channel currents after application of tetramethrin to the *internal* surface of the membrane. (**C**) Channel open time distribution in the control. (**D**) Channel open time distribution after application of tetramethrin. *Inset* shows the distribution of short open times. From Yamamoto *et al.*[33]

tion. This suggests that the individual sodium channels are modified by tetramethrin in an all-or-none manner, the same conclusion obtained by tail current measurements as described before.

As would be expected from the result of voltage clamp experiments with axons, type II pyrethroids have been found to prolong the open time of individual sodium channels in a very drastic manner. In the presence of fenvalerate or deltamethrin, the

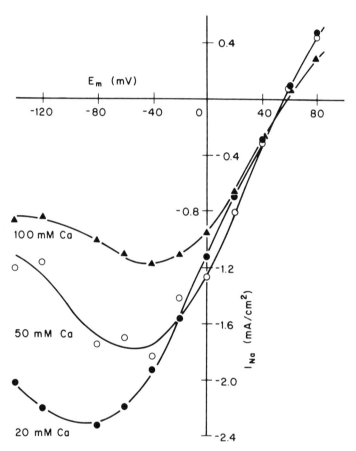

FIGURE 13. Effects of the external calcium concentration on the instantaneous sodium current (I_{Na})-membrane potential relationship in a squid giant axon. Three curves were obtained in solution containing 20 mM, 50 mM, and 100 mM Ca. From Yamamoto *et al.*[36]

individual channels were seen to remain open for a few hundred milliseconds to several seconds during and after a depolarizing step.[34,35] Such a sustained opening of a channel has made it possible to plot the current-voltage curve of a single open channel. By applying a ramp voltage pulse, single channel current could be recorded as a function of membrane potential. Type II pyrethroids are expected to become useful tools for the study of sodium channels because of their unique action in maintaining the channel at its open state for a long period of time.

Mechanism and Site of Action

From the result of experiments described in foregoing sections, it is clear that pyrethroids, both type I and type II, modify the kinetics of both the activation (m) and inactivation (h) gates. Despite such drastic changes in the gating kinetics, the modified sodium channel, once opened, exhibits normal characteristics.

The normal sodium channels of both squid axons and neuroblastoma cells were blocked at their open state by divalent cations such as calcium and magnesium and by permeant monovalent cations such as sodium, lithium, and guanidine.[36] The block was voltage dependent and was shown by rectification of the current-voltage curve at large negative membrane potentials. FIGURE 13 illustrates the current-voltage curves of a squid axon in the presence of various concentrations of calcium. As the calcium concentration was increased from 20 mM to 100 mM, rectification became more pronounced, indicating that calcium blocked the open sodium channels at potentials more negative than -40 mV. The cation block was also observed in the tetramethrin-modified open sodium channels of squid axons.[37]

The open sodium channel of the squid axon shows a certain degree of cation selectivity. The channel is highly permeable to sodium and lithium, less permeable to guanidine, formamidine, and ammonium, and negligibly permeable to cesium, methylguanidine, and methylamine.[13] The permeability (P) ratios remained unchanged after exposure to tetramethrin. The ratios $P_{Na}:P_{Li}:P_{ammonium}:P_{guanidine}:P_{formamidine}$ were 1:1.19:0.21:0.28:0.20 before application of tetramethrin and 1:1.18:0.29:0.29:0.25 after application.[37]

The above two observations indicate that the energy profile in the sodium channel is not modified by tetramethrin. Unlike BTX, tetramethrin may not occupy a site within the sodium channel. Since tetramethrin is highly hydrophobic, the molecule will be able to reach anywhere in the lipid phase of the membrane. It is likely that the tetramethrin molecule is dissolved in the lipid phase of the membrane and reaches the gating machinery that controls both the activation and inactivation mechanisms. In support of this hypothesis, octylguanidine and pyrethroids did not interact with each other in the sodium channel (unpublished observation).

SUMMARY

A variety of toxins and chemicals has been shown to modulate the gating kinetics of the sodium channel. Studies of batrachotoxin, grayanotoxins and pyrethroids are summarized here as examples. Batrachotoxin and grayanotoxins eliminate the sodium channel inactivation thereby causing a prolonged, steady-state sodium current to flow during a depolarizing step. The sodium channel activation kinetics are not affected markedly. Batrachotoxin appears to bind to a site in the sodium channel to which the inactivation gate normally binds, thus causing an inhibition of sodium inactivation. Single channel recording experiments have shown that the mean open time of individual sodium channels is greatly prolonged by batrachotoxin. It appears that individual sodium channels are modified by batrachotoxin in an all-or-none manner.

Pyrethroids which are synthetic derivatives of pyrethrins also modify the kinetics of sodium channels in a very drastic manner. In the presence of type I pyrethroids which lack a cyano group at the α position (*e.g.,*allethrin and tetramethrin), a large steady-state sodium current appears during a step depolarization and a large slowly decaying sodium tail current appears upon repolarization. Thus both the activation and inactivation kinetics are slowed. Type II pyrethroids which contain an α-cyano group (*e.g.,* deltamethrin, cyphenothrin, and fenvalerate) exert effects on sodium channels qualitatively similar to those of type I pyrethroids. However, the amplitudes of the steady-state sodium current and sodium tail current are smaller and the time constant of tail current decay is much longer. The mean open time of single sodium channels is greatly prolonged by the pyrethroids, and the effect is much more pronounced in type II than in type I pyrethroids. A high degree of stereospecificity has been found among four isomers of tetramethrin, (+)-*trans* and (+)-*cis* isomers being highly active and (–)-*trans* and (–)-*cis* isomers almost totally inactive. The inactive isomers bind to the sodium channel sites, thus preventing the action of the active isomers. Because of the unique action of pyrethroids in modulating the sodium channels, they are becoming useful tools for channel physiology and pharmacology.

ACKNOWLEDGMENT

I would like to thank Regina Kareiva for secretarial assistance.

REFERENCES

1. NARAHASHI, T., J. W. MOORE & W. R. SCOTT. 1964. Tetrodotoxin blockage of sodium conductance increase in lobster giant axons. J. Gen Physiol. **47:** 965–974.
2. NARAHASHI, T. 1974. Chemicals as tools in the study of excitable membranes. Physiol. Rev. **54:** 813–889.
3. ALBUQUERQUE, E. X., J. DALY & B. WITKOP. 1971. Batrachotoxin: Chemistry and pharmacology. Science **172:** 995–1002.
4. NARAHASHI, T., E. X. ALBUQUERQUE & T. DEGUCHI. 1971. Effects of batrachotoxin on membrane potential and conductance of squid giant axons. J. Gen. Physiol. **58:** 54–70.
5. ALBUQUERQUE E. X., I. SEYAMA & T. NARAHASHI. 1973. Characterization of batrachotox-in-induced depolarization of the squid giant axons. J. Pharmacol. Exp. Ther. **184:** 308–314.
6. SEYAMA, I. & T. NARAHASHI. 1973. Increase in sodium permeability of squid axon membranes by α-dihydrograyanotoxin II. J. Pharmacol. Exp. Ther. **184:** 299–307.
7. NARAHASHI, T. & I. SEYAMA. 1974. Mechanism of nerve membrane depolarization caused by grayanotoxin I. J. Physiol. **242:** 471–487.
8. HIRONAKA, T. & T. NARAHASHI. 1977. Cation permeability ratios of sodium channels in normal and grayanotoxin-treated squid axon membranes. J. Membr. Biol. **31:** 359–381.
9. KHODOROV, B. I. 1978. Chemicals as tools to study nerve fiber sodium channels; effects of batrachotoxin and some local anesthetics. *In* Membrane Transport Processes, vol. 2. D. C. Tosteson, A. O. Yu & R. Latorre, Eds. 153–174. Raven Press. New York.
10. KHODOROV, B. I. & S. V. REVENKO 1979. Further analysis of the mechanisms of action of batrachotoxin on the membrane of myelinated nerve. Neuroscience **4:** 1315–1330.
11. KHODOROV, B. I., E. M. PEGANOV, S. V. REVENKO & L. D. SHISHKOVA. 1975. Sodium currents in voltage clamped nerve fiber of frog under the combined action of batracho-toxin and procaine. Brain Res. **84:** 541–546.
12. KHODOROV, B. I. 1985. Batrachotoxin as a tool to study voltage-sensitive sodium channels of excitable membranes. Prog. Biophys. Mol. Biol. **45:** 57–148.
13. SEYAMA, I. & T. NARAHASHI. 1981. Modification of sodium channels of squid nerve membranes by grayanotoxin I. J. Pharmacol. Exp. Ther. **219:** 614–624.

14. QUANDT, F. N. & T. NARAHASHI. 1982. Modification of single Na⁺ channels by batrachotoxin. Proc. Natl. Acad. Sci. **79:** 6732–6736.
15. TANGUY, J., J. Z. YEH & T. NARASHASHI. 1984. Interaction of batrachotoxin with sodium channels in squid axons. Biophys. J. **45:** 184a.
16. TANGUY, J., J.Z. YEH & T. NARAHASHI. 1985. Gating charge movement and Na current kinetics of batrachotoxin-modified Na channels. Biophys. J. **47:** 437a
17. ARMSTRONG, C. M., F. BEZANILLA & E. ROJAS. 1973. Destruction of sodium conductance in squid axons perfused with pronase. J. Gen. Physiol. **62:** 375–391.
18. ROJAS, E. & B. RUDY. 1976. Destruction of the sodium conductance inactivation by a specific protease in perfused nerve fibres from *Loligo*. J. Physiol. **262:** 501–531.
19. KIRSCH, G. E., J. Z. YEH, J. M. FARLEY & T. NARAHASHI. 1980. Interaction of *n*-alkylguanidines with the sodium channels of squid axon membrane. J. Gen. Physiol. **76:** 315–335.
20. NARAHASHI, T. 1985. Nerve membrane ionic channels as the primary target of pyrethroids. Neurotoxicology **6:** 3–22.
21. NARAHASHI, T. 1971. Efects of insecticides on excitable tissues. *In* Advances in Insect Physiology, Vol. 8. J. W. L. Beament, J. E. Treherne & V. B. Wigglesworth, Eds.: 1–93, Academic Press. London and New York.
22. NARAHASHI, T. 1976. Effects of insecticides on nervous conduction and synaptic transmission. *In* Insecticide Biochemistry and Physiology. C. F. Wilkinson, Ed.: 327–352. Plenum. New York.
23. LUND, A. E. & T. NARAHASHI. 1983. Kinetics of sodium channel modification as the basis for the variation in the nerve membrane effects of pyrethroids and DDT analogs. Pestic. Biochem. Physiol. **20:** 203–216.
24. NARAHASHI, T. & N. C. ANDERSON. 1967. Mechanism of excitation block by the insecticide allethrin applied externally and internally to squid giant axons. Toxicol. Appl. Pharmacol. **10:** 529–547.
25. WANG, C. M., T. NARAHASHI & M. SCUKA. 1972. Mechanism of negative temperature coefficient of nerve blocking action of allethrin. J. Pharmacol. Exp. Ther. **182:** 442–453.
26. LUND, A. E. & T. NARAHASHI. 1981. Modification of sodium channel kinetics by the insecticide tetramethrin in crayfish giant axons. Neurotoxicology **2:** 213–229.
27. LUND, A. E. & T. NARAHASHI. 1981. Kinetics of sodium channel modification by the insecticide tetramethrin in squid axon membranes. J. Pharmacol. Exp. Ther. **219:** 464–473.
28. NARAHASHI, T. & A. E. LUND 1980. Giant axons as models for the study of the mechanism of action of insecticides. *In* Insect Neurobiology and Pesticide Action (Neurotox 79). Soc. Chem. Industry. London. pp. 497–505.
29. DE WEILLE, J. R., L. D. BROWN, H. P. M. VIJVERBERG & T. NARAHASHI. 1986. Kinetics of deltamethrin modification of squid axon sodium channels. Fed. Proc. **45**(3): 513.
30. NARAHASHI, T., K. NISHIMURA, J. L. PARMENTIER, K. TAKENO & M. ELLIOTT. 1977. Neurophysiological study of the structure-activity relation of pyrethroids. Synthetic pyrethroids. Am. Chem. Soc. Symp. Ser., no. 42. M. Elliott, Ed.: 85–97.
31. NISHIMURA, K. & T. NARAHASHI. 1978. Structure-activity relationships of pyrethroids based on direct action on nerve. Pestic. Biochem. Physiol. **8:** 53–64.
32. LUND, A. E. & T. NARAHASHI. 1982. Dose-dependent interaction of the pyrethroid isomers with sodium channels of squid axon membranes. Neurotoxicology **3:** 11–24.
33. YAMAMOTO, E., F. N. QUANDT & T. NARAHASHI. 1983. Modification of single sodium channels by the insecticide tetramethrin. Brain Res. **274:** 344–349.
34. HOLLOWAY, S. F., V. L. SALGADO, C. H. WU & T. NARAHASHI. 1984. Maintained opening of single Na channels by fenvalerate. Fourteenth Annual Meeting of Society for Neuroscience. **10:** 864. Abstract.
35. CHINN, K. & T. NARAHASHI. 1986. Stabilization of sodium channel states by deltamethrin in mouse neuroblastoma cells. J. Physiol. In press.
36. YAMAMOTO, D., J. Z. YEH & T. NARAHASHI. 1985. Interactions of permeant cations with sodium channels of squid axon membranes. Biophys. J. **48:** 361–368.
37. YAMAMOTO, D. & T. NARAHASHI. 1986. Ion permeation and selectivity of squid axon sodium channels modified by tetramethrin. Brain Res. **372:** 193–197.

Single-Channel Studies of TTX-Sensitive and TTX-Resistant Sodium Channels in Developing Rat Muscle Reveal Different Open Channel Properties[a]

RICHARD E. WEISS AND RICHARD HORN

Department of Physiology
University of California at Los Angeles
Los Angeles, California 90024

INTRODUCTION AND METHODS

Tetrodotoxin (TTX) and saxitoxin (STX) are specific blockers that bind with high affinity to sodium (Na) channels of adult nerve and muscle. The action of these toxins has been used both to identify Na channels and to study the molecular nature of the channel protein. We have used TTX to distinguish two different classes of Na channels in primary cultures of rat myoblasts and myotubes. The two classes of channels have been described previously to be about 100 to 1000 times different in their sensitivity to TTX[1-6] and are called TTX-sensitive and TTX-resistant Na channels. The equilibrium dissociation constant (K_d) for TTX-sensitive channels is between one and ten nanomolar at 4°C. Our single channel measurements show that these Na channels also have different open channel properties. Tetrodotoxin binding to TTX-sensitive Na channels has been studied intensely and it has been proposed that a carboxyl oxygen is a principal component of the TTX binding site.[7-15] The effects of chemical modification of TTX-sensitive Na channels by trimethyloxonium (TMO) support this hypothesis and also suggest that the carboxyl oxygen affects the local accumulation of cations, which affects in turn the open channel conductance and block of the channels by Ca^{2+}.[16,17] We find that there is similarity between the open channel properties of TTX-resistant Na channels and the reported properties of TMO-treated Na channels. The possibility is discussed that some of the altered open-channel properties that occur after O-methylation exist naturally in TTX-resistant Na channels.

The coexistence of the two types of Na channels with different TTX and STX binding affinities has been studied in rat primary myotubes using radioisotope binding, flux assays, and macroscopic current recordings,[5,6,18-22] and in denervated muscle of adult rat using macroscopic current recordings.[4] More recently it has been reported that only a single class of functional Na channels with an intermediate TTX affinity exists in rat myoblasts and myotubes.[19] We have performed whole cell and single channel measurements from both myoblasts and myotubes to identify individual TTX-sensitive and TTX-resistant channels and found differences in the open channel and kinetic properties (see also ref. 23).

Experimental methods were similar to those previously described.[24] Primary

[a]This work was supported by NIH grants NS 00703 and NS 18608, NSF grant BNS84-11033, and an NIH postdoctoral training grant to REW.

152

cultures of rat myoblasts and myotubes were prepared from thigh muscle of neonatal rats.[25] Growth medium consisted of Dulbecco's medium enriched with 10% horse serum, 1% chick embryo extract, 1% glutamine, 6 g/1 glucose, 100 U/1 penicillin and 100 μg/ml streptomycin. Cells were preplated onto plastic flasks for 45 min on the day after dissection to remove fibroblasts. The myoblasts were then plated onto collagen-coated glass coverslips. Cytosine arabinoside was added to the cultures on day 4 to further inhibit fibroblasts. Myoblasts were discriminated from fibroblasts in experiments by their bipolar shapes. Single channel measurements were made on outside-out patches using a List EPC-7 patch clamp (Medical Instruments, Great Neck, N.Y.) which was interfaced with a VAX-11/730 computer (Digital Equipment Corp., Marlboro, Ma.). Pipettes were made from Corning 8161 glass, coated with Sylgard (Dow-Corning, Midland, Mich.) and filled with a solution containing 140 mM CsF, 10 mM NaCl, 5 mM EGTA, and 10 mM Hepes at pH 7.2. The bath solution contained 160 mM NaCl, 2 mM $CaCl_2$, 1 mM $MgCl_2$, 10 mM Hepes, and 5 mM glucose at pH 7.3. When [Ca] was varied, Ca acetate was used. Experiments were performed at $9.5° \pm 0.3°C$. Tetrodotoxin was premixed in vials and added to the bath in small, concentrated aliquots.

TTX SENSITIVITY OF MYOBLASTS AND MYOTUBES

FIGURE 1A shows macroscopic Na currents from a myoblast before and after TTX was added to the bath. A small dose (11.6 nM, trace 2) of TTX decreased peak Na current to 61% of the control level (trace 1). A 100-fold greater TTX concentration (1.05 μM, trace 3) reduced peak Na current to only 43% of the control level. If the Na channels in this cell had a single affinity for TTX, the response to the small dose would indicate that the K_d is in the range of 18 nM. However, the response to the 1.05 μM TTX indicates a K_d of 0.8 μM. Therefore, it may be concluded that the Na channels in this cell were not a homogeneous population with respect to TTX binding affinity and that channels with at least two different affinities were present. In the experiment shown in FIGURE 1A, Na currents were blocked completely and reversibly in 15 μM $[TTX]_o$ (trace 4). Our whole cell voltage clamp experiments showed myoblasts could exist with (1) no excitable Na currents, (2) Na currents that required micromolar concentrations of TTX to be blocked, or (3) Na currents of which a large fraction could be blocked by nanomolar concentrations of TTX.

Macroscopic currents from myotubes were obtained by averaging single channel records from excised outside-out patches. FIGURE 1B shows that the sensitivity of the Na current to TTX is much greater than in the myoblast in FIGURE 1A. The dose of TTX, 156 nM, decreased peak Na current to less than 5% of the control level, which calculates to a K_d of less than 10 nM. This estimate of the K_d may reflect the true affinity of the TTX-sensitive channel for TTX, because there appeared to be very few TTX-resistant channels in this patch according to the analysis of single channels described below.

In general, myoblasts rarely showed measurable Na current less than 2 days after preplating. Currents began to appear at 2 days and the proportion of cells with measurable Na current progressively increased up to 5 days, the oldest myoblasts studied (data not shown). In patch experiments on myotubes, TTX-sensitive Na current usually predominated, and also seemed to increase in absolute density as the myotubes aged. Although measurement of Na current from individual cells, and in particular from membrane patches, is not the optimal method by which to study the TTX sensitivity of a large population of cells, our results are consistent with the coexistence of two classes of functional Na channels with different affinities for TTX.

Open-channel properties of Na channels were studied by single-channel current measurements from excised patches. FIGURE 2A shows that, in an outside-out patch from a myotube, not all channels had the same current amplitudes at a given transmembrane voltage. There appeared to be two classes of channels, distinguished by different open-channel current amplitudes. Small-current events are indicated by arrows. For transmembrane voltages of −40 mV (inside negative), small- and large-current events appeared to have amplitudes of about 1.0 and 1.4 pA, respectively. FIGURE 2B shows current records from a myoblast outside-out patch. Both sizes of channels were also seen. When TTX was added to the bath (final concentration: 156 nM), however, the large-current events disappeared, and only the small-current events remained (lower half of FIGURE 2A). Increasing $[TTX]_o$ above about 5μM blocked all events (single channel data not shown, but see FIGURE 1A), indicating that small-

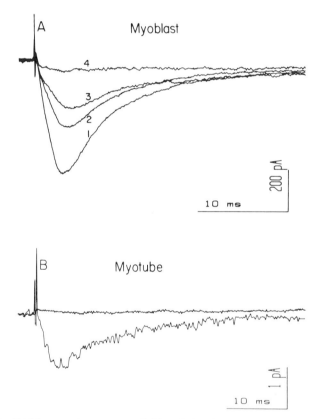

FIGURE 1. (A) Macroscopic traces recorded by whole cell voltage clamp from a myoblast in TTX-free conditions (trace 1) and in the presence of 11.6 nM (trace 2), 1.04 μM (trace 3), and 15.6 μM (trace 4) TTX. The effect of TTX was reversible. The conditions were as follows: holding voltage, −90 mV; prepulse, −110 mV (100 ms); test voltage, −20 mV; temperature, 9.6°C; filter, 8 kHz. Experiment: TTX030. (B) Average currents from an outside-out myotube patch in the absence and presence of 156 nM TTX. Conditions were as follows: holding voltage, −100 mV; prepulse, −120 mV (100 ms); test voltage, −40 mV; temperature, 9.7°C; filter, 2.0 kHz. Experiment: TTX033.

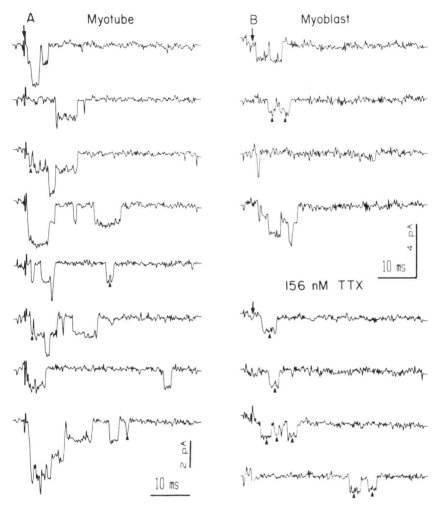

FIGURE 2. Single-channel currents from outside-out patches recorded at a test voltage of -40 mV, filtered at 2.0 kHz. The temperature was 9.5° C. (**A**) Records from a myotube patch in TTX-free solution. *Upward-pointing arrowheads* mark small-current channel openings. The *downward-pointing arrows* show the beginning of the test pulse. The holding voltage was -100 mV and the prepulse -120 mV for 100 ms. Experiment: TTX033. (**B**) Records obtained from a myoblast patch in the absence and presence of TTX. *Arrows* and *arrowheads* are used as in FIGURE 2A. TTX (156 nM) abolishes large-current events. The holding voltage was -90 mV, the prepulse -110 mV for 100 ms, and the temperature 9.5°C. Experiment: TTX035.

current events also represent Na channels. These effects of TTX were seen consistently and led us to conclude that in developing muscle, the Na channels with larger open channel currents were also TTX-sensitive channels. There are other reports of large- and small-current Na channels in the literature,[26-29] but differences in the TTX sensitivity of these channels has not been previously described.

The question arises whether there are really two distinct populations of channels, or perhaps just one population of channels with a continuum of open-channel current amplitudes (within a bounded range). To distinguish between these possibilities, amplitude distributions were calculated from the single-channel records. Typical examples are shown in FIGURES 3A and 3B for data obtained respectively from a myotube and a myoblast at a test voltage of -40 mV. In FIGURE 3A (upper panel) there are two peaks with about 0.4 pA separating them. The positions of the two peaks in the distributions were remarkably similar in all of our experiments. At -40 mV the large peak was always about 1.4 pA and the small peak about 1.0 pA. There were very few events in the 1.1–1.3 pA range, indicating that two populations of Na channels can account for the distribution. In a few experiments where the distribution showed only one peak (e.g., see FIG. 3B), the peak was centered either at 1.0 or 1.4 pA (at -40 mV) and was shaped similarly to the corresponding peak in a bimodal distribution.

If the two peaks in FIGURE 3A (upper panel) represent independent populations of Na channels, we might expect that the amplitude distributions would be best approximated by a linear combination of Gaussian curves. The smooth curve in FIGURE 3A (upper) is the weighted sum of two Gaussian distributions. The 5 parameters for the double Gaussian (2 means, 2 standard deviations, and a weighting factor) were obtained by maximum likelihood estimation from the current amplitudes of the individual events. The means are labeled μ_S and μ_L, the standard deviations σ_S and σ_L, and the weighting factor, w_L, where the subscripts S and L denote respectively small and large conductance events. In all records where individual amplitudes were measured to be both greater than 1.2 pA and less than 1.1 pA at -40 mV, the amplitude distributions were better approximated by the sum of two rather than one Gaussian(s). In a few experiments where the amplitude distributions had single peaks, a double Gaussian distribution did not improve the fit significantly, as indicated by a likelihood ratio test. FIGURE 3B (upper panel) is an example of an experiment in which there was only a single appearance of a large-current channel. The Gaussian curve that is shown was obtained by maximum likelihood estimation of a single Gaussian (the large event was omitted). The standard deviation of the single Gaussian distribution is comparable to σ_S in FIGURE 3A, suggesting that large- and small-current channels are distinct populations.

The lower panels of FIGURE 3 show the effects of 156 nM TTX on the distributions of single channel amplitudes. In FIGURE 3A, the large-current events disappeared when TTX was added to the bath. The mean and standard deviations of the single Gaussian distribution are very similar to those of the small-current channel part of the two-peaked distribution seen in the upper panel. Similarly, the lower panel of FIGURE 3B shows that when a single Gaussian distribution represents the small-current events, TTX does not change the essential features of the distribution. TTX also has no effect on the mean or standard deviation of the large-current channels. The results shown above suggest that TTX-resistant single channels pass less current than TTX-sensitive channels but that TTX does not affect the open channel properties of either class of Na channels.

EFFECTS OF VARYING EXTERNAL [Ca²⁺]

In addition to the correlation of the open channel current amplitudes with the TTX affinity, we have also begun to investigate the effects of external Ca^{2+} on both types of channel. The current through Na channels is known to be reduced by increasing $[Ca^{2+}]_0$, and this is thought to occur by a very rapid block-unblock reaction[17,30,31]; Ca^{2+} is also known to interfere with the binding of TTX and STX to (TTX-sensitive) Na channels. Previous studies on Na channels from nerve and muscle and on chemically

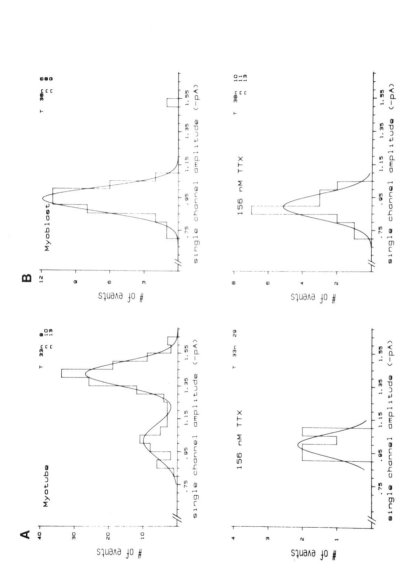

FIGURE 3. Amplitude distributions of single-channel currents from outside-out patches at a test voltage of −40 mV. The holding voltage was −100 mV, the prepulse −120 mV for 100 ms, and the temperature 9.6°C. The smooth curves are Gaussian distributions fit to the data (see text). (**A**) Distributions from a myotube outside-out patch in the absence (*upper panel*) and presence (*lower panel*) of 156 nM TTX. This dose blocks all large-current events. Experiment: TTX033. (**B**) Distributions from a myoblast membrane patch. TTX (156 nM) does not significantly affect the distribution of the small-current events. Experiment: TTX038.

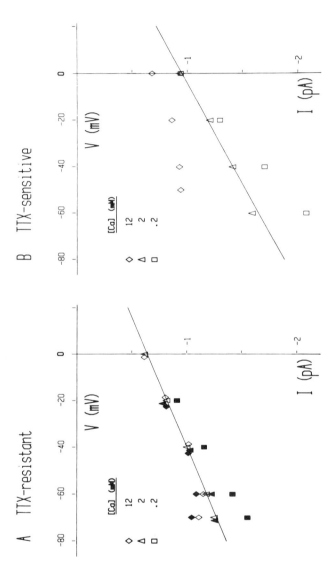

FIGURE 4. The effect of external Ca^{2+} (0.2–12 mM) on the single-channel currents of TTX-resistant and TTX-sensitive Na channels. Each current value plotted is the average of all single-channel currents measured in an experiment under the same conditions. SEMs are all smaller than the symbols. Graph points are offset laterally where they would otherwise be obscured due to overlap. The straight lines are linear regressions through the 2.0 mM Ca^{2+} points. Experimental conditions were as follows: holding voltage, -110 mV; prepulse, -130 mV (100 ms); temperature, 9.3°C. (**A**) TTX-resistant channels. The linear regression gives a slope of 9.0 pS. Filled and open symbols represent different experiments. (**B**) TTX-sensitive channels. The linear regression gives a slope of 11.7 pS.

modified Na channels have suggested that an anionic group near the mouth of the channel is required for high-affinity TTX binding.[7-17] These studies suggest that the anionic group includes a carboxyl oxygen. O-methylation of this group by trimethylox-onium (TMO) causes loss of normal TTX sensitivity, reduction of the single channel conductance, and reduction of Ca^{2+} block of Na channels. Both Ca^{2+} and the toxins protect channels against TMO modification.[17] Since TTX-resistant and TMO-treated channels both have reduced current amplitudes, we also wanted to investigate the effects of external Ca^{2+} on TTX-resistant and TTX-sensitive channels.

The Ca^{2+} sensitivity of the single channel conductance of both TTX-resistant and TTX-sensitive Na channels is shown respectively in FIGURES 4A and 4B. FIGURE 4A shows data from two experiments from myoblast membrane patches in which more than 99% of the channel openings were small-current events. FIGURE 4B was obtained from one experiment on a myotube membrane patch in which large-current events accounted for more than 95% of the channel openings. The linear regression line through the filled circles represents average single channel amplitudes obtained with a standard (2mM) concentration of external Ca^{2+}. The slope conductance of the TTX-resistant channels is $\gamma_s = 9.0$ pS in 2 mM Ca^{2+} (FIG. 4A). Under the same conditions, the slope conductance of TTX-sensitive Na channels is greater ($\gamma_s = 11.7$ pS, (FIG. 4B). This result is comparable with those obtained from 13 other experiments where the linear regression of all data points gave $\gamma_s = 9.8$ pS ± 0.6 pS (95% confidence level) for TTX-resistant channels and $\gamma_s = 12.1$ pS ± 1.3 pS for TTX-sensitive channels (see also FIG. 3 in ref. 23).

The effect of changing external Ca^{2+} on the TTX-sensitive channel is shown in FIGURE 4B. With 0.2 or 2.0 mM external Ca^{2+} the current-voltage (I–V) relationships are reasonably straight lines, with a somewhat greater conductance at the lower Ca^{2+} concentration. In 12 mM external Ca^{2+}, the single channel currents become markedly smaller and the I–V relationship becomes nonlinear. The reduction of the current is expected of a blocker that rapidly binds and dissociates from the channel, thus reducing the apparent conductance of an open channel. The curvature in 12 mM external Ca^{2+} suggests that Ca^{2+} blocks at a site within the electrical field of the membrane.[30,31] By comparison, the TTX-resistant channel I–V relationships (FIG. 4A) show much smaller dependence on external Ca^{2+}. At 12.0 mM Ca^{2+}, only the values at -60 mV and below deviate from the values for 2.0 mM Ca^{2+}. With lower Ca^{2+} concentrations (0.2 mM), a small but consistent increase in the single channel currents occurs at all voltages.

Our results indicate that the open channel properties of naturally occurring TTX-resistant Na channels show a close resemblance to those of TMO-modified Na channels. The similarities between TMO-modified and TTX-resistant channels suggest that a carboxyl oxygen which is O-methylated by TMO in TTX-sensitive channels is either not present or is in some way neutralized or shielded in TTX-resistant channels. The electrical presence of the carboxyl oxygen may be required for high affinity TTX binding. Although experimental conditions were not identical, it does appear that TMO-treated channels are less affected by low Ca^{2+} concentrations. This may be an indication that the carboxyl oxygen is not as essential for cation accumulation near the mouth of the channel as it is for TTX binding. It could also be that there exist other important differences between TTX-resistant and TTX-sensitive channels.

REFERENCES

1. HARRIS, J. B. & S. THESLEFF. 1971. Studies on tetrodotoxin resistant action potentials in denervated skeletal muscle. Acta Physiol. Scand. **83:** 382–388.

2. REDFERN, P. & S. THESLEFF. 1971. Action potential generation in denervated rat skeletal muscle. II. The action of tetrodotoxin. Acta Physiol. Scand. **82:** 70–78.
3. HARRIS, J. B. & M. W. MARSHALL. 1973. Tetrodotoxin-resistant action potentials in newborn rat muscle. Nature New Biol. **243:** 191–192.
4. PAPPONE, P. 1980. Voltage-clamp experiments in normal and denervated mammalian skeletal muscle fibres. J. Physiol. **306:** 377–410.
5. LAWRENCE, J. C. & W. A. CATTERAL. 1981. Tetrodotoxin-insensitive sodium channels. Binding of polypeptide neurotoxins in primary cultures of rat muscle cells. J. Biol. Chem. **256:** 6223–6229.
6. LAWRENCE, J. C. & W. A. CATTERALL. 1981. Tetrodotoxin-insensitive sodium channels. Ion flux studies of neurotoxin action in a clonal rat muscle cell line. J. Biol. Chem **256:** 6213–6222.
7. KAO, C. Y. & A. NISHIYAMA. 1965. Actions of saxitoxin on peripheral neuromuscular systems. J. Physiol. **180:** 50–66.
8. HILLE, B. 1968. Pharmacological modifications of the sodium channel of frog nerve. J. Gen. Physiol. **51:** 199–219.
9. SHRAGER, P.-C. PROFERA. 1973. Inhibition of the receptor for tetrodotoxin in nerve membranes by reagents modifying carboxyl groups. Biochim. Biophys. Acta **318:** 141–146.
10. HENDERSON, R., J. M. RITCHIE & G. R. STRICHARTZ. 1974. Evidence that tetrodotoxin and saxitoxin act at a metal cation binding site in the sodium channels of nerve membrane. Proc. Natl. Acad. Sci. **71:** 3936–3940.
11. BAKER, P. F. & K. A. RUBINSON. 1975. Chemical modification of crab nerves can make them insensitive to the local anesthetics tetrodotoxin and saxitoxin. Nature **257:** 412–414.
12. HILLE, B. 1975. The receptor for tetrodotoxin and saxitoxin: A structural hypothesis. Biophys. J. **15:** 615–619.
13. SPALDING, B. C. 1980. Properties of toxin-resistant sodium channels produced by chemical modification in frog skeletal muscle. J. Physiol. **305:** 485–500.
14. KAO, P. N., M. R. JAMES-KRACKE & C. Y. KAO. 1983. The active guanidinium group of saxitoxin and neosaxitoxin identified by the effects of pH on their activities on squid axon. Pfluegers Arch. Eur. J. Physiol. **398:** 199–203.
15. STRICHARTZ, G. 1984. Structural determinants of the affinity of saxitoxin for neuronal sodium channels. Electrophysiological studies on frog peropheral nerve. J. Gen. Physiol. **84:** 281–305.
16. SIGWORTH, F. J. & B. C. SPALDING. 1980. Chemical modification reduces the conductance of sodium channels in nerve. Nature **283:** 293–295.
17. WORLEY, J. F., III, R. J. FRENCH & B. K. KRUEGER. 1986. Trimethyloxonium modification of single batrachotoxin-activated sodium channels in planar bilayers: Changes in unit conductance and in block by saxitoxin and calcium. J. Gen. Physiol. **87:** 327–329.
18. FRELIN, C., P. VIGNE, H. SCHWEITZ & M. LAZDUNSKI. 1984. The interaction of sea anemone and scorpion neurotoxins with tetrodotoxin-resistant Na$^+$ channels in rat myoblasts. Mol. Pharmacol. **26:** 70–74.
19. FRELIN, C., H. P. M. VIJVERBERG, G. ROMEY, P. VIGNE & M. LAZDUNSKI. 1984. Different functional states of tetrodotoxin sensitive and tetrodotoxin resistant Na$^+$ channels occur during in *in vitro* development of rat skeletal muscle. Pfluegers Arch. **402:** 121–128.
20. SHERMAN, S. J., J. C. LAWRENCE, D. J. MESSNER, K. JACOBY & W. A. CATTERALL. 1983. Tetrodotoxin-sensitive sodium channels in rat muscle cells developing *in vitro*. J. Biol. Chem. **258:** 2488–2495.
21. GONOI, T., S. J. SHERMAN & W. A. CATTERAL. 1985. Voltage clamp analysis of tetrodotoxin-sensitive and -insensitive sodium channels in rat muscle cells developing *in vitro*. J. Neurosci. **5:** 2559–2564.
22. HAIMOVICH, B., J. C. TANAKA & R. BARCHI. 1986. Developmental appearance of functional sodium channel subtypes in rat skeletal muscle cultures. J. Neurochem. In press.
23. WEISS, R. E. & R. HORN. 1986. Functional differences between two classes of sodium

channels in developing myoblasts and myotubes in rat skeletal muscle. Science **233:** 361–364.

24. HORN, R. & C. A. VANDENBERG. 1984. Statistical properties of single sodium channels. J. Gen. Physiol. **84:** 505–534.

25. HORN, R. & M. S. BRODWICK, 1980. Acetylcholine-induced current in perfused rat myoballs. J. Gen. Physiol. **75:** 297–321.

26. CACHELIN, A. B., J. E. DEPEYER, S. KOKUBUN & H. REUTER. 1983. Sodium channels in cultured cardiac cells. J. Physiol. **340:** 389–401.

27. NAGY, K., T. KISS & D. HOFF. 1983. Single Na channels in mouse neuroblastoma cell membrane: Indications for two open states. Pfluegers Arch. Eur. J. Physiol. **399:** 302–308.

28. DECINO, P. & Y. KIDOKORO. 1985. Development and subsequent neural tube effects on the excitability of cultured xenopus myocytes. J. Neurosci. **5:** 1471–1482.

29. KUNZE, D. L., A. E. LACERDA, D. L. WILSON & A. M. BROWN. 1985. Cardiac Na currents and the inactivating, reopening, and waiting properties of single cardiac Na channels. J. Gen. Physiol. **86:** 691–719.

30. WOODHULL, A. M. 1973. Ionic blockage of sodium channels in nerve. J. Gen. Physiol. **61:** 687–708.

31. YAMAMOTO, D., J. Z. YEH, & T. NARAHASHI. 1984. Voltage-dependent calcium block of normal and tetramethrin-modified single sodium channels. Biophys. J. **45:** 337–344.

PART III. BIOCHEMICAL CHARACTERIZATION OF ISOLATED CHANNELS

The Sodium Channel from *Electrophorus electricus*[a]

S. R. LEVINSON,[b] D. S. DUCH,[b] B. W. URBAN,[c]
AND E. RECIO-PINTO[c]

[b]*Department of Physiology*
University of Colorado Medical School
Denver, Colorado 80262

[c]*Departments of Anesthesiology and Physiology*
Cornell University Medical College
New York, New York 10021

INTRODUCTION

The purification of the sodium channel from excitable tissues has been a crucial step toward the elucidation of channel mechanism and molecular biology. In turn, this advance required the development of assays for channels during their fractionation from disrupted and solubilized membranes (which obviously could not be based on their normal physiological role as voltage-gated mediators of ion transport into intact cells). Fortunately, such precise and sensitive assays have been achieved through the channel-specific, high affinity binding of tetrodotoxin (TTX) and saxitoxin.[1,2] In addition, when bound to the channel these toxins prevent their own binding site from denaturing during the lengthy purification procedures employed, allowing a high proportion of channel protein to be purified which retains the ability to bind toxin.[3] Thus both TTX and saxitoxin have played a vital role in the study of the molecular biology of the sodium channel.

Naturally successful purification of sodium channels also requires a rich tissue source which is readily available and amenable to biochemical isolation techniques. To the naive reader the use of the electric eel *Electrophorus electricus* as a source of channel material may seem unnecessarily exotic, but in fact these beasts are endowed with amazingly large quantities of sodium channels at high density.[4] As a result, the eel electroplax channel has played a prominent role in channel studies, having now been purified,[3,5] chemically characterized[5] and sequenced,[6] and visualized both by electron microscopy[7] and immunocytochemical techniques.[8] In addition, the function and pharmacology of the eel channel appear to be very similar to channels from other animals, so that there is reason to suppose that molecular information derived from electroplax channels will be broadly applicable to those from other sources.

The success of the electric organ preparation is probably due as much to the richness of the tissue in sodium channels as to the skill (and luck!) of the investigators. A crude fraction of electroplax membranes has about 0.5% sodium channel relative to

[a]The authors gratefully acknowledge support from the following sources: NIH Training Grants to E. E. Windhager (ERP) and A. R. Martin (DSD), a Whitaker Foundation grant and NIH grant NS22602 (to BWU), a Muscular Dystrophy Association grant, NIH grant NS15879, and an NIH Research Career Development Award (to SRL).

other protein present, thus requiring only a 200-fold enrichment to achieve homogeneity.[3] Thus we have been able to purify the sodium channel from this source using the relatively routine procedures of detergent solubilization and crude ion exchange fractionation, followed by gel filtration chromatography.[3,5] However, it should be realized that this purification approach isolates the *tetrodotoxin and saxitoxin binding component* (TTXR) of the sodium channel. This naturally raises the question whether the component thus isolated also contains the other molecular structures required for channel function (*e.g.*, the ion pore and gating structures). In addition, TTXRs in detergent solutions exhibit some rather unusual physicochemical characteristics in their micellar form that allow their ready separation from other electroplax proteins.[3] In one sense these properties are important for the purification of the electroplax sodium channel, although they are perhaps more significant in that they are manifestations of a highly unusual composition and structure which presumably underlies the molecular mechanism of the channel itself.

In the paper we outline our thesis that compositional components other than protein may be part of the sodium channel apparatus from electroplax. In order to do this we first describe the evidence for the existence of extensive nonprotein domains in association with a monomeric protein core, followed by a description of the properties of reconstituted electroplax sodium channels as observed in lipid vesicles and planar bilayers. Finally, we discuss several hypotheses on the role of compositional domains in channel mechanism and biology and their implications for future channel studies.

PROPERTIES OF THE TETRODOTOXIN BINDING COMPONENT FROM ELECTROPLAX

Physicochemical Characteristics of the Native TTXR

The first hints of the unusual physical nature of the TTXR were obtained in early purification studies. Thus, data obtained from gel filtration, sedimentation, and temperature denaturation experiments suggested that the molecule solubilized in nondenaturing detergents was intimately associated with a very large lipid-detergent micellar phase.[3,9] In addition, the solubilized TTXR was found to be very negatively charged, as evidenced both by its high electrophoretic mobility on nondenaturing electrophoresis and its tenacious binding to anion exchange resins at high ionic strength.[10] This combination of unusual micellar size (Stokes radius = 95 Å) and high negativity (*e. g.,* six times greater than the fairly acidic acetylcholine receptor) are the basis for the efficient purification protocol devised for the electroplax TTXR.[3,5]

Polypeptide Composition of the Purified Electroplax TTXR

An equally unexpected feature of the eel TTXR was the finding that it consists of only a single large polypeptide species ($M_r \approx 250,000$, but see below). As this point is discussed at length elsewhere,[5] we only briefly describe the supporting evidence here. First, exhaustive purification of eel TTXRs yielded preparations which demonstrated only a single band on sodium dodecyl sulfate-polyacrylamide gel electrophoresis (SDS-PAGE). Second, even in less pure preparations the fractionation of TTX binding activity was quantitatively correlated only to the presence of this large band, and to no other peptides.[5,10] Third, antibodies raised to highly purified native material specifically coimmunoprecipitated only the large polypeptide along with TTX binding activity when mixed into crude detergent extracts of electroplax membranes.[8] Thus in all cases TTX binding activity was associated only with the large polypeptide, and a requirement for other species could be excluded.

Anomalous Behavior of the TTXR Peptide on Reducing SDS Gels

Although the electroplax TTXR banding pattern on SDS-PAGE showed only a single peptide, the electrophoretic behavior of the protein in this system was found to be highly anomalous in two different respects.[5] First, values for the molecular size of the TTXR peptide determined by SDS-PAGE were highly variable and depended on the porosity of the separating polyacrylamide gel. When analyzed for this behavior by a Ferguson experiment,[11] the TTXR peptide migrated as if it had four times the electrophoretic free mobility of the standard proteins on SDS-PAGE. The second anomaly was seen in the highly diffuse nature of the single TTXR band on SDS-PAGE (known as "microheterogeneity"), which was shown to be due to a slight variability in the size of the TTXR peptides.[5] Thus, in addition to the properties described above, the behavior of the purified TTXR peptide on SDS-PAGE was also suggestive of a highly unusual physical character.

COMPOSITIONAL COMPLEXITY OF THE ELECTROPLAX TTXR: EXTENSIVE NONPROTEIN DOMAINS ACCOUNT FOR ANOMALOUS PHYSICOCHEMICAL BEHAVIOR

Similar anomalous behavior on SDS-PAGE to that described above has been reported for a number of other peptides.[12,13] Generally, microheterogeneity seems to arise from variable glycosylation of these peptides, whereas abnormally high free mobilities are thought to arise from unusually hydrophobic regions of a polypeptide which increase its binding of amphipathic dodecyl sulfate anions, resulting in an increased charge-to-mass ratio for the protein on SDS-PAGE. Since these anomalies are usually related to the biochemical composition of the molecule, we have subjected the purified TTXR peptide to amino acid, carbohydrate, and fatty acid analysis.

Amino Acid Composition Does Not Explain Anomalous Properties

As we have reported,[5] the amino acid composition of the eel TTXR is rather typical of integral membrane proteins generally, being somewhat enriched in hydrophobic residues. However, the extent of this enrichment was actually less than other integral membrane proteins from the eel which do not display any of the anomalous properties mentioned above. In addition, the amount of negatively charged residues was normal, thus failing to account for the high intrinsic charge of the native protein or the elevated free mobility on SDS-PAGE. Thus we concluded that the cause of the highly unusual properties of the purified electroplax TTXR must lie elsewhere.

The TTXR Is Heavily Glycosylated

Analysis of the carbohydrate composition revealed an unusually high degree of glycosylation (30% by weight, TABLE 1), certainly sufficient to account for the microheterogeneity seen. In addition, deglycosylation of the peptide tends to increase the band sharpness on SDS-PAGE dramatically.[14] Also noteworthy is the high proportion of sialic acid attached to the peptide, which adequately explains the highly acidic character of the native protein on ion exchange resins and nondenaturing electrophoresis. However, these charges still cannot account for the high free solution mobility deduced from Fergusion analysis on SDS-PAGE, because they only represent about 1% of the additional charge needed to explain this anomaly. Rather, it seemed more likely that the association of large amounts of SDS with the peptide was the explanation of its behavior on SDS gels.

Fatty Acids Are Associated with the Eel TTXR in Unprecedented Amounts

We have recently measured the binding of ^{35}S-SDS to the eel TTXR, and find that it does indeed associate with very large amounts of SDS compared with well-behaved proteins (see Thornhill and Levinson, this volume[45]). The amount of this binding is close to that expected to account for the anomalous free solution mobility on SDS-PAGE; moreover, the mode and degree of association suggest that the TTXR contains extensive hydrophobic regions which are *posttranslationally* attached to the

TABLE 1. Carbohydrate Composition of the TTXR Sodium Channel Polypeptide from Electroplax.[a]

| | Carbohydrate Composition | |
	% Total Weight	% of Carbohydrate
Fucose	0.5 ± 0.2	1.5 ± 0.5
Mannose	2.4 ± 0.5	8.3 ± 1.1
Galactose	1.5 ± 0.3	5.2 ± 0.6
N-Acetylhexosamine	13.3 ± 0.4	45.3 ± 2.6
Sialic Acid	11.8 ± 1.2	39.7 ± 1.6
Total	29.5 ± 2.4	

[a]Data taken from ref. 5.

protein core of the TTXR (see Thornhill and Levinson, this volume,[45] for further details). Recent literature has shown that many proteins are fatty acylated or covalently lipidated[15]; thus we have analyzed the purified eel TTXR for the presence of fatty acid moieties.

In order to do this, the TTXR was purified to apparent homogeneity on a SDS-Sepharose 4B column, followed by extensive dialysis to remove SDS as described.[5] The peptide was then exhaustively extracted with chloroform/methanol (2:1) to remove noncovalently attached lipid, and then transesterified in acid methanol.[16] The resultant methyl esters of fatty acids were then separated, identified, and quantitated by combined gas chromatography and mass spectrometry. Results of such an analysis are shown in FIGURE 1, in which palmitate (C16:0, 2.1% protein weight, FIG. 1, peak A) and stearate (C18:0, 0.7%, peak B) were the major species. Although the total proportion of fatty acid (about 3% by weight relative to protein) may appear small, it represents about 25 fatty acyl chains per TTXR molecule, an unprecedented number and proportion (see discussion in Thornhill and Levinson, this volume[45]). In addition, we have analyzed the dialyzed protein before chloroform/methanol extraction, and find that it contains 6% to 8% fatty acid. This additional 3% to 5% over the extracted protein represents noncovalently attached lipid. However, we suspect that the interaction with the TTXR molecule in this case is likely to be rather tight because this material was purified in SDS, which would have been expected to dissociate loosely bound lipid during chromatographic isolation.

Thus we propose that the intense hydrophobicity of the electroplax TTXR arises from the posttranslational covalent attachment of fatty acyl moieties which then organize free lipids into a stable hydrophobic core. At present we do not know the nature of the covalent linkages to the TTXR protein core, *e.g.*, the points of attachment or whether fatty acids are esterified directly through the protein or are part of linked phospholipid.[15] Nonetheless, it now appears likely that these lipids create an extensive, hydrophobic nonprotein domain which dramatically affects the physical behavior of the molecule.

RECONSTITUTION OF EEL SODIUM CHANNELS IN LIPID VESICLES AND PLANAR BILAYERS

The Large Polypeptide Appears to Contain the Entire Sodium Channel Mechanism in the Electroplax

As noted above, it is a point of considerable interest whether the highly unusual properties of the eel TTXR are related to the molecular mechanism of the sodium channel as a whole. An effective approach to this problem is to reconstitute highly purified material which consists of only the large TTXR peptide into artificial membranes, and then ask whether such a system is capable of demonstrating channel-mediated transport of sodium ions. In our laboratory we have developed procedures that allow the reconstitution of highly purified TTXRs into lipid vesicles with a minimum of loss of TTX binding activity.[22] With this system one can quantitatively relate polypeptide composition and TTX binding activity to channel-dependent isotopic sodium fluxes.

FIGURE 2 shows the results of a typical experiment. Here the vesicles, loaded with a high concentration of NaCl, were placed in a medium containing the sodium channel activator veratridine and a trace amount of ^{22}Na. In such a system, if the vesicles contain channels that can be opened by veratridine, then a sodium diffusion potential will result; this potential will cause tracer sodium to be accumulated in the vesicles at a concentration higher than that in the external solution. This results in an enhancement of the channel-dependent sodium uptake over systems in which sodium concentrations are equal on both sides of the membrane, and allows one to detect the activity of reconstituted channels with greater sensitivity.[25] The biphasic behavior observed in such systems is a consequence of the lower chloride permeability in the vesicles, which eventually causes the sodium gradient to dissipate.

The experiment shown in FIGURE 2 supports assignment of substantial channel behavior to the large polypeptide. First, veratridine did cause a substantial exhancement of sodium flux in these vesicles, indicating the presence of sodium channels. Further evidence is provided by the fact that TTX in the external solution blocked much of this veratridine-activated flux (the flux remaining after TTX block probably represents "inside-out" channels). Secondly, the material reconstituted in this experiment displayed only the large polypeptide on SDS-PAGE (FIG. 3), yet was about 50% active with respect to TTX binding activity (as judged by the specific activity of about 2400 pmol toxin bound per mg protein *after* reconstitution). Finally, we estimate that nearly all of these toxin-binding channels mediate sodium fluxes after reconstitution (as determined according to Tamkun *et al.*[23]). This makes it highly unlikely that flux activity is caused by a small fraction of channels (*e.g.*, less than 10%) which contain polypeptides undetected by SDS-PAGE other than the single large species. Therefore, since most of the highly purified TTXRs show these functional and pharmacological characteristics, one can conclude that the large polypeptide alone contains the underlying molecular structures involved in these phenomena, and that other polypeptide species are not required. This is in contrast to channels purified and reconstituted from mammalian excitable membranes, in which small peptides have been implicated

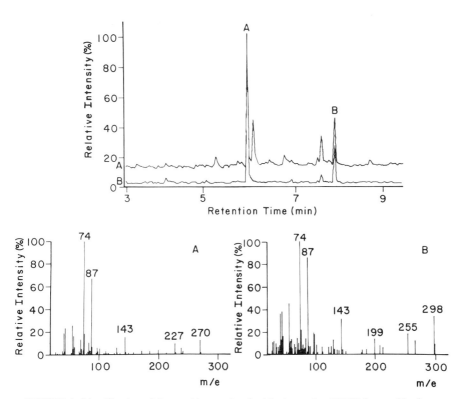

FIGURE 1. Identification of fatty acids associated with electroplax TTXR by combined gas chromatography and mass spectrometry. *Top panel*, Gas chromatogram; trace *A*, total ion current; trace *B*, current for m/e=74 (base peak for rearrangement ion of fatty acyl methyl esters). Note only peaks *A* and *B* have significant current at m/e=74. *Lower panels*, Mass spectra of peak *A* (*left*) and peak *B* (*right*). Note peaks at m/e=74, 87, and 143 (diagnostic of fatty acid methyl esters). The molecular ion of 270 in spectra *A* identifies palmitic acid methyl ester (C16:0), while the high ion at 298 in spectra *B* identifies stearic acid methyl ester (C18:0).

as part of the sodium channel structure.[23,24] At present the possible functional role of these smaller subunits in the mammalian channel is unknown.

Rationale for Toxin-modified Sodium Channels in Planar Bilayers

The vesicle fluxes observed above suffer from the fact that channel gating kinetics and voltage dependences are not readily obtainable. Thus, if one wishes to determine if

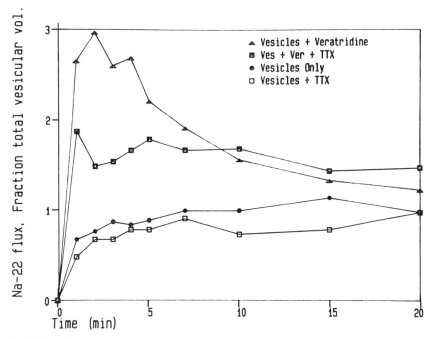

FIGURE 2. Sodium flux activity of the reconstituted TTX polypeptide. Polypeptide was purified in the zwitterionic detergent CHAPS supplemented with a 1:1 mixture of asolectin/phosphatidyl choline. The detergent was then removed by dialysis in 100 mM sodium phosphate (pH 6.8) to form liposomal vesicles containing reconstituted TTXR polypeptide. To test for channel-dependent sodium fluxes, the vesicles were placed in iso-osmotic 100 mM Trisphosphate-Tris Cl (pH 6.8) containing a trace of ^{22}Na and 100 micromolar veratridine. The accumulation of radiotracer sodium was then determined as previously described.[25] When added, TTX was mixed to a final concentration of 2.5 micromolar in the external solution. The TTX inhibition of sodium flux in vesicles alone without veratridine (*lower two curves*) is significant and has been shown to represent noninactivated channels which apparently "flicker" (Duch and Levinson, in preparation).

reconstituted channels are altered in their gating behavior from normal channels in situ (*e.g.,* if the reconstituted channels lost a modulating gating element during purification), it is necessary to observe the sodium fluxes with an electrical recording system which has both voltage-control and fast time resolution. Such a system is the planar lipid bilayer.[26–28]

It is not easy to judge the success of a functional reconstitution of purified sodium channels from the eel electroplax because of the lack of information on the behavior of native sodium channels in the voltage-clamped eel preparation. The high resting membrane conductance and large membrane time constant[29] have so far prevented adequate space-clamp and the faithful recording of sodium channel kinetics in the eel electroplax. Electrophysiological comparisons between purified and native eel sodium channels are therefore quite incomplete. A comparison of purified eel channels with native sodium channels of other preparations introduces at least two unknowns: the differences between sodium channel proteins, and the role of membrane environment in modifying channel function. One unknown is removed if, on the other hand, we are able to study different sodium channels under identical conditions in the same (though not native) membranes. This is why we chose to study toxin-modified (batrachotoxin, veratridine) purified eel sodium channels in planar lipid bilayers, as a great deal of information is available for similarly modified and reconstituted sodium channels from rat[26,30] and dog[28] brain and rat muscle.[27]

Purified eel electroplax sodium channels have been reconstituted into bilayers before using somewhat different techniques. This makes some comparisons with existing planar bilayer data more difficult and may account for some of the following observed discrepancies. For unmodified channels, Rosenberg *et al.*[31] measured single channel conductances of the order of 11.2 pS in patch-clamped liposomes, whereas Hanke *et al.*[32] reported values close to 150 pS; Rosenberg *et al.*[31] observed batracho-toxin (BTX) modified sodium channels that remained mainly closed, unlike other BTX-modified sodium channels in planar bilayers.[26–28,30] In addition to addressing these questions, we have used BTX modification to study the steady-state activation of eel channels which can be compared with other BTX-modified sodium channels.[26–28,30]

Bilayer Methods

The highly purified, large molecular weight TTX-binding polypeptide (2000–2900 pmol TTX bound/mg protein) from eel electroplax was reconstituted into liposomes as

TOP

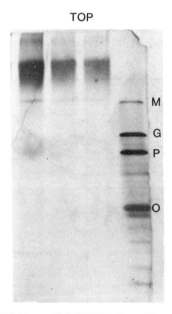

FIGURE 3. SDS-PAGE of highly purified TTXR polypeptide used for reconstitution in both FIGURE 2 and bilayer experiments. *Left two lanes,* TTXR at two different protein concentrations before reconstitution. *Third lane,* TTXR after reconstitution. *Right lane,* Molecular weight standards. From the top, the four darkest bands are myosin (200 kDa), β-galactosidase (116 kDa), phosphorylase B (93 kDa), and ovalbumin (45 kDa). Gradient gel, 3–30% acrylamide, 0.1% bis. The sharp band directly under the diffuse TTXR peptide is a product of TTXR degradation (Thornhill and Levinson, unpublished).

previously described.[22] From measurements of sodium fluxes in the presence of veratridine it was estimated that 85% to 100% of the TTX-binding polypeptides conducted sodium ions. Other polypeptides present constituted less than 10% of the total purified protein (SDS-PAGE).

In the presence of 1 μM BTX or 100 μM veratridine, vesicles containing the purified TTX-binding polypeptide were added to the bilayer chamber[26,28] or directly to planar bilayers made from neutral phospholipid solutions containing phosphatidylcholine/phosphatidylethanolamine (4:1) in decane.[33] Channel activity incorporated spontaneously and did not require prior freeze-thawing of channel-containing vesicles,[30,31] nor the presence of osmotic gradients,[30] divalent cations,[30-32] or cholesterol.[32] The following sections describe the properties of this channel activity using the electrophysiological sign convention.[33]

Current-Voltage Relationship

In FIGURE 4 the inset shows the single channel activity at +60 mV that developed after purified TTX-binding polypeptide was added to the cis chamber of the bilayer while the trans chamber contained 1 μM BTX. The height of the current transitions increased linearly and symmetrically with the magnitude of the applied potential over a wide range of membrane potentials. In symmetrical 500 mM NaCl the single channel conductance was constant with a value of 23.7 pS (FIG. 4, filled circles, two-channel membrane). This value is comparable to that of rat brain (25 pS, ref. 30, 29 pS, ref. 26), dog brain (25 pS, ref. 28), and rat muscle (21 pS, ref. 27) measured under similar conditions. When channels were observed for more than five hours they showed no detectable change in the I/V curve.

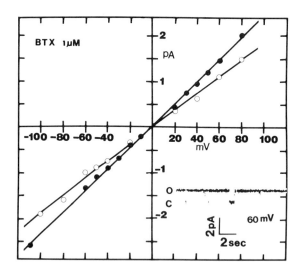

FIGURE 4. BTX-modified single channel currents as function of membrane potential in symmetrical 100 mM (*open circles*) and 500 mM (*closed circles*) NaCl electrolyte solutions (10 mM Hepes, pH 7.4, $T = 24°-25°C$). The inset shows the corresponding single channel transitions (500 mM NaCl) at 60 mV (Bessel filter set at 50 Hz). The straight lines have been fitted by linear regression and yield slopes of 23.7 pS (correlation $r = 0.999$) in 500 mM NaCl and 18.9 pS ($r = 0.998$) in 100 mM NaCl.

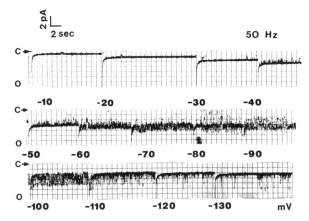

FIGURE 5. Gating of BTX-modified channels in symmetrical 500 mM NaCl (Bessel filter set at 50 Hz, 10 mM Hepes, pH 7.4, T = 24°–25°C). The membrane contains two different channels which begin to gate at different membrane potentials. At − 10 mV both channels are mostly open, at − 130 mV they are mostly closed.

The I/V curve in symmetrical 100 mM NaCl looked very similar except for a slightly lower single channel conductance of 18.9 pS (FIG. 4, open circles, two-channel membrane). The observation of symmetrical and linear behavior and a rather small reduction in single channel conductance between symmetrical 500 mM and 100 mM NaCl agrees well with findings from rat brain,[26] dog brain,[36] and rat muscle.[27] The value of 24.2 pS reported by Rosenberg *et al.*[31] for eel is comparable considering the quite different experimental conditions, which included a sodium gradient (90 mM/10 mM NaCl) and the use of membranes carrying a surface charge.

Apart from the predominant single channel conductances shown in FIGURE 4, we also observed smaller current transitions. Some of these may be similar to the subconductance states observed in sodium channels from dog brain.[36] We did not detect large single channel conductances of 150 pS reported by Hanke *et al.* for eel (symmetrical 140 mM NaCl) in the absence of BTX.[32]

Steady-State Activation

At + 60 mV the channels were open most of the time with a fractional open time of 0.98 (see FIG. 4 inset). This is characteristic of other BTX-modified sodium channels in planar lipid bilayers,[26–28] and is in contrast to patch-clamped liposomes where the BTX-modified eel sodium channels remained mainly closed even at very depolarized potentials.[31] Whereas in the latter preparation the activation behavior of purified eel channels has not yet been assessed, it can be done in the planar bilayer. FIGURE 5 shows that, at − 10 mV, the two channels contained in this membrane were mostly open, whereas beyond − 120 mV they remained predominantly closed. When the fractional open time is plotted against membrane potential (FIG. 6b, see legend for details) a steady-state activation curve is obtained which has a midpoint, in this example, at a membrane potential of − 77 mV. It is considerably more negative than that of unmodified sodium channels in other preparations where it has been shown that BTX modification typically shifts activation by 50 mV.[37] This eel midpoint potential is close to but approximately − 10 mV less than values reported in other preparations under

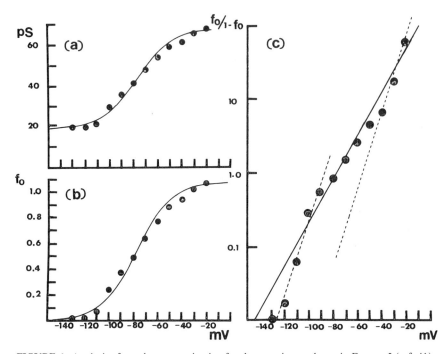

FIGURE 6. Analysis of steady-state activation for the experiment shown in FIGURE 5 (ref. 41). All continuous lines represent the results of a numerical curvefit to the equation $f_o = 1/(1 + \exp(qF[V - V_a])/RT)$ (ref. 38) with an apparent gating charge of 1.74 electronic charges and a midpoint potential $V_a = -76.8$ mV; f_o, fractional open time, q, apparent gating charge, F, Faraday constant, V, membrane potential, R, gas constant, T, absolute temperature. (a) Time averaged (filter set at 1 Hz, ref. 41) total conductance, including background, as a function of membrane potential. The unusually large background conductance was present before the addition of any polypeptide and resulted most likely from a slight leak in the septum seal. (b) Fractional open time, f_o, versus membrane potential. Data points as in above, corrected for the background conductance, divided by the single channel conductance and the number of channels (2) in the membrane. (c) Plot of $f_o/(1 - f_o)$ as function of membrane potential, with the slope yielding the apparent gating charge (1.74 electronic charges). The *dotted lines* are fitted by eye for regions of the membrane potential where the gating of a single channel dominates; the resulting slopes (lines are parallel) correspond to an apparent gating charge of 3.4 electronic charges.

similar ionic conditions.[28,38] The slope of this activation curve is rather shallow, corresponding to an apparent gating charge of 1.7 electronic charges (FIG. 6c). This is considerably lower than the range of 4 to 6 reported for other preparations.[27,33,38]

A closer inspection of FIGURE 6 reveals that the two channels appeared to be gating at quite different potentials; one channel began to gate at -60 mV. It was already mostly closed at -80 mV when the other channel began to gate. Correspondingly FIGURE 6c, which represents the slope of the activation curve,[38] becomes quite shallow in the region where the two gating behaviors overlap. In regions where the gating of just one channel dominates, the slopes (dashed lines) are similar for both channels, but much higher, corresponding to an apparent gating charge of approximately 3.4 electronic charges. Almost all membranes contained more than one channel, and in most cases at least two channels in a given membrane differed in their midpoints for steady-state activation. This spread was larger than in the dog brain preparation[33] and has also been observed for another purified sodium channel.[30] In addition, a number of channels showed the spontaneous shifts in the gating activity reported for other sodium channel preparations.[27,33]

In experiments with dog sodium channels, decreasing the sodium concentration (and thereby ionic strength) leads to a shift of the activation curve in a hyperpolarized direction.[33] At symmetrical 100 mM NaCl eel steady-state channel activation had an average midpoint potential of −71 mV, different from dog brain channels.[33]

Ion Selectivity

The experiment in FIGURE 7 shows the single channels to be sodium selective. One bilayer chamber was filled with 500 mM NaCl, the other with a mixture of 450 mM KCl and 50 mM NaCl. The single channel currents reversed when the chamber containing 500 mM NaCl had become 30.8 mV more negative than the other chamber. From this reversal potential, using the Goldman-Hodgin-Katz equation, a permeability ratio of 4.5 was calculated. Under the same experimental conditions, Andersen *et*

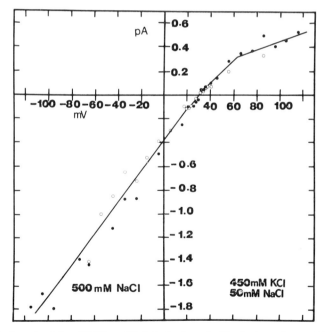

FIGURE 7. Ion selectivity of BTX-modified single channels. Single channel current is plotted as a function of membrane potential. One bilayer chamber was filled with 500 mM NaCl, the other with a mixture of 450 mM KCl + 50 mM NaCl. The single channel currents reversed when the chamber containing 500 mM NaCl had become 30.8 mV more negative than the other chamber. Two different membranes contained 10 (*open circles*) and 4 (*filled circles*) channels; 10 mM Hepes buffer, pH 7.4, T = 24°–25°C. The line between +20 and +40 mV was fitted by linear regression (reversal potential 30.8 mV, r = 0.958), and the other lines have been drawn by eye.

al.[36] reported a permeability ratio of 5.6 for dog brain. Under different conditions, Rosenberg et al.[31] obtained a permeability ratio of 7 for unmodified eel channels, whereas a value of 14 has been measured for BTX-modified sodium channels from both rat brain and muscle.[26,27] Although Andersen et al. have determined that the permeability ratio did not change with varying mole fraction at constant ionic strength,[36] it is not yet clear how the presence of divalent cations, a change in ionic strength, and different membrane lipids would affect the permeability ratio.

Tetrodotoxin Block

Addition of submaximal concentrations of tetrodotoxin (TTX) to the extracellular aspect of the sodium channel (as defined by its gating characteristics) led to long duration closures without changing the single channel conductance of open channels (data not shown). The block (fractional closed time) increased with increasing TTX concentration (data not shown). The block was voltage dependent as demonstrated in FIGURE 8, where the K_d has been plotted as a function of membrane potential. Furthermore, interaction between Na^+ and TTX was observed as the K_d decreased when the sodium concentration was lowered from 500 mM to 100 mM (FIG. 8). This

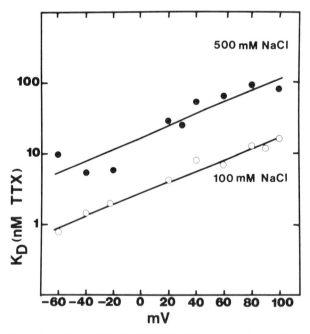

FIGURE 8. Voltage dependence of block by TTX. The K_d has been calculated from the fractional close time, f_c, as follows: $f_c = [TTX]/(K_d + [TTX])$.[27,28] The K_d has been fitted by linear regression to the equation $K_d(V)/K_d(0) = \exp[aFV/(RT)]$; a, fraction of the applied potential that affects the TTX block; F, Faraday constant; V, membrane potential; R, gas constant; T, absolute temperature.[28] The values in symmetrical 100 mM (500 mM) NaCl are, respectively: $K_d(0) = 2.8$ nM (17.1 nM), $a = 0.71$ (0.75), correlation $r = 0.987$ (0.929); 10 mM Hepes buffer, pH 7.4, $T = 24°–25°C$.

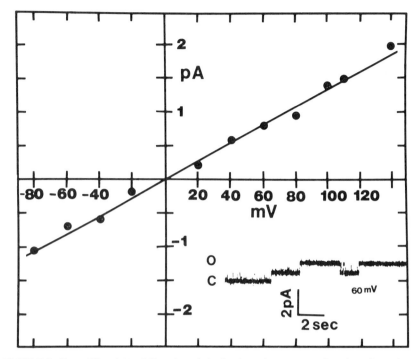

FIGURE 9. Veratridine (100 μM) activated single channel currents as function of membrane potential in symmetrical 500 mM NaCl electrolyte solutions (10 mM Hepes, pH 7.4, T = 24°–25°C). The inset shows the corresponding single channel transitions at 60 mV (Bessel filter 50 Hz). The straight line has been fitted by linear regression and yields a slope of 13.5 pS (correlation r = 0.998).

behavior parallels reports for rat muscle[21] and dog brain,[28,39] and the observed values for $K_d(V)$ and the voltage dependence (see legend of FIG. 8) are very similar to those reported for dog brain under identical conditions.[28,39]

Veratridine-modified Sodium Channels

Ideally one would like to compare purified and bilayer reconstituted sodium channels in the absence of modifying toxins in order to establish similarities and differences between them. This has not yet been accomplished although it has been possible to move away from the specificity of a batrachotoxin modification by using veratridine, another alkaloid toxin.[40] The purified eel sodium channel could also be incorporated into planar bilayers using veratridine, shown in FIGURE 9. Under the same conditions as in FIGURE 4 (symmetrical 500 mM NaCl) the veratridine-activated channels remained open for briefer periods of time, and long closing events were observed even at very depolarized potentials. The I/V characteristic was again linear over a wide range of potentials, but the resulting single channel conductance of 13.5 pS was almost half that observed for the batrachotoxin modified channel, analogous to observations made on the rat muscle sodium channel.[40]

Conclusions from Planar Bilayer Work

The present studies confirm and add to the work begun by Rosenberg et al.[31] on identifying, on the single channel level, the purified large molecular weight TTX-binding polypeptide as a major component of the eel electroplax sodium channel. The similar behavior of sodium channels of quite different origins is indeed remarkable, and the purified eel TTX-binding component does not form an exception. Quantitative differences are relatively small. At present it is impossible to judge whether they are introduced during the purification procedure or whether they reflect the true properties of the unpurified eel electroplax sodium channel.

POSSIBLE FUNCTIONAL ROLES FOR NONPROTEIN DOMAINS IN SODIUM CHANNEL MECHANISMS

The large number of sialic acid residues and high hydrophobicity of the molecule prompt one to speculate whether they are in some way related to the specific molecular mechanisms of the sodium channel. In the case of channel carbohydrate one can consider that glycosylation of membrane proteins is nearly always localized to the outside of the cell membrane. Thus it can be estimated that about 100 sialic acid residues will reside in a volume roughly 75 Å in diameter around the external mouth of the sodium pore. The most likely implication for such a high concentration of negative charge lies in its effects on the conductance of sodium ions through the pore. For example, it has been shown that placement of three negative charges near the opening of the pore-forming substance gramicidin A raises the cation conductance of the channel threefold over that of underivatized gramicidin.[17] Furthermore, a similar group apparently exists near the mouth of the sodium channel which can be chemically neutralized, resulting in a threefold decrease in channel conductance.[18] Although the precise placement of the sialic acid residues relative to the mouth of the eel channel is unknown, the sheer number of such charges suggests that at least several of them will be close enough to the pore to affect sodium transport rates significantly. If this is true, the sialic acid groups may represent modifications which would ultimately enhance the discharge from the electric organ, thus aiding the eel in predation and defense. In addition, the presence of such a cloud of charge might be expected to influence the magnitude of the surface membrane potential sensed by gating charges.[19] Although the possible functional significance of this latter effect is unclear, it may provide an explanation for the well-known effects of calcium on gating behavior.[20]

One must be even more speculative regarding the role of the hydrophobic domain. However, based on several lines of evidence, it is widely believed that the voltage-sensing structures of the gates reside in the lipid surrounding the channel.[21] The hydrophobic domain of the channel may serve to organize this lipid environment, precisely regulating its physical characteristics (such as viscosity, thickness, and surface tension) which are thought to be important to gating kinetics and voltage dependence. Thus the need for such regulation could be to maintain consistent channel operation in the face of significant differences in bulk membrane lipid composition and properties that are found in the variety of tissues in which sodium channels exist.

Additional or alternative roles for these domains have been suggested by the observation that posttranslational modifications appear to be a general feature of membrane protein biosynthesis.[15,43] A number of lines of evidence suggest that glycosylation serves as a sorting signal that allows the cellular machinery to properly transport and insert a given membrane protein in its proper location on the cell surface.[42] In addition, hydrophobic domains may serve to aid in the insertion or anchoring of a membrane protein in the lipid bilayer, although the evidence for this role is not conclusive.[15]

IMPLICATIONS FOR FUTURE STUDIES OF SODIUM CHANNEL MECHANISMS

Finally, what are the implications of our findings for future studies of sodium channel structure and mechanism? If, as we speculate, extensive nonprotein domains have significant functional roles in sodium channel mechanisms, then it might be difficult to understand the operation of the sodium channel from approaches which only consider protein structure. For example, methods which attempt to elucidate mechanism by perturbing protein conformation, such as site-directed mutagenesis,[44] will be harder to interpret if nonprotein domains are involved in channel function.

An alternative approach to the study of sodium channel mechanism may be possible throuth the study of channel biosynthesis. Both glycosylation and acylation-lipidation appear to occur during posttranslational modification of the core channel protein.[45] Substances have been discovered which modify or inhibit posttranslational synthesis; alternatively, it is possible to remove or modify posttranslational domains by chemical or enzymatic means and determine the functional consequences using the reconstitution techniques described above. With these methods, it should be possible to assess the role of these posttranslational domains in the expression of functional sodium channels in the cell membrane.

ACKNOWLEDGMENTS

We very much wish to thank A. W. Pike and P. V. Fennessey for performing the gas chromatography and mass spectrometry analyses, W. N. Green and O. S. Anderson for freely sharing their experimental expertise and results, and Mary Poranicas, Ellen Connole and George Tarver for technical assistance. We are grateful to Dr. J. W. Daly for kindly providing batrachotoxin.

REFERENCES

1. RITCHIE, J. M. & R. B. ROGART. 1977. Rev. Physiol. Biochem. Pharmacol. **79:** 1–50.
2. LEVINSON, S. R., C. J. CURATALO, J. REED & M. A. RAFTERY. 1979. Anal. Biochem. **99:** 72–84.
3. AGNEW, W. S., S. R. LEVINSON, J. S. BRABSON & M. A. RAFTERY. 1978. Proc. Natl. Acad. Sci. U. S. A. **75:** 2606–2610.
4. LEVINSON, S. R. 1981. *In* Molecular Basis of Drug Action. T. J. Singer & R. Ondarza, Eds.: 315–331. Elsevier-North Holland. Amsterdam and New York.
5. MILLER J. A., W. S. AGNEW & S. R. LEVINSON. 1983. Biochemistry **22:** 462–470.
6. NODA, M., S. SHIMIZU, T. TANABE, T. TAKAI, T. KAYANO, T. IKEDA, H. TAKAHASHI, H. NAKAYAMA, Y. KANAOKA, N. MINAMINO, K. KANGAWA, H. MATSUO, M. A. RAFTERY, T. HIROS, S. INAYAMA, H. HAYASHIDA, T. MIYATA, S. NUMA. 1984. Nature **312:** 121–127.
7. ELLISMAN, M. H., J. A. MILLER & W. S. AGNEW. 1983. J. Cell Biol. **97:** 1834–1840.
8. ELLISMAN, M. H. & S. R. LEVINSON. 1982. Proc. Natl. Acad. Sci. U. S. A. **79:** 6707–6710.
9. AGNEW, W. S. & M. A. RAFTERY. 1979. Biochemistry **10:** 1912–1919.
10. AGNEW, W. S., A. C. MOORE, S. R. LEVINSON & M. A. RAFTERY. 1980. Biochem. Biophys. Res. Comm. **92:** 860–866.

11. FERGUSON, K. A. & A. L. C. WALLACE. 1961. Nature **190:** 629.
12. HOROWITZ, M. I. 1977. *In* Glycoconjugates, vol. 1. M. I. Horowitz & W. Pigman, Eds: 15–34. Academic Press. New York.
13. LEACH, B. S., J. F. COLLAWN & W. W. FISH. 1980. Biochemistry **19:** 5734–5741.
14. AGNEW, W. S., J. A. MILLER, M. H. ELLISMAN, R. L. ROSENBERG, S. A. TOMIKO & S. R. LEVINSON. 1983. Cold Spring Harbor Symp. Quant. Biol **XLVIII:** 165–179.
15. SCHMIDT, M. F. G. 1983. Curr. Top. Microbiol. Immunol. **102:** 101–129.
16. CHRISTIE, W. W. 1982. Lipid Analysis. Pergamon. Elmsford, N. Y.
17. APELL, H. J., E. BAMBERG, H. ALPES & P. LÄUGER. 1977. J. Membr. Biol. **31:** 171–188.
18. SIGWORTH, F. J. & B. C. SPALDING. 1980. Nature **238:** 293–295.
19. LEVINE, S., M. LEVINE, K. A. SHARP & D. E. BROOKS. 1983. Biophys. J. **42:** 127–135.
20. FRANKENHAEUSER, B. & A. L. HODGKIN. 1957. J. Physiol. **169:** 431–437.
21. HILLE, B. 1984. Ionic Channels of Excitable Membranes, chaps. 13 and 16. Sinauer Associates. Sunderland, Mass.
22. DUCH, D. S. & S. R. LEVINSON. 1985. Biophys. J. **47:** 192a.
23. TAMKUN, M. M., J. A. TALVENHEIMO & W. A. CATTERALL. 1984. J. Biol. Chem. **259:** 1676–1688.
24. BARCHI, R. L. 1983. J. Neurochem. **40:** 1377–1385.
25. GARTY, H., B. RUDY & S. J. KARLISH. 1983. J. Biol. Chem. **258:** 13094–13099.
26. KRUEGER, B. K., J. F. WORLEY & R. J. FRENCH. 1983. Nature **303:** 172–175.
27. MOCZYDLOWSKI, E., S. S. GARBER & C. MILLER. 1984. J. Gen. Physiol. **84:** 665–686.
28. GREEN, W. N., L. B. WEISS & O. S. ANDERSEN. 1984. Ann. N.Y. Acad. Sci. **435:** 548–550.
29. RUIZ-MANRESA, F. & H. GRUNDFEST. 1976. Proc. Natl. Acad. Sci. U. S. A. **73:** 3554–3557.
30. HARTSHORNE, R. P., B. U. KELLER, J. A. TALVENHEIMO, W. A. CATTERALL & M. MONTAL. 1985. Proc. Natl. Acad. Sci. U. S. A. **82:** 240–244.
31. ROSENBERG, R. L., S. A. TOMIKO & W. S. AGNEW. 1984. Proc. Natl. Acad. Sci. U. S. A. **81:** 5594–5598.
32. HANKE, W., G. BOHEIM, J. BARHANIN, D. PAURON & M. LAZDUNSKI. 1984. EMBO J. **3:** 509–515.
33. WEISS, L. B., W. N. GREEN & O. S. ANDERSEN. 1984. Biophys. J. **45:** 167a.
34. GREEN, W. N., L. B. WEISS & O. S. ANDERSEN. J. Gen. Physiol. Submitted.
35. GREEN, W. N., L. B. WEISS & O. S. ANDERSEN. J. Gen. Physiol. Submitted.
36. ANDERSEN, O. S., W. N. GREEN & B. W. URBAN. 1985. *In* Ion Channel Reconstitution. C. Miller, Ed. Plenum. New York. pp. 385–404.
37. KHODOROV, B. I. & S. V. REVENKO. 1979. Neuroscience **4:** 1315–1330.
38. FRENCH, R. J., J. F. WORLEY & B. K. KRUEGER. 1984. Biophys. J. **45:** 301–310.
39. GREEN, W. N., L. B. WEISS & O. S. ANDERSEN. 1984. Biophys. J. **45:** 168a
40. GARBER, S. S. & C. MILLER. 1985. J. Gen. Physiol. **86:** A14–A15.
41. ANDERSEN, O. S. & R. U. MULLER. 1982. J. Gen. Physiol. **80:** 403–426.
42. FARQUHAR, M. G. 1983. Methods Enzymol. **98:** 1–13.
43. LENNARZ, W. 1983. Methods Enzymol. **98:** 91–97.
44. MISHINA, M., T. TOBIMATSU, K. IMOTO, K. TANAKA, Y. FUJITA, K. FUKUDA, M. KURASAKI, H. TAKAHASHI, Y. MORIMOTO, T. HIROSES, S. INAYAMA, T. TAKAHASHI, M. KUNO & S. NUMA 1985. Nature **313:** 364–369.
45. THORNHILL, W. B. & S. R. LEVINSON. 1986. Biosynthesis of electroplax sodium channels. This volume.

Biochemistry of Sodium Channels from Mammalian Muscle

ROBERT L. BARCHI

Mahoney Institute of Neurological Sciences
University of Pennsylvania School of Medicine
Philadelphia, Pennsylvania 19104

Mammalian skeletal muscle, like most nerve and muscle cells, generates action potentials mainly through transient changes in the sodium conductance of its surface membranes. The voltage-sensitive sodium channel that controls these time- and potential-dependent currents has been isolated from the surface membranes of rat skeletal muscle and from the T-tubular membranes of rabbit skeletal muscle.[1-3] In its physiological and biophysical properties, this sodium channel closely resembles that found in most nerve membranes, and recent work suggests that this resemblance holds for many of the molecular properties of the isolated channel protein as well.[4]

MOLECULAR PROPERTIES OF THE ISOLATED MUSCLE CHANNEL

When solubilized in nonionic detergents such as NP-40 or Lubrol PX, the sodium channels from rat sarcolemma and rabbit T-tubular membranes are similar in overall molecular size ($\approx$300,000 MW) and Stokes radius (8.6 nm).[3,5] In its highly purified form, the rabbit T-tubular sodium channel contains one large glycoprotein of $\approx$260 kDa and one smaller subunit of 38 kDa (FIG. 1).[3] The sodium channel from rat sarcolemma is very susceptible to proteolytic cleavage during the isolation of the sarcolemmal membranes[2,6] and with standard purification methods the large subunit of this channel is obtained as a smaller fragment of 150 kDa.[7] This cleavage occurs during the isolation of the muscle sarcolemmal membrane fraction and has proved difficult to control even with complicated cocktails of protease inhibitors. More recently, we have used immunoaffinity purification techniques to isolate the sodium channel directly from whole rat muscle without the intervening preparation of sarcolemmal membranes.[6] With this approach, it can be shown that the rat sarcolemmal channel also contains a single large 260 kDa glycoprotein subunit as well as a smaller 38 kDa component. The latter is occasionally resolved as two distinct bands of 37 and 39 kDa.

The presence or absence of a small beta subunit of $\approx$38 kDa in preparations of the mammalian sodium channel has been a point of some controversy. We consistently see this subunit in rat and rabbit skeletal muscle isolated with standard biochemical techniques,[3,7] but this observation is open to criticism on the grounds that proteolysis might occur during the 36 h interval required for the isolation of membranes and the purification of the channel protein. We have used monoclonal antibodies directed against the rat sarcolemmal large subunit to address this question. These antibodies recognize the 260 kDa subunit of the channel in Western blots of total glycoproteins prepared from fresh skeletal muscle, but show no immunoreactivity with the 38 kDa subunit either in these preparations or in blots of the purified channel itself.

Antibodies recognizing the 260 kDa subunit were coupled to Sepharose and used as an immunoaffinity matrix to isolate the sodium channel under nondenaturing condi-

179

Mol. Wt.

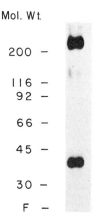

200 —

116 —
92 —

66 —

45 —

30 —

F —

FIGURE 1. Purified sodium channel from rabbit T-tubular membranes. In this preparation the 260 kDa α subunit is associated with a single diffuse band at 38 kDa. In other preparations (see FIG. 2) this broad 38 kDa band can be resolved as two bands of molecular weight 39 kDa and 37 kDa. SDS-PAGE had a 7% to 15% gradient. Proteins were iodinated prior to electrophoresis and visualized by autoradiography.[3]

tions from rat skeletal muscle homogenized directly in detergent and protease inhibitors. The protein complex that was specifically retained by this immunoaffinity column contained as expected the 260 kDa α subunit but invariably also contained either one broad band at 38 kDa or two closely spaced bands at 37 and 39 kDa[2] (FIG. 2). These small subunits coeluted with the 260 kDa subunit when gradients of thiocyanate were used to dissociate bound proteins from the antibody column. The 38 kDa protein must be tightly associated with the 260 kDa subunit in the muscle channel in order to remain attached to the antibody column during the extensive high ionic strength washes used to remove nonspecifically bound material. Our studies support the position that this 38 kDa component is a true subunit of the muscle sodium channel.

The 260 and 38 kDa subunits of the purified rabbit T-tubular sodium channel have

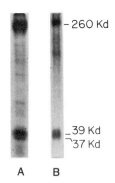

— 260 Kd

— 39 Kd
— 37 Kd

A   B

FIGURE 2. Comparison of sodium channel purified with immunoaffinity techniques from (A) rat skeletal muscle and (B) sodium channel purified with standard biochemical techniques from rabbit T-tubular membrane. For the rabbit channel, monoclonal antibodies directed against the 260 kDa subunit were immobilized on Sepharose and used as an immunoaffinity matrix to isolate the channel from a crude glycoprotein fraction prepared directly from whole skeletal muscle. In this example, two components of molecular weight 39 kDa and 37 kDa are resolved in the β region of both preparations.

been isolated separately under denaturing conditions and their chemical properties examined. Both are heavily glycosylated. The large subunit is 26% by weight carbohydrate; of this, the predominant sugars are N-acetylhexosamines (46%) and N-acetylneuraminic acid (34%).[8] The 38 kDa subunit is even more extensively glycosylated (32% by weight carbohydrate) with a higher percentage of sugar present as N-acetylhexosamines (71%). Again, N-acetylneuraminic acid constitutes most of the remainder (22%).

The rabbit 38 kDa subunit can be enzymatically deglycosylated by treatment with endoglycosidase F (Endo F), either alone or in conjunction with neuraminidase. Treatment with neuraminidase increases the mobility of the broad glycoprotein band but does not sharpen it appreciably. Treatment with the endoglycosidase produces a stepwise reduction in apparent molecular mass, the limit being a sharp band migrating at 26.5 kDa corresponding to the core polypeptide.[8] The 260 kDa subunit is less easily deglycosylated, but after treatment with neuraminidase and Endo F approaches an apparent mobility of ≈ 210 kDa on SDS-PAGE.

Amino acid analysis of both the large and small subunits of the rabbit channel has yielded no surprises. The overall amino acid compositions of both differ little from those of typical large soluble proteins and are comparable to analyses previously reported for the rat brain channel.[9] Both the 260 kDa subunit and the 38 kDa subunit are NH_2-terminally blocked.

The stoichiometry of the large and small subunits of the channel has been examined in both the immunoaffinity purified rat preparation and in the standard channel preparation from rabbit T-tubular membranes.[2,8] Isolated, purified α and β subunits from the rabbit channel were used to calibrate our gel system for relative labeling efficiency of the two proteins; in each case the absolute amount of protein was determined directly by total amino acid analysis rather than by colorometric or fluorometric assays relative to a standard protein. With the iodination procedure that we use for identifying proteins on SDS-PAGE, β subunit is more efficiently labeled than the α-subunit on a molar basis. Subsequent quantitation of autoradiograms of SDS-PAGE profiles of the purified channels yielded apparent subunit stoichiometries of 1:1 for the two subunits in both rat and rabbit muscle.

Although it is possible that the relative contribution of the β subunit(s) to the total channel complex is underestimated because of dissociation or degradation during the purification process, this stoichiometry suggests that the muscle channel may differ from the brain channel in regard to the number of small subunits associated with each large subunit.

FUNCTIONAL RECONSTITUTION OF THE MUSCLE CHANNEL

Both the rat sarcolemmal channel and the rabbit T-tubular channel have been functionally reconstituted into liposomes prepared from egg phosphatidylcholine.[3,10,11] Both purified channels gate the influx of monovalent cations in response to activation by veratridine or batrachotoxin, and in both cases these activated fluxes are specifically blocked by tetrodotoxin (TTX) or saxitoxin (STX). Pharmacological activation and block are produced by concentrations of these toxins that correspond to those that are active on the channel in its native environment. Of interest from a mechanistic point of view is the observation that activation with veratridine reaches a maximal level very rapidly, whereas batrachotoxin, although ultimately a more potent agonist, requires prolonged incubation to achieve full effect even with channels reconstituted into small vesicles.

By using an adaptation of classical quenched flow techniques, the relative rates of influx for various monovalent cations have been determined through the reconstituted rat and rabbit channels after activation by batrachotoxin and veratridine.[3,11] With batrachotoxin-activated channels, specific initial rates could be easily resolved for K^+, Rb^+, and Cs^+, and an upper limit ascribed to the initial influx rate for Na^+. For both the rat and the rabbit channels, the cation selectivity sequence and the relative influx rates were comparable, with a lower limit for the Na^+/K^+ selectivity of 0.15. Rb^+ and Cs^+ influx rates that were no greater than 0.02 and 0.005 respectively relative to that for Na^+, and the relative rates of influx for all cations were consistent with the conductance ratios measured for the muscle sodium channel in situ.

The rabbit T-tubular channel has also been successfully incorporated into planar lipid bilayers for single channel measurements by the fusion of liposomes containing the channel with a preformed bilayer in a teflon oriface. After exposure to batrachotoxin, single purified channels exhibited voltage-dependent activation over a narrow range of potentials with the half-maximal opening probabilities falling between -95 and -115 mV (FIG. 3).[12] The single channel conductance averaged 20 ± 1 pS and was independent of voltage over the range of -130 to -60 mV. Single conductance events were blocked by TTX applied to the appropriate side of the bilayer. Similar results have been obtained with the purified rat muscle channel using patch clamp of frozen-thawed liposomes.[13]

We have been able to confirm the presence of voltage-dependent activation in populations of purified rabbit T-tubular channels reconstituted into liposomes. In this approach, the randomly inserted channels were functionally oriented by trapping TTX within the vesicles during their formation in order to block inward-facing channels. Subsequent removal of external TTX by gel filtration allows outward-facing channels to function normally. A membrane potential was established in the vesicles with a potassium concentration gradient after rendering the membrane permselective to potassium with valinomycin, and the potential was rapidly changed by alteration of the external potassium concentration. In these experiments, all the channels that could be activated by batrachotoxin were also turned off with hyperpolarizing potentials and activated by depolarization (FIG. 4), confirming that the voltage dependence observed with the single channel measurements in planar bilayers was a characteristic of the population of purified channels and not of only a small fraction of the purified material.[12]

ANTIBODIES AND SODIUM CHANNEL LOCALIZATION

Monoclonal antibodies and polyclonal antisera have been prepared against the purified rat muscle sodium channel. These antibodies are being used to probe the channel's structure and to assist in channel localization at the light and electron microscopic level.

Monoclonal antibodies raised against the purified rat skeletal muscle sodium channel in its mixed micellar form have, to date, exclusively recognized epitopes on the 260 kDa subunit or on its 150 kDa proteolytic fragment.[6] No monoclonals have been found that bind only to the 38 kDa subunit on Western blots and none of the antibodies against the 260 kDa subunit cross-react with epitopes on the small subunit. Antibodies against the large subunit seem to recognize preferentially a limited number of sites on the basis of binding competition studies. Of 23 fully characterized antibodies, 18 fall into three groups each having overlapping binding characteristics. Antibodies in each of these groups appear to recognize epitopes that are spatially related on the quarternary structure of the channel protein.

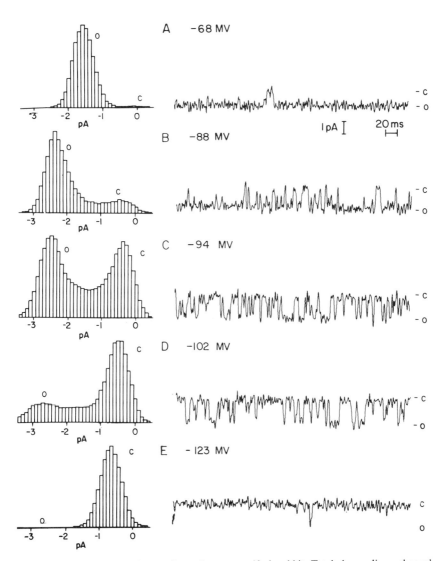

FIGURE 3. Single channel recordings from a purified rabbit T-tubular sodium channel reconstituted into a planar bilayer (see ref. 12 for details). A single channel is seen which activates abruptly between −100 and −90 mV. The single channel conductance in this example was 20 pS. Current histograms are shown in the left-hand column and representative current traces from the primary data on the right.

We have used immunocytochemical techniques and polyclonal and monoclonal antibodies against the channel to yield evidence of multiple sodium channel subtypes in mature rat skeletal muscle. For example, on immunofluorescence at the light microscopic level one group of antibodies recognizes sodium channels on the surface membrane of both fast and slow skeletal muscle fibers, but shows no staining of the T-tubular system. Another group of antibodies labels predominantly internal membranes in slow fibers but not in fast fibers within the same muscle. Electron immunocytochemistry confirms that this internal labeling is associated with the T-tubular system.[14,15]

Of interest is the fact that antibodies which recognize surface channels on muscle fibers detect high concentrations of channels at the endplate region of the neuromuscu-

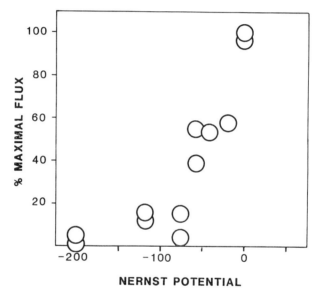

NERNST POTENTIAL

FIGURE 4. Sodium influx into vesicles containing purified rabbit T-tubular sodium channels activated by batrachotoxin. A potential was imposed across the vesicle membrane with a potassium concentration gradient in the presence of valinomycin. The batrachotoxin-activated sodium influx is voltage sensitive; influx is shut off by hyperpolarizing potentials and activated by depolarization.

lar junction. At the ultrastructural level, this staining is associated with all regions of the junctional folds and is not restricted to either the superficial or the deep regions of these structures.

Some of the antibodies that recognize mature muscle surface channels also stain the surface membranes of rat primary skeletal muscle in culture.[16] At the myoblast stage, this staining is patchy and unevenly distributed across the cell surface. As the myoblasts fuse to form myotubes, the staining becomes diffuse and homogeneous over the cell surface, decreasing in density only in the terminal portions where the myotubes spread to attach to the substrate. In the same preparations, antibodies that bind to the T-tubular membranes in the adult muscle show no staining of primary rat myoblasts. After fusion begins, selected myotubes show internal staining when their membranes are permeabilized with saponin. A few days after the completion of fusion, virtually all tubes demonstrate this internal staining pattern. It may be that these antibodies will provide insight into the development of the T-tubular elements in this culture system.

SUMMARY

Sodium channels from rat and rabbit skeletal muscle have been isolated, characterized, and functionally reconstituted. These channel proteins closely resemble those purified from the eel electroplax and from rat brain. Work now in progress on the determination of the primary sequence of the 260 kDa subunit through the cloning and sequencing of the muscle message should shed further light on the relationship between these unique voltage-sensitive sodium channels.

REFERENCES

1. BARCHI, R. L., S. A. COHEN & L. E. MURPHY. 1980. Proc. Natl. Acad. Sci. U. S. A. 77: 1306–1310.
2. CASADEI, J. M., R. D. GORDON & R. L. BARCHI. 1986. J. Biol. Chem. 261: 4318–4323
3. KRANER, S. D., J. C. TANAKA & R. L. BARCHI. 1985. J. Biol. Chem. 260: 6341–6347.
4. BARCHI, R. L. 1984. Trends Biochem. Sci. 9: 358–361.
5. BARCHI, R. L. & L. E. MURPHY. 1981. J. Neurochem. 36: 2097–2100.
6. CASADEI, J. M., R. D. GORDON, L. A. LAMPSON, D. S. SCHOTLAND & R. L. BARCHI. 1984. Proc. Natl. Acad. Sci. U. S. A. 81: 6227–6231.
7. BARCHI, R. L. 1983. J. Neurochem. 40: 1377–1388.
8. ROBERTS, R. & R. L. BARCHI. J. Biol. Chem. In press.
9. GRISHIN, E. V., V. A. KOVALENKO, V. N. PASHKOV & O. G. SHAMOTIENKO. 1984. Biological Membrane (U. S. S. R.). 1: 858–866.
10. WEIGELE, J. B. & R. L. BARCHI. 1982. Proc. Natl. Acad. Sci. U. S. A. 79: 3651–3655.
11. TANAKA, J. C., J. F. ECCLESTON & R. L. BARCHI. 1983. J. Biol. Chem. 258: 7519–7526.
12. FURMAN, R. E., J. C. TANAKA, P. MUELLER & R. L. BARCHI. 1986. Proc. Natl. Acad. Sci. U. S. A. 83: 488–492.
13. BARCHI, R. L., J. C. TANAKA & R. E. FURMAN. 1984. J. Cell. Biochem. 26: 135–146.
14. HAIMOVICH, B., E. BONILLA, J. CASADEI & R. BARCHI. 1984. J. Neurosci. 4: 2259–2268.
15. HAIMOVICH, B., D. SCHOTLAND & R. L. BARCHI. 1985. J. Cell. Biol. 101: 188a.
16. HAIMOVICH, B., A. HORWITZ & R. BARCHI. 1984. Biophys. J. 45: 182a.

Structure and Biosynthesis of Neuronal Sodium Channels

WILLIAM A. CATTERALL, JOHN W. SCHMIDT,
DONALD J. MESSNER, AND DANIEL J. FELLER

Department of Pharmacology
University of Washington
Seattle, Washington 98195

INTRODUCTION

Sodium channels in neurons initiate the conducted action potential at the axon initial segment and mediate its propagation along the axon to the nerve terminal. They are the pharmacological receptors for local anesthetics and certain anticonvulsant drugs as well as the molecular targets for tetrodotoxin, saxitoxin, and a wealth of other biological toxins. In the past decade, the sites of interaction of these several classes of neurotoxins with the sodium channel have been defined and these toxins have been used as molecular probes to identify, purify, and characterize the protein components of the sodium channel as described in this volume. Recent experiments have extended these studies to analysis of the biosynthesis and molecular biology of the sodium channel protein. This paper reviews experiments from our laboratory that have contributed to the emerging molecular view of neuronal sodium channels.

Neurotoxins as Molecular Probes of Sodium Channels

The neurotoxins that have been useful to date in revealing new aspects of sodium channel structure and function act at four separate receptor sites as outlined in TABLE 1. Assignment of toxins to these separate sites of action has been based upon assessment of competitive and synergistic interactions as analyzed in studies of neurotoxin binding and neurotoxin-activated $^{22}Na^+$ flux. These studies have been extensively reviewed.[1-4]

Neurotoxin receptor site 1 binds the water-soluble heterocyclic guanidines tetrodotoxin and saxitoxin. These toxins inhibit sodium channel ion transport by binding to a common receptor site that is thought to be located near the extracellular opening of the ion-conducting pore of the sodium channel, as discussed in other papers in this volume. In addition, neurotoxin receptor site 1 is the site of action of certain conotoxins, novel polypeptide toxins that preferentially block muscle sodium channels.[5,35]

Neurotoxin receptor site 2 binds several lipid-soluble toxins including grayanotoxin and the alkaloids veratridine, aconitine, and batrachotoxin. The competitive interactions of these four toxins at neurotoxin receptor site 2 that were first demonstrated in ion flux experiments have been confirmed by direct measurements of specific binding of ^3H-labeled batrachotoxinin A 20α-benzoate to sodium channels.[6] These toxins cause persistent activation of sodium channels at the resting membrane potential by blocking sodium channel inactivation and shifting the voltage dependence of the channel activation to more negative membrane potentials. Therefore, neurotoxin receptor site 2 is likely to be localized on a region of the sodium channel involved in voltage-dependent activation and inactivation.

Neurotoxin receptor site 3 binds polypeptide toxins purified from North African scorpion venoms or sea anemone nematocysts. These toxins slow or block sodium channel inactivation. They also enhance persistent activation of sodium channels by the lipid-soluble toxins acting at neurotoxin receptor site 2. The affinity for binding of ^{125}I-labeled derivatives of the polypeptide toxins to neurotoxin receptor site 3 is reduced by depolarization. These data indicate that neurotoxin receptor site 3 is located on the part of the sodium channel that is involved in coupling of activation to inactivation.

Neurotoxin receptor site 4 binds a new class of scorpion toxins that has also proved valuable in studies of sodium channels. Venom of the American scorpion *Centruroides sculpturatus* modifies sodium channel activation rather than inactivation. Pure toxins from several American scorpions have a similar action. These toxins bind to a new receptor site on the sodium channel and have been designated β scorpion toxins.

These several neurotoxins provide specific high affinity probes for distinct regions of the sodium channel structure. They have been used to study sodium channel function in intact excitable membranes, to identify and purify the protein components of sodium channels that bind these toxins, and to analyze their structural and functional properties.

TABLE 1. Neurotoxin Receptor Sites on the Sodium Channel

Site	Neurotoxin	Physiological Effect
1	tetrodotoxin saxitoxin geographutoxin	inhibit ion transport
2	veratridine batrachotoxin grayanotoxin aconitine	cause persistent activation
3	North African α scorpion toxins sea anemone toxins	slow inactivation
4	American β scorpion toxins	enhance activation

MOLECULAR PROPERTIES OF SODIUM CHANNEL

Identification of Polypeptide Components by Photoaffinity Labeling

Direct chemical identification of sodium channel components in situ was first achieved by specific covalent labeling of neurotoxin receptor site 3 with a photoreactive azidonitrobenzoyl derivative of the α scorpion toxin from *Leiurus quinquestriatus*. The photoreactive toxin derivative is allowed to bind specifically to sodium channels in the dark. Irradiation with ultraviolet light then chemically activates the arylazide group, which covalently reacts with the scorpion toxin receptor site on the sodium channel. Analysis of covalently labeled synaptosomes by polyacrylamide gel electrophoresis under denaturing conditions in sodium dodecyl sulfate (SDS) to separate synaptosomal proteins by size revealed specific covalent labeling of two polypeptides that were subsequently designated the α and β subunits of the sodium channel.[7] These proteins, as assessed by polyacrylamide gel electrophoresis in SDS, have molecular sizes of 260,000 Da and 36,000 Da, respectively.

The covalent labeling of these two polypeptides in synaptosomes was shown to be specific by inhibition by competition with excess unlabeled scorpion toxin or by blockade of voltage-dependent binding of scorpion toxin by membrane depolarization.[7]

The 260,000 Da α subunit of the sodium channel could also be covalently labeled with azidonitrobenzoyl scorpion toxin in electrically excitable neuroblastoma cells. In contrast, in mutant neuroblastoma cells that are neurotoxin-resistant and lack functional voltage-sensitive sodium channels, the 260,000 Da polypeptide corresponding to the α subunit is not present.[7,8] These data provided additional evidence for the specificity of photoaffinity labeling.

Specific labeling of both the α and β subunits by azidonitrobenzoyl scorpion toxin suggests that neurotoxin receptor site 3 is located near the contact regions of these two subunits such that azidonitrobenzoyl groups attached to different points on the toxin surface can react covalently with one or both nearby subunits. Evidence in favor of this conclusion has been derived from experiments with purified isomeric derivatives of azidonitrobenzoyl scorpion toxin.[9] Two different mono-substituted isomers of the toxin derivative were resolved by ion-exchange chromatography. As illustrated in FIGURE 1, one of these isomers preferentially labels the α subunit whereas the other preferentially

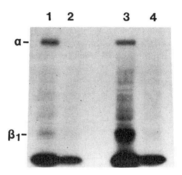

FIGURE 1. Specific photoaffinity labeling of the α and β1 subunits of the sodium channel by isomers of azidonitrobenzoyl scorpion toxin. Rat brain synaptosomes were prepared and covalently labeled as described (ref. 9) using 1 nM of isomer I in the absence (*lane 1*) or the presence (*lane 2*) of 200 nM unlabeled *Leiurus* scorpion toxin or using 1 nM of isomer II in the absence (*lane 3*) or presence (*lane 4*) of unlabeled *Leiurus* scorpion toxin. The labeled synaptosomes were dissolved in sodium dodecyl sulfate and β-mercaptoethanol; the labeled proteins were separated by polyacrylamide gel electrophoresis and detected by autoradiography.

labels the β subunit. Different regions of specifically bound scorpion toxin molecule must therefore be located within a few angstroms of appropriate reactive groups on the α and β subunits of the sodium channel, suggesting a role for both of these subunits in the binding of the toxin.

Subunits of membrane proteins are often damaged by proteolysis during solubilization and purification. Could the α and β subunits of the sodium channel have been derived from a larger native form? Identification of these subunits by covalent labeling in intact synaptosomes as described above makes this unlikely. Further evidence that these subunits are the native components of the sodium channel is derived from photoaffinity labeling of sodium channel subunits in freshly prepared brain homogenates.[9] Total brain particulate preparations were prepared at 4°C in the presence of 12 protease inhibitors and photoaffinity labeled within 45 minutes of sacrifice of the rat. The preparations were immediately denatured by boiling in sodium dodecyl sulfate and β-mercaptoethanol and resolved by gel electrophoresis. The α and β1 subunits were clearly identified under these conditions, indicating that they are components of the sodium channel in situ.

Molecular Size of the Neuronal Sodium Channel

The molecular size of the intact sodium channel protein has been measured by hydrodynamic studies of the detergent-solubilized channel. The saxitoxin and tetrodotoxin binding component of sodium channels was solubilized with retention of high affinity and specificity of toxin binding by treatment with nonionic detergents such as Triton X-100.[10]

In contrast to the ease of solubilization of the sodium channel with retention of saxitoxin and tetrodotoxin binding activity at neurotoxin receptor site 1, both neurotoxin receptor site 2 and neurotoxin receptor site 3 lose their high affinity neurotoxin binding activity on solubilization.[10] The molecular size of the solubilized sodium channel from rat brain has been estimated by hydrodynamic studies to be 601,000 Da.[11] Since the detergent-channel complex contains 0.9 g of Triton X-100 and phosphatidylcholine per gram of protein, the size of the sodium channel protein solubilized from rat brain is 316,000 Da.[11] This represents the size of the entire sodium channel as solubilized in detergents and corresponds to a complex of three nonidentical protein subunits as described below. If the channel protein is spherical in shape, the diameter indicated by these results is 118 Å. Thus the channel protein is much larger than the postulated transmembrane pore through which Na^+ moves, which is proposed to be 3 by 5 Å at its narrowest point, the ion selectivity filter.[12]

Protein Subunits of the Purified Sodium Channel from Mammalian Brain

The ability to solubilize the sodium channel from brain membranes in a well-defined monomeric form with retention of binding activity for saxitoxin and tetrodotoxin has allowed purification by a sequence of conventional protein separation procedures.[13-15] The current purification scheme developed in this laboratory consists of anion exchange chromatography on DEAE-Sephadex, adsorption chromatography on hydroxylapatite gel, affinity chromatography on wheat germ agglutinin covalently attached to Sepharose 4B, and velocity sedimentation through sucrose gradients.[15] The purified sodium channel preparation binds 0.9 mole of saxitoxin per mole of sodium channel of 316,000 Da. If the sodium channel binds only one saxitoxin molecule, these data indicate that at least 90% of the protein in the purified preparation must be associated with the sodium channel.

Analysis of the purified sodium channel preparation by gel electrophoresis in sodium dodecyl sulfate and β-mercaptoethanol reveals three protein subunits: α of 260 kDa, β1 of 36 kDa, and β2 of 33 kDa (FIGURE 2[13-16]). Comparison of SDS gels of samples denatured with or without reduction of disulfide bonds by β-mercaptoethanol shows that the α and β2 subunits are covalently linked through disulfide bonds as illustrated diagrammatically in FIGURE 2.[14,16] The three polypeptides quantitatively comigrate as a complex under native conditions.[13-15] They appear to be present in 1:1:1 stoichiometry,[14,15] to give a complex with a total size of 329 kDa in close agreement with the oligomeric size of 316 kDa estimated from hydrodynamic studies[11] as summarized in TABLE 2.

Unlike the α and β1 subunits, β2 subunits are not covalently labeled by scorpion toxin derivatives. Analysis of covalently labeled synaptosomes or freshly prepared brain homogenates by SDS gel electrophoresis with or without reduction of disulfide

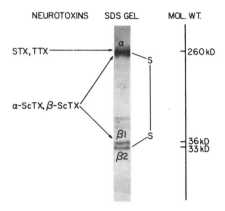

FIGURE 2. Properties of the sodium channel subunits. Purified sodium channels were depolymerized in sodium dodecyl sulfate and β-mercaptoethanol and the subunits were resolved by polyacrylamide gel electrophoresis as described (ref. 16). Molecular weights, intersubunit disulfide bonds, and sites of covalent labeling by neurotoxins are illustrated.

bonds with β-mercaptoethanol, however, reveals the presence of the disulfide-linked β2 subunit as a decrease of 30 kDa in the apparent molecular weight of the photoaffinity labeled α subunit upon reduction of disulfide bonds to β2.[9] Thus, a complex of α, β1, and β2 subunits is present in intact synaptosomes and native brain membranes as well as in purified sodium channel preparations.

The β1 and β2 subunits are similar in size but differ in several other respects. β2 is disulfide-linked to α whereas β1 is not; β1 is photoaffinity labeled by scorpion toxin derivatives and β2 is not. Finally, limited proteolytic maps of the two subunits using four different proteases show characteristic differences.[16] Considered together, these properties indicate that the β1 and β2 subunits are distinct polypeptide subunits of similar size.

Posttranslational Modification of the Neuronal Sodium Channel

Membrane proteins are often covalently modified after biosynthesis of their polypeptide chains. Glycosylation at asparagine residues and proteolytic cleavage accompany insertion into membranes and transport to the cell surface. Phosphorylation by specific protein kinase is a common mediator of cellular regulatory process. The sodium channel for rat brain is specifically adsorbed and eluted from chromatographic columns containing immobilized wheat germ agglutinin, a carbohydrate-binding protein with specificity for N-acetylglucosamine and sialic acid residues in

TABLE 2. Subunits of the Purified Sodium Channel

Component	Native Mol. Weight	Carbohydrate-Free Mol. Weight	Probable Stoichiometry
native complex	316,000		
α	260,000	220,000	1.0
β1	36,000	22,000	1.0
β2	33,000	21,000	1.0

glycoproteins.[13] These results indicate that the sodium channel is a glycoprotein. Further analyses have shown that all three of the subunits of the sodium channel from rat brain are glycosylated. They bind wheat germ agglutinin after separation by SDS gel electrophoresis.[16] Their apparent molecular weights are reduced by hydrolysis of carbohydrate residues with HF or trifluoromethane sulfonic acid or by enzymatic cleavage with neuraminidase and endoglycosidase F under conditions where no proteolysis occurs.[16] The apparent molecular weights of the three subunits following removal of carbohydrate (TABLE 2) indicate that the native α, $\beta 1$ and $\beta 2$ subunits are 20%, 36%, and 36% carbohydrate by weight.[16]

There is no evidence at present of an essential role of the carbohydrate moieties in the function of sodium channels in neuronal surface membranes. Blockade of protein glycosylation with the specific inhibitor tunicamycin, however, reduces the level of functional sodium channels in cultured neuroblastoma cells to less than 20% of control levels.[17] These results indicate that glycosylation is required for the normal biosynthesis, membrane insertion, and maintenance of functional sodium channels in neural cells.

Protein phosphorylation is one of the most important mechanisms of cellular regulation[18] and has been implicated in the long-term regulation of neuronal excitability.[19] The rat brain sodium channel is also modified by phosphorylation and dephosphorylation. The purified sodium channel is phosphorylated at four sites on the α subunit by cyclic-AMP dependent protein kinase added *in vitro*.[20] Kinetic analysis of the rate and extent of phosphorylation indicates that the sodium channel is a physiological substrate for cyclic-AMP-dependent protein kinase. Similarly, sodium channels in purified preparations and in synaptosomal surface membranes are phosphorylated by the calcium-activated, phospholipid-dependent protein kinase at multiple sites, some of which are different from those phosphorylated by cAMP-dependent protein kinase.[21]

The development of specific antiserum to the purified sodium channel has allowed measurement of phosphorylation of the α subunit of the sodium channel in intact synaptic nerve ending particles (synaptosomes). We found that addition of the 8-bromo derivative of cyclic AMP causes complete phosphorylation of the sodium channel in synaptosomes in 15 seconds.[22] Phosphorylation occurred at the same sites that were phosphorylated on the α subunit of the purified sodium channel.[22] These results show that the sodium channel is phosphorylated in situ in nerve terminals when intracellular cyclic AMP increases. Phosphorylation is associated with a decrease in the maximum rate of toxin-activated $^{22}Na^+$ influx and possibly a small increase in the concentration of neurotoxins required for half-maximal activation.[22] These results indicate that phosphorylation reduces persistent activation of sodium channels by neurotoxins. Electrophysiological experiments are required to determine whether this reflects either a reduced probability of sodium channel activation or an increased probability of inactivation by membrane depolarization. Small changes in the voltage dependence of either of these channel functions would be expected to have important effects on the threshold and frequency of action potential generation in neurons and on the extent of impulse-induced release of neurotransmitters from nerve terminals. Such changes may serve to modulate the response of neurons to their synaptic inputs on a long-term basis.

Topology of Sodium Channel Subunits

A number of lines of evidence indicate that the α subunit of the sodium channel is exposed to the extracellular environment: it is glycosylated[16] and it is covalently labeled by photoreactive scorpion toxin derivatives[7,9] which act only on the extracellular side of the channel. The α subunit is also exposed on the intracellular side of the membrane since it is phosphorylated on four sites by cAMP-dependent protein kinase within intact synaptosomes[21] and intact brain neurons in cell culture.[1] Thus, the α subunit is a transmembrane polypeptide. Its size allows numerous membrane-spanning segments.

Both the $\beta1$ and $\beta2$ subunits of the sodium channel appear to be exposed at the extracellular surface. Each is heavily glycosylated with more than 30% of the apparent mass made up of carbohydrate.[22] The $\beta1$ subunit is composed of covalently labeled scorpion toxin derivates which act on the extracellular surface of the sodium channel.[7,9] These two subunits have not been shown to be exposed at the intracellular surface. Since their protein mass is small (23 kDa and 21 kDa, respectively) and much of their mass must be extracellular to accommodate attachment of carbohydrate, they may not have major regions which protrude to the cytoplasmic surface of the membrane.

RECONSTITUTION OF SODIUM CHANNEL FUNCTION FROM PURIFIED COMPONENTS

The purified sodium channel preparations bind [³H]saxitoxin and tetrodotoxin with the same affinity as the native sodium channel and therefore contain neurotoxin receptor site 1 of the sodium channel in an active form. The purified channel also contains the α and $\beta1$ subunits that were identified as components of neurotoxin receptor site 3 by photoaffinity labeling with scorpion toxin, although after solubilization the binding activity for scorpion toxin is lost. Purified channels do not, however, have binding activity for neurotoxins at receptor site 2 and cannot transport sodium in the detergent-solubilized state. Reconstitution of these sodium channel functions from purified components is the only rigorous proof that the proteins identified and purified on the basis of their neurotoxin binding activity are indeed sufficient to form a functional voltage-sensitive ion channel. In addition, successful reconstitution will provide a valuable experimental preparation for biochemical analysis of the structure and function of sodium channels.

Neurotoxin-activated Ion Flux

Sodium channel ion transport was first successfully reconstituted from sodium channels substantially purified from rat brain and skeletal muscle.[23,24] We have now applied these methods to essentially homogeneous preparations of sodium channels from rat brain.[25] Purified sodium channels in Triton X-100 solution are supplemented with phosphatidylcholine dispersed in Triton X-100, and the detergent is removed by adsorption to polystyrene beads. As the detergent is removed, phosphatidylcholine vesicles with a mean diameter of 1800 Å are formed containing an average of 0.75 to 2 sodium channels per vesicle. The functional activities of the sodium channel can then be assessed in neurotoxin binding and ion flux experiments.

The time course of $^{22}Na^+$ influx into phosphatidylcholine vesicles containing purified sodium channels from rat brain is illustrated in FIGURE 3. The vesicle preparation was incubated for 2 minutes with veratridine to activate sodium channels and then diluted into medium containing $^{22}Na^+$ to give an outward-oriented Na^+ gradient which enhances $^{22}Na^+$ accumulation and slows the approach to equilibrium. Influx into vesicles under control conditions was slow. Incubation with veratridine increased the initial rate of influx 10 to 15 times. When tetrodotoxin was present in both the intravesicular and extravesicular phases, the veratridine-dependent increase in initial rate of ^{22}Na$^+$ influx was nearly completely blocked. Half-maximal activation was observed with 28 μM veratridine and half-maximal inhibition with 14 nM tetrodotoxin, in close agreement with the corresponding values for the action of these toxins on native sodium channels. These results show that the purified sodium channel regains the ability to mediate neurotoxin-stimulated ion flux after incorporation into phosphatidylcholine vesicles. Evidently, the purified channel retains neurotoxin receptor site 2 and the ion-conducting pore of the sodium channel.

The above results show that at least some of the sodium channels in our most highly purified preparations can mediate selective neurotoxin-activated ion transport after incorporation into phospholipid vesicles. We have attempted to estimate how many of

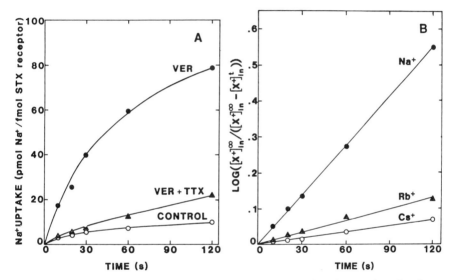

FIGURE 3. Neurotoxin-activated ion flux mediated by purified and reconstituted sodium channels. Sodium channels were purified from rat brain as described in ref. 15 and incorporated into single-walled phosphatidylcholine vesicles as described in ref. 25. (**A**) Reconstituted vesicles were incubated for the indicated times in the absence of neurotoxins (O), in the presence of 100 μM veratridine (●), or in the presence of 100 μM tetrodotoxin both inside and outside of the vesicles (▲) and ^{22}Na$^+$ influx was measured as described in ref. 25. (**B**) Veratridine-stimulated ion flux was measured as in **A** with ^{22}Na$^+$, ^{86}Rb$^+$, or ^{137}Cs$^+$ as the permeant cation.

the reconstituted sodium channels contribute to our ion flux measurements. First, the ion transport rates in purified and reconstituted sodium channel preparations were compared to those of veratridine-activated sodium channels in neuroblastoma cells and synaptosomes.[25] This comparison shows that the transport rate measured in ions per minute per saxitoxin receptor site is 33% to 70% of that in native membranes, suggesting that at least 33% to 70% of the reconstituted sodium channels are active. Second, we have compared the proportion of vesicles that contain sodium channels to the proportion of vesicles whose internal volume is accessible to veratridine-activated sodium channels. If sodium channels are distributed among vesicles according to a Poisson distribution, this comparison leads to a range of 30% to 70% for the fraction of active channels, depending on whether active vesicles containing more than one channel are assumed to have one active channel or all active channels. Both of these estimates indicate that a minimum of 30% of the reconstituted sodium channels are active. Since the sodium channel preparation is 90% pure and no single contaminant composes as much as 2% of the protein, we conclude that the purified complex of α, $\beta1$, and $\beta2$ is sufficient to mediate selective neurotoxin-activated ion flux.

Voltage-Dependent Scorpion Toxin Binding

Although sodium channels reconstituted into phosphatidylcholine vesicles can transport sodium, these channels do not bind α-scorpion toxin at neurotoxin receptor site 3.[25] In contrast, if purified sodium channels are incorporated into vesicles composed of a mixture of phosphatidylcholine and brain lipids, scorpion toxin binding is recovered.[25] The toxin binding reaction is of high affinity (K_d = 57 nM) and a mean of 0.76 ± 0.08 mole of scorpion toxin is bound per mole of purified sodium channel. In order to determine which phospholipids in the brain lipid fraction are required for restoration of scorpion toxin binding, purified sodium channels were reconstituted into vesicles composed of phosphatidylcholine and different individual brain lipids. Phosphatidylethanolamine and phosphatidylserine, the other two major lipids of brain plasma membranes, were found to enhance high affinity binding of scorpion toxin to the purified sodium channel in reconstituted phosphatidylcholine vesicles to a similar extent as brain lipid when added at levels comparable to those in synaptic plasma membranes. Optimum restoration of toxin binding was obtained with 35% to 50% phosphatidylethanolamine and 20% to 40% phosphatidylserine (FIGURE 4 and ref. 26). Phosphatidylethanolamine restored toxin binding more effectively at all ratios tested and further addition of phosphatidylserine to vesicles having an optimum ratio of

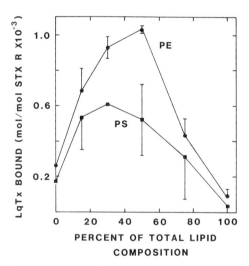

FIGURE 4. Phospholipid dependence of reconstitution of voltage-dependent scorpion toxin binding. Purified sodium channels were incorporated into phospholipid vesicles composed of phosphatidylcholine and the indicated ratios of phosphatidylserine (*PS*) or phosphatidylethanolamine (*PE*). Specific binding of ^{125}I-labeled *Leiurus* scorpion toxin and [3H]saxitoxin was then measured as described (ref. 26).

TABLE 3. Voltage Dependence of Scorpion Toxin Binding to Purified and Reconstituted Sodium Channels

$[Na^+]out/[Na^+]in$	Voltage (mV)	^{125}I-labeled LqTx Bound (mol/mol × 10^{-3})
0.07	−70	3.31
0.15	−50	2.27
0.32	−30	1.32
1	0	0.87

phosphatidylethanolamine to phosphatidylcholine did not improve scorpion toxin binding. Minor brain lipids including sphingomyelin, gangliosides, and cholesterol did not increase scorpion toxin binding when added at levels similar to those in synaptic plasma membranes. Thus, incorporation of purified sodium channels into phospholipid vesicles with an appropriate ratio of phosphatidylethanolamine and phosphatidylcholine is sufficient to satisfy the lipid requirement for high affinity binding of scorpion toxin.

Binding of α-scorpion toxins to sodium channels in intact neuronal membranes is voltage-dependent with K_d values in the range of 1 to 2 nM at resting membrane potentials of −40 to −50 mV. If a membrane potential of −50 mV is generated by diluting reconstituted vesicles containing 135 mM Na^+ into Na^+-free choline medium to give a 10-fold outward sodium gradient, scorpion toxin binding is increased three-fold at 0.5 to 2 min after dilution but then decays back to the value in the absence of a Na^+ gradient over 30 to 60 min.[26] Measurements of membrane potential show that it follows a similar time course, indicating that the increase in scorpion toxin binding caused by the Na^+ gradient is due to the potential generated. More stable membrane potentials can be generated by dilution into a sucrose-substituted Na^+-free medium. TABLE 3 illustrates the results obtained when the concentration of Na^+ within the vesicles is varied during reconstitution and the resulting vesicles are diluted to a constant final concentration of 13.5 mM Na^+ outside. Binding of scorpion toxin is progressively reduced as the membrane potential changes from −60 to 0 mV, consistent with an increase in K_d upon depolarization. At −60 mV, the K_d is 1.9 nM, in close agreement with values measured in intact synaptosomes or neuroblastoma cells. These results show that the purified sodium channel mediates high affinity, voltage-dependent binding of scorpion toxin when incorporated into phospholipid vesicles of appropriate composition. Because the voltage dependence of scorpion toxin binding is closely correlated with the voltage dependence of activation of sodium channels,[2] these data indicate that the purified channels retain voltage-dependent gating as well as selective ion transport. Thus the purified sodium channel preparation from rat brain consisting of a stoichiometric complex of the α, $\beta1$, and $\beta2$ subunits is sufficient to mediate most of the functions of the sodium channel that can be measured biochemically.

Single Channel Recording of Purified Sodium Channels

In excitable membranes, sodium channels are normally activated and inactivated by changes in membrane potential. Electrical recording of sodium conductance mediated by the purified sodium channel on the ms time scale is required to demonstrate the full functional integrity of the sodium channel. In order to record ionic currents mediated by single purified sodium channels, reconstituted phospholipid vesicles of phosphatidylcholine and phosphatidylethanolamine containing purified sodium channels were incorporated into planar phospholipid bilayer membranes by vesicle fusion and single channel currents were recorded under voltage clamp in collaboration with Drs. Robert Hartshorne, Bernard Keller, and Mauricio Montal of the University of California at San Diego.[27] These results, described by R. Hartshorne in another paper of this volume,[36] show that the purified sodium channel from rat brain retains all the functional properties of native sodium channels.

Functional Properties of Subunit-Deficient Sodium Channel Complexes

The next phase of analysis of sodium channel function by resolution and reconstitution is to develop methods for selective dissociation of $\beta1$ and $\beta2$ subunits and determination of the functional properties of such subunit-deficient complexes. Incubation of purified sodium channels at 0°C in Triton X-100 solutions of high ionic strength causes dissociation of the $\beta1$ subunit.[28] Dissociation is accompanied by a stoichiometric loss of high affinity binding of saxitoxin (ref. 28 and TABLE 4). Thus, the state of the sodium channel having high affinity for saxitoxin and tetrodotoxin may require noncovalent association of the α and $\beta1$ subunits. If this interpretation is correct, tetrodotoxin and saxitoxin should stabilize the complex of α and $\beta1$ subunits against dissociation through free energy coupling. As expected, tetrodotoxin (10 μM) prevents dissociation of the α and $\beta1$ subunits in 1.0 M $MgCl_2$ and prevents loss of high affinity saxitoxin binding (TABLE 4). Evidently, a complex of α and $\beta1$ subunits is required for maintenance of a sodium channel state having high affinity for tetrodotoxin and saxitoxin.

The $\beta2$ subunit of the sodium channel can be specifically dissociated by reduction of intersubunit disulfide bonds with dithiothreitol at physiological ionic strength in the presence of tetrodotoxin to stabilize the noncovalent $\alpha\beta1$ complex.[28] In contrast to results with the $\beta1$ subunit, dissociation of $\beta2$ subunits has no effect on saxitoxin binding (TABLE 4). Thus it appears that $\beta2$ subunits are not required for high affinity saxitoxin binding.

In recent preliminary experiments, we have examined the functional properties of these subunit-deficient complexes in reconstituted phospholipid vesicles (Messner and Catterall, unpublished). As for saxitoxin binding, $\alpha\beta1$ complexes are fully functional in mediating neurotoxin stimulated ion flux whereas $\alpha\beta2$ complexes are not functional. These data point to a critical role for the $\beta1$ subunit, but not the $\beta2$ subunit, in establishing and maintaining the functional state of the purified neuronal sodium channel.

BIOSYNTHESIS OF THE NEURONAL SODIUM CHANNEL

The sodium channel in rat brain is a heterotrimeric complex of three glycoprotein subunits and the α and $\beta2$ subunits are linked by disulfide bonds. The three subunits must therefore undergo several steps of posttranslational processing before a structurally mature sodium channel can be produced. Initial evidence for the importance of these posttranslational processing events has been derived from studies of the effects of tunicamycin on sodium channel levels in cultured neuroblastoma cells.[17] Inhibition of N-linked protein glycosylation with tunicamycin reduces the level of functional sodium channels as measured by saxitoxin binding to less than 20% of normal in 48 hours of treatment. The number of saxitoxin binding sites is reduced with a half-life of 18 to 22 hours, suggesting that the mature sodium channels present on the cell surface before treatment with tunicamycin have a half-life in this range.

TABLE 4. Role of β1 and β2 Subunits in Saxitoxin Binding

Treatment	Percent Recovery		Saxitoxin Binding
	β1	β2	
None	100	100	100
1.0 M MgCl$_2$	8	96	2
1.0 M MgCl$_2$ + 10 mM TTX	92	98	89
1.65 mM DTT + 10 mM TTX	89	12	82

More recently, the biosynthesis and precursor forms of the sodium channel in primary cultures of embryonic rat brain neurons have been studied with isotopic labeling methods and specific antisera directed primarily against the α subunits.[29,30] Labeling of the entire sodium channel population of rat brain neurons with [γ-^{32}P]ATP and cAMP-dependent protein kinase followed by immunoprecipitation reveals that approximately two-thirds of the α subunits in these cells, and in neonatal rat brain *in vivo*, are not linked to β2 subunits by disulfide bonds.[29] Further analysis showed that these free α subunits are full-sized, membrane-associated, and have complex carbohydrate chains like mature α subunits. However, they are located in the intracellular compartment and are inactive in binding saxitoxin. Free α subunits are not observed in adult rat brain. Thus, it was proposed that they form an inactive reserve of sodium channels for incorporation into the cell surface during periods of rapid membrane assembly in development.[29]

The first form of the newly synthesized α subunits, detected after a 5 min pulse of [^{35}S]methionine, has an apparent size of 224 kDa.[30] In the presence of tunicamycin to block cotranslational glycosylation, the newly synthesized α polypeptide is 203 kDa.[30] The amino acid sequence of the α subunit does not reveal a cleavable hydrophobic leader sequence (see below). Consistent with this, the size of this initial translation product increases progressively during further processing. The time course of the intermediates in this process is illustrated in FIGURE 5. Over 2 hours, this initial precursor undergoes a single-step increase in apparent size to 250 kDa followed by a slow increase to the mature apparent size of 260 kDa. During this time, the

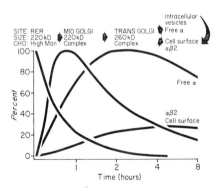

FIGURE 5. Time course of biosynthesis and processing of the α subunit. Primary cultures of rat brain neurons were incubated with [^{35}S]methionine for 30 min and then in medium containing excess unlabeled methionine for the times indicated. Newly synthesized α subunits were isolated by immunoprecipitation with affinity purified polyclonal antibodies, resolved by SDS gel electrophoresis, and quantitated by autoradiography and liquid scintillation counting. The smooth curves drawn represent a fit by eye to a composite of data from several separate experiments.

carbohydrate chains are processed to give complex structures containing N-acetylgly-cosamine and sialic acid as indicated by binding to the carbohydrate binding protein wheat germ agglutinin.[30] After 1 h, newly synthesized α subunits begin to be linked to $\beta2$ subunits by disulfide bonds and this process continues for approximately 8 h until an average maximum of one-third of the newly synthesized α subunits have been linked to $\beta2$ subunits.[30] Only α subunits disulfide-linked to $\beta2$ subunits appear on the cell surface, suggesting that disulfide bond formation is a late event in sodium channel processing and assembly. Since two-thirds of newly synthesized α subunits do not form a disulfide bond with $\beta2$ and remain in an inactive intracellular pool, it appears that posttranslational processing and assembly are rate-limiting steps in biosynthesis of functional cell surface sodium channels in developing brain neurons.

STRUCTURAL MODELS FOR SODIUM CHANNEL FUNCTION

Topographical Model of the Sodium Channel Subunits

Data summarized above indicate that the α subunit is a transmembrane polypeptide, whereas the $\beta1$ and $\beta2$ subunits are present at the extracellular surface but perhaps not at the intracellular surface. Since dimeric $\alpha\beta1$ and $\alpha\beta2$ complexes can be isolated as described above, the primary contacts among these three subunits must be $\beta1$-α-$\beta2$. These experimental observations are summarized in the form of a topographical model illustrating the disposition of the sodium channel polypeptides across the membrane (FIGURE 6, top).

Primary Structure of the α Subunit

The availability of highly purified, functional preparations of sodium channels from rat brain has provided the necessary tools to undertake the isolation of cDNA clones encoding the primary structure of protein components of the sodium channel. Specific antisera directed primarily against the α subunit of the sodium channel were used to identify cDNA clones in a library of mRNA transcripts from membrane-bound polysomes of neonatal rat brain in the bacteriophage expression vector λ gt11.[31] Clones which reacted specifically with the antibodies were used to identify additional clones by hybridization. The nucleotide sequence of a series of these clones has now been determined and the corresponding amino acid sequence representing approximately 90% of the α subunit of the sodium channel has been deduced and compared with the sequence of the sodium channel from electric eel electroplax defined by Noda *et al.*[32] The overall amino acid sequences of these two molecules are approximately 60% homologous.

As for the electroplax sodium channel, homology matrix comparison of the deduced sequence reveals the presence of four internal repeated domains of approximately 250 residues having greater than 50% homology in the sequence from rat brain. This high degree of sequence homology is strong evidence that these four domains arose from a common ancestor by gene duplication and that they adopt similar secondary structures in pseudosymmetric orientations in the channel structure.

The amino acid sequence of the α subunit also supports the view that it is a transmembrane polypeptide with multiple membrane-spanning segments. Analysis of the repeated domains for hydropathy and probable secondary structure indicate that each contains six regions of predicted α helix named S1 through S6 by Noda *et al.*[32] S5 and S6 are completely hydrophobic in all four domains and therefore are assigned as transmembrane segments. S1 and S2 contain occasional charged residues but are still sufficiently hydrophobic to warrant tentative designation as transmembrane segments. S3 and S4 are more hydrophilic. Segment S4 contains unique sequences of 22 to 32 residues in which repeated positively charged amino acids are separated by 2 or 3 hydrophobic residues. These are the most highly conserved regions of the α subunit with essentially complete homology between rat brain and eel electroplax.

Formation of a Transmembrane Pore

All of the highly hydrophobic segments of the sodium channel α subunit which are likely to be membrane-spanning segments are located in the four homologous domains of the polypeptide.[31,32] Thus it is probable that these four homologous domains form a pseudosymmetric array of homologous transmembrane structural units of the sodium channel. Noda *et al.*[32] proposed that the transmembrane pore of the sodium channel is formed in the center of this array of transmembrane units, with each domain contributing one-quarter of the wall of the channel. The strong retention of this domain structure in the α subunit of the rat brain sodium channel suggests that it too may form a transmembrane pore in the center of a square array of structurally homologous units. This proposal is illustrated diagrammatically in FIGURE 6 (bottom).

A Sliding Helix Model of Voltage-Dependent Gating

Activation of the sodium channel is considered to be a voltage-driven conformational change in which the equivalent of approximately six positive charges in the channel structure move outward across the membrane permeability barrier or a larger number of charges move a shorter distance across the membrane. The movement of protein-bound charge gives rise to gating current.[33] The requirement for such large charge movements within the sodium channel protein focuses attention on the four highly conserved positively charged S4 segments of the homologous domains of the sodium channel. Noda *et al.*[32] suggested that these regions might be involved in channel gating. Their topological model, however, placed these segments on the cytoplasmic side of the membrane where they would be little affected by the membrane electrical field and no specific suggestions of gating mechanism were made. Based upon their unique structure and the high degree of homology between electroplax and brain, we have proposed that these α helical segments span the membrane and function as voltage sensors in responding to changes in membrane potential with an outward movement which transfers gating charge across the membrane and initiates conformational changes leading to activation.[34]

The requirement for movement of six charges across the membrane places critical restraints upon the underlying structural mechanisms. Mechanisms in which individual amino acid residues are translocated all the way across the permeability barrier seem excluded. Mechanisms in which full charge transfer is postulated to result from simultaneous neutralization of one positive charge at the inner membrane surface and exposure of a different positive charge at the extracellular surface are plausible. For these mechanisms, a process by which simultaneous charge exposure and neutralization is coupled to protein conformational change must be proposed. The structural features of the S4 segments of the sodium channel seem well designed for such a charge transfer model.

In considering how gating charge might be transferred across the membrane, Armstrong[33] suggested a model in which each gating element contains a row of paired positive and negative charges that extends across the membrane and acts as a charge transfer mechanism. Changes in electric field cause translocation of the negative charges relative to the positive charges resulting in loss of a positive charge on the intracellular side of the protein and appearance of a positive charge on the extracellular side. Full charge translocation is thus achieved without movement of individual charged species fully across the bilayer. If the segments S4 are postulated to span the membrane, this helix forms a rigid structural element placing positive charges at regular intervals across the permeability barrier (FIGURE 7). Negative charges from other regions of the protein structure are postulated to form ion pairs with each of the positive charges of the helices. FIGURE 7 illustrates a hypothetical voltage-sensing element. Depolarization alters the electrical force on the intramembranous charges

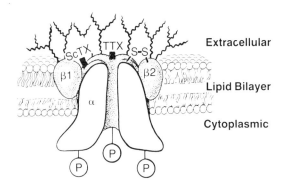

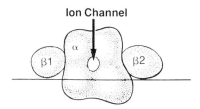

FIGURE 6. Structural model of the sodium channel.

causing negative charges to move inward and positive charges to move outward. An outward spiral movement of the α-helix with respect to the array of negative charges causes an exchange of ion pair partners and creates an unneutralized positive charge in the extracellular compartment and an unneutralized negative charge in the intracellular compartment for a gating charge movement of $+1$. Movement of amino acid residues over similar distances have been observed in studies of conformational changes in much smaller proteins and therefore seem plausible. This movement of the S4 α-helix then initiates a conformational change in its domain as one step in channel activation.

Activation of the sodium channel follows a sigmoidal time course indicating that the channel protein must pass through multiple (at least three) nonconducting states

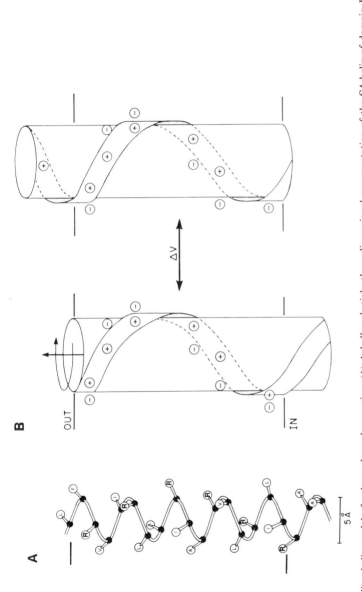

FIGURE 7. A sliding helix model of voltage-dependent gating. (A) A ball-and-stick, three-dimensional representation of the S4 helix of domain IV. *Darkened circles* represent the α-carbon of each amino acid residue. *Open circles* show the direction of projection of the side chain of each residue away from the core of the helix. Nonpolar residues are illustrated in thin letters by their single letter code: *F,* Phe; *A,* Ala; *I,* Ileu; *L,* Leu; *V,* Val. Positively charged amino acids are illustrated in bold letters: *R,* Arg. (B) The spiral path made by the positively charged arginine residues is illustrated in the form of a ribbon wrapped around the central core of the helix. *Right,* Movement of the S4 helix in response to membrane depolarization. The proposed transmembrane S4 helix is illustrated as a cylinder with a spiral ribbon of positive charge. At the resting membrane potential *(left),* all positively charged residues are paired with fixed negative charges on other transmembrane segments of the channel and the transmembrane segment is held in that position by the negative internal membrane potential. Depolarization reduces the force holding the positive charges in their inward position. The S4 helix is then proposed to undergo spiral motion through a rotation of approximately 60° and an outward displacement of approximately 5 Å. This movement leaves an unpaired negative charge on the inward surface of the membrane and reveals an unpaired positive charge on the outward surface to give a net charge transfer of +1.

before channel activation.[33] Analysis of gating current data suggests there are five transitions before activation occurs and the last requires movement of twice as much gating charge.[33] If each of the four homologous domains contains a voltage-sensing element analogous to that in FIGURE 7 and undergoes an independent voltage-driven conformational change, a sequence of four changes of state is expected before activation. The *sliding helix* model of voltage-sensing therefore provides a mechanism to connect the sigmoid time course of channel activation with the presence of four homologous domains.

Movement of six positive charges outward through the membrane permeability barrier accompanies activation of the sodium channel.[4] The voltage-sensing element depicted in FIGURE 7 mediates a movement of gating charge of $+1$. In fact, the S4 segments of domains I and II contain only four or five positive charges whereas those in domains III and IV contain six that would be membrane associated.[31,32] The total gating charge of $+6$ may arise from progressive voltage-driven transitions of the four domains yielding $+1$, $+1$, $+2$, and $+2$ charges transferred.

The sliding helix model attempts to define a workable structure for the voltage-sensing elements of the sodium channel. Each of these elements is proposed to initiate a conformational change in its own domain. The structure of each individual domain defines the energetic barrier to its voltage-driven conformational change and therefore the sequence of conformational transitions that occurs during the sigmoid time course of activation. Additional structural information is needed to construct a mechanism for coupling of the conformational changes in each domain to opening of a high conductance transmembrane pore and to eventual inactivation of the ion conductance mechanism.

REFERENCES

1. RICHIE, J. M. & R. B. ROGART. 1977. Rev. Physiol. Biochem. Pharmacol. 79: 1–50.
2. CATTERALL, W. A. 1980. Ann. Rev. Pharmacol. 20: 15–43.
3. CATTERALL, W. A. 1984. Science 223: 653–661.
4. LAZDUNSKI, M. & J. F. RENAUD. 1982. Ann. Rev. Physiol. 44: 463–473.
5. OHIZUMI, Y., H. NAKAMURA, J. KOBAYASHI & W. A. CATTERALL. 1986. J. Biol. Chem. 261: 6149–6152.
6. CATTERALL, W. A., C. S. MORROW, J. W. DALY & G. B. BROWN. 1981. J. Biol. Chem. 256: 8922–8927.
7. BENESKI, D., & W. A. CATTERALL. 1980. Proc. Natl. Acad. Sci. U. S. A. 77: 639–642.
8. COSTA, M. R. C. & W. A. CATTERALL. 1982. Mol. Pharmacol. 22: 196–203.
9. SHARKEY, R. G., D. A. BENESKI & W. A. CATTERALL. 1984. Biochemistry 23: 6078–6086.
10. CATTERALL, W. A., C. S. MORROW & R. P. HARTSHORNE. 1979. J. Biol. Chem. 254: 11379–11387.
11. HARTSHORNE, R. P., J. COPPERSMITH & W. A. CATTERALL. 1980. J. Biol. Chem. 255: 10572–10575.
12. HILLE, B. 1972. J. Gen. Physiol. 58: 599–619.
13. HARTSHORNE, R. P. & W. A. CATTERALL. 1981. Proc. Natl. Acad. Sci. U. S. A. 78: 4620–4624.
14. HARTSHORNE, R. P., D. J. MESSNER, J. C. COPPERSMITH & W. A. CATTERALL. 1982. J. Biol. Chem. 257: 13888–13891.
15. HARTSHORNE, R. P. & W. A. CATTERALL. 1984. J. Biol. Chem. 259: 1667–1675.
16. MESSNER, D. J. & W. A. CATTERALL. 1985. J. Biol. Chem. 260: 10597–10604.
17. WAECHTER, C. J., J. SCHMIDT & W. A. CATTERALL. 1983. J. Biol. Chem. 258: 5117–5123.
18. KREBS, E. G. & J. A. BEAVO. 1979. Ann. Rev. Biochem. 48: 923–959.
19. NESTLER, E. J. & P. GREENGARD. 1983. Nature 305: 583–588.

20. COSTA, M. R. C., J. E. CASNELLIE & W. A. CATTERALL. 1982. J. Biol. Chem. **257:** 7918–7921.
21. COSTA, M. R. C. & W. A. CATTERALL. 1984. Cell. Mol. Neurobiol. **4:** 291–297.
22. COSTA, M. R. C. & W. A. CATTERALL. 1984. J. Biol. Chem. **259:** 8210–8218.
23. WEIGELE, J. B. & R. L. BARCHI. 1982. Proc. Natl. Acad. Sci. U. S. A. **79:** 3651–3655.
24. TALVENHEIMO, J. A., M. M. TAMKUN & W. A. CATTERALL. 1982. J. Biol. Chem. **257:** 11868–11871.
25. TAMKUN, M. M., J. A. TALVENHEIMO & W. A. CATTERALL. 1984. J. Biol. Chem. **259:** 1676–1688.
26. FELLER, D. J., J. A. TALVENHEIMO & W. A. CATTERALL. 1985. J. Biol. Chem. **260:** 11542–11547.
27. HARTSHORNE, R. P., B. U. KELLER, J. A. TALVENHEIMO, W. A. CATTERALL & M. MONTAL. 1985. Proc. Natl. Acad. Sci. U. S. A. **82:** 240–244.
28. MESSNER, D. J. & W. A. CATTERALL. 1986. J. Biol. Chem. **261:** 211–215.
29. SCHMIDT, J. W., S. R. ROSSIE & W. A. CATTERALL. 1985. Proc. Natl. Acad. Sci. U. S. A. **82:** 4847–4851.
30. SCHMIDT, J. W. & W. A. CATTERALL. 1986. Cell **46:** 437–445.
31. AULD, V., J. MARSHALL, A. GOLDIN, A. DOWSETT, W. CATTERALL, N. DAVIDSON & R. DUNN. 1985. J. Gen. Physiol. **86:** 10a–11a.
32. NODA, M., S. SHIMIZU, T. TANABE, T. TAKAI, T. KAYANO, T. IDEDA, H. TAKAHASHI, H. NAKAYAMA, Y. KANAOKA, N. MINAMINO, K. KANGAWA, H. MATSUO, M. A. RAFTERY, T. HIROOSE, S. INAYAMA, H. HAYASHIDA, T. MIYATA & S. NUMA. 1984. Nature **312:** 121–127.
33. ARMSTRONG, C. M. 1981. Physiol. Rev. **61:** 644–683.
34. CATTERALL, W. A. 1986. Trends Neurosci. In press.
35. MOCZYDLOWSKI, E., A. UEHARA, X. GUO & J. HEINY. 1986. Isochannels and blocking modes of voltage-dependent sodium channels. This volume.
36. HARTSHORNE, R. P., B. U. KELLER, J. A. TALVENHEIMO, W. A. CATTERALL & M. MONTAL. 1986. Functional reconstitution of purified sodium channels from brain in planar lipid bilayers. This volume.

Polypeptide Toxins as Tools to Study Voltage-Sensitive Na$^+$ Channels[a]

MICHEL LAZDUNSKI, CHRISTIAN FRELIN,
JACQUES BARHANIN, ALAIN LOMBET,
HAMUTAL MEIRI,[b] DAVID PAURON,
GEORGES ROMEY, ANNIE SCHMID,
HUGUES SCHWEITZ, PAUL VIGNE,
AND HENK P. M. VIJVERBERG[c]

*Centre de Biochimie du Centre National
de la Recherche Scientifique
Parc Valrose 06034 Nice, France*

The Na$^+$ channel is now known to be the receptor of numerous natural toxins which can be classified in six different categories, presented in TABLE 1. Each toxin type is associated with a different type of receptor. This paper describes two types of polypeptide toxins that have been of particular interest in recent studies devoted to the molecular analysis of the properties of the Na$^+$ channel.

TITYUS γ TOXIN

Mechanism of Action and Affinity for the Na$^+$ Channel

The *Tityus* γ toxin (TiTxγ) has been isolated from the venom of a Brazilian scorpion, *Tityus serrulatus*.[1,2] It is 61 amino acids long and its structure is represented in FIGURE 1. The mechanism of action of this toxin on the Na$^+$ channel has been extensively studied using electrophysiological techniques.[3,4] The main effect of the toxin is to shift the voltage dependence of the Na$^+$ channel towards negative potentials (FIG. 1). As a result of this effect, Na$^+$ currents are created at membrane potentials as low as -70 mV at which the Na$^+$ channel is normally in the resting state, that is, in a closed form. The TiTxγ-induced Na$^+$ current is more resistant to the local anaesthetic procaine than the control Na$^+$ current.[3] The voltage dependence of the inactivation of the TiTxγ-induced Na$^+$ current is different from that of the control Na$^+$ current in the absence of the toxin.[3,4] Because of this action on both the activation and inactivation of the Na$^+$ channel, TiTxγ appears to be an excellent marker of the gating system of this channel.

[a]This work was supported by the Centre National de la Recherche Scientifique, the Ministère de la Recherche et de la Technologie (grant 83.C.0918), the Association des Myopathes de France, the Fondation sur les Maladies Vasculaires, and the Fondation pour la Recherche Médicale.

[b]Present address: Rappaport Family Institute for Research in the Medical Sciences, Technion Israel Institute of Technology, Efron St., P.O. Box 9697, Haifa 31096, Israel.

[c]Present address: Institute of Veterinary Pharmacology, Pharmacy and Toxicology, P.O. Box 80176, 3508 TD Utrecht, the Netherlands.

The other interest of the toxin is illustrated in FIGURE 2, which shows that ^{125}I-labeled TiTxγ binds with a high affinity to the Na^+ channel of *Electrophorus electricus* electroplaque and to the Na^+ channel of rat brain.[5] The dissociation constant of the TiTxγ-Na^+ channel complex is about 4 pM. TABLE 2 lists dissociation constants found with excitable membrane from very different types of tissues from different animal species. K_d values are in the pM range in most membranes. It is particularly remarkable to see that the affinity of the toxin for its receptor is nearly the same in the insect and in the mammalian nervous system. Respective stoichiometries of the tetrodotoxin (TTX) and of the TiTxγ receptor in the different preparations tested are 1:1. Affinities of TTX, en-TTX (the ethylenediamine derivative of TTX) and TiTxγ are compared in TABLE 2. Even in the system having the best affinity for TTX and its derivative, *i.e.,* the insect Na^+ channel, the affinity of TiTxγ remains higher than that of TTX. It is only in neuroblastoma cells which have a Na^+ channel that is less sensitive to TiTxγ (although the K_d value is still 7.5×10^{-10} M) that the two types of

TABLE 1. A Summary of the Different Classes of Toxins Acting on the Na^+ Channel

Toxin	Physiological Effect
tetrodotoxin and saxitoxin	block Na^+ currents
Lipid-Soluble Molecules veratridine batrachotoxin aconitine grayanotoxins	cause persistent activation of Na^+ channels
North American or North African scorpion toxins and polypeptide toxins from sea anemone	specifically slow down Na^+ current inactivation

Central or South American Scorpion
  Toxins
Centruroides suffusus suffusus
  (CssII)
Tityus serrulatus (*Tityus* γ)
pyrethroids
	block partially the early Na^+
	current and create a new type of
	channel activated at lower
	potentials
	modify the closing of fast Na^+
	channels

ciguatoxin	increases Na^+ permeability

toxins (TiTxγ and TTX) have the same type of affinities. *Centruroides suffusus* toxin II,[5-9] as well as several other *Centruroides* toxins,[10] share the same site as TiTxγ. However the affinity of *Centruroides* toxins for their site is lower than that of TiTxγ, corresponding to K_d values of about 1 nM.[5-10]

Use of TiTxγ for Affinity Labeling and Purification of the Na^+ Channel

TiTxγ is an excellent toxin to purify the Na^+ channel protein from different sources. FIGURE 3 summarizes different types of data concerning the elucidation of the subunit structure of the Na^+ channel from rat brain and from the electric organ of *Electrophorus electricus*. Affinity labeling of the TTX receptor in the *Electrophorus electricus* Na^+ channel[11] with a TTX derivative identifies a polypeptide chain with an

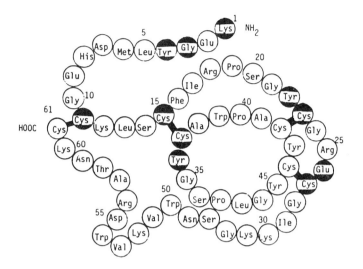

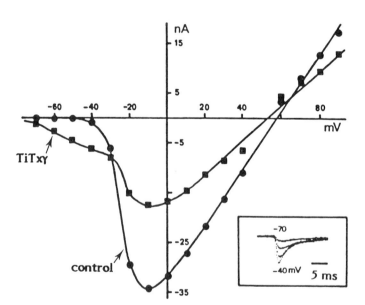

FIGURE 1. *Top*, Structure of *Tityus* γ toxin assuming that disulfide bridges have the same pairing as in other scorpion neurotoxins.[39,40] Amino acids common to *Tityus* γ toxin, to *Androctonus australis* Hector toxin II, and to *Centruroides suffusus suffusus* toxin II are indicated. *Bottom*, I/V curves relative to the effect of TiTxγ (53 nM) on Na$^+$ channels in neuroblastoma cells (N1E 115). All membrane depolarizations were preceded by a 100 ms conditioning hyperpolarization at −110 mV. The inset shows superimposed traces of TiTxγ-induced Na$^+$ current evoked by membrane depolarizations to −70, −60, −50, and −40 mV.

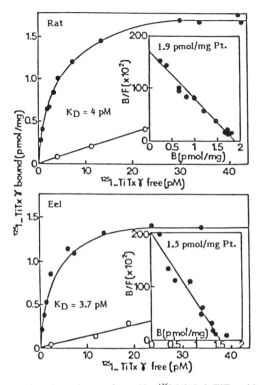

FIGURE 2. Concentration dependence of specific ^{125}I-labeled TiTxγ binding to rat brain synaptosomes and to eel electroplaque membranes. Specific (●) and nonspecific (○) binding. *Insets,* Scatchard plots of the data with indications of maximal binding capacities.

TABLE 2. Affinity of TiTxγ, TTX, and a TTX Derivative for Na$^+$ Channels in Different Excitable Membranes

Preparation	Dissociation Constant (M)		
	^{125}I-labeled TiTxγ	[^{3}H]en-TTX	TTX
Rat synaptosomes	4×10^{-12}	1.5×10^{-9}	1.8×10^{-9}
E. electricus electroplax	4×10^{-12}	1.0×10^{-9}	2.5×10^{-9}
Neuroblastoma cells (N1E 115)	7.5×10^{-10}	5×10^{-10}	6.0×10^{-10}
Frog skeletal muscle (sarcolemma)	1.2×10^{-11}	8×10^{-9}	4.0×10^{-9}
Rabbit skeletal muscle (sarcolemma)	3×10^{-10}	2×10^{-9}	2.0×10^{-9}
Chick cardiac muscle	3×10^{-12}	1.4×10^{-9}	3.0×10^{-9}
Insect nervous system (fly head membranes)	6×10^{-12}	3×10^{-11}	7.7×10^{-11}

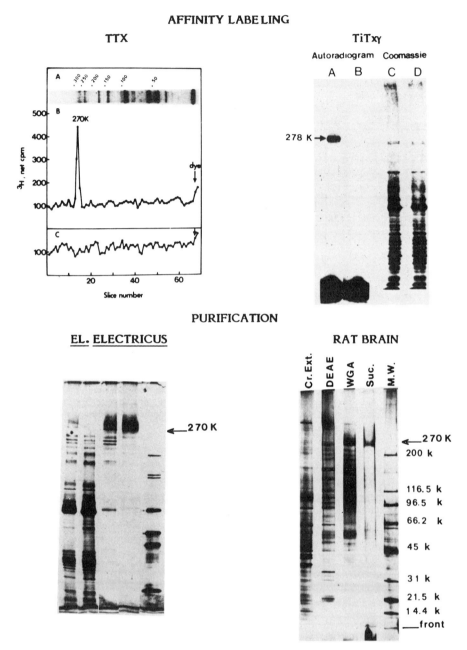

FIGURE 3. Affinity labeling (*top*) and purification (*bottom*) of Na$^+$ channels from eel electroplaque membranes and from rat brain. *Upper left*, identification on gel electrophoresis of the high M_r polypeptide (270,000) which has covalently and specifically incorporated an ethylenediamine derivative of TTX cross-linked with disuccinimidyl suberate.[11] (A) SDS gel

M_r of 270,000. Purification of the ^{125}I-labeled TiTxγ receptor complex in the same system leads to the same type of identification since it results in the isolation of a single polypeptide chain of 270,000 daltons.[12] Moreover at each purification step there is a parallel enrichment of TiTxγ and TTX receptors. The conclusion that the Na$^+$ channel protein in *Electrophorus electricus* electric organ is made of a single large polpeptide chain is consistent with independent evidence obtained by other authors using saxitoxin and reconstitution techniques.[13-15]

The same types of conclusions have been obtained for the Na$^+$ channel from rat brain. Affinity labeling incorporates ^{125}I-labeled TiTxγ (M_r = 8000) into a large polypeptide of M_r 270,000 (FIG. 3).[16] Purification of the TiTxγ-Na$^+$ channel complex results in the isolation of a single chain of M_r 270,000 with a copurification at each step of both the TiTxγ and the TTX receptor.[17] These results are consistent with those obtained by radiation inactivation experiments which have indicated an M_r of 260,000 for both the TiTxγ and the TTX receptor.[16] Moreover the Na$^+$ channel preparation from rat brain has been successfully reconstituted into bilayers and is sensitive to the different toxins known to alter the function of the Na$^+$ channel.[18,19]

FIGURES 4–6 indicate the main properties of interaction of TiTxγ with the Na$^+$ channel in chick heart cells of the high affinity type for TTX. Here again the purification using ^{125}I-labeled TiTxγ results in the final isolation of a single polypeptide chain of M_r 230,000–270,000 with a parallel enrichment of the TTX and TiTxγ receptors throughout the purification.[9] In the cardiac membrane as in the synaptic membrane, affinity labeling with ^{125}I-labeled TiTxγ using cross-linking with disuccinimidyl suberate incorporates the polypeptide toxin into a 230,000–240,000 M_r chain.

All these results taken together strongly suggest that the large molecular weight polypeptide chain (230,000–270,000), which contains the receptor site for TTX and STX[20] that is somehow related to Na$^+$ recognition by the Na$^+$ channel[21] and the receptor site for TiTxγ that is related to the activation-inactivation machinery of the gating component of the Na$^+$ channel, is the only peptide necessary to ensure Na$^+$ channel function.

A Monoclonal Antibody against the Na$^+$ Channel Having Properties Similar to Those of TiTxγ

One of the monoclonal antibodies obtained against the Na$^+$ channel[4] has the interesting property of preventing ^{125}I-labeled TiTxγ from binding to its receptor (FIG. 7), and this inhibition is of the competitive type. This monoclonal antibody has the following properties: (1) it permits a cytoimmunochemical localization of Na$^+$ channels[4]; (2) it acts as an "agonist" on Na$^+$ channel function with properties that are very similar to those of TiTxγ itself[4] (FIG. 8); (3) it binds with a relatively high affinity

---

electrophoresis of a DEAE-purified fraction (Coomassie staining) labeled with [^{3}H]en-TTX in the (B) absence or (C) presence of 10 μM TTX. *Lower left,* SDS gel electrophoresis of the purified TiTxγ receptor from *Electrophorus electricus* electroplax at different stages of purification. Lane 1 (numbered from left) is the Lubrol PX extract; lane 4 is the most purified fraction.[12] *Upper right,* Covalent cross-linking of ^{125}I-labeled TiTxγ to its receptor in rat brain synaptosomes with disuccinimidyl suberate.[16] Lanes A and C, cross-linking after incubation with ^{125}I-labeled TiTxγ (8 nM). Lanes B and D, cross-linking after incubation with ^{125}I-labeled TiTxγ plus 30 nM unlabeled toxin. Autoradiographies are shown in A and B and the corresponding gels stained with Coomassie blue in C and D. *Lower right,* SDS polyacrylamide gel electrophoresis of rat brain Na$^+$ channel preparations.[17] Lane 1 (numbered from left), Coomassie blue staining of the membrane preparation. Lanes 2 and 3, silver staining of wheat germ agglutinin and sucrose gradient steps, respectively. Lane 4 corresponds to the most purified material.

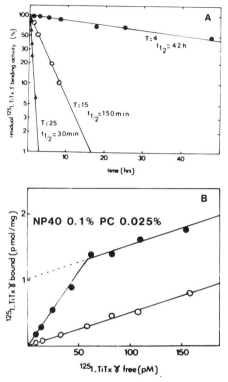

FIGURE 4. The solubilized cardiac TiTxγ receptor. The TiTxγ receptor from chick heart sarcolemma was solubilized with 1% Nonidet P-40 in the presence of protease inhibitors. (**A**) Temperature dependence of the stability of the solubilized TiTxγ receptor. The half-lives of the TiTxγ receptor were measured at 4°C (●), 15°C (○), and 23°C (▲). (**B**) Total binding (●) of ^{125}I-labeled TiTxγ to Nonidet P-40 extract of heart sarcolemma incubated with increasing concentrations of ^{125}I-labeled TiTxγ at 4°C. Nonspecific binding (○) was measured in the presence of 0.1 μM unlabeled toxin.

to Na$^+$ channels from rat brain ($K_d = 1.5$ nM). *Electrophorus electricus* electroplax ($K_d = 1.5$ nM), chick heart ($K_d = 0.6$ nM), and rat heart ($K_d = 8$ nM) affinities are of the same order of magnitude as those found for *Centruroides* toxins.

SEA ANEMONE TOXINS

Structure-Function Relationships and Mechanism of Action

This family of toxins is now well known to be selective for the Na$^+$ channel, whose inactivation it slows down.[22] This effect is observed in a variety of preparations including nerve, muscle, cardiac, and nonexcitable cells such as glial cells and fibroblasts.[23] FIGURE 9 indicates that the true effect of sea anemone toxins might be to reveal a slow Na$^+$ channel instead of slowing down inactivation of the standard fast Na$^+$ channel.

A number of sequences of sea anemone toxins active on Na$^+$ channels are now known and a comparison of primary structures is presented in FIGURE 10. Among the different toxins listed in FIGURE 10, some such as ASI and RpII are inactive on Na$^+$ channels of mammalian systems, whereas others such as ASV, AXI, and AXII are both active on crustacean Na$^+$ channels and very active on mammalian Na$^+$ channels. ASII, the most popular (but not the most active) of sea anemone toxins has intermediate properties. Toxins extracted from the sea anemone *Radianthus paumotensis,* such as RpII, differ from other sea anemone toxins by their antigenic properties.[24] A comparison of sequence presented in FIGURE 10 suggests that amino acids which determine the "mammalian" character of the toxins may be His-39 and Pro-41, which are found in all "mammalian" toxins sequenced so far and are absent in toxins with no activity for mammalian Na$^+$ channels.

Among the amino acids which are common to all these toxins, besides Gly, Pro, and Cys residues, the most interesting residues are Asp-9, Arg-4, Trp-33, and Lys-48. Little is known about Trp-33, which probably has a structural role. More information is available about the function of other residues.[25] Chemical modification of Arg-14

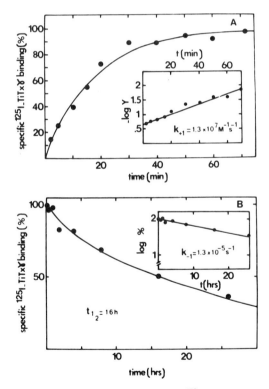

FIGURE 5. (A) Association kinetics for the binding of ^{125}I-labeled TiTxγ to chick cardiac sarcolemma at 4°C. Association was started by addition of ^{125}I-labeled TiTxγ (65 pM) to membrane receptor (15 pM). The same data are presented semilogarithmically in the *inset.* (B) Dissociation kinetics for the binding of ^{125}I-labeled TiTxγ to cardiac sarcolemma at 4°C. After 1 h of association in the same conditions as described above, the dissociation was started by the addition of 0.1 μM unlabeled TiTxγ. A semilogarithmic plot of the data is given in the *inset.*

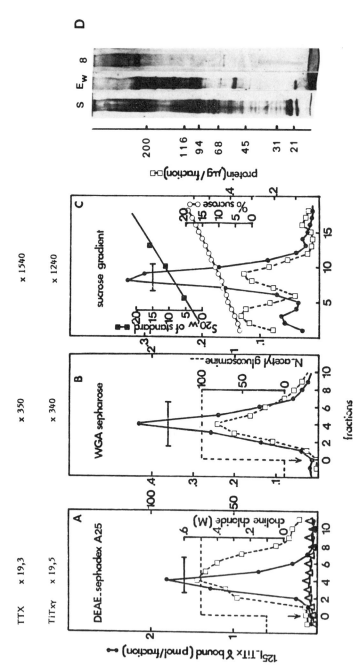

FIGURE 6. Analysis of a sodium channel purification from chick heart sarcolemma. Elution profiles for the **(A)** DEAE-Sephadex A25, **(B)** WGA-Sepharose column, and **(C)** sucrose density gradient are shown. In each panel, picomoles of ^{125}I-labeled TiTxγ binding sites in pmol/fraction are indicated by the left axis (●) and nonspecific binding is presented in **A** (△). The total amount of protein per fraction is given on the right axis (□). Overlaid curves give the concentration gradient of the component used for elution (*dashed line* in **A** and **B**) or the density of sucrose (○, **C**) in each fraction, and sedimentation coefficient of standards (■, **C**). **(D)** SDS polyacrylamide gel electrophoresis was carried out in gels containing 4%–12% polyacrylamide gradient under reducing conditions after denaturation of samples for 1 h at 30°C in 75 mM Tris/Cl, pH 6.8, 2% SDS, 7.5% sucrose, 2.5% 2-mercaptoethanol. Lanes: S, Nonidet P-40 extract (1 µg of protein); E_w, peak fraction from WGA-Sepharose column (0.5 µg of protein); 8, most active fraction from sucrose gradient (0.1 µg of protein). Numbers over panels A–C represent the respective enrichment factors in TTX and TiTxγ receptors.

with 1,2-cyclohexanedione abolishes both the toxicity and the binding activity of the toxin to the Na$^+$ channel. This residue is clearly an essential element of the active site of the toxin. Chemical modification of positively charged lysine side chains into positively charged homoarginine side chains preserved the activity of the toxin, whereas acetylation of the ϵ-amino groups of lysine side chains abolished toxicity.

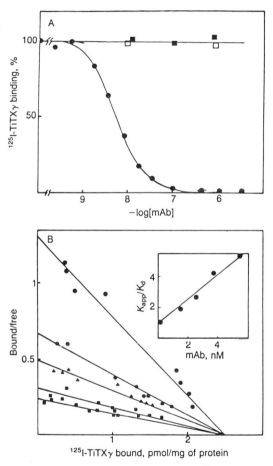

FIGURE 7. (A) Inhibition by monoclonal antibody 72.38 of ^{125}I-labeled TiTxγ binding to the Na$^+$ channel of rat brain membranes (●). Control antibodies (■, □). (B) Scatchard plots for ^{125}I-labeled TiTxγ binding at different concentrations of mAb 72.38. *Top to bottom:* zero, 1.4 nM, 2.5 nM, 3.6 nM, and 5.4 nM. *Inset,* K_{app}/K_d is plotted as a function of the concentration of 72.38. $K_{app} = K_d(1 + \text{mAb } 72.38/K_i)$, where K_i is the true equilibrium constant of 72.38.

Therefore it seems probable that Lys-48 also plays an important role in the biological activity of the polypeptide. Chemical modification (esterification) of glutamic and aspartic side chains abolished biological activity. However it was shown[25] that the modified toxin could still bind to its receptor site on the Na$^+$ channel protein while it had lost all capacity to modify the electrophysiological properties of this channel. The modified toxin behaved as an antagonist of the native toxin. Therefore Asp-9 is probably directly involved in the modification of the gating properties of the channel by sea anemone toxins.

Sea anemone toxins have been ^{125}I-iodinated and their receptor site has been

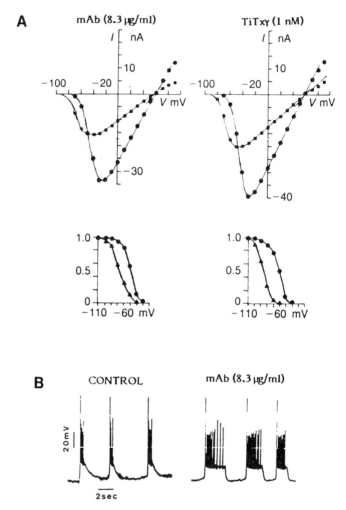

FIGURE 8. (A) I/V curves of peak Na$^+$ current in rat myoballs in the absence (●) and in the presence (■) of 72.38 (8.3 μg/ml) and TiTxγ (1 nM). The lower part of the figure presents the inactivation of the Na$^+$ current in control experiments (●) and the inactivation of the remaining Na$^+$ current after the external application of 72.38 and TiTxγ (▲). (B) Spontaneous patterns of burst activity induced by the monoclonal antibody 72.38 in rat myotubes.

identified on synaptosomes.[26] Unlike binding of scorpion toxins from *Androctonus australis* or from *Leiurus quinquestriatus*[26,27] that also slows down Na$^+$ channel inactivation, binding of sea anemone toxins can be easily detected on depolarized synaptosomes, that is, when the Na$^+$ channel is in the inactivated state. Stoichiometry

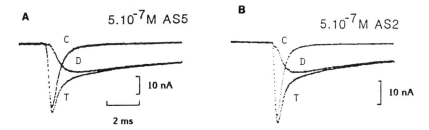

FIGURE 9. Effects of sea anemone toxins on Na^+ currents. *C*, control; *T*, at equilibrium after toxin application; *D*, difference between total Na^+ current after addition of the polypeptide toxin and control current. A slowly activating and inactivating Na^+ current component remains both in (**A**) neuroblastoma (N1E/115) cells and (**B**) rat myoballs.

determinations suggest that the sea anemone toxin and TTX binding sites are in a 1:1 to 2:1 stoichiometry.[26]

It is often assumed that toxins from the scorpions *Androctonus australis Hector* or *Leiurus quinquestriatus* share the same receptor as sea anemone toxins even though the respective sequences of these different polypeptides have no homologies. This view, however, may not be completely correct because (1) the number of sites titrated with

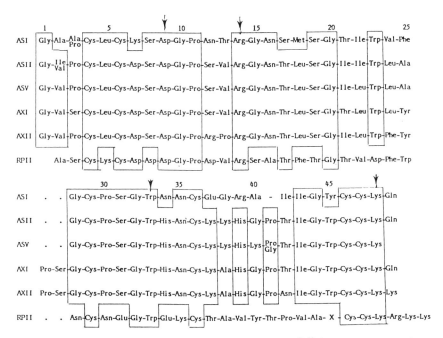

FIGURE 10. Comparative sequences of sea anemone toxins[41-46] from *Anemonia sulcata*, *Anthopleura xanthogrammica*, and *Radianthus paumotensis*. The guanidine function of Arg-14 was modified with 1,2-cyclohexanedione. Carboxyl groups were modified with glycine ethyl ester and a soluble carbodiimide; ε-amino groups of lysines were modified with *o*-methylisourea or with acetic anhydride.[25]

[125]I-labeled sea anemone toxins far exceeds (by a factor of about 10) the number of sites found with ^{125}I-labeled *Androctonus* toxins,[26] and (2) if sea anemone toxins prevent the binding of ^{125}I-labeled *Androctonus* toxin, the binding of ^{125}I-labeled sea anemone toxins is unaffected by the *Androctonus* toxin.[26] It is interesting to observe that one of the *Radianthus paumotensis* sea anemone toxins, which does not react with antibodies against *Anemonia sulcata* or *Anthopleura xanthogrammica* toxins, behaves similarly to the *Androctonus* toxin.[24]

Sea anemone toxins have not been particularly useful in characterizing the subunit structure of Na$^+$ channels. We have successfully synthesized photoaffinity (azido)

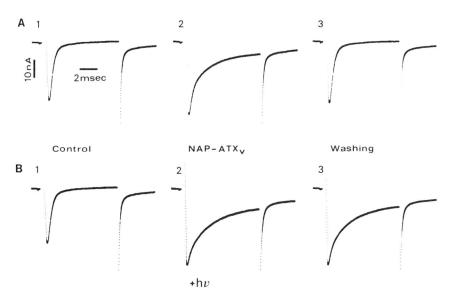

FIGURE 11. Irreversible effect of a photoactivable derivative of toxin V from *Anemonia sulcata* (2-nitro-4-azidophenyl ATXV : NAP-ATXV) on Na$^+$ current of NIE 115 neuroblastoma cells. (**A**) *1*, control, *2*, five min after addition of 0.1 μM NAP-ATXV, *3*, washing under dim light, which completely restores the control current. (**B**) *1*, control, *2*, five min after addition of 0.1 μM NAP-ATXV followed by photoirradiation of the cells by 50 flashes of visible light; *3*, the toxin effect persists after the washing step. Holding potential at − 100 mV; test pulse to − 20 mV.

derivatives of ASV which irreversibly block Na$^+$ channel inactivation after irradiation (FIG. 11). However these derivatives do not permit successful identification of the polypeptide chain which carries the toxin binding site (unpublished results). The Na$^+$ channel from rat brain which only contains the 270,000 M_r subunit has been reconstituted in planar bilayers and responds to sea anemone toxins.[18]

Use of Sea Anemone Toxins to Identify Subtypes of Na$^+$ Channels

One of the interesting characteristics of sea anemone toxins is that they permit the identification of subtypes of Na$^+$ channels. The existence of subtypes of Na$^+$ channels had first been detected from their TTX sensitivity. It is now well known that there are

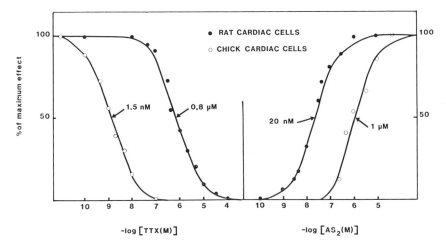

FIGURE 12. Concentration dependence of the effects of TTX and of the sea anemone ASII on Na^+ channel activity in chick and rat heart cells in culture. Measurements have been carried out using $^{22}Na^+$ flux experiments.[30,33]

TTX-sensitive and TTX-resistant Na^+ channels (see for example ref. 28). TTX-sensitive Na^+ channels are blocked at toxin concentrations in the nanomolar range (10–100 nM), whereas TTX-resistant Na^+ channels are blocked in the micromolar range (1–10 μM). Well-known examples of TTX-resistant Na^+ channels are those which are found in mammalian cardiac cells.[29] The coexistence of high affinity and low affinity binding sites for TTX has been observed in both mammalian cardiac cells and in noninnervated mammalian skeletal muscle cells.[30–32]

FIGURE 12 shows that Na^+ channels in chick cardiac cells which have a high affinity for TTX ($K_{0.5} = 1.5$ nM) have a relatively low affinity for anemone toxins (ASII), ($K_{0.5} = 1$ μM). Conversely, Na^+ channels of rat cardiac cells in culture which are resistant to TTX ($K_{0.5} = 0.8$ μM) have a high affinity for ASII ($K_{0.5} = 20$ nM).

TABLE 3 extends this observation to a variety of sea anemone toxins and a variety of cellular types in culture. Clearly, in all systems investigated, resistance to TTX action is accompanied by a high sensitivity to sea anemone toxins and vice versa. Although

TABLE 3. Dissociation Constants (nM) for Sea Anemone Toxins and Androctonus Toxin II on Different Cell Preparations

	TTX-Resistant Na^+ Channels		TTX-Sensitive Na^+ Channels	
	Rat Myoblasts	N1E 115	Fibroblasts	Chick Myotubes
ASII[a]	5	150	600	1000
ASV	2	15	100	500
AXI[b]	3	47	400	1000
AXII	0.15	7	60	300
AaII[c]	0.20	0.20	—	1

[a]AS = *Anemonia sulcata*.
[b]AX = *Anthopleura xanthogrammica*.
[c]Aa = *Androctonus australis*.

TTX receptor sites and sea anemone toxin receptor sites are clearly distinct,[26,28] changes of affinity for TTX are clearly correlated to changes of affinity for sea anemone toxins.

Interestingly, *Androctonus australis* Hector toxin II, which is the most active scorpion toxin acting on Na^+ channel inactivation, does not discriminate between Na^+ channels having high and low affinity sites for TTX (TABLE 3).

Sea anemone toxins have also been particularly useful tools for following the ontogenesis of Na^+ channels in various tissues.[33-35] One recent example of the use of these toxins in differentiation studies concerns the mammalian skeletal muscle system.[35] Early myoblasts are unable to fire action potentials. At first sight they do not seem to have functional Na^+ channels. Na^+ channels are revealed in the presence of sea anemone toxins, however. They are of the TTX-resistant type with a high affinity for sea anemone toxins. In fact patch-clamp recording of single Na^+ channel activity (H.P.M. Vijverberg, unpublished data) as well as $^{22}Na^+$ flux studies[35] show that Na^+ channels are present at this early stage. They are, however, present in an amount which is too low to produce an inward current capable of generating an action potential. The contribution of the new inward Na^+ current is largely increased by sea anemone toxins which slow down inactivation, and this increase is high enough to generate electrical activity. Late myoblasts generate action potentials with a TTX-resistant and sea anemone toxin-sensitive Na^+ channel. Myotubes generate action potentials which are faster than those found in late myoblasts. The Na^+ channel in these cultured muscle fibers is TTX resistant and sensitive to sea anemone toxin as in myoblasts, although the fusion of myoblasts into myotubes is accompanied by the synthesis of another category of TTX receptor site which has a high affinity for TTX and does not seem to be functionally expressed. The amount of Na^+ channels with a low affinity for TTX seems to be the same in late myoblasts (just prior to fusion) and in myotubes. After innervation, the electrically expressed muscle Na^+ channel becomes TTX sensitive and sea anemone toxin resistant.[35,36] Denervation brings back the properties of the Na^+ channel[36] to the stage identified in noninnervated myotubes.

In chick skeletal muscle cells, in culture and *in vivo*, the situation is more simple. The Na^+ channel is absent in myoblasts, is expressed in noninnervated myotubes, and is then TTX sensitive and of a low affinity for sea anemone toxins.[34,35] Innervation does not change the toxin sensitivity of the channel.

When sea anemone toxins have a higher affinity for Na^+ channels, their effect is very voltage dependent. They are much more active at more polarized membrane potentials[28] than at depolarized potentials.

Finally it should be recalled that sea anemone toxins are very efficient cardiotonic molecules.[29] It has now been shown very clearly[37,38] that this property is linked to the following sequence of events: (1) slowing down of Na^+ channel inactivation which produces an increased Na^+ entry into the cardiac cells which results in an increase of the internal Na^+ concentration, and (2) an entry of Ca^{2+} through the Na^+/Ca^{2+} exchange system due to the increased $[Na^+]_i$. The activity of sea anemone toxin on the mammalian cardiac cell is seen at concentrations of the toxin in the nanomolar range due to the presence of a Na^+ channel with a high affinity for these polypeptide toxins in these heart cells.

ACKNOWLEDGMENTS

We wish to thank Drs. R. I. Norman, K. P. Wheeler, J. R. Giglio and S. V. Sampaio for fruitful collaboration. We are grateful to C. Roulinat-Bettelheim for expert technical assistance.

REFERENCES

1. POSSANI, L. D., A. C. ALAGON, P. L. FLECHTER, JR. & B. W. ERICKSON. 1977. Arch. Biochem. Biophys. **180:** 394–403.
2. SAMPAIO, S. V., C. J. LAURE & J. R. GIGLIO. 1983. Toxicon **21:** 265–277.
3. VIJVERBERG, H. P. M., D. PAURON & M. LAZDUNSKI. 1984. Pfluegers Arch. **401:** 297–303.
4. BARHANIN J., H. MEIRI, G. ROMEY, D. PAURON & M. LAZDUNSKI. 1985. Proc. Natl. Acad. Sci. U. S. A. **82:** 1842–1846.
5. BARHANIN, J., J. R. GIGLIO, P. LEOPOLD, A. SCHMID, S. V. SAMPAIO & M. LAZDUNSKI. 1982. J. Biol. Chem. **257**(21): 12553–12558.
6. WHEELER, K. P., J. BARHANIN & M. LAZDUNSKI. 1982. Biochemistry **21:** 5628–5634.
7. JAIMOVICH, E., M. ILDEFONSE, J. BARHANIN, O. ROUGIER & M. LAZDUNSKI. 1982. Proc. Natl. Acad. Sci. U. S. A. **79:** 3896–3900.
8. JOVER, E., F. COURAUD & H. ROCHAT. 1980. Biochem. Biophys. Res. Commun. **95:** 1607–1614.
9. LOMBET, A. & M. LAZDUNSKI. 1984. Eur. J. Biochem. **141:** 651–660.
10. WHEELER, K. P., D. D. WATT & M. LAZDUNSKI. 1983. Pfluegers Arch. **397:** 164–165.
11. LOMBET, A., R. I. NORMAN & M. LAZDUNSKI. 1983. Biochem. Biophys. Res. Commun. **114:** 126–130.
12. NORMAN, R. I., A. SCHMID, A. LOMBET, J. BARHANIN & M. LAZDUNSKI. 1983. Proc. Natl. Acad. Sci. U. S. A. **80:** 4164–4168.
13. AGNEW, W. S., S. R. LEVINSON, J. S. BRABSON & M. A. RAFTERY. 1978. Proc. Natl. Acad. Sci. U. S. A. **75:** 2606–2611.
14. MILLER, J. A., W. S. AGNEW & S. R. LEVINSON. 1983. Biochemistry **24:** 462–470.
15. ROSENBERG, R. L., S. A. TOMIKO & W. S. AGNEW. 1984. Proc. Natl. Acad. Sci. U. S. A. **81:** 5594–5598.
16. BARHANIN, J., A. SCHMID, A. LOMBET, K. P. WHEELER, M. LAZDUNSKI & J. C. ELLORY. 1983. J. Biol. Chem. **258:** 700–702.
17. BARHANIN, J., D. PAURON, A. LOMBET, R. I. NORMAN, H. P. M. VIJVERBERG, J. R. GIGLIO & M. LAZDUNSKI. 1983. EMBO J. **2:** 915–920.
18. HANKE, W., G. BOHEIM, J. BARHANIN, D. PAURON & M. LAZDUNSKI. 1984. EMBO J. **3:** 509–515.
19. HARTSHORNE, R. P., B. U. KELLER, J. A. TALVENHEIMO, W. A. CATTERALL & M. MONTAL. 1985. Proc. Natl. Acad. Sci. U. S. A. **82:** 240–244.
20. TALVENHEIMO, J. A. 1985. J. Membr. Biol. **87:** 77–91.
21. FRELIN, C., P. VIGNE & M. LAZDUNSKI. 1981. Eur. J. Biochem. **119:** 437–442.
22. ROMEY, G., J. P. ABITA, H. SCHWEITZ, G. WUNDERER & M. LAZDUNSKI. 1976. Proc. Natl. Acad. Sci. U. S. A. **73:** 4055–4059.
23. BERGMAN, C., J. M. DUBOIS, E. ROJAS & W. RATHMAYER. 1976. Biochim. Biophys. Acta **455:** 173–184.
24. SCHWEITZ, H., J. N. BIDARD, C. FRELIN, D. PAURON, H. P. M. VIJVERBERG, D. M. MAHASNEH & M. LAZDUNSKI. 1985. Biochemistry **24:** 3554–3561.
25. BARHANIN, J., M. HUGUES, H. SCHWEITZ, J. P. VINCENT & M. LAZDUNSKI. 1981. J. Biol. Chem. **256:** 5764–5769.
26. VINCENT, J. P., M. BALERNA, J. BARHANIN, M. FOSSET & M. LAZDUNSKI. 1980. Proc. Natl. Acad. Sci. U. S. A. **77:** 1646–1650.
27. CATTERALL, W. A., R. RAY & C. S. MORROW. 1976. Proc. Natl. Acad. Sci. U. S. A. **73:** 2682–2686.
28. FRELIN, C., P. VIGNE, H. SCHWEITZ & M. LAZDUNSKI. 1984. Mol. Pharmacol. **26:** 70–74.
29. LAZDUNSKI, M. & J. F. RENAUD. 1982. Ann. Rev. Physiol. **44:** 463–473.
30. RENAUD, J. F., T. KAZAZOGLOU, A. LOMBET, R. CHICHEPORTICHE, E. JAIMOVICH, G. ROMEY & M. LAZDUNSKI. 1983. J. Biol. Chem. **258**(14): 8799–8805.
31. LOMBET, A., C. FRELIN, J. F. RENAUD & M. LAZDUNSKI. 1982. Eur. J. Biochem. **124:** 199–203.
32. FRELIN, C., P. VIGNE & M. LAZDUNSKI. 1983. J. Biol. Chem. **258**(12): 7256–7259.
33. RENAUD, J. F., G. ROMEY, A. LOMBET & M. LAZDUNSKI. 1981. Proc. Natl. Acad. Sci. U. S. A. **78:** 5348–5352.

34. FRELIN, C., A. LOMBET, P. VIGNE, G. ROMEY & M. LAZDUNSKI. 1981. J. Biol. Chem. **256:** 12355–12361.
35. FRELIN, C., H. P. M. VIJVERBERG, G. ROMEY, P. VIGNE & M. LAZDUNSKI. 1984. Pfluegers Arch./Eur. J. Physiol. **402:** 121–128.
36. ERXLEBEN, C. & W. RATHMAYER. 1984. Toxicon **22:** 387–399.
37. ROMEY, G., J. F. RENAUD, M. FOSSET & M. LAZDUNSKI. 1980. J. Pharm. Exp. Ther. **213:** 607–615.
38. RENAUD, J. F., M. FOSSET, H. SCHWEITZ & M. LAZDUNSKI. 1985. Eur. J. Pharmacol. In press.
39. BECHIS, G., F. SAMPIERI, P. M. YUON, T. BRANDO, M. F. MARTIN, C. R. DINIZ & H. ROCHAT. 1984. Biochem. Biophys. Res. Commun. **3:** 1146–1153.
40. ROCHAT, H., P. BERNARD & F. COURAUD. 1979. *In* Advances in Cytopharmacology, vol. 3. B. Ceccarelli & F. Clementi, Eds: 325–334. Neurotoxins: Tools in Neurobiology. Raven. New York.
41. WUNDERER, G. & M. EULITZ. 1978. Eur. J. Biochem. **89:** 11–17.
42. WUNDERER, G., H. FRITZ, E. WACHTER & W. MACHLEIDT. 1976. Eur. J. Biochem. **68:** 193–198.
43. SCHEFFLER, J. J., A. TSUGITA, G. LINDEN, H. SCHWEITZ & M. LAZDUNSKI. 1982. Biochem. Biophys. Res. Commun. **107:** 272–278.
44. TANAKA, M., M. HANIU, K. T. YASUNOBU & T. R. NORTON. 1977. Biochemistry **16:** 204–208.
45. REIMER, N. S., C. L. YASUNOBU, K. T. YASUNOBU & T. R. NORTON. 1985. J. Biol. Chem. **260:** 8690—8693.
46. KUMAR, N. V., D. E. WEMMER, R. METRIONE, H. SCHWEITZ, M. LAZDUNSKI & N. R. KALLENBACH. 1986. Biophysical Society Meeting. Abstract.

Spatial Relations of the Neurotoxin Binding Sites on the Sodium Channel[a]

KIMON ANGELIDES,[b] SUSUMU TERAKAWA,[c] AND
GEORGE B. BROWN[d]

[b]Department of Physiology and Molecular Biophysics
Baylor College of Medicine
Texas Medical Center
Houston, Texas 77030

[c]National Institute for Physiological Sciences
Okazaki, Japan

[d]Neurosciences Program
University of Alabama at Birmingham
Birmingham, Alabama 35294

INTRODUCTION

The electrical excitability of nerve and muscle cell membranes is a result of rapid and precisely controlled voltage-dependent changes in the permeability to Na^+ and K^+ ions. The selective permeability of these ions is in part modulated by the action of the Na^+ channel protein that forms an actual pore that traverses the membrane. This channel is gated by a transmembrane voltage through a sequence of resting, open, and closed states during excitation.

Pharmacological dissection of the Na^+ channel with neurotoxins has revealed at least four separate receptor sites for neurotoxins.[1,2] Among these the neurotoxins tetrodotoxin and saxitoxin bind to a receptor at or near the ion selectivity filter and reversibly block sodium conductance, presumably by occluding the external surface of the channel and thereby preventing Na^+ ions from passing. Batrachotoxin and veratridine associate with a second receptor site, and alter the voltage dependence of activation and inactivation and elicit persistent activation of Na^+ channels. The scorpion toxins from *Leiurus quinquestriatus quinquestriatus* and *Centruroides suffusus suffusus* act on the gating properties of the channel, the *Leiurus* toxin modulating the inactivation kinetics (α scorpion toxins), and the *Centruroides* toxin (β scorpion toxin) inducing repetitive firing because of the appearance of abnormal sodium channel activation without affecting the inactivation kinetics of the channel. These toxins which bind to distinct receptor sites on the channel have been extremely useful in probing the structure, function, and development of Na^+ channels at the molecular level.

Because of the extensive work on neurotoxin action and the high affinity of these neurotoxins for the Na^+ channel, we have placed spectroscopic and ultrastructural tags on these molecules to investigate the molecular structure and cellular dynamics of the Na^+ channel. Fluorescence spectroscopy in particular is an exquisitely sensitive and versatile method for obtaining structural and conformational information. We have

[a]This work was supported by research grants from the National Institutes of Health (NS 18268 and NS 15617) and the Muscular Dystrophy Association.

prepared biologically active fluorescent and photoactivable fluorescent derivatives of these neurotoxins specific to the Na^+ channel in order to elucidate the spatial relationship between neurotoxin binding and functional sites on the Na^+ channel and to describe the steady-state conformational coupling and transitions between these sites. The microenvironments of the receptors as well as the dynamic conformational motion of actively gating channels in excitable cells have been explored. These probes have also been used to examine the organization and lateral mobility of Na^+ channels in nerve and muscle fibers.

PREPARATION AND CHARACTERIZATION OF FLUORESCENT Na^+ CHANNEL NEUROTOXINS

In order to use chemically derivatized neurotoxins as spectroscopic molecular probes of the Na^+ channel confidently, there are several features that must be designed into the fluorescent toxin. First, the biological activity and high affinity of the toxin must be preserved after chemical derivatization. This necessitates the incorporation of a fluorophore that can either substitute for a functional moiety, be nonperturbing, or generally small. The probe should be appropriately chemically reactive so that the modification can be carried out under mild conditions. Additional functionality is desirable for further derivatization (e.g., to alter an amino group to an azido). Furthermore, the length between the neurotoxin and the probe moiety is minimized so that the spectroscopic properties reflect events at the neurotoxin receptor site. Secondly, because of the low density of Na^+ channels in excitable membranes, the fluorescent probe should have a high extinction coefficient ($>15,000$ $M^{-1}cm^{-1}$) and a high quantum yield ($\phi > 0.2$). In order to report on the environmental features of the receptor sites the probe should also demonstrate a Stokes shift of at least 20 nm (thus it should have an excited state dipole moment). The latter can be predicted on the basis of the chemical functionality substituted on the aromatic ring. Together with the probe's environmental sensitivity, an excited state lifetime that can be conveniently measured by either phase-demodulation techniques or pulse sampling should also be considered if the rotational relaxation and motion of the neurotoxin probe at the receptor will be measured. Thirdly, both the wavelengths of absorption and fluorescence emission of the probe should be selected for use as donor-acceptor pairs as well as for long-wavelength characteristics where suitable microscopic filters and gas ion laser lines can be found. Keeping these general properties in mind, we have designed and constructed several fluorescent derivatives of the Na^+ channel neurotoxins that can be utilized for a variety of molecular and cellular studies.

This first section describes the synthesis of channel-specific neurotoxin derivatives, the characterization of these derivatives chemically, biologically, and spectrally, and their use in structural studies of the Na^+ channel.

Tetrodotoxin

Tetrodotoxin (TTX) and saxitoxin (STX) have been most widely used as molecular and cellular markers for voltage-dependent Na^+ channels. TTX and STX bind at or near the ion selectivity filter and the binding selectively eliminates the transient inward Na^+ current but does not affect channel gating. TTX can be oxidized either at C-6 or C-11 to form a C-6 ketone or C-11 aldehyde and subsequently reacted with hydrazides to form hydrazones or reductively aminated with amines to form a primary amine at C-6 (amino-TTX, FIG. 1).[3,4] This latter derivatization is particularly useful because it

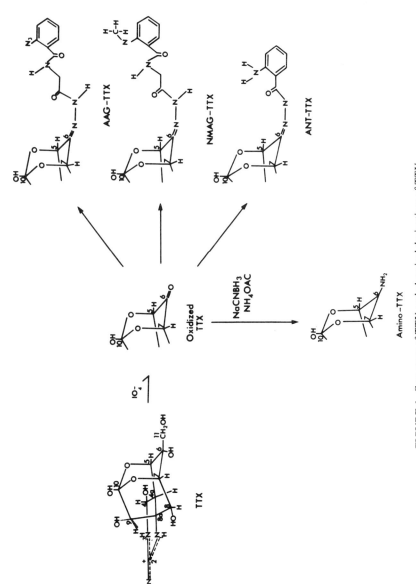

FIGURE 1. Structure of TTX and chemical derivatives of TTX.

allows coupling to N-succinimidyl esters that bear either radioactive alkyl groups or a variety of fluorescent groups, for example 7-dimethylamino-coumarin-4-acetate, N-methylanthranilate, or dinitrophenylamino-propionate. Purification is subsequently carried out by high-performance liquid chromotography using reverse phase on a SIL-C_{18} or SIL-C_8 and a cation exchange column of Partisil SCX/10. Chemical characterization by 300 MHz proton NMR and mass spectral analysis of the HPLC purified compounds is consistent with the structures. Unreacted TTX is eliminated by these procedures and does not therefore mask the biological properties of the derivatives. 7-Azidocoumarin-4-[2,3-hydroxybutyrl]amide-TTX is a unique reagent in that a photoactivable fluorescent moiety is attached to TTX which can be cleaved via the vic diol (see FIG. 6). This has been used as an active-site-directed probe[5] on rat neuronal membranes where TTX, after photolysis followed by low concentrations of periodate, which cleave the reagent and regenerate an active channel, delivers covalently the fluorescent moiety to the receptor. The spectroscopic properties of this reporter group, now attached to the channel matrix at or near the ion selection site, can monitor the binding of cations, TTX, or conformational events during the action potential (see below).

After oxidation of TTX at C-6 or C-11 and further modification the biological activity and high affinity are conserved. A detailed comparison of the effect of TTX and the fluorescent and photoactivable fluorescent derivatives on the action potential of rat sciatic nerve show that the derivatives are only about two to five times less active than TTX itself. Similar results are obtained by measurement of binding affinity based on the ability of the derivatives to displace [^{3}H]TTX or [^{3}H]STX from specific receptor sites on rat brain synaptosomes or from equilibrium binding isotherms obtained by spectroscopic analyses.

Batrachotoxin Derivatives

Of all the alkaloid neurotoxins that act as depolarizing agents by altering the voltage dependence of both activation and inactivation, batrachotoxin (BTX) is the most potent and selective, activating more than 95% of the channels. Fortunately chemical studies on BTX derivatives have revealed important details about the structure-activity relationships. The oxygen bridge between the A and B rings and the dimethylpyrrole carboxylate ester moiety are essential for activity in the naturally occurring compound. Elimination of the pyrrole rings results in a biologically inactive derivative, BTX-A. Given this structure-activity information we chose a fluorescent moiety whose structure would be sterically compatible with the native toxin. This of course places constraints on the size of the fluorophore and as a result on the spectral properties. A fluorophore with the suitable size and spectral properties is N-methylanthranilate, which has a reasonable extinction coefficient and high quantum yield. It suffers, however, from an excitation maximum at 350 nm, which is at the lower end of the visible spectrum. Batrachotoxinin-A-N-methylanthranilate (BTX-A-NMA), an analogue of the potent depolarizing agent BTX, was prepared by selective esterification of the 20-α hydroxyl of naturally occurring BTX-A with N-methylanthranilic acid using ethyl chloroformate. Purification was accomplished on TLC and the identity and purity of the product was determined by mass spectral analysis.[6]

When exposed to either BTX or BTX-NMA, the surface fibers from frog sartorius muscle are depolarized at similar rates and there is no observable difference in the ability of either toxin to depolarize these fibers. Within 20 min of application of a solution of 80 nM BTX-NMA, the resting membrane potential rose from -78 to -31

mV, with a reduction in the spike amplitude and rate of rise of the action potential. After 15 min, the membrane potential was at -37 mV and the ability to generate an action potential was completely lost despite polarization of the membrane to -78 mV, although end-plate potentials could still be recorded upon indirect stimulation of BTX-NMA-depolarized muscle fibers. The frequency of miniature end-plate potentials increased from about 10–20 Hz to more than 400 Hz, and finally disappeared at a membrane potential of -33 mV as the muscle fiber continued to depolarize.[6] Equilibrium binding of BTX-NMA to rat synaptosomes indicates a K_d of 78 nM compared to 44 nM for BTX with an average receptor site capacity of 2 pmol/mg protein in the presence of 1 μM α-ScTX. The BTX derivative maintains the same allosteric coupling as the native toxin between the α-ScTX site and the BTX receptor. Thus, electrophysiological and equilibrium binding measurements indicate that BTX-NMA retains high affinity for voltage-dependent Na$^+$ channels. The fluorescence emission of the toxin upon addition to rat brain synaptosomes indicates that BTX-NMA is initially in a hydrophobic environment.[6] Binding of toxin V from *Leiurus quinquestriatus,* an allosteric activator, effects a 20 nm red shift in the spectrum of bound BTX-NMA and a fourfold enhancement in the quantum yield, disclosing a conformational change into a more hydrophilic environment.[6] These spectroscopic experiments and previous binding measurements indicate direct conformational coupling between these two sodium channel sites.

Scorpion Toxin Derivatives

Scorpion toxins are basic polypeptides with molecular weights of 7,000 that act on the gating properties of the Na$^+$ channel. Our efforts have focused on the chemical modification and biological characterization of two classes of scorpion neurotoxins: α scorpion toxins which modify the closing kinetics of the channel and bind in a voltage-dependent manner (*e.g.,* Lqq V) and β toxins which modify the kinetics of channel opening and bind in a voltage-independent fashion (*e.g.,* CssII).

Previous modification of these toxins indicated that acylation, alkylation, citraconylation of amino groups, carboxylate esterification, and acylation or alkylation of histidine lead to a loss of toxin activity.[7] However, guanididation of amino groups and limited iodination of tyrosine preserve the toxic activity. To us this suggested that the charge is critical, and a successful modification and introduction of fluorescent chromophores would necessitate preserving the peptide's net positive charge. Four different modification strategies were pursued in which selectively acylated, amidinylated, thio-amidinylated, and reductively alkylated scorpion toxins were prepared. Utilizing these methods a number of fluorescent derivatives have been prepared, purified, and chemically and biologically characterized.[8,9] Selective acylation of Lys-60 and Lys-13 in Lqq and Css respectively induced a loss of net positive charge on the toxin and the derivatives were therefore purified by preparative isoelectric focusing, ion-exchange chromatography, and HPLC.[9] Amidinylation and reductive alkylation preserved the protonation state of the toxin and thus the native tertiary structure of the toxin. Because the charge is not significantly altered in these derivatives, we developed immunoprecipitation/affinity purification methods using small amounts of modified toxin. In the first method, rabbit antibodies were raised against the fluorophore. Anti-fluorophore IgG was then used to precipitate the fluorescently modified toxin, separating any unmodified (native) toxin that would otherwise mask the biological properties of the modified toxin. Sequence analysis of the modification site shows that Lys-58 is modified in the α scorpion toxins and Lys-13 is modified in the β scorpion toxins, regions of the toxins which appear from the 1.4 Å toxin crystal maps to be on the putative toxin-channel surface.

A more versatile modification that we have used is the incorporation of a unique functional group onto the peptide for subsequent modification and use. Since the toxin does not contain cysteine, a new sulfhydryl was generated through amidination (which also preserves the toxin's net charge) by reaction with the cyclic imidoester, 2-iminothiolane.[8,9] In order to facilitate separation of modified from unmodified toxin,

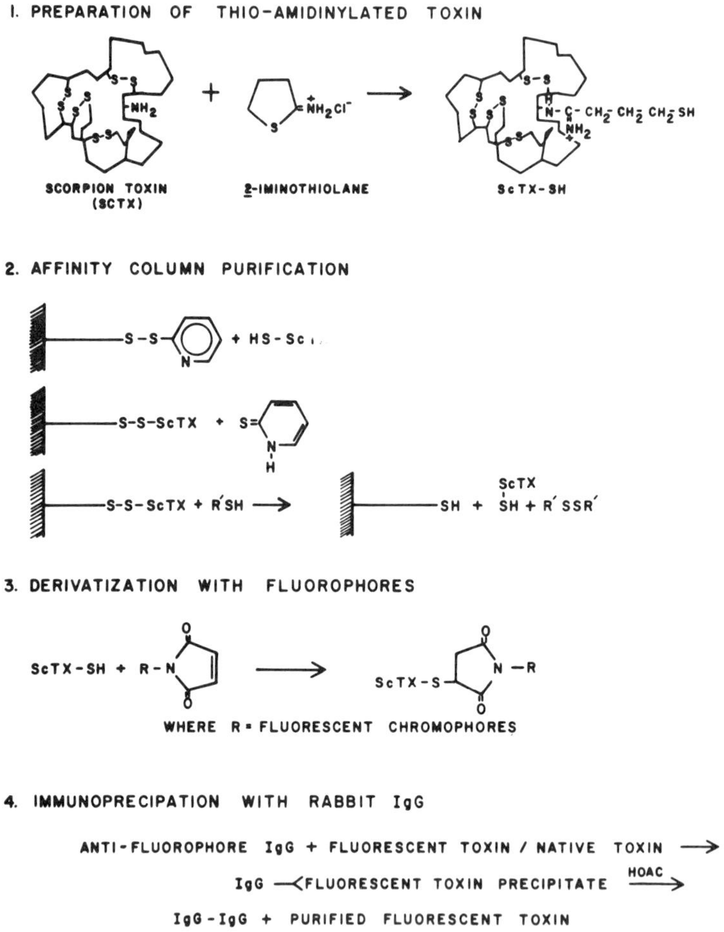

FIGURE 2. Preparation and affinity purification of fluorescent scorpion toxins.

we have employed a procedure with an affinity purification step. The method is shown schematically in FIGURE 2. Amidination of the toxin's lysine at high pH results in the concomitant generation of a new sulfhydryl group. The availability of a sulfhydryl-containing modified toxin permits purification through covalent thiol-disulfide interchange chromatography to separate modified toxin from unmodified toxin, which might otherwise mask the biological properties of the modified toxin. The unmodified toxin passes right through the column whereas the modified toxin undergoes covalent linkage. Release of modified toxin from the column takes place with low concentrations of cysteine. The sulfhydryl-bearing toxin is then modified with any number of fluorescent maleimides with the appropriate spectral characteristics. This has led to (1) the separation of modified from native toxin by thiol-disulfide exchange chromatography, (2) the preparation of a wide variety of fluorescent toxins using sulfhydryl specific fluorescent maleimides that can be changed as necessary for FRAP studies, and (3) the attachment of cleavable photoactivable fluorescent chromophores that can be incorporated into the channel protein to examine conformational fluctuations about these channel sites.

The biological activities of all modified scorpion toxin have been assessed electrophysiologically. The action potential of rat muscle after α scorpion toxin treatment presents a prolongation of the falling phase with a marked plateau. At high concentrations of toxin the resting membrane potential moves toward more positive potentials, accompanied by action potential durations up to 500 ms, and spontaneous firing of the fiber. As with the native α toxin, the binding is voltage dependent and can be enhanced by the binding of BTX. After modification β scorpion toxin derivatives retain their voltage-independent binding. The biological activities, equilibrium binding, and spectroscopic properties indicate that these derivatives retain high affinity for the sodium channel and are as active or only two or three times less active than *Leiurus q.* V or toxin II from *Centruroides suffusus* toxin itself.[8,9]

The fluorescent properties of the modified scorpion toxins in particular show excellent environmental sensitivity and are suitable for probing the molecular dynamics of their receptors and for topographic mapping of the sodium channel by fluorescence resonance energy transfer measurements. The fluorescence emission properties indicate that the α and β scorpion toxin sites are buried in hydrophobic domains of the channel and that the fluorescence properties of derivatized CssII are markedly altered in the presence of α scorpion toxin, indicating receptor site coupling and intrasubunit communication (see below).[8,9]

Other Toxins and Local Anesthetics

Quaternary or protonated forms of local anesthetics are effective in blocking Na^+ flux and seem to gain access to their Na^+ channel receptor under depolarizing conditions. We have prepared a fluorescent procaine analogue by condensation of isatoic anhydride and dimethylaminoethanol in dioxane. At high concentrations (100 μM) this procaine analogue blocks the inward Na^+ current in a frequency-dependent manner. The fluorescence emission of procaine is exquisitely sensitive to the environment and can distinguish readily between hydrophobic and hydrophilic components of the anesthetic binding site. We have examined the proposed phase partition mechanism of action of the local anesthetics because the fluorescence emission is able to report on the environment and kinetics of the partitioning as a result of the membrane potential and inactivation of the channel gates. Preliminary experiments have found the procaine fluorescence to be sensitive to applied voltages across the membrane and these changes can be antagonized by α scorpion toxins.

With the five TTX, seven LqqV, two CssII, and BTX derivatives that we have prepared, electrophysiological recordings from frog muscle or spinal cord neurons, equilibrium binding to neuronal membranes, and spectroscopic measurements indicate that these neurotoxin derivatives retain high affinity for the Na^+ channel and are as active or only two to five times less active than the native toxins themselves. The spectroscopic properties of these fluorescent derivatives cover the absorption range from 290 nm to 470 nm, and fluorescence emission ranges from 360 nm to 650 nm where suitable microscopic filters, gas ion laser lines, and spectral overlap for energy transfer can be found between all derivatives. For many which incorporate NBD or CPM, the fluorescence properties are suitable for dipolar relaxation measurements of channel conformation during ion conduction, cellular distribution, and lateral diffusion studies because the emissions are at long wavelengths (520 nm) and are highly efficient ($\phi = 0.2$ to 0.8). FIGURE 3 summarizes some of the fluorescent neurotoxin tools we have constructed, together with their spectral and biological properties. Several incorporate cleavable groups that deliver an "extrinsic-intrinsic" reporter group to the channel via the specificity of the toxin moiety.

STRUCTURAL MAPPING OF THE Na$^+$ CHANNEL BY FLUORESCENCE RESONANCE ENERGY TRANSFER

One advantage of utilizing fluorescent ligands, besides the low concentrations and sensitivity that is afforded by their use, is that the distances between the various probes or ligand can be determined.[10] Given these fluorescent toxin derivatives, we have determined the molecular arrangement between the functional sites on the Na$^+$ channel by fluorescence resonance energy transfer.

Distance Determinations

Fluorescence energy transfer is the nonradiative transfer of energy from a donor to an acceptor molecule after the donor has absorbed light at its characteristic absorption frequency. The Forster theory relates the efficiency of energy transfer, E, to the fluorescence lifetime of the donor in the presence and absence of the acceptor and to the distance between the donor and acceptor, R.[11] Equations 2, 3, and 4 give these relationships:

$$E = 1 - Q_{D \to A}/Q_D = 1 - \tau_{D \to A}/\tau_D \tag{2}$$

$$E = \frac{R^{-6}}{R^{-6} + R_o^{-6}}$$

$$R_o = 9.79 \times 10^3 \, (Q_D J^2 n^{-4})^{1/6} \, \text{Å}$$

$$R = R_o \cdot (1/E - 1)^{1/6} \, \text{Å}, \tag{3}$$

where τ_D and Q_D are the lifetime and quantum yield of the donor and $\tau_{D \to A}$ and $Q_{D \to A}$ are the lifetime and quantum yield of the donor in the presence of the acceptor. The Forster critical distance, in which the donor and acceptor must be separated to give 50% energy transfer is R_o, and is a characteristic of the $D \to A$ pair; J is the spectral overlap integral, n is the refractive index of the medium, and K^2 is a dipole-dipole orientation factor. The spectral overlap integral is a measure of how well the absorption spectrum of the acceptor overlaps the fluorescence emission of the donor and is given by

$$J = \frac{\sum_\lambda F_D(\lambda)\epsilon_A(\lambda)\lambda^4 \delta\lambda}{\sum_\lambda F_D(\lambda)d\lambda}, \tag{4}$$

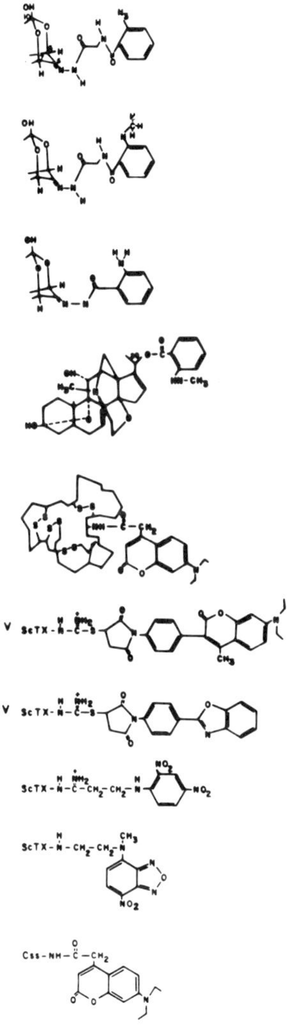

LIGAND	STRUCTURE	SPECTRAL CHARACTERISTICS			
		$\lambda_{ex,nm}$	$\lambda_{em,nm}$	Φ_{ROC}	K_D,nM
AAG-TTX		402			
NMAG-TTX		352	439	0.67	7.10
ANT-TTX		325	402	0.56	6.10
BTX-A-NMA		345	427	0.53	8.50
DACA-Lqq V		375	472	0.33	2.50
CPM-SH-Lqq V		392	468	0.58	5.80
NBPM-SH-Lqq V		308	456	0.83	8.60
DNP-Lqq V		360			
NBD-Lqq V		343 487	526	0.42	6.20
DACA-Css II		365	467	0.31	6.90

FIGURE 3. Fluorescent neurotoxins used to probe the voltage-dependent Na^+ channel.

where F is the donor fluorescence, ϵ is the molar extinction coefficient of the acceptor and λ is the wavelength. In general, when choosing acceptor-donor pairs for fluorescence energy transfer measurements, large overlap integrals are desirable since this results in a large value of R_o. The orientation factor, K^2, can range from 0 to 4.0. If the acceptor and donor rotate freely in a time-frame that is short relative to the donor excited-state lifetime the value of K^2 is $\frac{2}{3}$. This rotational mobility can be estimated by measuring the time dependence of the emission anisotropy. Bounds on K^2 can be estimated utilizing steady-state and dynamic polarization measurements. Careful consideration of these factors can generally limit the uncertainty in R due to K^2 to

10%–20%.[12] Statistical treatments can be used to narrow the range of K^2 for donors and acceptors which show depolarization due to local rotation during the excited state lifetime or due to a combination of mixed polarization and local rotation.[13]

Experimentally, steady-state efficiencies of energy transfer, E, are measured by both quenching of donor fluorescence and sensitized emission of the acceptor. To evaluate distances between multiple donor-acceptor pairs, the positions of the chromophores were exchanged.[6,9,14,15] Limits on the range of calculated distances between the sites were evaluated by using several donor-acceptor pairs and from the depolarization of the transferred excitation. The distance range is further narrowed to 5% to 10% because these probes show depolarization due to a combination of mixed polarization and local rotation.

In all experiments, samples for energy transfer were prepared with fluorescent donor, fluorescent donor plus unlabeled acceptor, fluorescent donor and fluorescent acceptor, and unlabeled donor plus fluorescent acceptor. Measurements were performed by the addition of the appropriate concentration of fluorescent donor to a suspension of synaptosomes or axolemma in which the scattering spectrum was first obtained, followed by the addition of either fluorescent acceptor or unlabeled acceptor. When fluorescent acceptor was added, the spectrum was recorded, followed by the addition of 1 μM unlabeled toxin to displace the specific fluorescent toxin from the receptor. The resulting spectrum was then recorded in which fluorescent donor,

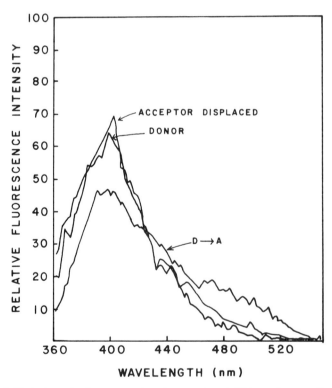

FIGURE 4. Typical result of an energy transfer experiment. Distance between the TTX and β-scorpion toxin receptors.

TABLE 1. Energy Transfer Distances between Neurotoxin Binding Sites on the Sodium Channel

Donor		Acceptor		Distance
Ligand	Channel Site	Ligand	Channel Site	Å
TTX	ion selection	LqqV (α-ScTX)	inactivation gate	35
		+ BTX		42
BTX	activation/inactivation	LqqV	inactivation gate	37
TTX	ion selection	CssII (β-ScTX)	activation gate	33
CssII (β-ScTX)	activation gate	LqqV (α-ScTX)	inactivation gate	22
LqqV (α-ScTX)	inactivation gate	Glu-PL	membrane surface	15
CssII (β-ScTX)	activation gate	Glu-PL	membrane surface	23
TTX	channel	TTX	channel	70

fluorescent acceptor, and unlabeled acceptor were present.[6,9,14] The spectra from a typical energy transfer experiment is shown in FIGURE 4 and is an experiment in which the distance from the TTX to β scorpion toxin receptor was measured.

Using these procedures, we observed an efficiency for the case presented in FIGURE 4 by donor quenching of 0.23 and by the sensitized emission of the acceptor of 0.25. Since the CssII receptor sites were not all occupied, the observed transfer efficiency is corrected to that which would be observed if all channels had acceptors. Under the conditions of these expriments the fraction of channels with bound DACA-CssII is 0.44. The corrected efficiencies are 0.52 and 0.57 by donor quenching and sensitized emission, respectively.

With the corrected transfer efficiencies and an R_o of 35 Å for the anthraniloyl coumarin pair, this translates into an intermolecular distance of 34 Å from the data presented in FIGURE 4 (TABLE 1).

The good agreement between efficiencies measured by donor quenching and measured by sensitized emission indicates that the observed quenching of the donor TTX is due to dipolar energy transfer to DACA-CssII, and not to other electronic deactivating mechanisms.

The results of a series of energy transfer experiments are summarized in TABLE 1, which lists the distances between neurotoxin sites on the Na^+ channel.

When the channel is activated by BTX the TTX to Lqq distance increases by 7 Å and indicates that conformational changes in the channel are effected over significant distances (37 Å). From equilibrium binding measurements it is known that the α scorpion toxin and BTX receptor are allosterically coupled. In order to construct a three-dimensional model of the intramolecular distances, the intramembrane positions of the LqqV and Css binding sites were measured from the fluorescence quenching of DACA-LqqV or DACA-Css as a function of the membrane surface acceptor density and analyzed with a parallel infinite planes model. The acceptor was NBD-*N*-methyl-D-glucosyl-phosphatidylglycerol, a lipid that bears a carbohydrate moiety in order to prohibit flip-flop motion across the bilayer. The α-SCTX site is embedded about 15 Å into the membrane and the β scorpion toxin site is 23 Å. This suggests that the scorpion toxins elicit their physiological effects by an internal Na^+ channel receptor.

When ANT-TTX (donor) is randomly mixed with increasing amounts of coumarin-TTX (acceptor) energy transfer between these two is observed (TABLE 1). The quenching of ANT-TTX fluorescence can be relieved by disruption of the bilayer, for example with detergents, indicating that the integrity of the membrane is required for these interactions. Calculation of the distance of separation indicates that two or more Na^+ channels lie within 50–70 Å of each other in neuronal membranes because there is one TTX site per channel, and that channels likely occur as oligomers or in patches on the cell surface. Energy transfer measurements between channel proteins reconstituted do not, however, give any experimental evidence that would indicate that the channels are organized as oligomers. Even though channels were reconstituted in various protein to lipid ratios, no energy transfer has been observed. Thus energy transfer measurements provided the first indications that Na^+ channels in synaptic and axonal membranes are organized into microclusters and assume a nonuniform distribution even though the underlying cytoskeleton has been detached from these membranes. These studies have been extended by direct quantitation of Na^+ channel density by a fluorescence microbeam and by measurement of the lateral mobility by FPR.[16,17] The hillock in particular contains a dense and immobile cluster of Na^+ channels which appears to be segregated to this region by direct cytoskeletal attachments. Together with preliminary data on the rotational diffusion of Na^+ channels in synaptosomes, it is becoming apparent that in some areas and systems Na^+ channel proteins are closely associated.

Microenvironments and Conformational Transitions of Channel Sites

The binding, spectroscopic, and energy transfer distance measurements indicate that the Lqq, Css, and BTX sites are sensitive to either voltage- or neurotoxin-dependent conformation changes. For example, when BTX is added to bound DACA-LqqV, a 10 nm change to the red in the emission spectrum is noted together with a large fluorescence enhancement.[14] Similar effects are noted on the spectral properties of BTX-NMA, in which addition of LqqV shifts the emission maximum more than 30 nm to the red, into an environment of greater polarity, and enhances the emission intensity 10-fold. Although binding measurements indicate allosteric interactions among channel receptor sites, the first direct indication of molecular conformational coupling between these receptors is shown in TABLE 1 where an alteration in the receptor site distance occurs between the TTX and LqqV receptors in the presence of BTX. In the presence of BTX, the TTX Lqq distance increases to 42 Å, indicating a neurotoxin-induced conformational change in one subunit of the channel or a change in the interaction between two subunits coupled to the BTX binding sites. In spite of the sensitivity of the fluorescence to ligand binding, the energy transfer measurements summarized in TABLE 1 indicate that the BTX and Lqq sites are quite far apart (e.g., 37 Å). Thus the binding of BTX must involve conformational changes that extend over large distances from the Lqq binding locus. In addition, the fluorescence properties of DACA-Css bound to the channel are blue-shifted 10 nm in the presence of LqqV.[9] This information together with the distance measurement of TTX to Lqq and Lqq to Css and the conformational transition associated with the distances upon ligand binding suggest a conformationally flexible channel with coupling of sites through the polyatomic framework of a single polypeptide chain (e.g., domain-domain interactions) or through alterations in subunit-subunit interactions.

Spatial Relationships and Molecular Topology of Neurotoxin Binding Sites on the Sodium Channel

From the fluorescence spectral information, resonance energy transfer between receptor sites on the channel, biochemical composition,[18–20] target face analysis,[21,22] and molecular morphology, we arrive at a map of the receptor sites shown in FIGURE 5. The TTX and STX binding site is placed in a highly polar environment at the extracellular face of the 270,000 α-component of the Na$^+$ channel complex. Affinity labeling with photoreactive Lqq and CssII derivatives specifically label the α-peptide as well as a smaller peptide, $\beta 1$ of molecular weight 39,000.[23,25] Radiation inactivation of the STX, Lqq, and BTX receptors indicate target sizes of 220,000 for TTX, 263,000 for Lqq,

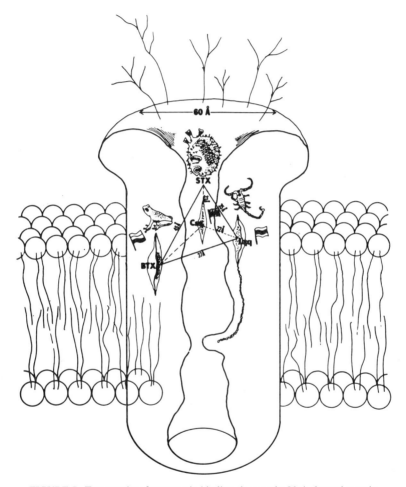

FIGURE 5. Topography of neurotoxin binding sites on the Na$^+$ channel protein.

45,000 for Css II, and 280,000 and 48,000 for the BTX receptors, in which the 45,000–48,000 unit appears to represent a domain of the α-peptide.[22] From the experimental distances and results using the purified peptide of the rat brain Na$^+$ channel,[22] most if not all of the functional neurotoxin receptors are on the α-peptide of the channel. Thus those spectroscopic changes associated with ligand binding at remote and spatially separated neurotoxin sites indicate a conformationally flexible single polypeptide that transmits and communicates these changes over significant distances. Measurement of the secondary structure by circular dicroism also shows that the α-peptide is a conformationally flexible polypeptide, which, although capable of binding STX with high affinity, contains mostly β-sheet and random coil in mixed detergent-phospholipid micelles and folds into a conformation that has 65% α-helix after reconstitution into phosphatidylcholine vesicles.[20] Together with the primary structure available from the cloned cDNA, the distances between receptor sites will be used in conjunction with the identification and sequencing of the peptides associated with the neurotoxin receptor sites and will lead to a model in which the three-dimensional folding of the polypeptide chain can be traced.

OPTICAL STUDIES OF THE Na$^+$ CHANNEL IN SITU

Dynamics of Probes and Neurotoxin Receptors on Live Axons: Changes in the Environment and Spatial Relationship During the Action Potential

Although the energy transfer measurements have provided a useful topographic map of the neurotoxin functional sites on the Na$^+$ channel, this is unfortunately a static representation. We have extended the use of these probes and techniques to monitor the conformational events of the channel by the placement of spectroscopic probes at these neurotoxin receptors and by simultaneous monitoring of electrical and spectroscopic signals during active propagation.

The intensities, polarization, and resonance energy transfer of fluorescent neurotoxins and photofluorescent moieties incorporated into the channel matrix at specific sites have been used to examine structural rearrangements at channel loci associated with channel opening and closing.

The application of optical techniques to the study of excitable membranes at the millisecond time scale was initiated approximately 10 years ago. By measuring birefringence, light scattering, and extrinsic fluorescence with covalent and noncovalent probes in squid and crab nerve fibers it was found possible to record optical signals of a rapid reversible nature which could be attributed to transient changes in the state of the membrane macromolecules or in the dye-membrane interaction during nerve excitation.[25] The major problem in all these studies has been the inability to relate these structural rearrangements directly to molecular properties of the Na$^+$ channel protein. The further aim of developing specific Na$^+$ channel probes utilizing the specificity of the neurotoxin moiety is to understand the molecular mechanisms of the Na$^+$ channel during impulse propagation using highly specific conformational probes of its structure, and to relate the observed optical changes directly to structural rearrangements of the channel protein during ion flux.

The optical probes and optical experiments that have been used in these studies have been of three types:

1. Fluorescent probes attached to neurotoxins that bind to the channel and whose fluorescent signals are monitored directly.
2. Fluorescent probes that are photoactivable fluorescent probes. These do not fluoresce until incorporated into a protein matrix. Specific toxins have been synthesized in which these photoactivable probes are brought to the channel through the affinity of the neurotoxin, and the toxin is subsequently cleaved to leave the fluorescent reporter group attached to the channel protein matrix. The characteristics of such a probe are shown in FIGURE 6.
3. Those optical experiments where two neurotoxins or two intrinsic labels will be

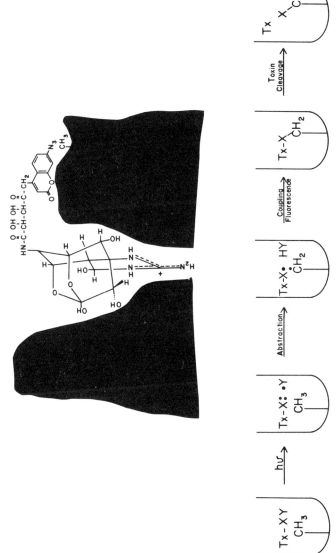

FIGURE 6. Photoactivable cleavable fluorescent neurotoxin probes that deliver a fluorescent reporter group onto the channel matrix.

used as an energy transfer pair, for example the energy transfer pair DACA-TTX and eosin-ScTX. With the former, squid giant axon was utilized in voltage-clamp experiments whereas with the latter crayfish axons were utilized because squid axons are relatively insensitive to scorpion toxin at the concentrations required for these experiments.

In all cases examined the optical arrangement and wavelength were configured in order to maximize the optical signal with the elimination of any other contaminating signals such as scattering and birefringence. FIGURE 7 shows signals obtained with DACA-TTX in the fluorescence mode and with eosin-ScTx in the absorption mode.

These experiments and others have demonstrated that a significant physiological optical signal can be obtained. Because these signals emanate from pharmacologically

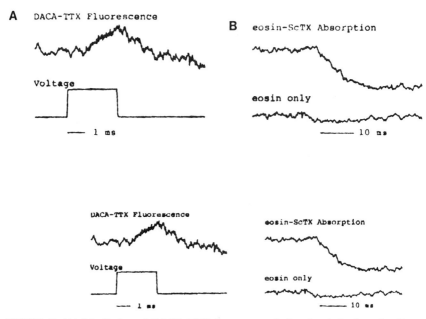

FIGURE 7. (A) Monitoring of DACA-TTX fluorescence during depolarization of voltage-clamped squid giant axon. (B) Optical monitoring of eosin-ScTX on crayfish axon.

modified channels, further work has been directed towards the introduction of optical probes alone onto the channel sites via the specificity of the neurotoxin. Photoactivable fluorescent derivatives of TTX and ScTX (in FIGURE 6) are being utilized to incorporate donor-acceptor chromophores onto the channel macromolecule, with subsequent cleavage of the neurotoxins to generate an active channel. Although the fraction of channels modified in this manner has been low due to the inefficiency of the photolysis reaction, preliminary measurements of donor quenching and sensitized emission during stimulation indicate that structural rearrangements occur within the time frame of channel opening and closing, with displacements of the peptide by about 9 Å during conduction. It is thus hoped that methods of detecting fluorescence signals utilizing Na^+-channel-specific fluorescent-neurotoxin incorporated at identified sequences on the channel protein during nerve conduction will provide insights into the dynamic molecular mechanisms of the action potential.

REFERENCE

1. CATTERALL, W. A. 1980. Ann. Rev. Pharmacol. Toxicol. **20**: 15–41.
2. LAZDUNSKI, M., M. BALERNA, J. BARHANIN, R. CHICHEPORTICHE, M., FOSSET, C. FRELIN, Y. JACQUES, A. LOMBET, J. POUYSSEGUR, J. F. RENAUD, G. ROMEY, H. SCHWEITZ & J. P. VINCENT. 1980. Ann. N. Y. Acad. Sci. **358**: 169–182.
3. CHICHEPORTICHE, R., M. BALERNA, A. LOMBET, G. ROMEY & M. LAZDUNSKI, 1980. Eur. J. Biochem. **104**: 617–623.
4. ANGELIDES, K. J. 1981. Biochemistry **20**: 4107–4118.
5. ANGELIDES, K. J. 1981. Biochem. Biophys. Acta **669**: 149–155.
6. ANGELIDES, K. J. & G. B. BROWN. 1984. J. Biol. Chem. **259**: 6117–6126.
7. HABERSETZER-ROCHAT, C. & F. SAMPIERI. 1976. Biochemistry **15**: 2254–2261.
8. ANGELIDES, K. J. & T. J. NUTTER. 1983. J. Biol. Chem. **258**: 11948–11957.
9. DARBON, H. & K. J. ANGELIDES. 1984. J. Biol. Chem. **259**: 6074–6084.
10. FAIRCLOUGH, R. H. & C. R. CANTOR. 1978. Methods Enzymol. **48**: 347–368.
11. FOSTER, T. 1965. Modern Quantum Chemistry. Lect. Istanbul Inst. Summer Sch. 1964. **3**: 93–103.
12. DALE, R. D., J. EISINGER & W. E. BLUMBERG. Biophys. J. **26**: 161–194.
13. HAAS, E., E. KATCHALSKI-KATZIR & I. Z. STEINBERG. 1978. Biochemistry **17**: 5064–5070.
14. ANGELIDES, K. J. & T. J. NUTTER. 1983. J. Biol. Chem. **258**: 11958–11967.
15. ANGELIDES, K. J. & T. J. NUTTER. 1984. Biophys. J. **45**: 31–34.
16. ANGELIDES, K. J., L. ELMER, D. LOFTUS & E. L. ELSON. 1986. J. Cell Biol. In press.
17. ANGELIDES, K. J. 1986. Nature **321**: 63–66.
18. HARTSHORNE, R. P. & W. A. CATTERALL. 1984. J. Biol. Chem. **259**: 1667–1676.
19. BARHANIN, J., D. PAURAN, A. LAMBET, R. I. NORMAN, H. P. M. VIJVERBERG, J. GIGLIO & M. LAZDUNSKI. 1983. EMBO J. **2**: 915–922.
20. ELMER, L. W., B. O'BRIEN, T. J. NUTTER & K. J. ANGELIDES. 1985. Biochemistry **24**: 8128–8136.
21. BARHANIN, J., A. SCHMID, A. LAMBET, K. P. WHEELER, M. LAZDUNSKI & J. C. ELLORY. J. Biol. Chem. **258**: 700–706
22. ANGELIDES, K. J., T. J. NUTTER, L. W ELMER & E. S. KEMPNER. 1985. J. Biol. Chem. **260**: 3431 3439.
23. BENESKY, P. A. & W. A. CATTERALL. 1980. Proc. Natl. Acad. Sci. U. S. A. **77**: 639–642.
24. DARBON, H., E. JOVER, F. COURAUD & H. ROCHAT. 1983. Biochem. Biophys. Res. Commun. **115**: 415–422.
25. COHEN, L. B. & D. LANDOWNE. 1971. Physiology and Biophysics of Excitable Membranes, W. J. Adelman, Ed.: 247. Van Nostrand-Reinhold. New York.

The Structure and Function of the Voltage-Sensitive Na Channel[a]

W. S. AGNEW, S. A. TOMIKO, R. L. ROSENBERG,
M. C. EMERICK, AND E. C. COOPER

Department of Physiology
Yale University School of Medicine
New Haven, Connecticut 06510

INTRODUCTION

The overriding objective of our research is to explain the molecular mechanisms of the voltage-sensitive sodium channel[1-3] (or channel*s*, as recent findings indicate there are distinct, though perhaps small, differences among channels from different sources[4]). The term "mechanism" refers specifically to the relationship between the protein structure and its biological functions. The incentive for doing this is that Na channels are the first example of voltage-gated proteins to be studied in detail with biochemical and molecular biological approaches. The search to understand the mechanisms whereby a protein is regulated by voltage provides the necessity for innovative technical advances.

In order to gain insight into Na channel behavior, it will be necessary first to provide a detailed description of its chemical structure. This, however, will yield only a static view of the molecule. It will therefore be important to be able to characterize the dynamic properties of the channel. We wish to be able to monitor channel function under defined conditions, both when the protein is in its normal form and after specific chemical modifications have been introduced. This report reviews some of the basic biochemical characteristics of the Na channel protein isolated from eel electric organ, and progress made in recreating from the purified protein an artificial electrically excitable membrane which may be studied with electrical and biochemical methods.

THE ISOLATED Na CHANNEL PROTEIN

Radioactive derivatives of tetrodotoxin (TTX) and saxitoxin (STX) are used in binding assays as markers during the isolation of the Na channel protein.[5-7] When solubilized in Lubrol-PX detergent, the TTX binding protein of the electroplax is a particle of protein, lipid, and detergent of 90 Å Stokes radius, and a molecular mass of 592,000 Da (TABLE 1). Of this, approximately 262,000 Da (35%) is detergent and lipid associated with the protein component independently estimated to be 295,000 Da. The protein appears to be formed of a single class of large molecular weight glycopeptide, as illustrated in FIGURE 1. The apparent size of the glycopeptide is 230,000–290,000

[a]This work was supported by the National Institutes of Health (grant NS17928) and a grant from the Multiple Sclerosis Society. SAT was supported by a postdoctoral fellowship from the Muscular Dystrophy Association.

Da, determined by gel electrophoresis.[6] This peptide behaves anomalously in gel studies,[6] in a manner which suggests it binds three-to-four times the amount of SDS as a conventional protein; this results in variations in the apparent size of the peptide, depending on the gel conditions used. Thus the native solubilized protein includes not more than one equivalent of the polypeptide. There is at present no firm evidence for smaller subunits which are found with the mammalian brain and skeletal muscle channels.[9,10,16]

The chemical composition of the peptide has been determined both by direct analysis[6] and deduced from the sequences of cloned cDNA derived from mRNA coding for the channel.[11] TABLE 2 reports the amino acid composition measured directly,[6] and deduced from the cDNA sequences. This composition is not dissimilar to that of the nicotinic acetylcholine receptor from the eel electroplax. The carbohydrate composition is dramatically different, however, constituting nearly 30% of the glyco-

TABLE 1. Hydrodynamic Parameters of Solubilized Na Channel Protein

Molecular mass (M_r) of the total protein-detergent-lipid complex	592,000 Da
Partial specific volume ($\bar{v}$) of the complex	0.847 g/cm^3
Partial specific volume of the detergent-lipid micelles	0.995 g/cm^3
Partial specific volume of the glycopeptide portion of the complex	0.73 g/cm^3
Native protein molecular mass	330,000 Da
Detergent-lipid bound per g protein	0.79
Stokes radius (Rs) of the complex	90 Å
Sedimentation coefficient ($S_{20,w}$, calculated)	8.9 S
Diffusion coefficient ($D_{20,w}$, calculated)	2.4 F
Frictional coefficient (f/f_o)	1.5
Mass of the (denatured) glycopeptide	295,000 Da

The Stokes radius was determined by gel filtration over Sepharose 4B, with catalase, β-galactosidase, thyroglobulin, and glutamic decarboxylase as standards (W. S. Agnew *et al.*, unpublished). The TTX binding protein was run in 0.1% Lubrol-PX:PC and also in 1% Na cholate:PC, with no difference in the elution position being detected. The $\bar{v}$ of the glycopeptide was calculated from the amino acid composition derived from the cDNA sequence, the carbohydrate composition, and the data of Cohn and Edsall.[38] The values of $\bar{v}$ (particle), M_r (particle), and M_r (protein) were derived from sedimentation equilibrium studies (W. S. Agnew, H. F. Rudnick, and M. C. Emerick, in preparation). The values of $S_{20,w}$, $D_{20,w}$, and f/f_o were calculated from M_r, Rs, and $\bar{v}$ (particle). The mass of the denatured glycopeptide was calculated from the primary amino acid sequence (208,321 Da) of Noda *et al.*[11] together with the average carbohydrate composition (29.5 wt %) of Miller *et al.*[6]

peptide mass (TABLE 3). These carbohydrates are of the complex variety, and are enriched both in N-acetylhexoseamines (uncharged at neutral pH) and in sialic acids; these contribute about 113 negative charges per molecule (TABLE 4). This accounts for the observation that the free electrophoretic mobility of native TTX binding protein (in agarose gels) is about four times as great as the acetylcholine receptor, despite having a hydrodynamic, frictional coefficient that is about 1.3 times larger. Consistent with this high degree of glycosylation is the presence in the amino acid sequence of ten consensus glycosylation sites for N-linked sugars.[11] Further, in deglycosylation experiments under SDS-PAGE conditions where the glycosylated protein migrated as a 285,000 Da species, the protein after deglycosylation with *endo-β-N*-acetylglucosaminadase F behaved as a 200,000-Da species.[12] Consistent with this, the deduced primary amino acid sequence predicts a peptide of 208,321 Da, which together with 29.5% carbohydrate yields a glycopeptide of 295,000 Da, also accounting for a distinct microhetero-geneity stemming from variations in glycosylation.[6]

FUNCTIONAL PROPERTIES OF THE ISOLATED PROTEIN

Demonstrating the functional activity of the purified protein is important, both because it is required to prove that the species isolated represents a complete molecular

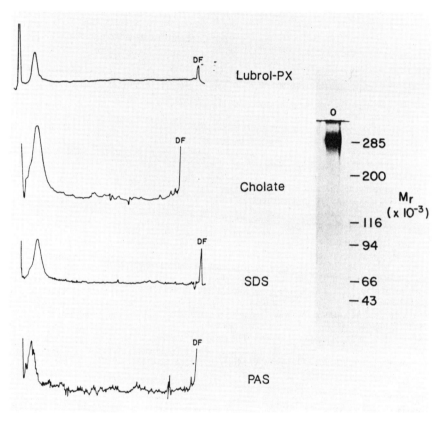

FIGURE 1. Densitometer scans of Na channel protein purified in Lubrol-PX- or in Na-cholate-containing buffers, and in denatured form in SDS, together with an actual gel photograph. The lowermost densitometer scan is of periodic acid Schiff-stained protein, illustrating the extensive glycosylation.

ensemble, and because domains of the protein responsible for different functions are explicitly the object of study. In this regard, the binding of channel-specific ligands such as TTX and STX represents the simplest category of "functional" behavior. With the electroplax protein, specific activities of approximately 3,000 pmol [³H]-TTX bound per mg protein (based on quantitative amino acid analysis) may be achieved.

TABLE 2. Amino Acid Composition of the Large Peptide of the Electroplax Na Channel[a]

Amino Acid	Miller et al.[6]	Noda et al.[11]
Asp	} 10.1	5.10 } 11.9
Asn		6.81
Thr	5.0	5.10
Ser	7.1	6.15
Glu	} 10.8	6.81 } 9.77
Gln		2.96
Pro	4.7	4.06
Gly	6.5	4.94
Ala	6.0	5.76
Cys	2.0	1.97
Val	5.3	7.41
Met	3.4	3.90
Ile	5.5	8.13
Leu	9.3	10.38
Tyr	2.8	3.39
Phe	5.9	6.97
His	2.8	0.93
Trp	3.5	1.70
Lys	5.0	5.10
Arg	4.3	4.17

[a]The amino acid composition arrived at by direct analysis (Miller et al.[6]) is compared with that deduced from the cDNA sequence of Noda et al.[11]

Given that the protein molecular mass is roughly 300,000 Da, a fully active preparation binding one equivalent of TTX might have been expected to have a specific activity of 3,300 pmol/mg protein. However, because a large proportion of the molecular mass is due to carbohydrate, the maximal value should be 4,800 pmol/mg protein, indicating that the best electroplax preparations are 60%–65% active. (Such revised estimates of maximal theoretical specific activity may also apply to the proteins from mammalian brain and muscle. These proteins have masses reported to be 314,000 ± 63,000 and 316,000 ± 32,000 Da, respectively.[13,14] Although both appear to be composed of one or two smaller peptides in addition to a ~260,000 Da species,[15–17] each subunit exhibits a high degree of glycosylation, yielding an underestimate of the maximal specific activity.)

The physiological function of the channel, of course, is to induce transient

TABLE 3. Carbohydrate Composition of the Large Peptide of the Electroplax Na Channel[a]

Glycoside	wt %	mol/mol Protein[b]
Fucose	0.5 ± 0.2	9 ± 3
Mannose	2.4 ± 0.3	39 ± 8
Galactose	1.5 ± 0.3	25 ± 5
N-Acetyl hexoseamines	13.3 ± 0.4	177 ± 5
Sialic acids	11.8 ± 1.2	113 ± 11
Total	29.5 ± 2.4	363

[a]From Miller et al.[6]
[b]Assuming a molecular weight of 295,000 Da.

TABLE 4. Estimated Net Charges per 295,000 Da Glycopeptide of Components of the Large Peptide[a]

Lys + Arg + ½ His[b]	+178
Glu + Asp	−217
Sialic acid	−113
Total	−152

[a]Estimates were made based on the balance of positively and negatively charged amino acids and carbohydrates.
[b]This assumes half of the histidines are protonated at neutral pH.

fluctuations in the membrane potential by opening a conducting pathway which is selective for Na^+. This conductance is governed by changes in conformation which depend kinetically and thermodynamically on voltage. The conductance state of the channel can be manipulated with a host of pharmacological compounds which can "block" the opened pathway, alter the gating mechanisms, or change the single channel conductance or permeation selectivity.[18,19,24] The influence of voltage, of drug binding, and chemical modification on the conductance state of the channel can then be measured with biochemical or electrophysiological methods, some of which are quite novel.

To study channel activity, the protein may be reconstituted into membranes which separate solvent compartments. The geometry of the membranes and the solvent compartments often determines the types of experiments which can then be carried out. The channel is purified as a solubilized protein dispersed in a phase of mixed lipid-detergent micelles (e. g., phosphatidylcholine and Lubrol-PX). By supplementing this suspension with sonicated liposomes (avoiding added detergent), and subsequently removing the detergent by adsorption to polystyrene beads (or, with detergent such as CHAPS or Na cholate, by dialysis or gel filtration; J. A. Miller, R. L. Rosenberg, and W. S. Agnew, unpublished observations), the micellar phase is progressively reduced. The proteins and lipid spontaneously form small vesicular particles, comparatively free of detergent. Liposomes formed in the manner described have high surface to volume ratios, usually being between 300 Å and 1000 Å in diameter. This makes them less than ideal for transport assays. In FIGURE 2 is illustrated a reconstitution protocol which permits both biochemical screening with either of two flux assays, and also single channel recording studies, all with the same preparation. The small vesicles formed during the initial reconstitution are fused, under appropriate conditions (lipid composition, lipid concentration, and ionic strength), by a freeze-thaw cycle to produce extremely large particles. These particles present surfaces of smooth bilayer membrane, suitable for patch-clamp recording. Because of their extreme size and heterogeneity they are not ideal for flux assays. However, mild sonication breaks these into intermediate sized particles that appear to be predominately unilamellar, and that are still large enough for flux assays carried out in the seconds time scale.[20,21]

Radiotracer flux assays[22] can be used to establish whether basic functional elements of the channel protein have been retained during isolation and reconstitution. Clearly it is difficult to control the normal regulatory parameter, transmembrane voltage, in a vesicle suspension. The task becomes even more challenging when it is considered that the channel responds to brief (~ms) changes in potential by opening and closing in an activity cycle completed in 1–10 ms. It is possible, however, to perturb the gating behavior with a variety of drugs and toxins, including alkaloid toxins (batrachotoxin, veratridine, grayanotoxin, and aconitine),[19] pyrethroids (allamethrin, tetramethrin, and fenvalerate),[24] or polypeptide toxins (α- and β-type toxins from venoms of scorpions and anemones).[19] These compounds bind to sites on the protein and can alter the gating mechanisms so as to produce chronic activation at potentials where the channel may normally be in resting, inactivated or slow-inactivated states. Such chemically activated channels are still subject to blockade by compounds such as tetrodotoxin and saxitoxin, or by local anesthetics. Thus, by using radiotracer flux to detect the average permeability, many drug and toxin receptor sites can be demonstrated and may be studied at the level of the chemistry of the protein.

The assays are carried out by equilibrating the vesicle suspension with the activating toxin, or the toxin together with a blocking compound, or with a vehicle control. After sufficient time, the vesicle suspension is diluted into a buffer containing high specific activity radioisotopes, usually $^{22}Na^+$, to begin the influx. At various times aliquots are rapidly eluted through a cation exchange resin (Dowex 50×8–100) to remove the external tracer, and to exchange permeant external cations for an impermeant ion, such as $Tris^+$.[22] This serves to trap the internal ion in the vesicle during the time it percolates through the column to be collected for counting. In FIGURE 3 are shown influx assays for reconstituted channels which have been activated

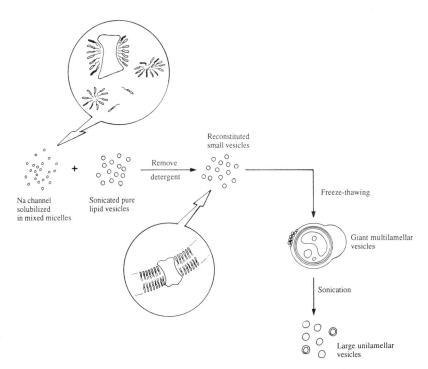

FIGURE 2. Reconstitution protocol. The purified Na channels in mixed lipid/detergent micelles are mixed with liposomes of defined composition (PE:PS:PC in 5:4:1 molar ratio to 10 mg/ml final). Detergent is removed by agitating the sample for 5 h at 0°C with polystyrene beads (0.3 g/ml). The small reconstituted liposomes that result are enlarged by freezing and thawing, to yield giant multilamellar vesicles (up to 30 μm). Brief sonication (2 to 10 s, depending on sample size) converts many of these to large (1–5 μm) unilamellar vesicles. Alternatively, the exogeneous liposomes can be added to the protein after the detergent has been removed.

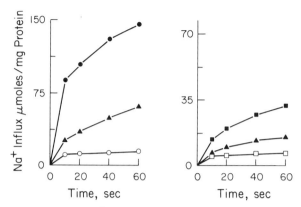

FIGURE 3. Neurotoxin-stimulated ^{22}Na$^+$ uptake. Purified Na channel samples ($\sim$100 pmol/ml) were pre-equilibrated in 84 mM Na$_2$SO$_4$, 1 mM EGTA, and 10 mM HEPES-NaOH, pH 7.4, before addition of exogenous lipid and removal of detergent to yield reconstituted vesicles. Samples were then frozen 1 min in dry ice/acetone, thawed at room temperature, and sonicated 10 s. *Left:* Vesicles were treated with 5 μM BTX (●) in ethanol (1% final, v/v), 5 μM BTX + 1 μM TTX external (▲), or ethanol vehicle alone (○, 1% final, v/v), and influx was measured as described in ref. 20 ($n = 1$). *Right:* Vesicles were treated with 100 μM veratridine (■), 100 μM veratridine + 1 μM TTX external (▲), or the veratridine vehicle alone (□, 175 mM Tris SO$_4$, pH 7.4), and influx was measured ($n = 1$).

with BTX or veratridine. As indicated, the influx activated by these toxins is blocked approximately by half with external TTX; when saturating concentrations of TTX are present on both sides of the membrane, blockade is complete (not shown). BTX is significantly more effective than veratridine, as expected from studies in synaptosomes and neuroblastoma cells.[35,36] An ion permeation pathway is therefore present, and this path can be activated by alkaloid neurotoxins and blocked by guanidinium toxins. Similarly, local anesthetics such as tetracaine, dibucaine, QX-314, and QX-222 retain sites of interaction on the reconstituted channel.[20]

Tracer assays can also be used to demonstrate the presence of functional ion-selectivity mechanisms. From studies described in more detail elsewhere,[21] it was deduced that the slow kinetics of ion influx results from the large vesicle size and comparatively low channel abundance. The extended time course represents equilibration of large vesicles by channels which are conducting at essentially normal rates. This makes it possible to resolve relative rates of influx of various radioisotopes of alkali cations.[23] In FIGURE 4 the influx time courses of Na$^+$, K$^+$, Rb$^+$, and Cs$^+$ are shown. The relative permeabilities, roughly estimated from these studies, are both in the expected sequence and approximately of the expected magnitude for Na channels characterized in physiological studies,[18] or in planar bilayer studies under the influence of BTX.[28] Thus, the mechanism for permeation selectivity has been preserved.

There are drawbacks in the use of radioisotope influx assays for screening Na channel preparations. The procedures have slow time resolution, employ harsh isotopes, generally provide few data points, and consume fairly large amounts of protein. Further, if one wishes quantitative information from such studies, the ability to collect data suitable for kinetic analysis from many experiments with the same preparation becomes important. To this end we have established a very efficient and quantitative fluorescence flux assay.[21] This method consumes between 1–10 fmol of Na channel protein per time course, which makes it approximately 1000 times more sensitive than the ³H-TTX binding assay. An average reconstituted preparation is fully active for 6 to 10 weeks, and comprises 350–700 pmol of ³H-TTX binding sites, or enough for thousands of experiments.

This assay employs three principles: (1) heavy metal quenching of the fluorescence from a water-soluble chromophore trapped within the vesicle by an ion which itself is poorly permeable to membrane bilayers, but which will pass through the activated channel,[18,25,26] (2) the use of the cation-selectivity of the activated channel to produce diffusion potentials which selectively concentrate the quenching ion above the concentration in the outside solution,[27,37] and (3) the use of the large vesicles produced during freeze-thaw sonication to slow the kinetics to the seconds time-scale.

As illustrated in FIGURE 5, during this freeze-thaw cycle a highly fluorescent water

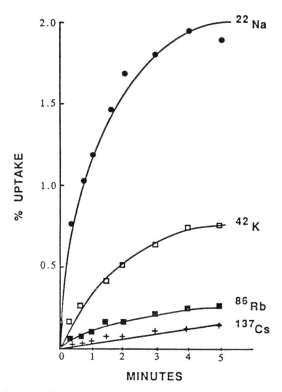

FIGURE 4. Cation selectivity of reconstituted channel. Vesicles as in FIGURE 3 (except 6 s sonication) were treated ±BTX (2.5 μM) for 45 min at 30°C. Before assay, samples were applied to Dowex columns and rinsed with 9 parts isomolar Tris SO_4, pH 7.4, to strip external Na^+ in exchange for $Tris^+$. Samples were supplemented with BTX (to 2.5 μM) or vehicle (1% ethanol), and with Na_2SO_4 to 8.4 mM final ($[Na^+]_{in}/[Na^+]_{out}$ = 10). Radiotracer uptake time courses were begun with the addition of $^{22}Na^+$ and $^{42}K^+$, $^{22}Na^+$ and $^{86}Rb^+$, or $^{42}K^+$ and $^{137}Cs^+$, at final concentrations of 5–10 μCi/ml. At the indicated times after the addition of radiotracer, uptake was stopped as in ref. 20. Internalized radioactivity was determined using a LKB Wallac 1219 Rackbeta liquid scintillation counter with correction made for dual labels and quench compensation. Net BTX-activated uptake (total uptake-control uptake) is plotted as percentage of total counts originally added. Relative initial rates of influx were $Na^+(1.0) > K^+(0.14) > Rb^+(0.045) > Cs^+(0.029)$.

soluble chromophore 8-amino-1,3,6-napthalenetrisulfonate (ANTS) is trapped in the vesicle interior. Following sonication, external dye (>99.9%) is removed by gel filtration. The dye fluorescence is quenched by collisional interactions with the heavy-metal cation Tl^+, which can pass through toxin-activated Na channels more easily than Na^+ itself.[41] The quench relationship is nonlinear, as described by the Stern-Volmer relationship

$$F_o = F(1 + K_s [Tl^+]), \qquad (1)$$

where K_s is the Stern-Volmer quench constant, equal to the reciprocal of the Tl^+ concentration causing 50% quenching. For this dye, K_s^{-1} is 20 mM Tl^+, which provides a very suitable sensitivity for the assay. The chromophore is readily capable of reporting influx into a vesicular volume representing less than 0.03% of the total suspension.

The cation selectivity is exploited to improve the net signal and the signal-to-background leak ratio. Vesicles containing high concentrations of Na_2SO_4 are

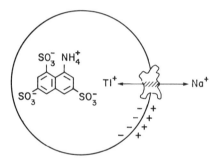

FIGURE 5. Basis for the fluorescence assay. The fluorophore, 8-amino-1,3,6-naphthalenetrisul-fonate (ANTS), is trapped by freeze-thaw-sonication inside reconstituted vesicles containing Na channels. Removal of external Na^+ leads to the creation of a negative-inside diffusion potential across those vesicles containing activated Na channels. The heavy metal cation Tl^+ will be transported into vesicles through activated Na channels in electroneutral exchange for Na_{inside}^+. Tl^+ concentrates above its ambient level and quenches dye fluorescence.

loaded with the chromophore during freeze-thaw-sonication. The vesicle suspension is then treated with the relevant activating or blocking pharmacological agent and then passed over a cation-exchange resin (Dowex-50) to exchange the external Na^+ for impermeant species (*e.g.*, $Tris^+$). This material is then rapidly mixed with a second solution containing low concentrations of $TlNO_3$, in a small glass mixing chamber which leads directly into a 28 μl quartz cell in a flow fluorimeter. In those vesicles which do not leak and which contain no Na channels, no effect on fluorescence is produced by the addition of the Tl^+. In vesicles which are somewhat leaky, the chromophore may be quenched, but only to the extent produced by the ambient Tl^+ concentration. In vesicles which are otherwise nonleaky, but which contain an activated Na channel, the ion-exchange step leads to loss of a small fraction (<1%) of the internal Na^+ content, at which point a large inside-negative diffusion potential is established, sufficient to prevent further net cation efflux. When Tl^+ is introduced to the external solution, however, Na^+ is lost to the vesicle exterior by electroneutral exchange with the Tl^+. By this means the Tl^+ is transiently concentrated to the initial

Na internal concentration, thereby producing enhanced quenching of the reporter groups in this vesicle subpopulation.

The kinetics of such a quench time course may be analyzed by first deducing the form of the Tl^+ influx, and transforming this concentration, by means of the Stern-Volmer equation, into a time course for the fluorescence signal. The basic form of the influx equation, under conditions where diffusion potentials are employed, is approximately

$$[Tl_t^+] = [Tl_\infty^+][1 - \exp(-t/\tau)], \tag{2}$$

where $[Tl_t^+]$ is the internal concentration at time t, $[Tl_\infty^+]$ is the concentration at infinite time (equal to the initial Na^+ concentration), and τ is a time constant, which under standard assay conditions is inversely proportional to the external Tl^+ concentration (for a detailed explanation, see ref. 21). When combined with equation 1, this yields a somewhat unusual quench relationship, which may be written in either of two ways:

$$F_t = F_\infty/[1 - (F_o - F_\infty)/F_o]\exp(-t/\tau) \tag{3}$$

or

$$\ln[(F_t - F_\infty)/F_t] = \ln[(F_o - F_\infty)/F_o] - t/\tau \tag{4}$$

The latter equation can be used to linearize the fluorescence time course. In effect, the kinetics are described by three terms which specify an amplitude and a time constant. The amplitude $(F_o - F_\infty)/F_o$ reflects the fraction of the vesicle population which participates in the quench reaction, whereas the time constant, τ, reflects the rate at which the average vesicle equilibrates. These two parameters may be obtained unambiguously (that is, there are no degrees of freedom) from a semi-log replot of the fluorescence data. A theoretical time course may then be reconstructed from these constants and equation 3 for comparison with the original data, to show the aptness of the fit. Thus, it is possible to extract two parameters, either of which under appropriate circumstances may provide measures of fractional channel activity. This makes it possible to construct undistorted dose-response curves, and to deduce information about relative channel abundance and vesicle dimensions.

In FIGURE 6 are shown the fluorescence quench timecourses for channels activated with batrachotoxin. In panel A are the quench time courses in the absence of activating toxin (*a*), in the presence of 5 μM BTX (*b*), in the presence of BTX with saturating external TTX (*c*), or with saturating TTX on both sides of the membrane (*i.e.*, added before freeze-thaw sonication, *d*). In panel B, these data have been plotted according to equation 4, to determine the kinetic parameters describing the time course. In panel C, points along the theoretical time course have been recalculated with equation 3 for comparison with the original data, showing a satisfactory fit.

Several things become apparent from an analysis of this type. First, in the linear replots it is clear that the slopes of the lines are not systematically affected by the addition of the activating or activating plus blocking toxin. This also is evident when quench signals for different doses of BTX are subjected to this kinetic analysis, as in FIGURE 7. The slopes of the lines vary little compared to the y-intercepts, as BTX varies from 0.01 μM to 5 μM. Therefore, the rate at which the average participating vesicle equilibrates is not greatly affected by the toxins, and τ would not be an appropriate parameter to plot in a dose-response curve. In contrast, the intercept at $t = 0$, representing the amplitude, or fraction of the vesicle population which participates in the reaction, is affected by toxin additions and does represent an appropriate variable

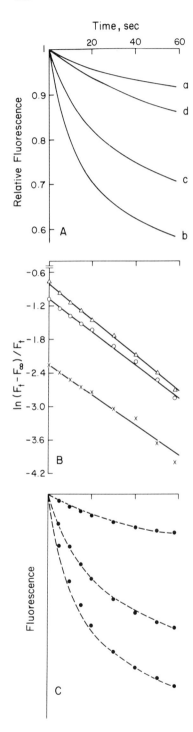

FIGURE 6. BTX-stimulated fluorescence quenching and kinetic analysis of the quench signals. (**A**) Vesicles containing fluorophore (3 mM ANTS) were treated with 1% ethanol vehicle (*a*), 5 μM BTX (*b*), 5 μM BTX + 1 μM TTX external (*c*), or 5 μM BTX + 1 μM TTX internal and external (*d*), *i.e.,* added before freeze-thaw-sonication (2 s sonication). Before assay, BTX-treated samples were applied to Dowex columns and rinsed with 6 parts isomolar Tris SO$_4$, pH 7.4, to strip external Na$^+$ in exchange for Tris$^+$. Fluorescence was measured in 40 mM TlNO$_3$. Curves represent chart recorder tracings from superimposed triplicate time courses. (**B**),(**C**) Kinetic analysis of quench signals. Data from **A** were linearized using equation 4 with $F_o = 1$. In **B**, $\triangle = 5$ μM BTX, $F_\infty = 0.535$, $\tau = 31.3$ s, $F_t = 0.574$ at $t = 58$ s; O = 5 μM BTX + 1 μM TTX external, $F_\infty = 0.660$, $\tau = 33.7$ s; × = 1% ethanol vehicle, $F_\infty = 0.895$, $\tau = 37.2$ s. (**C**) Data from **A** are replotted as *dashed lines* superimposed with theoretical F_ts (●) determined by inserting the values for F_∞ and τ, listed above, into equation 3.

for use in dose-response analysis. This sort of response is expected when the surface abundance of the channels is roughly comparable to the surface area per vesicle. Alternatively, if channel abundance were very high, even at low fractional channel activation, all vesicles would take part in the quench kinetics, because even a single active channel is sufficient to equilibrate a vesicle of average dimensions. In that case, only the number of channels per vesicle (and hence τ) would vary with toxin conditions.

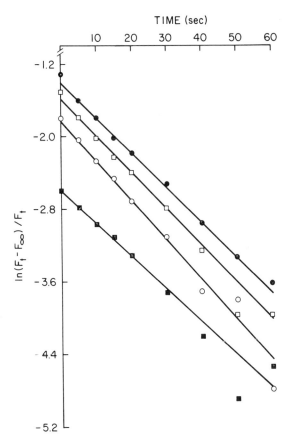

FIGURE 7. Linear replots of BTX dose-response data. Selected difference time courses from FIGURE 8 were analyzed at more time points and then linearized using equation 4 with $F_o = 1$; ● = 5 μM BTX, $F_\infty = 0.730$, $\tau = 26.0$ s; □ = 1 μM BTX, $F_\infty = 0.780$, $\tau = 24.9$ s; ○ = 0.25 μM BTX, $F_\infty = 0.835$, $\tau = 23.0$ s; ■ = 0.01 μM BTX, $F_\infty = 0.925$, $\tau = 27.8$ s.

Here, when channel abundance is so low that there are generally fewer than one or two per vesicle, only the intercept should vary systematically with toxin occupancy.

The parameter which should be used in order to construct an undistorted dose-response curve will vary depending on the above considerations. If one were to use only amplitude as a measure of fractional channel activation, at very high channel surface densities the $K_{1/2}$ for an activating drug would be underestimated, as activation

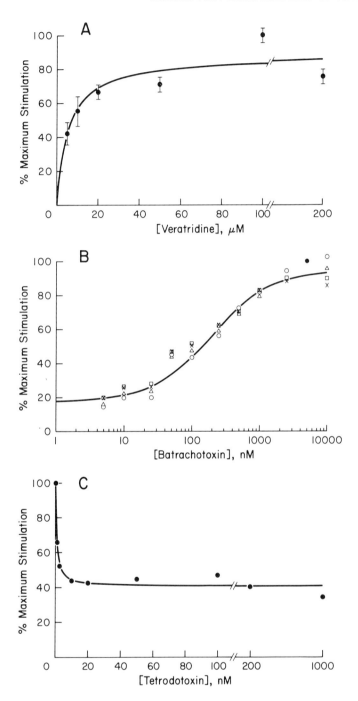

of only a few percent of the channels would be sufficient for a maximal signal. Similarly, the $K_{1/2}$ for a blocking neurotoxin would be severely overestimated. The complete analysis of flux kinetics reveals the parameter most likely to reflect a true sensitivity to the compound being studied. In FIGURE 8 are shown dose-response curves for activation of channels by veratridine and BTX and for the blockade of BTX-activated flux by external TTX. The $K_{1/2}$s for these compounds were 5.4 μM, 169 nM, and 4.3 nM, respectively, well within the expected pharmacological range.

Vesicles formed by the freeze-thaw-sonication procedures described are generally between 1 and 5 μm in diameter (ref. 21 and W. Bollinger and W. Agnew, unpublished observations). The large size of the vesicles, together with the comparatively low surface abundance, explains the slow time course of the quench reaction. A single active channel, with a conductance of 18 pS, would equilibrate a vesicle of 1000 Å diameter with 0.2 M cation, with a time constant of 22.2 ms. However, a vesicle of 1 μm equilibrated by the same channel would exhibit a time constant of approximately 22.2 s. A vesicle of 2 μm diameter has a surface of approximately 4 μm^2, which is approximately the size of an excised patch on the tip of a microelectrode. In studies aimed at increasing channel surface abundance, when many channels per vesicle are produced, τ rather than the amplitude should begin to vary with toxin occupancy. Because of the dimensions of the vesicles, the point at which one detects many more than one channel per vesicle represents precisely the conditions under which the frequency of encountering an active channel in an excised patch should become greater than unity. Thus, the vesicles being studied have the twin advantages of putting the time scale in a range convenient for measurement with standard recording devices, and providing information about channel abundance in the scale relevant to patch-recording studies.

The biochemical assays which have been briefly described provide indispensible tools in the study of sodium channel protein chemistry. However, only biophysical methods offer at present the time resolution (0.1 ms) and sensitivity (down to the single channel level) required to study this steeply voltage-dependent molecule. Biophysical studies of the channel in reconstituted membranes have been generally limited to the study of the protein in planar bilayers. The large membrane areas of painted bilayers, however, result in capacitance transients which seldom settle in the 1–10 ms of an Na-channel activity cycle. Thus, step depolarizations are of limited use with unmodified channels. In an ingenious strategy, Krueger *et al.*[28] surmounted the problem by using BTX, which functionally removes all inactivation mechanisms, permitting the study of the protein at steady-state potentials. These methods have now been exploited

---

FIGURE 8. Dose-response curves determined by fluorescence quench. Vesicles loaded with ~185 mM Na$^+$, 3 mM ANTS, were stripped of external Na$^+$ after incubation with toxins, and assayed in 40 mM TlNO$_3$. (A) Vesicles were incubated for 6 min at 30°C ± VTN. Difference curves were determined from triplicate averages after 60 s of Tl$^+$ influx. Stimulated quench in 100 μM VTN was set to 100%. *Bars* denote standard propagated error of the means. An Eadie-Hofstee fit of the data yielded K_d = 5.4 μM and maximum stimulation of 87.8%. These parameters were used to generate the Langmuir isotherm shown. (B) Vesicles were incubated for 36 min at 30°C ± BTX. Difference curves were determined from triplicate averages at 10 s (O), 20 s (△), 40 s (□), and 60 s (×) of Tl$^+$ influx. Stimulated quench in 5 μM BTX at all times was set to 100% (●). Data were best fit by a Langmuir isotherm with maximum stimulation set to 95%, baseline effect in absence of BTX set to 18%, and K_d = 200 nM, to yield the curve shown. (C) Vesicles were incubated for 12 min at 0°C with TTX, and then 36 min at 30°C ± 5 μM BTX. Difference curves from triplicate averages were linearized by equation 4 to determine F_∞. An Eadie-Hofstee fit of the F_∞ data yielded K_d = 0.7 nM and maximum inhibition of 59.3%. These parameters were used to generate the Langmuir isotherm shown.

by a number of laboratories and have yielded a great deal of information about Na channels in defined environments. This approach suffers, however, in that most of the basic properties of the channel seem to be altered by the action of this powerful neurotoxin, including voltage-dependence and kinetics of activation, single channel conductances, ion selectivity, and interactions with blocking neurotoxins such as TTX and STX.[18,29–31]

We have used an approach first advocated by Tank et al.[33] in studies with the Torpedo Cl channel and nicotinic acetylcholine receptor, which involves patch-clamping reconstituted liposomes.[34] When the Na channel is reconstituted with phosphatidylethanolamine:phosphatidylserine:phosphatidylcholine and freeze-thawed, the multilamellar liposomes which form are large enough for patching.[32] Thin, apparently unilamellar blebs may be accentuated on these liposomes by slight osmotic challenge (D. Landowne and W. Agnew, unpublished observations). High resistance seals are obtained with polished microelectrodes by gentle suction onto the vesicle surface. Patches are excised by retraction and passing the tip of the microelectrode through the air-water interface. The patch may then be tested for activity with voltage pulses, either in the presence or absence of neurotoxins.

FIGURE 9 illustrates unitary current events recorded from such a patch held at −100 mV and pulsed to −25 mV in 28 ms epochs. We used the cellular convention that the bath is cytoplasmic and the electrode interior is extracellular. These currents exhibit a number of characteristics that indicate they are Na-channel-mediated events.[32] First, the events are seldom observed at −100 mV, a potential at which Na channels would be expected to be in the resting state. Upon depolarization, the probability of observing an event is markedly increased. Summation of many such depolarizing epochs reveals that the probability distribution of openings is greatest immediately after the depolarizing pulse, indicating voltage activation. Subsequently the probability declines, just as would be expected for inactivating Na channels. The inactivation time course in the illustrated experiments was approximately 6 ms, which is in keeping with physiological studies. Mean channel lifetimes follow a single exponential distribution, with a time constant of 1.9 ms. The single channel conductance recorded from such patches are uniform, as exemplified by data presented in TABLE 5. At a sodium concentration of 100 mM, conductances of 11 pS have been consistently observed. When Na^+ concentration is raised to higher levels, the events increase to about 16 pS. Although single channel data from native electroplax are not available for comparison, these values are consistent with those reported for other cell types. Other experiments (cf. ref. 32) also demonstrate these currents are selective for Na^+ or K^+.

These initial studies demonstrate the feasibility of patch-recording the reconstituted Na channel. An essential objective at present is to optimize the channel surface abundance, thereby improving the encounter frequency of channels in excised patches. As discussed above, the fluorescence assay can be used to identify preparations which have many channels per vesicle, and thus many per patch.

SUMMARY AND COMMENTARY

The study of the ion transport, permeation selectivity, and gating mechanisms of Na channel molecules requires information about structure as well as dynamic behavior. A fully defined, normally behaved reconstituted system—in effect, a "synthetic nerve"—will prove to be an extremely useful preparation. We have summarized here some observations demonstrating that the single-peptide protein

A

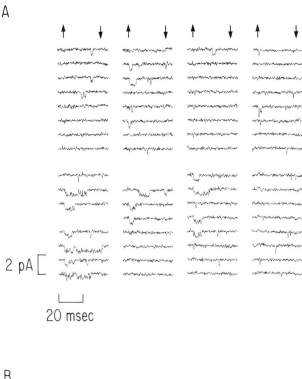

2 pA

20 msec

B

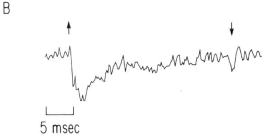

5 msec

FIGURE 9. Single-channel currents of an excised patch containing the reconstituted purified channel. Purified Na channel sample was agitated for 5 h at 0°C with polystyrene beads to remove detergent. Exogenous lipid (PE:PS:PC in 5:4:1 molar ratio) was then added to 10 mg/ml final and the sample was frozen and thawed to create large multilamellar vesicles. These records are from a patch excised from one such vesicle. The patch was held at -100 mV and depolarizations to -25 mV lasting 30 ms were made at 0.75 s intervals. The bath solution was 10 mM NaCl:80 mM KCl:5 mM MgCl$_2$:10 mM Hepes-KOH, pH 7.4, and the electrode solution was 90 mM NaCl:5 mM MgCl$_2$:10 mM Hepes-NaOH, pH 7.4. (**A**) A collection of depolarization epochs are presented (*arrows*) above in the sequence in which they were obtained. Channel opening is a downward deflection. (**B**) Summated currents, scaled arbitrarily, to show the statistical probability of channels being opened during the depolarization epoch.

from eel electroplax may be isolated on the basis of TTX binding activity, and reincorporated into a defined membrane environment, with recovery of a constellation of expected pharmacological and biophysical properties. Thus, to a first approximation, the stage is set technically for a systematic assault on the mechanisms of this protein. It is worth mentioning, however, some unresolved problems which still must be considered.

Reconstituted preparations may not be entirely normal. It is possible that the reassembly of purified proteins may not leave the molecules in exactly the same arrangement as in the native membrane. This may cause subtle but important differences in channel function. For example, with the electroplax protein we have

TABLE 5. Single Channel Conductances from Excised Patches[a]

11.2 pS	$T = 20°C$	
	$E_{rev} = 37$ mV	(3 voltages)
	bath (mM)	electrode (mM)
	10 NaCl	100 NaCl
	90 KCl	5 MgCl$_2$
	5 MgCl$_2$	10 Na Hepes, pH 7.4
	10 Na Hepes, pH 7.4	
11.1 ± 0.9	$T = 20°C$	
	symmetrical solutions	
	100 NaCl	
	5 MgCl	
	10 Na Hepes, pH 7.4	
11.2 ± 1	$T = 20°C$	
	symmetrical solutions	
	100 NaCl	
	5 MgCl	
	10 Na Hepes, pH 7.4	
16.1	$T = 20°C$	
	$E_{rev} \simeq -55$ mV	(6 voltages)
	bath (mM)	electrode (mM)
	250 NaCl	25 NaCl
	5 MgCl$_2$	5 MgCl$_2$
	10 Na Hepes, pH 7.4	10 Na Hepes, pH 7.4

[a]Estimates of single channel conductance were based on patch recording measurements of reconstituted Na channel proteins. Each determination is the average of ten or more well-resolved openings, under the conditions indicated.

failed to demonstrate functional interactions with the peptide toxin ATXII, either by itself or in conjunction with veratridine or batrachotoxin (ref. 20 and unpublished data). Similar difficulties have been reported by Catterall and colleagues with the analogous peptide toxin from *Leiurus quinquestriatus* (ref. 15 and references therein). Binding of that toxin was found to be lost on solubilization, but could be restored when the protein was reconstituted with the appropriate mixture of lipids, some of the same lipids which we normally employ with the electroplax channel. Although those authors found that the voltage dependence of toxin binding could be restored, at least to a small fraction of the channels, the toxin has no effects on flux activation either by itself or in conjunction with the alkaloid neurotoxins. In that case, however, the "malfunction" could be due to a problem with the alkaloid toxin binding site, because BTX, normally a more powerful activator than veratridine in synaptosomes, is a weak activator in the reconstituted brain preparation. This cannot be an issue with the electroplax protein because here BTX is far more effective than veratridine.

Another concern which has been raised, in particular by Catterall,[15] is the existence of two small peptide subunits in the brain protein which have not surfaced in studies with the electroplax channel. This presents several issues which will have to be resolved. While it is possible that the electroplax protein has lost a small subunit during isolation, it appears not to be necessary for channel function. In simple biochemical flux studies, the electroplax protein is fully as active as the brain protein when activated by veratridine; when treated with BTX it is several times more active. With respect to biophysical studies, the electroplax protein remains the only reconstituted channel in which normal gating, in absence of neurotoxins, has been described.[32] Thus, although arguments have been advanced that the small subunits of the brain channels are essential for some aspects of that channel function, the experiments suggesting this have alternative interpretations and it should be perhaps considered that the question remains open.

An additional concern which must be borne in mind as channel mechanisms are investigated with biochemical methods is that of heterogeneity of the channels under study. In the interesting findings of Numa and colleagues,[4,39] it is clear that there are at least three distinct, though structurally similar, Na channel genes expressed in mammalian brain. The differences may explain functional anomalies reported by others. For example, in a report by Catterall *et al.*,[40] binding studies with STX and *Leiurus* toxin showed that in synaptosomes there were consistently more STX binding sites than peptide toxin binding sites ($\sim$3.7:1), whereas the purified protein shows a stoichiometry of $\sim$1:1. It is possible that there are differences in the binding of peptide toxins to the channels, and that purification has resulted in enrichment of one iso-form of the channel. This potential heterogeneity, which can be an issue with material isolated from any source, could produce confusing results in site-specific chemical modification studies.

In conclusion, it is clear that a most exciting phase of the study of mechanisms of regulation by the first biochemically isolated voltage-regulated ion channel has begun. It is also apparent that while novel approaches are emerging, nevertheless the imperfections of the experimental preparations must be carefully considered.

REFERENCES

1. HODGKIN, A. L. & A. F. HUXLEY. 1952. J. Physiol. (London) **116:** 500–544.
2. ARMSTRONG, C. M. 1981. Physiol. Rev. **61:** 644–682.
3. AGNEW, W. S. 1984. Ann. Rev. Physiol. **46:** 517–530.
4. NUMA, S. & M. NODA. 1986. Molecular structure of sodium channels. This volume.
5. AGNEW, W. S., S. R. LEVINSON, J. S. BRABSON & M. A. RAFTERY. 1978. Proc. Natl. Acad. Sci. U. S. A. **75:** 2606–2611.
6. MILLER, J. A., W. S. AGNEW & S. R. LEVINSON. 1983. Biochemistry **22:** 462–470.
7. LEVINSON, S. R., C. CURATALO, J. K. REED & M. A. RAFTERY. 1979. Anal. Biochem. **99:** 72–84.
8. AGNEW, W. S., A. C. MOORE, S. R. LEVINSON & M. A. RAFTERY. 1980. Biochem. Biophys. Res. Commun. **92:** 860–866.
9. HARTSHORNE, R. P., D. J. MESSNER, J. C. COPPERSMITH & W. A. CATTERALL. 1982. J. Biol. Chem. **257:** 13888–91.
10. BARCHI, R. L. 1983. J. Neurochem. **40:** 1377–1385.

11. NODA, M., S. SHIMIZU, T. TANABE, T. TAKAI, T. KAYANO, T. IKEDA, H. TAKAHASHI, H. NAKAYAMA, Y. KANAOKA, N. MINAMINO, K. KANGAWA, H. MATSUO, M. A. RAFTERY, T. HIROSES, S. INAYAMA, H. HAYASHIDA, T. MIYATA & S. NUMA. 1984. Nature 312: 121–127.
12. AGNEW, W. S., J. A. MILLER, M. H. ELLISMAN, R. L. ROSENBERG, S. A. TOMIKO & S. R. LEVINSON. 1983. Cold Spring Harbor Symp. Quant. Biol. Molec. Neurobiol. 48: 165–179.
13. HARTSHORNE, R. P., J. C. COPPERSMITH & W. A. CATTERALL. 1980. J. Biol. Chem. 255: 10572–75.
14. BARCHI, R. L. & L. E. MURPHY. 1981. J. Neurochem. 36: 2097.
15. CATTERALL, W. A., J. W. SCHMIDT, D. J. MESSNER & D. J. FELLER. 1986. Structure and biosynthesis of neuronal sodium channels. This volume.
16. BARCHI, R. L. 1986. Biochemistry of sodium channels from mammalian muscle. This volume.
17. GRISHIN, E. V., V. A. KOVALENKO, V. N. PASHIKOV & G. SHAMAOTIEN. 1984. Biol. Membranes (Moscow) 1: 858.
18. KHODOROV, B. I. 1981. Prog. Biophys. Molec. Biol. 37: 49–89.
19. CATTERALL, W. A. 1980. Ann. Rev. Pharmacol. Toxicol. 20: 15–43.
20. ROSENBERG, R. L., S. A. TOMIKO & W. S. AGNEW. 1984. Proc. Natl. Acad. Sci. U.S.A. 81: 1239–1243.
21. TOMIKO, S. A., R. L. ROSENBERG, M. C. EMERICK & W. S. AGNEW. 1986. Biochemistry 25: 2162–2174.
22. GASKO, O. D., A. F. KNOWLES, H. G. SHERTZER, E.-M. SUOLINNA & E. RACKER. 1976. Anal. Biochem. 72: 57–65.
23. COOPER, E. C., S. A. TOMIKO & W. S. AGNEW. 1986. In preparation.
24. NARAHASHI, T. 1981. J. Physiol. (Paris) 77: 1093–1101.
25. MOORE, H.-P. & M. A. RAFTERY. 1980. Proc. Natl. Acad. Sci. U.S.A. 77: 4509–4513.
26. WU, W. C.-S., H. P. MOORE & M. A. RAFTERY. 1981. Proc. Natl. Acad. Sci. U. S. A. 8: 775–779.
27. TALVENHEIMO, J. A., M. M. TAMKUN & W. A. CATTERALL. 1982. J. Biol. Chem. 257: 11868–11871.
28. KRUEGER, B. K., J. F. WORLEY, III & R. J. FRENCH. 1983. Nature 303: 172–175.
29. KRUEGER, B. K., J. F. WORLEY, III & R. J. FRENCH. 1986. Block of sodium channels in planar lipid bilayers by guanidinium toxins and calcium: Are the mechanisms of voltage dependence the same? This volume.
30. HARTSHORNE, R. P., B. U. KELLER, J. A. TALVENHEIMO, W. A. CATTERALL & M. MONTAL. 1985. Proc. Natl. Acad. Sci. U.S.A. 82: 240–244.
31. MOCZYDLOWSKI, E., S. HALL, S. S. GARBER, G. S. STRICHARTZ & C. MILLER. 1984. J. Gen. Physiol. 84: 687–704.
32. ROSENBERG, R. L., S. A. TOMIKO & W. S. AGNEW. 1984. Proc. Natl. Acad. Sci. U. S. A. 81: 5594–5598.
33. TANK, D., C. MILLER & W. W. WEBB. 1982. Proc. Natl. Acad. Sci. U.S.A. 79: 7749–7754.
34. HAMILL, O. P., A. MARTY, E. NEHER, B. SAKMANN & F. J. SIGWORTH. 1981. Pfluegers Arch. 391: 85–100.
35. TAMKUN, M. M. & W. A. CATTERALL. 1981. Molec. Pharmacol. 19: 78–86.
36. CATTERALL, W. A. 1977. J. Biol. Chem. 252: 8669–8676.
37. GARTY, H., B. RUDY & S. J. D. KARLISH. 1983. J. Biol. Chem. 258: 13094–13099.
38. COHN, E. J. & J. T. EDSALL. 1943. Proteins, Amino Acids, and Peptides. Van Nostrand-Reinhold. Princeton, N.J.
39. NODA, M., T. IKEDA, T. KAYANO, H. SUZUKI, H. TAKESHIMA, M. KURASAKI, H. TAKAHASHI & S. NUMA. 1986. Nature 320: 188–192.
40. CATTERALL, W. A., C. S. MORROW & R. P. HARTSHORNE. 1979. J. Biol. Chem. 254: 11379–11387.
41. TOMIKO, S. A. & W. S. AGNEW. 1986. Soc. Neurosci. Abstr. In press.

Block of Sodium Channels in Planar Lipid Bilayers by Guanidinium Toxins and Calcium

Are the Mechanisms of Voltage Dependence the Same?[a]

BRUCE K. KRUEGER, JENNINGS F. WORLEY, III,[b]
AND ROBERT J. FRENCH[c,d]

Department of Physiology
[c]Department of Biophysics
University of Maryland School of Medicine
Baltimore, Maryland 21201

INTRODUCTION

Voltage-dependent sodium channels underlie the generation and propagation of action potentials in most nerve and muscle cells.[1] Previous work from this[2,3] and other[4,5] laboratories has established that these sodium channels can be incorporated into planar lipid bilayer membranes and studied electrophysiologically at the single channel level. Purified sodium channels have recently been reconstituted in artificial membranes and studied by similar methods.[6-9] These sodium channels, which were studied after activation by the frog neurotoxin batrachotoxin (BTX), display properties expected for sodium channels from nerve including voltage-dependent activation, selectivity for sodium over divalent and other monovalent cations, and block by nanomolar concentrations of tetrodotoxin (TTX) and saxitoxin (STX).

It is of interest that block of BTX-activated sodium channels by STX and TTX was dependent on membrane potential, with hyperpolarizing potentials favoring block.[2-5] This could be due to (1) the toxins binding at a site located within the membrane electric field, or (2) a voltage-dependent conformational change in the three-dimensional structure of the channel protein resulting in an alteration of the toxin binding site and the affinity for toxins. For mechanism 1, the voltage dependence of block by TTX (a monovalent cation) should be less than that for STX (a divalent cation). For mechanism 2, the voltage dependence should be independent of the toxin's charge. In addition, for mechanism 1, the ln K_i for toxin block should be linearly related to membrane potential, whereas for mechanism 2, the K_is should go asymptotically to limiting values at very positive and negative potentials.

External calcium and other multivalent cations are also capable of blocking open

[a]This work was supported by grants from the National Institutes of Health to BKK (NS16285) and RJF (NS20106), by contracts DAMD17–82–C–2188 and DAMD17–85–C–5283 from the U.S. Army Medical Research and Development Command (to BKK and RJF), and by a University of Maryland Fellowship (to JFW).
[b]Present address: Department of Pharmacology, University of Vermont College of Medicine, Burlington, Vt. 05405.
[d]Present address: Department of Medical Physiology, University of Calgary, Alberta T2N4N1 Canada.

sodium channels. This block is also voltage dependent, with hyperpolarizing potentials increasing the degree of block.[10-13] Unlike STX and TTX, calcium ions probably have access to binding sites deep within the channel pore, suggesting that the voltage dependence could arise from binding within the membrane field. In this paper, we argue that the voltage dependence of block by STX and TTX is due to a different mechanism than is the voltage dependence of block by divalent ions, and suggest additional experiments that may provide more information about these blocking mechanisms.

MATERIALS AND METHODS

Materials

STX was provided by J. E. Gilchrist (Food and Drug Administration, Cincinnati, Ohio). BTX was a generous gift of Dr. John Daly (NIH-National Institute of Arthritis, Metabolism and Digestive Diseases). Phosphatidylethanolamine was obtained from Avanti Polar Lipids, Birmingham, Ala. Trimethyloxonium tetrafluoroborate was obtained from Alfa Products, Danvers, Ma.

Methods

All experiments were done with sodium channels from membrane vesicles prepared by differential centrifugation of rat forebrain homogenates.[14] The channels were incorporated into planar bilayers formed on 250 μm holes from a solution of bovine brain phosphatidylethanolamine in decane.[2] The solutions on both sides of the bilayer contained 125 mM NaCl, 0.15 mM $CaCl_2$, 0.1 mM $MgCl_2$, and 0.05 mM EGTA, pH 7; 120 nM BTX was present on the intracellular side. Single channel currents across the bilayer were measured using a homemade voltage clamp circuit.[15] All experiments were performed at ambient temperature (22°–24°C). Where indicated, additional calcium was added to the extracellular side of the channels. The channels incorporated into the bilayers with their STX binding sites facing the side of vesicle addition, allowing us to define that as the extracellular side. The voltage convention used is the normal cell physiological convention of $E_{mem} = E_{in} - E_{out}$, with the outside of the bilayer defined as the side from which STX or TTX blocked. With this convention, channels tend to close with increasingly negative potentials. See refs. 2, 3, and 13 for further details of the methods and data analysis.

In those experiments in which the channels were modified with trimethyloxonium tetrafluoroborate (TMO), the reagent was added in solid form to the extracellular side of the channel and quickly mixed with stirring. The pH was maintained at approximately 7 by addition of NaOH. Modification (see FIG. 4) usually occurred within 1 minute of addition, often before completion of stirring. Control experiments established that the products of TMO hydrolysis (dimethyl ether and methanol) were not responsible for the observed alterations in channel properties.[13]

RESULTS

The block of a single rat brain sodium channel by STX is shown in FIGURE 1. In the presence of BTX and the absence of toxin, the channel remained open most of the time at −60 mV and more depolarized potentials. Addition of 5 nM STX to the

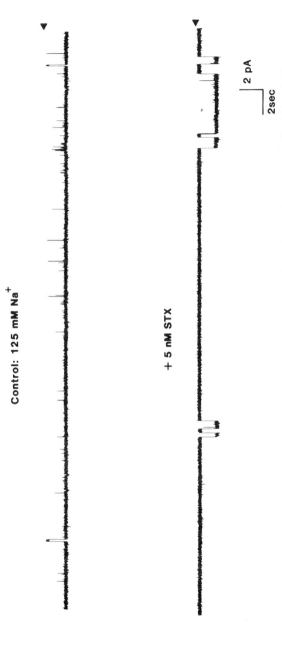

FIGURE 1. Current at −60 mV through a single BTX-activated sodium channel in a planar bilayer in symmetric 125 mM NaCl. The zero-current levels are indicated by *arrowheads*, so that upward current deflections represent channel closings. When 5 nM STX was added to the extracellular side of the channel (*bottom*), the channel was blocked most of the time with only infrequent openings. Records were filtered at 100 Hz on playback. (From Worley *et al.*[13] Reprinted by permission from the *Journal of General Physiology*.)

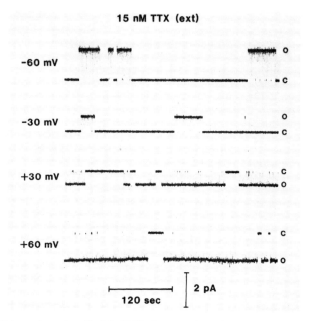

FIGURE 2. Voltage-dependent block by TTX of current through a single BTX-activated sodium channel. Conditions were as in FIGURE 1 except that 15 nM TTX was present on the extracellular side. The closed (blocked) and open (unblocked) levels are indicated by c and o at the right of each trace. Records were filtered at 30 Hz on playback.

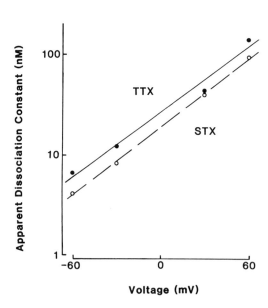

FIGURE 3. Semilog plot of K_i vs. membrane potential for STX and TTX. K_i was calculated from the mean fraction of current blocked (f_b) by the following equation: $K_i = (1 - 1/f_b)[TX]$, where [TX] is the concentration of TTX or STX. The voltage dependence of block was 39 mV/e-fold for STX and 41 mV/e-fold for TTX.

extracellular side caused the appearance of long-lived nonconducting (blocked) periods that result from binding of an STX molecule to the channel. Within the time resolution of these experiments, block by STX is an all-or-none event. The apparent dissociation constant for STX was about 2 nM at -60 mV and increased with membrane depolarization at about 40 mV/e-fold (c.f. refs. 3, 5, and 16). Intracellular addition of STX had no effect on the channel.

TTX also blocks these sodium channels with similar kinetics and slightly lower affinity. The voltage dependence of block by TTX is illustrated in FIGURE 2. The unblocked times increased and the blocked times decreased with membrane depolarization, reflecting a decrease in the blocking rate and an increase in the unblocking rate (c.f. refs. 3, 5, and 16).

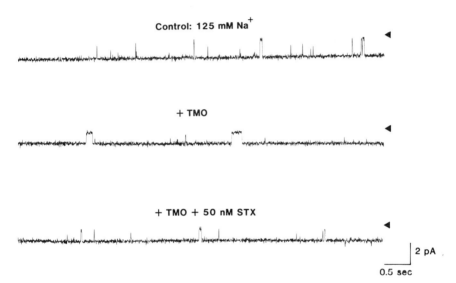

FIGURE 4. Effect of TMO on single sodium channels. Current through a single BTX-activated sodium channel in symmetric 125 mM NaCl. *Top:* Control record at -60 mV; the channel was open more than 95% of the time. *Middle:* One minute after addition of 50 mM TMO to the external solution; note reduction in single channel current. *Bottom:* Addition of 50 nM STX to the TMO-treated channel; channel is insensitive to 50 nM STX. Records were filtered at 150 Hz on playback. (From Worley *et al.*[13] Reprinted by permission from the *Journal of General Physiology.*)

The voltage dependence of block of the rat brain sodium channels by STX and TTX is shown in FIGURE 3. The apparent dissociation constant was calculated from the mean fraction of current remaining following addition of toxin as described in the legend to FIGURE 3. The slope of both curves was about 40 mV/e-fold despite the fact that STX is a divalent cation and TTX is monovalent under these conditions. This result is very similar to those reported by Moczydlowski *et al.*[4,16] and Green *et al.*[5] for rabbit skeletal muscle and dog brain sodium channels, respectively, and strongly suggests that the toxins do not sense a significant fraction of the membrane electric field as they enter their binding site.

Sensitivity to STX and TTX was eliminated by treating the channels with external trimethyloxonium[17,18] (TMO) as shown in FIGURE 4. TMO, which methylates protein carboxyl residues, reduced the single channel conductance by about one-third (see also FIG. 6), and rendered the channel insensitive to STX, indicating that a carboxyl residue is associated with the toxin binding site[18-23] and may play a role in the movement of permeant ions through the channel.[17] TMO always caused both changes concomitantly, suggesting that a single site modification is responsible for the reduced conductance and toxin insensitivity. Extracellular STX and calcium protect the channels from modification by TMO and inhibit TMO-induced reduction in ^{3}H-STX binding in the membrane vesicle preparation.[13]

Two effects of external calcium on BTX-activated sodium channels are illustrated in FIGURE 5. Calcium relieved block by STX, as indicated by the increased unblocked times, and also inhibited sodium current through the open, unblocked channel. The effect of calcium on toxin block was seen primarily as an increase in the unblocked dwell times (reflecting a decrease in the effective blocking rate constant), as would be expected if calcium were competing with STX for the same binding site. This is illustrated by the data given in TABLE 1. Extracellular calcium (10 mM) caused about a sevenfold increase in the apparent K_i for STX, and this was due mainly to a decrease in the on-rate for toxin block.

The block of open sodium channels by calcium was also voltage dependent, as illustrated by the relation of the single channel current to voltage (FIGURE 6). External calcium caused a voltage-independent block of outward currents (upper right quadrant) but a strongly voltage-dependent block of inward currents (lower left) which, like block by STX and TTX, was favored by hyperpolarizing potentials. TMO-modifica-

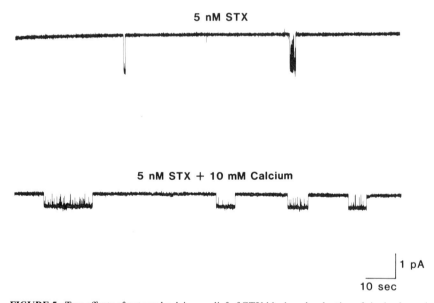

5 nM STX

5 nM STX + 10 mM Calcium

1 pA

10 sec

FIGURE 5. Two effects of external calcium: relief of STX block and reduction of single channel current. *Top:* Current through a planar bilayer containing a single sodium channel in the presence of 5 nM STX. Channel is blocked most of the time with occasional unblocked conducting periods (two shown in this record). *Bottom:* Same channel after addition of 10 mM external calcium. Note that unblocked periods are longer and that single channel current is reduced because of calcium block of the open channel. Records were filtered at 30 Hz on playback. See TABLE 1 for data. (From Worley *et al.*[13] Reprinted by permission from the *Journal of General Physiology.*)

TABLE 1

$[Ca^{2+}]_o$	k_{on} 10^8 $M^{-1}s^{-1}$	k_{off} s^{-1}	K_i (nM) from: Rate Constants	K_i (nM) from: Mean Current (f_b)
0 mM	0.310 ± 0.010	0.034 ± 0.020	1.3 ± 0.3	1.5 ± 0.4
10 mM	0.065 ± 0.010	0.058 ± 0.020	9.6 ± 0.4	9.8 ± 0.6

Data show that calcium decreases the on-rate (blocking) constant without significantly changing the off-rate (unblocking) constant as expected for competition and simple block. These determinations were obtained at -60 mV from three separate single channel membranes. K_i was calculated from the ratio of the rate constants, k_{off}/k_{on}, for each experiment and from the mean reduction in current, f_b (see legend to FIGURE 3). See ref. 13 for details.

tion dramatically altered these current-voltage relations (FIG. 6B). First, there was a 37% reduction in the single channel conductance in the absence of calcium. Secondly, there was no voltage-independent block of outward currents by calcium. Thirdly, there was a dramatic reduction in the block of inward current, as if calcium were much less potent.

DISCUSSION

It appears very likely that for BTX-activated sodium channels from rat brain, the voltage dependence of STX and TTX block arises from a voltage-dependent conformational change in the molecular structure of the channel's binding site, because the voltage dependence of block by STX and TTX is virtually identical. A similar conclusion has been drawn by Moczydlowski et al.[16] and Green et al.[5] Additional data provide more information on this point. For example, if the toxins bind to a site deep within the channel pore, it might be expected that the concentration of internal cations, including sodium, would affect the apparent affinity for externally applied toxins. This seems unlikely because Moczydlowski et al.[4] showed that toxin block was independent of internal sodium from 40 to 600 mM; moreover, the voltage dependence of block was not affected by variations in the concentration of external sodium,[4] eliminating the possibility that competition with a voltage-dependent sodium binding reaction is the basis for voltage-dependent toxin block.

If a voltage-dependent conformational change in the sodium channel's structure is responsible for the voltage dependence of toxin block, it would be expected that the apparent affinities should reach limiting levels at large positive and negative potentials.[16] No such deviation from linearity of the ln K_i vs. E relations has been observed[3–5,16] (c.f. FIG. 3). If observed changes in K_i with potential reflected the relative occupancies of a high and a low affinity state as determined from a Boltzmann distribution, then the ln K_i vs. E relation (FIG. 3) should be described by one of a family of curves illustrated in FIGURE 7. For limiting dissociation constants of about 1 and 100 nM, significant deviation from linearity should be observed over ± 60 mV (dotted curve) in contrast to the experimental results. For K_i ranges of 0.3–500 nM and greater, the relationships would appear linear over about ± 100 mV or more (dashed curve). It should be noted that for extreme ranges of limiting dissociation constants (solid line) the relation is identical to that describing voltage-dependent block due to the blocker's entry into a portion of the membrane electric field.[10]

In principle, either of the two mechanisms considered above for the voltage dependence of toxin block could be responsible for the voltage dependence of calcium block. Although calcium competes with STX and TTX for the binding site (FIG. 4), it

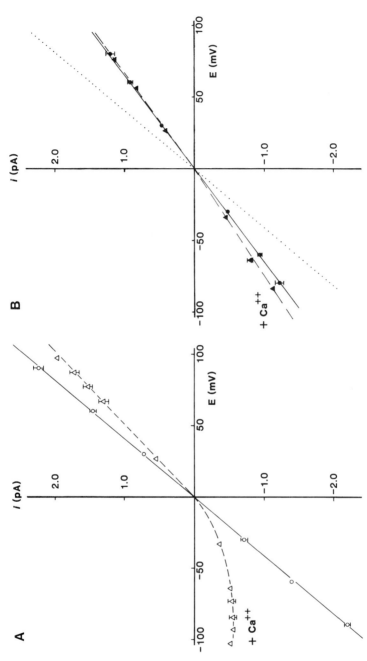

FIGURE 6. Effect of calcium on single sodium channel current-voltage relations before and after TMO. (A) Control. Single channel current is plotted as a function of membrane potential, O = symmetrical 125 mM NaCl, no divalents; Δ =same as control plus 10 mM extracellular calcium. Error bars give SEM (n = 6) when larger than the symbol. The *smooth curve* was drawn by eye. (B) TMO-modified channels. ●=symmetrical 125 mM NaCl, no divalents; ▲ = plus 10 mM extracellular calcium. Error bars give SEM (n = 9 for no calcium and n = 4 for plus calcium) when larger than the symbols. The *smooth curve* was drawn by eye. The *dotted line* gives the current-voltage relation for unmodified channels in the absence of calcium from A.

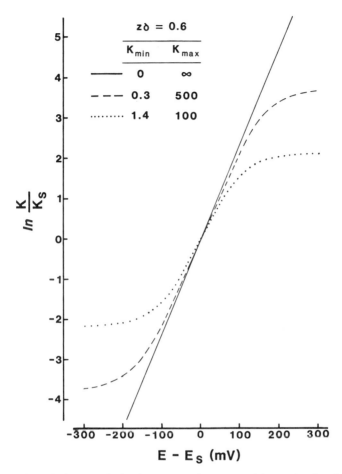

FIGURE 7. Theoretical curves plotting $\ln K_i$ vs. membrane potential assuming that the channel can undergo a voltage-dependent transition between two conformational states, one with a high affinity for toxin ($K = K_{min}$) and the other with a low affinity ($K = K_{max}$). The fractional occupancy (f_{max}) of the low affinity state is given by a Boltzmann distribution: $f_{max} = 1/[1 + \exp(z\delta FE/RT)]$, where $z\delta = 0.6$ (from the voltage dependence of STX and TTX block) and R, T, and F have their usual meanings. K was determined as $f_{max}(K_{max} - K_{min}) + K_{min}$. The three curves have been forced through the origin by plotting $\ln K/K_s$ vs. $E - E_s$, where K_s is equal to K at the midpoint of each curve and $E_s = E$ at $K = K_s$. Curves are shown for three arbitrarily selected pairs of K_{min} and K_{max} for which $K_s = 12$.

seems unlikely that the complex bonding interactions between the toxins (MW 300) and the channel, which result in dissociation constants in the nanomolar range, would also occur between calcium (at. wt 40) and the channel. It is therefore unlikely that the conformational change that underlies the voltage dependence of toxin binding would confer a similar voltage dependence on calcium block. A more reasonable mechanism is that calcium ions bind and block at a site deep within the channel pore and experience a substantial fraction of the membrane electric field as they approach the site.[10,11] If the site were about 20% of the distance into the membrane electric field,

such a mechanism would account for the voltage-dependent block seen in FIGURE 6A.
Protons may also block sodium channels at this internal site[10,24] in some systems (see
ref. 25 for a possible exception).

We have been able to modify the channel with an agent (TMO) that methylates
protein carboxyl residues and found that this treatment eliminates STX binding and
block, and reduces, but does not completely eliminate, calcium block (FIG. 6). We
interpret this to mean that both sodium and calcium interact with the STX and TTX
binding site as they enter the channel. Both can then reach the second, deeper site at

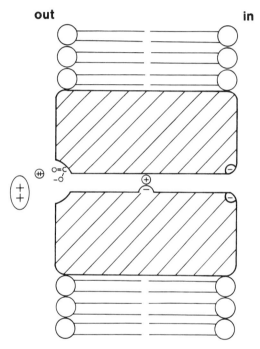

FIGURE 8. Diagram showing a cross section of the sodium channel embedded in a phospholipid
bilayer, indicating the proposed locations of the carboxyl group at the STX and TTX binding site
near the channel mouth and a deeper binding site accessible to Na$^+$ and Ca^{2+} but not to toxins. A
third cation binding site, near the internal mouth of the channel, has been identified on the basis
of voltage-independent block by internal calcium (Worley, Krueger, and French, in preparation).
The external dimensions of the channel are approximately those of a 300 kDa protein in the shape
of a cylinder that just spans the membrane. Saxitoxin and a calcium ion are shown schematically
by the *oval* and *circle* in the extracellular space. A sodium ion is indicated in the middle binding
site.

which calcium block is voltage dependent. Methylation of the external toxin binding
site by TMO impedes access of both calcium and sodium to the channel, resulting in
reduced single channel conductance (FIG. 6 and refs. 13 and 17) and reduced potency
of block by calcium (FIG. 6). Additional experiments, similar to that shown in FIGURE
6B, involving larger hyperpolarizations and/or higher external calcium, will be
necessary to determine if the residual calcium block after TMO has the same voltage
dependence as before. It has also been reported that calcium can slightly permeate

sodium channels,[26] indicating that calcium has access to virtually all sites within the channel pore. This access to deeper sites provides the most plausible explanation for the voltage dependence of block by calcium.

In summary, we believe that the sodium channel pore contains at least three binding sites for cations (FIG. 8): an external, toxin binding site containing a carboxylic acid (which can undergo a voltage-dependent change in toxin affinity), a deeper site, inaccessible to toxins, at which calcium blocks in a voltage-dependent manner, and an internal site at which voltage-independent block by calcium occurs (Worley, Krueger and French, in preparation). This differs from previous multisite models[11,27] of the channel in that the internal and external sites are placed superficially (at the entrances to the pore), and there is a substantial component of calcium block at these sites in the unmodified channel. Application of rate theory to this model accurately predicts the available experimental data; alterations in only the parameters for the external site satisfactorily account for the effects of TMO on single channel conductance and calcium block shown in FIGURE 6.

SUMMARY

The block of single, batrachotoxin-activated sodium channels by saxitoxin (STX), tetrodotoxin (TTX), and Ca^{2+} has been investigated in planar bilayers. All three substances block in a voltage-dependent manner with hyperpolarizing potentials favoring block. Extracellular Ca^{2+} competitively inhibits binding of STX and relieves STX block. Trimethyloxonium, a carboxyl-methylating agent, eliminates block by STX and TTX and dramatically reduces block by Ca^{2+}. These results suggest that STX, TTX, and Ca^{2+} compete for a negative site on the outside of the channel. The voltage dependence of block by STX (divalent cation) and TTX (monovalent) was similar (40 mV/e-fold), suggesting that voltage dependence is due to a conformational change in the channel rather than to the toxins entering the membrane electric field to block. A physical model, with an external binding site for toxins and Ca^{2+} and another site deeper within the electric field (associated with the "selectivity filter") that is accessible to Ca^{2+} but not toxins, predicts voltage-dependent Ca^{2+} block without invoking the conformational change needed to explain the voltage dependence of block by TTX and STX.

REFERENCES

1. HODGKIN, A. L. & A. F. HUXLEY. 1952. A quantitative description of membrane current and its application to conduction and excitation in nerve. J. Physiol. **117:** 500–544.
2. KRUEGER, B. K., J. F. WORLEY, III & R. J. FRENCH. 1983. Single sodium channels from rat brain incorporated into planar lipid bilayer membranes. Nature **303:** 172–175.
3. FRENCH, R. J., J. F. WORLEY, III & B. K. KRUEGER. 1984. Voltage-dependent block by saxitoxin of sodium channels incorporated into planar lipid bilayers. Biophys. J. **45:** 301–310.
4. MOCZYDLOWSKI, E., S. S. GARBER & C. MILLER. 1984. Batrachotoxin-activated Na^+ channels in planar lipid bilayers. Competition of tetrodotoxin block by Na^+. J. Gen. Physiol. **84:** 665–686.
5. GREEN, W. N., L. B. WEISS & O. S. ANDERSEN. 1984. Batrachotoxin-modified sodium channels in lipid bilayers. Ann. N.Y. Acad. Sci. **435:** 548–550.
6. ROSENBERG, R. L., S. A. TOMIKO & W. S. AGNEW. 1984. Single-channel properties of the reconstituted voltage-regulated Na channel isolated from the electroplax of *Electrophorus electricus*. Proc. Natl. Acad. Sci. U.S.A. **81:** 5594–5598.

7. HARTSHORNE, R. P., B. U. KELLER, J. A. TALVENHEIMO, W. A. CATTERALL & M. MONTAL. 1985. Functional reconstitution of the purified brain sodium channel in planar lipid bilayers. Proc. Natl. Acad. Sci. U.S.A. **82:** 240–244.

8. BARCHI, R. L., J. C. TANAKA & R. E. FURMAN. 1984. Molecular characteristics and functional reconstitution of muscle voltage-sensitive sodium channels. J. Cell. Biochem. **26:** 135–146.

9. HANKE, W., G. BOHEIM, J. BARHANIN, D. PAURON & M. LAZDUNSKI. 1985. Reconstitution of highly purified saxitoxin-sensitive Na^+ channels into planar lipid bilayers. EMBO J. **3:** 509–515.

10. WOODHULL, A. M. 1973. Ionic blockage of sodium channels in nerve. J. Gen. Physiol. **61:** 687–708.

11. YAMAMOTO, D., J. Z. YEH & T. NARAHASHI. 1984. Voltage-dependent calcium block of normal and tetramethrin-modified single sodium channels. Biophys. J. **45:** 337–344.

12. YAMAMOTO, D., J. Z. YEH & T. NARAHASHI. 1985. Interactions of permeant cations with sodium channels of squid axon membranes. Biophys. J. **48:** 361–368.

13. WORLEY, J. F., R. J. FRENCH & B. K. KRUEGER. 1986. Trimethyloxonium modification of single batrachotoxin-activated sodium channels in planar bilayers: Changes in unit conductance and in block by saxitoxin and calcium. J. Gen. Physiol. **87:** 327–349.

14. KRUEGER, B. K., R. W. RATZLAFF, G. R. STRICHARTZ & M. P. BLAUSTEIN. 1979. Saxitoxin binding to synaptosomes, membranes, and solubilized binding sites from rat brain. J. Membr. Biol. **50:** 287–310.

15. FRENCH, R. J., J. F. WORLEY, III, M. B. BLAUSTEIN, W. O. ROMINE, JR., K. K. TAM & B. K. KRUEGER. 1986. Gating of batrachotoxin-activated sodium channels in lipid bilayer membranes. *In* Ion Channel Reconstitution. C. Miller, Ed.: 363–383. Plenum. New York.

16. MOCZYDLOWSKI, E., S. HALL, S. S. GARBER, G. R. STRICHARTZ & C. MILLER. 1984. Voltage-dependent blockade of muscle Na^+ channels by guanidinium toxins. Effect of toxin charge. J. Gen. Physiol. **84:** 687–704.

17. SIGWORTH, F. J. & B. C. SPALDING. 1980. Chemical modification reduces the conductance of sodium channels in nerve. Nature **282:** 293–295.

18. SPALDING, B. C. 1980. Properties of toxin-resistant sodium channels produced by chemical modification in frog skeletal muscle. J. Physiol. **305:** 485–500.

19. SHRAGER, P. & C. PROFERA. 1973. Inhibition of the receptor for tetrodotoxin in nerve membranes by reagents modifying carboxyl groups. Biochim. Biophys. Acta **318:** 141–146.

20. BAKER, P. F. & K. A. RUBINSON. 1975. Chemical modification of crab nerves can make them insensitive to the local anaesthetics tetrodotoxin and saxitoxin. Nature **257:** 412–414.

21. REED, J. K. & M. A. RAFTERY. 1976. Properties of the tetrodotoxin binding component in plasma membranes isolated from *Electrophorus electricus*. Biochemistry **15:** 944–953.

22. BAKER, P. F. & K. A. RUBINSON. 1977. TTX-resistant action potentials in crab nerve after treatment with Meerwein's reagent. J. Physiol. **206:** 3–4P.

23. GULDEN, K.-M. & W. VOGEL. 1985. Three functions of sodium channels in the toad node of Ranvier are altered by trimethyloxonium ions. Pfluegers Arch. **403:** 13–20.

24. BEGENISICH, T. & M. DANKO. 1983. Hydrogen ion block of the sodium pore in squid giant axons. J. Gen. Physiol. **82:** 599–618.

25. CAMPBELL, D. T. 1982. Do protons block Na^+ channels by binding to a site outside of the pore? Nature **298:** 165–167.

26. MEVES, H. & W. VOGEL. 1973. Calcium inward currents in internally perfused giant axons. J. Physiol. **235:** 225–265.

27. HILLE, B. 1975. Ionic selectivity, saturation, and block in sodium channels. J. Gen. Physiol. **66:** 535–560.

Isochannels and Blocking Modes of Voltage-Dependent Sodium Channels[a]

EDWARD MOCZYDLOWSKI,[b] AKIRA UEHARA,[c]
XIAOTAO GUO,[d] AND JUDITH HEINY

Department of Physiology and Biophysics
[d]Department of Pharmacology and Cell Biophysics
University of Cincinnati College of Medicine
Cincinnati, Ohio 45267

INTRODUCTION

This paper addresses two questions in current research on voltage-dependent sodium channels: the possible heterogeneity of channel structure among excitable tissues, and the diverse mechanisms of channel block by small molecules and ions.

The role of Na channels in the firing of fast action potentials would seem to require only one type of Na-channel protein in various nerve and muscle tissues. Indeed, early studies of macroscopic Na-channel currents suggested that most of the functional properties of Na channels were similar from tissue to tissue. For example, in conclusion to a careful comparison of Hodgkin-Huxley parameters, and effects of H^+, Ca^{2+}, and saxitoxin on Na currents of frog myelinated nerve and skeletal muscle fibers, Campbell and Hille[1] wrote: "The results show an overwhelming similarity in the two tissues, and we conclude that the channels may comprise the same molecular species." To account for observed differences in the temperature dependence and absolute rates of gating between muscle and nerve, these authors suggested that differences in "the surrounding membrane material" (*e.g.*, the lipid environment) could explain these functional differences.

In contrast to the close similarity of nerve and skeletal muscle Na^+ currents, the fast Na^+ spike in cardiac muscle has long been known to be rather insensitive to tetrodotoxin. Whereas 5 nM tetrodotoxin is sufficient to produce half-maximal block in normal rat skeletal muscle,[2] about 1–5 μM tetrodotoxin is required to produce a similar effect in mammalian cardiac muscle.[3–5] This large difference in toxin sensitivity led several groups to suspect that the toxin receptor of heart Na channels might be intrinsically different from that of nerve or skeletal muscle. Na currents of denervated mammalian muscle[2,6,7] and mammalian muscle cells in culture[8] also exhibit an insensitive component that requires about 1 μM tetrodotoxin for half-maximal

[a]This work was supported by grants from the Muscular Dystrophy Association and the National Institutes of Health (AM 35128), and the Searle Scholars Program/Chicago Community Trust.
[b]EM is an Established Investigator of the American Heart Association. Present address: Department of Pharmacology, Yale University School of Medicine, New Haven, Conn. 06510.
[c]Present address: Department of Physiology, Fukuoka University School of Medicine, 34 Nanakuma, Jonan-Ku, Fukuoka 814–01, Japan.

269

inhibition, a case analogous to that of the heart. Recent biochemical studies have followed up on these early observations and suspicions regarding multiple types of Na channels by employing various toxin probes to distinguish different classes of Na channels in skeletal muscle and heart cell membranes on the basis of high or low affinity toxin receptor sites.[9-21]

Electrophysiological studies of block by toxins and small molecules have been used to characterize specific properties of diverse sites of blocker action. For example, block by external H^+ and Ca^{2+} ions exhibits an apparent voltage dependence, with enhancement of block at hyperpolarizing voltages.[22-25] Block by internal organic cations such as QX-314 and tetramethylammonium is also voltage dependent, with enhancement of block at depolarizing voltages.[26-29] These cases of external and internal block have been considered to result from entry of the blocking ion into the channel pore, so that the rates of blocker entry and exit fall under the direct influence of the transmembrane electric field. In addition to voltage dependence, the binding of local anesthetics has also been proposed to be state dependent, with different affinities of the blocker for open, closed, and inactivated channels.[26,30,31]

In order to pursue these questions of channel heterogeneity and blocking mechanisms, we have studied batrachotoxin-activated currents of single Na channels in planar lipid bilayers, a system introduced by Krueger et al.[32] with Na channels from rat brain synaptosomes. This system is well suited to the study of these questions because slow rates of block can be measured at equilibrium as discrete blocking events of open channels and the action of fast blockers can be measured directly as a decrease in the apparent single-channel conductance. Also, the behavior of channels from different tissues can be compared after incorporation in the same lipid bilayer environment. We have found that native vesicles of rat skeletal muscle plasma membrane are an especially favorable preparation for this technique, because channel incorporation can be routinely observed and single-channel membranes can be obtained with good frequency from day to day.[33,34]

In this article, we summarize recent work showing that dramatic differences exist in the molecular properties of the guanidinium toxin receptor of various Na-channel subtypes after transfer from native membranes to artificial planar membranes. The peptide μ-conotoxin GIIIA is shown to block Na-channel currents in skeletal muscle and also to inhibit ^3H-saxitoxin binding in this tissue. In contrast to these results in skeletal muscle, Na channels from brain, heart, and lobster axons are virtually unaffected by GIIIA. We also find that the low sensitivity to tetrodotoxin in heart and denervated skeletal muscle can be directly observed at the single channel level as a decreased dwell time of this toxin on the channel and as an increased waiting time for toxin binding to the channel.

Other blocking modes of small molecules are also explored with the batrachotoxin-activated Na channel of rat skeletal muscle. The local anesthetics benzocaine and procaine produce discrete blocking events when added to either side of the channel. This blocking mode appears to be a preferential interaction with certain closed states of the channel, because the duration of the closing events increases with procaine concentration. We find that guanidinium and quaternary ammonium cations produce a voltage-dependent block from the inside of the channel but are weak blockers on the extracellular side. Block by external methylguanidine is rather unusual, in that its blocking action appears to be voltage independent; however, inward Na^+ current is blocked more effectively than outward Na^+ current. In contrast to organic cations, divalent inorganic cations such as Ca^{2+} and Co^{2+} are more effective blockers from the outside, exhibiting about a threefold steeper voltage dependence from the outside than the inside.

μ-CONOTOXINS RECOGNIZE A DISTINCT Na-CHANNEL SUBTYPE

Over the past several years Cruz, Gray, Olivera, and their colleagues have isolated and sequenced three groups of small peptide toxins from the venom of *Conus geographus*, a fish-eating snail of the Pacific.[35-37] These toxins constitute a potent cocktail directed against various channels: α-conotoxins, which block acetylcholine receptor, channels of skeletal muscle, ω-conotoxins, which appear to block certain presynaptic Ca channels at nerve terminals, and μ-conotoxins, which block muscle Na channels.

The μ-contoxins are single chains of 22 amino acids with amidated carboxy termini that also contain *trans*-4-hydroxproline (Hyp). The following sequence is that of GIIIA, a predominant peptide of this group[37,38]:

1   5   10
Arg-Asp-Cys-Cys-Thr-Hyp-Hyp-Lys-Lys-Cys -

15   20
Lys-Asp-Arg-Gln-Cys -Lys-Hyp-Gln-Arg-Cys-Cys -Ala-NH$_2$

Micromolar concentrations of this peptide block action potentials of skeletal muscle in various amphibian and mammalian preparations. In similar experiments with nerve preparations, however, GIIIA has little effect.[37]

FIGURE 1 shows the effect of 2 μM GIIIA on macroscopic Na currents of a single frog semitendinosus muscle fiber as measured by a vaseline gap voltage-clamp method.[39] Trace *a* in FIGURE 1A shows a control record of inward Na current evoked by a depolarization to −10 mV from a holding potential of −110 mV. This record exhibits a typical rapidly activating and inactivating phase followed by a slightly delayed hump. This latter hump, which is commonly observed under these conditions, is primarily due to the lack of adequate voltage control in the transverse tubular system. Within minutes of exchanging the external Ringers solution for one containing 2 μM GIIIA, the Na currents began to decline. Traces *b* and *c* show the currents recorded from the fiber at about 10–15 and 25–30 minutes after the introduction of toxin. By 30 minutes, the peak current was reduced by 95%, including an elimination of the delayed hump. Inspection of the time courses of the declining currents in the presence of toxin suggested that there were no significant alterations in the kinetics of the remaining channels. A comparison of the voltage dependence of the Hodgkin-Huxley h_{∞} inactivation parameter before and 15 minutes after toxin addition revealed that this property was also unaffected (not shown). FIGURE 1B is a plot of the peak current-voltage relation, which is proportionately depressed at all potentials in the presence of GIIIA. These observations are quite similar to the published effects of tetrodotoxin on macroscopic Na-channel currents in muscle.[20] One difference is that the effect of nanomolar concentrations of tetrodotoxin is generally complete within about 5 minutes after perfusion, whereas 2 μM GIIIA seemed to require about 20 minutes for equilibration. This slowness of GIIIA action could be related to the large number of positive charges on the GIIIA molecule which might cause increased nonspecific association with the cell surface and could potentially slow the kinetics of equilibration with whole cells or tissue.

FIGURE 2 illustrates the blocking action of GIIIA at the level of a single Na channel from rat skeletal muscle. The top two traces are a consecutive control record at +25 mV of a single batrachotoxin-activated Na channel in a planar bilayer cast from a solution of neutral phospholipids in decane according to the Mueller-Rudin tech-

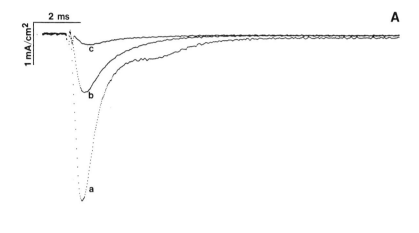

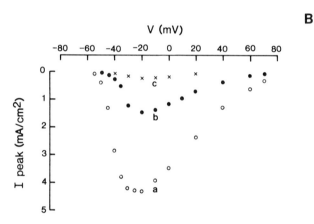

FIGURE 1. Effect of 2 μM μ-conotoxin GIIIA on macroscopic Na^+ current in a frog muscle fiber. Voltage-clamped ionic current from a single fiber of the semitendinosus muscle of *Rana catesbiana* was measured using a vaseline gap method.[39] Linear leak and capacity currents were eliminated using hyperpolarizing subtracting pulse protocols. A gap = 100 μ. The external solution bathing the fiber was 115 mM NaCl, 2.5 mM KCl, 1.8 mM $CaCl_2$, 5 mM Na-MOPS, pH 7. The cut ends of the fiber were equilibrated with 110 mM Cs-glutamate, 5 mM Cs-EGTA, 5 mM Cs-MOPS, 2 mM $MgCl_2$, 1.7 mM $CaSO_4$, 0.5 mM Na_2ATP, pH 7. Temperature = 5°C. (**A**) Current records evoked by a 20 ms step pulse to −10 mV from a holding potential of −110 mV:trace *a*, control taken before the addition of toxin; trace *b*, 10–15 minutes after perfusion with external solution containing 2 μM GIIIA; trace *c*, 25–30 minutes after perfusion with toxin. (**B**) Peak current is plotted for various step potentials for control (*a*), 10–15 minutes (*b*), and 25–30 minutes (*c*) after perfusion with GIIIA.

nique.[40] Under these conditions, the channel is open nearly all of the time with occasional brief closing events, as has been previously described.[32,33] When GIIIA is added to the external side (defined as the extracellular side) of the channel in the bilayer, discrete blocking events are observed. The bottom five traces in FIGURE 2 are a continuous record from a single channel membrane in the presence of 1 μM GIIIA and

0.2 M symmetrical NaCl. An analysis of the probability distributions of the durations of these events and their concentration dependence showed that the action of GIIIA on single Na channels is well described by reversible binding to a single site.[37] The equilibrium dissociation constant of GIIIA at 0 mV and 22°C was found to be 100 nM, with an exponential voltage dependence that increases the K_d e-fold for 34 mV of depolarization.

This blocking action of GIIIA is quite similar to the previously described action of tetrodotoxin and saxitoxin derivatives on single batrachotoxin-activated Na channels,[32,33,41] and led us to suspect that the μ-conotoxin peptides might recognize part of the same receptor site as these classical Na-channel toxins. In order to test this possibility, we recently carried out an extensive investigation of the effect of GIIIA on the binding of ^{3}H-saxitoxin in various membrane preparations.[42] FIGURE 3 shows the results of an experiment in which increasing concentrations of GIIIA were added to rat muscle and rat brain membranes in the presence of 4.5 nM ^{3}H-saxitoxin at 0°C. This experiment shows that specific saxitoxin binding in rat muscle membranes is inhibited by increasing GIIIA concentrations in the range of 10–100 nM. In contrast to this situation in muscle, ^{3}H-saxitoxin binding to rat brain membranes is unaffected in this same range of GIIIA concentration, but does show some slight inhibition at GIIIA

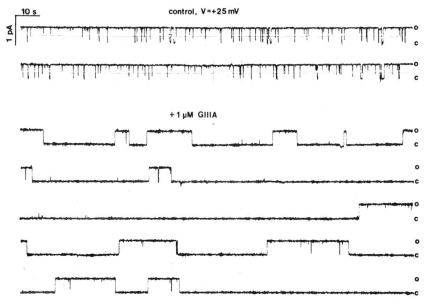

FIGURE 2. Effect of μ-conotoxin GIIIA on a single Na channel. Signal channel currents of batrachotoxin-activated Na channels from rat skeletal muscle were recorded after incorporation into planar bilayers as described previously.[33] The planar bilayer was cast from a solution of 17.5 mg/ml phosphatidylethanolamine and 7.5 mg/ml phosphatidylcholine in decane. The solution on both sides of the bilayer was 200 mM NaCl, 10 mM MOPS-NaOH, 0.1 mM EDTA, pH 7.4. Temperature = 22°C. The upper two records show typical control behavior of a single channel at a constant holding voltage of +25 mV (physiological convention for the sign of the voltage). The lower 5 records are a continuous trace recorded after the addition of 1 μM GIIIA to the side of the bilayer corresponding to the extracellular face of a single channel at +25 mV; *c*, closed state current level, *o*, open state current level. Filter = 100 Hz.

concentrations greater than 10 μM. In experiments to be published elsewhere, we found that ^{3}H-saxitoxin binding in eel electroplax membranes is also inhibited by GIIIA in the 10–1000 nM range, but ^{3}H-saxitoxin binding in membranes from lobster axon and rat heart is unaffected by GIIIA concentrations up to 40 μM. These results demonstrate that GIIIA interacts with the tetrodotoxin and saxitoxin receptor site in Na channels from skeletal muscle and Electrophorus electroplax, but weakly recog-

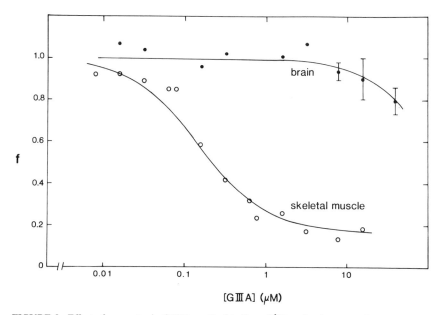

[GⅢA] (μM)

FIGURE 3. Effect of μ-conotoxin GIIIA on the binding of ^{3}H-saxitoxin to membrane preparations from rat muscle and rat brain. The membrane preparation from rat skeletal muscle was a low density fraction obtained after sucrose density centrifugation of crude microsomes layered over 32% (w/v) sucrose as described.[43] A crude membrane preparation from rat brain was isolated from the supernatant obtained after centrifugation at 2,000 × g of a homogenate of whole brains in 0.3 M sucrose, 10 mM MOPS-NaOH, pH 7.4. Specific binding of ^{3}H-saxitoxin to these preparations was measured after rapid separation of the bound ligand on 1 ml columns of Dowex 50X-200 as described previously.[43] Binding at 0°C was measured after incubation for 30–60 minutes in a solution containing 200 mM choline Cl, 10 mM MOPS-NaOH, pH 7.4, 0.5 mg/ml bovine serum albumin, 4.5 nM ^{3}H-saxitoxin, 2 mg protein/ml muscle membranes, or 0.4 mg/ml brain membranes and the indicated concentration of μ-conotoxin GIIIA. These results are expressed as the fraction (f) of bound ^{3}H-saxitoxin to that measured initially in the absence of GIIIA. The initial levels of binding were 2.3 nM bound ^{3}H-saxitoxin for the muscle preparation and 3.0 nM for the brain preparation.

nizes (if at all) the same receptor site in Na channels from nerve axons, brain, and heart.

   In other experiments, we have also found that the effect of GIIIA on ^{3}H-saxitoxin binding in eel electroplax can be described as simple competition for a common site[44]; however, in membrane preparations from rat skeletal muscle, the situation is slightly more complicated. FIGURE 3 shows that high concentrations of GIIIA (1–20 μM) did not inhibit the residual 10%–15% of specific saxitoxin binding under these conditions.

This consistently observed phenomenon suggested that a small fraction of saxitoxin sites in the muscle preparation might be insensitive to GIIIA. FIGURE 4 shows the results of a Scatchard plot analysis of ^{3}H-saxitoxin binding to a rat muscle membrane preparation in the absence and presence of 240 nM GIIIA. In the absence of GIIIA, ^{3}H-saxitoxin binding is fairly well described by a single-site binding curve with a K_d of about 0.85 nM, in agreement with previous studies.[45,46] However, in the presence of GIIIA, deviations from single-site behavior were consistently observed. For example, the data of FIGURE 4 in the presence of 240 nM GIIIA were fit by a sum of two independent saxitoxin binding sites with apparent K_ds of 0.25 and 16 nM. Our present interpretation of this result is that the skeletal muscle preparation contains a small fraction (~5%–15%) of saxitoxin binding sites that are insensitive to μ-contoxin, such as those of brain, whereas the remaining sites are competitively inhibited by GIIIA. The insensitive sites could conceivably represent contamination of the muscle preparation with nerve terminals or could be due to two distinct classes of Na channels in the adult rat muscle cell. Further work will be required to investigate these alternatives.

INCORPORATION OF TETRODOTOXIN-INSENSITIVE Na CHANNELS FROM HEART AND DENERVATED SKELETAL MUSCLE INTO PLANAR BILAYERS

The preceding μ-conotoxin studies distinguish a Na channel subtype specific for skeletal muscle (or related tissue such as electroplax) from that of nerve and heart. In order to characterize the toxin receptor of low-affinity channels from heart and denervated skeletal muscle, we screened various membrane preparations for the possible incorporation of tetrodotoxin-insensitive Na channels into planar bilayers. We found that such Na channels can be consistently incorporated from canine heart sarcolemma membranes (prepared according to Jones *et al.*[47]) and from plasma membranes of denervated muscles of the rat (prepared according to the methods of Moczydlowski and Lattore[43]).

FIGURE 5 shows an example of current records from a bilayer containing a single batrachotoxin-activated Na channel from dog heart. Most characteristics of this channel are grossly similar to those described previously for batrachotoxin-activated Na channels from rat[32,48] and dog brain[41] and normal rat muscle[33] in planar bilayers. From −50 to +50 mV, the channel is open nearly all of the time with occasional brief closing events. However, the conductance of this heart channel is 23–24 pS at 0.2 M NaCl, which is consistently about 10% larger than the conductance (20–21 pS) of the Na channel from normal rat muscle under these conditions. Also, concentrations of tetrodotoxin (20–100 nM) that produce effective block of brain and muscle channels result in few blocking events for the heart channel. Higher concentrations of tetrodotoxin do result in the appearance of frequent blocked states. This behavior is illustrated in FIGURE 5 by the records at +50 and −50 mV in the presence of 1 μM external tetrodotoxin. This discrete blocking behavior exhibits a voltage dependence similar to that of brain[41,48] and muscle channels,[33] as noted by a lengthening of the blocked times and a shortening of the unblocked times at −50 mV compared to +50 mV. The major difference exhibited by the dog heart channel is that the average duration of the tetrodotoxin blocked states is only about 20%–25% as long as those observed under similar conditions in rat muscle[33] or dog brain (W. Green, personal communication).

In studies to be presented elsewhere, a stochastic analysis of the blocking events induced in the heart channel by various guanidinium toxins revealed that this behavior

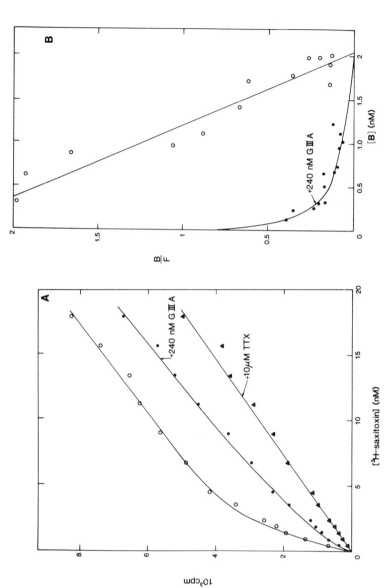

FIGURE 4. Titration of ^{3}H-saxitoxin binding to a rat muscle membrane preparation in the absence and presence of 240 nM GIIIA. ^{3}H-saxitoxin binding was measured at 0°C in the presence of 1 mg/ml rat muscle preparation, 200 mM choline Cl, 10 mM MOPS-NaOH, pH 7.4 and increasing ^{3}H-saxitoxin concentrations. (**A**) Raw binding data in cpm is plotted as a function of total ^{3}H-saxitoxin present in the assay: O = control; ● = 240 nM GIIIA; ▲ = 10 μM tetrodotoxin. Solid curves in A are drawn by eye. (**B**) Scatchard plot analysis of the data in **A**. Specific binding in the absence of GIIIA (O) was fit to a single site with a K_d of 0.85 nM and a binding capacity of n = 2.05 nM. Specific binding in the presence of GIIIA (●) was fit to a sum of two independent sites with a high affinity K_d = 0.25 nM and n = 0.17 nM and a low affinity K_d = 15.7 nM and n = 1.88 nM.

closely follows that expected of reversible binding to a single site, as also previously shown for other Na channels in artificial bilayers. The voltage dependence of tetrodotoxin binding to the heart channel is presented in FIGURE 6, where the derived association and dissociation rate constants and the equilibrium dissociation constants are plotted as functions of voltage. These functions can all be described adequately by a simple exponential dependence on voltage. The voltage dependence of each parameter is related to the slope of the log-linear plots of FIGURE 6. A comparison of these slope parameters indicates that the voltage dependence of toxin binding to heart Na channels is quite similar to that measured for various toxins in the high affinity channel from normal rat skeletal muscle (TABLE 1).

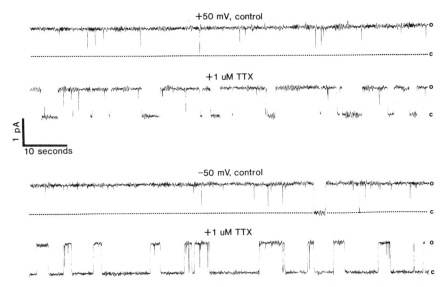

FIGURE 5. Effect of tetrodotoxin on a single batrachotoxin-activated Na channel from canine heart. A plasma membrane preparation from canine heart ventricular muscle was isolated according to Jones *et al.*[47] Incorporation of cardiac Na channels into planar bilayers was observed when this preparation was used in the presence of 0.2 μM batrachotoxin under the same conditions given in the legend of FIGURE 2. Representative records of a single heart channel at +50 mV and −50 mV are shown in the absence and presence of 1 μM tetrodotoxin on the external side of the channel.

Recently, we have also been able to observe single tetrodotoxin-insensitive Na channels from plasma membranes of denervated rat skeletal muscle.[49] An example of a recording from a bilayer containing one batrachotoxin-activated Na channel from this preparation is shown in FIGURE 7. The experiment of FIGURE 7 was carried out in the presence of 2 μM external tetrodotoxin to induce discrete blocking events. The unit conductance (23–24 pS) and other properties of such channels appear to be quite similar to that of the cardiac Na channel of FIGURE 5. A similar analysis of the tetrodotoxin blocking rate constants for this channel is summarized in TABLE 1, where values for the normal rat muscle channels are also listed. The data in TABLE 1 indicate that the kinetic constants for tetrodotoxin block of the dog cardiac and rat denervated muscle channel are practically indistinguishable within the accuracy of these measure-

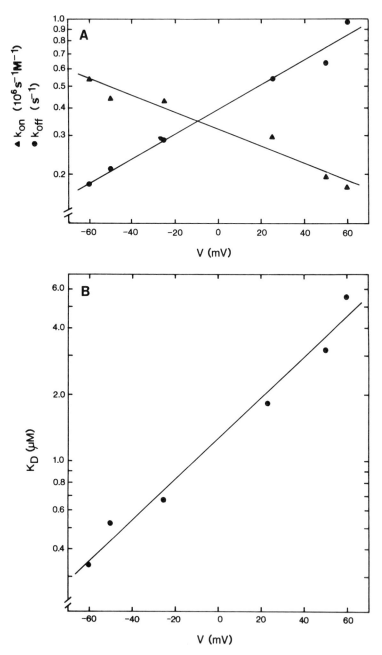

FIGURE 6. Rate and equilibrium constants of tetrodotoxin blocking of a canine heart Na channel measured as a function of voltage. (**A**) Dissociation (●) and association (▲) rate constants were measured from single channel records at 1 μM tetrodotoxin similar to that shown in FIGURE 5. Rate constants at the indicated voltage were calculated from the arithmetic mean of populations of 80–120 blocking events as described previously. (**B**) The equilibrium dissociation constant was calculated as the ratio of k_{off}/k_{on} on data in **A**. Solid lines represent fits to exponential functions of voltage with parameters given in TABLE 1.

TABLE 1. Single Channel Conductance and Tetrodotoxin Blocking Rate Constants of Various Na Channel Subtypes in Planar Bilayers

Channel Type	Single Channel Conductance g (pS)	Dissociation Rate $k_{-1}(V) = k_{-1}(0) \exp(A_{-1}V)$		Association Rate $k_{i1}(V) = k_{i1}(0) \exp(A_1 V)$		Equilibrium Dissociation Constant $K_d(V) = K_d(0) \exp(AV)$	
		$k_{-1}(0)$ (s^{-1})	A_{-1} (mV^{-1})	$k_{i1}(0)$ ($s^{-1}M^{-1}$)	A_1 (mV^{-1})	$K_d(0)$ (nM)	A (mV^{-1})
Rat skeletal muscle	20–21	0.12	0.013	4.5×10^6	−0.010	27	0.023
Denervated rat skeletal muscle	23–24	0.46	0.011	0.45×10^6	−0.011	1020	0.022
Canine heart ventricular muscle	23–24	0.39	0.013	0.32×10^6	−0.0088	1250	0.021

ments (standard error = ± 10%). The Na channels from all three sources exhibit nearly the same voltage dependence for tetrodotoxin block, indicating that this property is a conserved feature of various channel subtypes. TABLE 1 also shows that the low affinity for tetrodotoxin in heart and denervated muscle is due to the combined effects of an approximately fourfold faster dissociation rate constant and a twelvefold slower association rate constant, as compared to the Na channel from normal rat muscle. We have also found that such tetrodotoxin-insensitive channels from dog heart and denervated muscle are insensitive to 1 μM GIIIA in planar bilayers. These results lead us to propose that the tetrodotoxin-insensitive Na channels that appear in mammalian skeletal muscle after denervation are of the same toxin-insensitive Na-channel subtype that is normally expressed in mammalian heart. A similar conclusion was also reached by Catterall and Coppersmith[10] in Na$^+$ flux studies using cultured cells.

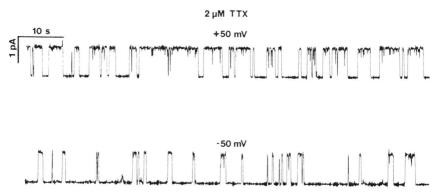

FIGURE 7. Current records from a bilayer containing a single toxin-insensitive Na channel from denervated rat skeletal muscle. Denervated skeletal muscle was prepared by surgical removal of a 1-cm piece of right sciatic nerve from 11 rats. On the seventh day after surgery, a plasma membrane fraction was isolated from 30 g of right lower hind limb muscle using methods similar to those described previously.[43] Incorporation of batrachotoxin-activated Na channels from this preparation into planar bilayers was observed under the same condition as described in FIGURE 2. Representative records are shown from a bilayer containing a single toxin-insensitive Na channel in the presence of 2 μM tetrodotoxin.

These results point to distinct molecular differences between Na channels of different tissues. These differences are preserved after the transfer of channels from native membranes into artificial bilayers of the same lipid composition. This result implies that the wide variation in toxin sensitivities among the three different channel subtypes cannot be explained by differences in tissue accessibility, lipid surface charge, membrane fluidity, or extrinsic soluble factors. We believe that the most likely explanation for these differences is the existence of multiple types of isochannels in analogy to multiple isozymes of soluble enzymes. The nerve-, muscle-, and heart-specific isochannels would presumably be coded for by three different structural genes that would be under developmental regulation. The only other likely explanation for our results would be specific posttranslational modification of a common Na channel polypeptide. Recent advances in the cloning and sequencing of a Na-channel gene from

Electrophorus electricus[50] may permit the existence of isochannel genes to be verified by molecular biological approaches.

A SLOW BLOCKING MODE OF BENZOCAINE AND PROCAINE

In screening the effects of various local anesthetics on single batrachotoxin-activated Na channels, we found that benzocaine and procaine exhibit a unique type of blocking behavior. Both of these agents induce the appearance of long-lived closing events of about 1 to 20 seconds in duration. This phenomenon is shown in comparison with control records in FIGURE 8. Because a detailed description of block by these agents was presented previously,[51,52] these results will only be summarized here.

Although the effect of benzocaine and procaine shown in FIGURE 8 may superficially resemble the action of tetrodotoxin, the actual mechanisms appear to be quite different. For example, the kinetics of tetrodotoxin and saxitoxin block have been shown to conform to a reversible binding interaction with the open channel.[33,48] Such behavior is indicated by the linear dependence of the reciprocal of the mean open or unblocked dwell times on blocker concentration and concentration independence of the blocked state dwell times. In contrast to this behavior, the duration of the procaine-induced closed states increases with procaine concentrations and the open-state dwell time is essentially independent of procaine concentration (see FIGURE 13 and TABLE 3 in ref. 52). This dependence of the closed state duration on blocker concentration suggests that procaine binds preferentially to closed instead of open conformations of the channel. In this mode of action, procaine appears to affect channel gating by modulating a shift of the gating equilibrium toward closed channel conformations.

In addition to the dependence of the closed state duration on anesthetic concentrations, several other observations are noteworthy. We find that benzocaine and procaine produce discrete blocking events with similar efficiency when added to either the external or internal side of the channel. This observation simply confirms the appreciable membrane solubility of benzocaine and the neutral form of procaine, which is a tertiary amine. The site of action of such drugs cannot easily be localized to either the internal or external surface because the addition of the drug to one side of a bilayer results in an unstirred layer of drug on the other side after diffusion of the neutral species across the membrane.[53] The fact that the neutral benzocaine molecule is effective in this blocking mode, however, suggests that the site of action may be quite hydrophobic and may perhaps be accessible from within the hydrophobic interior of the bilayer. Another feature of this blocking mode is its voltage dependence. We consistently find that the frequency of blocking events increases with increasing negative voltage. This dependence is qualitatively shown in the records of FIGURE 8, where an increased number of blocking events is observed at -50 mV compared to $+50$ mV. This voltage dependence may indicate that the particular closed states which bind the drug are favored by hyperpolarization, or it may indicate a voltage-dependent modulation of drug binding rates of the type observed with guanidinium toxins such as tetrodotoxin.

A final notable feature of the action of benzocaine and procaine is an apparent "disappearance" of channels at random intervals after the addition of drug. This behavior is qualitatively shown in the record of FIGURE 8B at -50 mV. In this particular record real time proceeds from right to left. The longest closing event at the left-hand portion of the record is an instance when channel opening events suddenly ceased and could not be elicited by depolarization to $+50$ mV. We have previously interpreted this disappearance phenomenon as the dissociation of batrachotoxin from

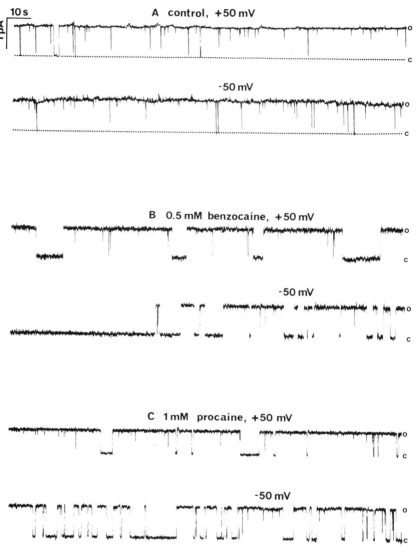

FIGURE 8. Effect of benzocaine and procaine on single batrachotoxin-activated Na channels from rat muscle. The bilayer composition and ionic conditions are the same as described in FIGURE 2. (**A**) Representative control records of a single channel from normal rat muscle at +50 and −50 mV. The open state current level at −50 mV exhibits more noise than at +50 mV because of the incorporation of an unidentified channel of very low conductance between the two records. (**B**) Records from a single channel bilayer in the presence of 0.5 mM external benzocaine. In the record at −50 mV, real time proceeds from right to left. After the last opening event at the left of this trace, the channel suddenly "disappeared" as described in the text. (**C**) Records from a single channel bilayer in the presence of 1 mM external procaine. Note the lower apparent single channel conductance at +50 mV compared to −50 mV.

the channel, resulting in a return to normal inactivation behavior.[51,52] We believe that this phenomenon reflects an increased dissociation rate constant of batrachotoxin in the presence of local anesthetics, as previously shown by direct binding studies with ³H-batrachotoxinin A 20-α-benzoate.[54]

FAST BLOCKING MODES OF ORGANIC CATIONS AND Ca²⁺

FIGURE 9 summarizes the effect of various organic cations when they are added to the internal side (defined as the intracellular side) of bilayers containing batrachotoxin-activated Na channels of normal rat skeletal muscle. Most of these molecules produce what has been referred to as a fast block, that is, an apparent reduction in the unitary current flowing through open channels. This effect is illustrated in FIGURE 9A where current records from a bilayer containing four Na channels in the presence of 50 nM external tetrodotoxin at +50 mV are shown before and after the addition of 2 mM internal methylguanidine. In this experiment it can be seen that the apparent single channel conductance is reduced by about 60% after the addition of methylguanidine. This effect also exhibits an apparent voltage dependence, because the fraction of blocked current increases with increasing depolarization. Thus the ohmic current-voltage relation of the channel in the absence of blockers is converted to a rectifying I-V relation in the presence of blocker. FIGURE 9B illustrates this behavior for single channel data taken in the absence and presence of 200 mM internal tetramethylammonium chloride (TMA).

This fast blocking mode definitely also appears to require a charged molecule because benzocaine, which has no protonable group at pH 7.4, does not produce this type of block. Tertiary amines, such as procaine and lidocaine, do however produce a fast block that increases with depolarization. This behavior of procaine is evident in the records of FIGURE 8C, where it can be seen that the channel conductance at +50 mV is about 20% less than that at −50 mV. Procaine is thus unique in that it causes both a slow blocking effect that increases with negative voltage and a fast blocking effect that increases with positive voltage.

To analyze fast blocking behavior, we have used a simple blocking model that has been commonly employed since a similar analysis of the effect of external H⁺ on macroscopic Na⁺-currents was presented by Woodhull.[22] This model assumes that the effect of the blocker, B, corresponds to rapid reversible binding to a single site, O, that can be characterized by a dissociation constant for the blocker, K_B:

$$O + B \underset{}{\overset{K_B}{\rightleftharpoons}} OB$$
$$\text{open} \qquad\qquad \text{blocked} \cdot$$

To take account of the effect of voltage, the blocker is assumed to traverse a fractional distance, δ, of a constant electric field across the membrane. The following expression then gives the ratio of the single channel current observed in the presence of blocker, i_B to that in the absence of blocker, i_0:

$$\frac{i_B}{i_0} = \left[1 + \frac{[B]}{K_B(0)\exp(z\delta FV/RT)} \right]^{-1}, \tag{1}$$

where $[B]$ is the blocker concentration, $K_B(0)$ is the apparent blocker dissociation constant at 0 mV, z is the valence of the blocker, V is the applied voltage, and F/RT has its usual meaning. This model makes the predictions that the fractional current, i_B/i_0, will follow a single site titration curve and that the apparent blocker dissociation

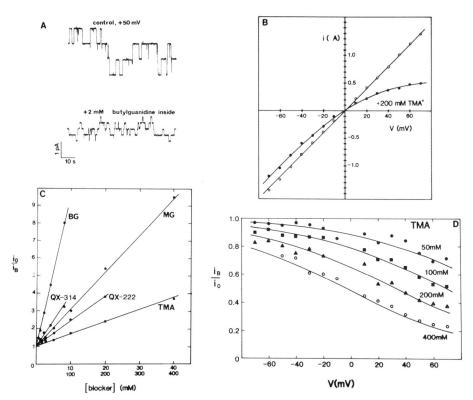

FIGURE 9. Fast block by organic cations on the internal side of Na channels in planar bilayers. Single channel currents of batrachotoxin-activated Na channels from rat skeletal muscle were recorded under conditions given in the legend of FIGURE 2. (A) Current records from a bilayer containing four channels oriented in the same direction in symmetrical 0.2 M NaCl and 50 nM tetrodotoxin present on the external side to induce discrete closing events. Channel opening is in the upward direction. Two records are shown at +50 mV, before and after the addition of 2 mM butylguanidine on the internal side. (B) Single channel current-voltage data is plotted for a control record in the presence of 200 mM symmetrical NaCl (O) and after the addition of 200 mM tetramethylammonium chloride (●) to the internal side. (C) The ratio of single channel current at +50 mV in the absence of blocker, i_0, to that in the presence of blocker, i_B, is plotted according to equation 1 as a function of the concentration of various internal blockers: BG, butylguanidine sulfate; MG, methylguanidine sulfate; TMA, tetramethylammonium chloride. QX-314 and QX-222 are quaternary ammonium derivatives of lidocaine whose structures are given in Hille.[56] The lower concentration scale refers to TMA; the upper scale refers to all the other blockers. (D) The ratio of single channel current in the presence of internal TMA, i_B, to that in the absence of blocker, i_0, is plotted as a function of voltage and internal TMA concentration. The solid lines are fits of the data to equation 2 with best-fit parameters given in TABLE 2.

constant is a simple exponential function of voltage. These two requirements of the model can be tested by examining the linearity of replots of i_0/i_B vs. $[B]$ and $\log(i_0/i_B - 1)$ vs. V, which are simple transformations of equation 1.

We have found that such a model closely approximates the real behavior of the batrachotoxin-activated Na channel in the presence of a variety of internal organic cations. FIGURE 9C illustrates the linearity of i_0/i_B vs. $[B]$ for several different guanidinium and quaternary ammonium compounds, and FIGURE 9D illustrates that voltage-dependent block by internal TMA closely follows equation 1. The blocking parameters of $K_B(0)$ and effective valence, $z\delta$, derived from studies of various internal blockers are summarized in TABLE 2.

These data can be used to speculate on structural characteristics of the internal mouth of the channel. For example, methylguanidine, butylguanidine, and TMA exhibit a significantly greater effective valence ($z\delta$ = 0.48–0.59) than procaine, QX-222 and QX-314 ($z\delta$ = 0.34–0.38). If this parameter can be taken to reflect the depth of penetration of the applied field, then perhaps procaine and the QX-compounds cannot enter the channel's mouth as deeply as the other ions, because of steric restrictions imposed by the bulky aromatic groups. The $K_B(0)$ values also indicate that increasing hydrophobic surface area (from methylguanidine to butyl-guanidine and methylation [QX-222] to ethylation [QX-314]) results in an increased binding affinity. Such behavior is usually taken to imply that favorable hydrophobic interactions between the walls of the channel mouth and the blocker contribute to the binding energy. These results also corroborate previous blocking studies of various internally applied organic cations with inactivating Na channels using macroscopic or microscopic current-recording techniques. The major structural conclusion of these studies is that the open Na channel has a wide internal vestibule that lies partly within the transmembrane field.[26–29]

In contrast, the structure of the external aspect of the open Na channel appears to be quite different. The same organic cations of FIGURE 9 are inefficient blockers when applied to the external side of the channel. FIGURE 10 illustrates this behavior with external methylguanidine (MG). Although high external concentrations of MG reduce the single channel current in the manner of a fast blocker (FIG. 10A), the complete

TABLE 2. Characteristics of Fast Block by Various Organic Cations, Ca^{2+} and Co^{2+}

Blocker (*n*)	Side	Effective Valence ($z\delta$)	Dissociation Constant $K_B(0)$ (mM)
methylguanidine (5)	internal	0.59 ± 0.04	15 ± 1.3
butylguanidine (4)	internal	0.53 ± 0.01	3.1 ± 0.16
TMA (4)	internal	0.48 ± 0.08	370 ± 30
QX-222 (9)	internal	0.34 ± 0.04	14 ± 1
QX-314 (5)	internal	0.36 ± 0.03	5.8 ± 1.5
procaine (3)	internal	0.38 ± 0.02	26 ± 4
Ca^{2+} (4)	internal	0.15 ± 0.02	54–110[a]
Co^{2+} (4)	internal	0.15 ± 0.03	14–33[a]
methylguanidine (5)	external	—	83 (at $-$V)[b]
Ca^{2+} (4)	external	-0.40 ± 0.02	30 ± 3.2[c]
Co^{2+} (3)	external	-0.50 ± 0.06	10–15 mM[a]

Current-voltage data at various blocker concentrations in experiments similar to those of FIGURES 9–13 were analyzed according to equation 1. Best fit values of $z\delta$ and $K_B(0)$ were found by linear regression. The values given are the mean and standard deviation from *n* experiments.

[a]For internal Ca^{2+} and Co^{2+} and external Co^{2+}, the range of lowest-highest $K_B(0)$ is given, because the apparent $K_B(0)$ appears to increase with increasing blocker concentration for these cations.

[b]Block by external methyl guanidine does not appear to be voltage dependent as discussed in the text.

[c]For external Ca^{2+}, $K_B(0)$ is given in activity rather than concentration as discussed in the text.

requirements of the preceding blocking model are not satisfied. Though MG titrations at a constant voltage appear to follow a single site titration (*e.g.*, FIG. 10B), the apparent binding constant cannot be fit to a simple exponential function of voltage. It rather appears that a low affinity-dissociation constant ($K_B = 1.04$ M) is exhibited at

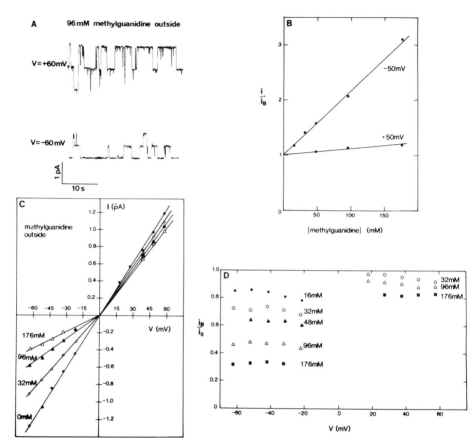

FIGURE 10. Fast block by methylguanidine on the external side of Na channels in planar bilayers. (**A**) Current records from a bilayer containing two channels oriented in the same direction in 0.2 M symmetrical NaCl plus 20 nM decarbamoylsaxitoxin and 96 mM methylguanidine on the external side. Channel opening is in the upward direction. (**B**) The ratio of single channel current in the absence of blocker to that in the presence of blocker, i_0/i_B, is plotted as a function of external methylguanidine concentration at -50 and $+50$ mV. (**C**) Single channel current-voltage data is plotted in the presence of 200 mM symmetrical NaCl ($\bullet$, g = 20.4 pS) and after the addition of 32 mM (O), 96 mM (▲), or 176 mM (△) methylguanidine sulfate to the external side. *Solid lines* through the data in the presence of methylguanidine are drawn by eye and are not meant to hold theoretical significance. (**D**) The ratio, i_B/i_0, is plotted as a function of voltage and the indicated concentrations of external methylguanidine.

all positive voltages tested ($+20$ to $+60$ mV) and a higher affinity dissociation constant ($K_B = 0.083$ M) is exhibited at all negative voltages tested (-20 to -60 mV). This behavior is illustrated by the constant slopes at positive and negative voltages in FIGURE 10C and by the replots of i_B/i_0 in FIGURE 10D at different MG concentrations.

To our knowledge, such behavior has not yet been described for blocking of any other ion channel, although certain diaminoalkanes appear to exhibit similar behavior with the sarcoplasmic reticulum K channel (Chris Miller, personal communication).

The behavior described in FIGURE 10 implies that the MG^+ cation cannot bind within the transmembrane electric field because the fraction of blocked current is essentially constant from -20 to -60 mV and from $+20$ to $+60$ mV (FIG. 10D). It appears that the apparent affinity for the blocker changes by a factor of ~12 as the direction of current shifts at 0 mV. If blocking by MG^+ strictly depends only on the direction of current through the channel, it should be possible to demonstrate a dependence of blocking action on the reversal potential. At present, we have not yet performed these experiments.

Although further theoretical and experimental work is needed to model block by external MG, it seems apparent that the external aspect of the open Na channel does not permit the entry of organic cations into the deepest portion of the permeation path. Hille's studies of permeant cations in the Na channel have previously defined the dimensions of the channel's narrowest region as a 3×5 Å^2 cross-sectional area.[55,56] Hille also proposed that molecules containing a single methyl group are impermeant because this substituent is too large to cross this region. Because methylguanidine seems to be unable to enter the electric field from the external side, it is possible that there is a constriction of the channel's outer mouth that lies outside the field. This may be the narrow region identified in Hille's permeation studies. This site could be considered as simply a "sieving site" that selects molecules on the basis of size. In addition to this outer sieve region, much evidence supports the existence of selectivity sites that do reside within the field and discriminate between small inorganic cations, as depicted in recent permeation models for the Na channel.[57,58] The finding of a voltage-dependent internal block and a voltage-independent external block by organic cations suggest a structural theme that also appears to be shared by certain K channels.[59,60]

Since organic cations do not appear to enter the electric field from the outside of the channel, it was of interest to examine the blocking modes of inorganic cations such as Ca^{2+}, because such small ions can sometimes be used to define blocking sites not accessible to larger molecules. The blocking behavior of external and internal Ca^{2+} on the batrachotoxin-activated Na channel from rat muscle is presented in FIGURES 11–13. In these experiments we found that equation 1 provides a good description of the reduction in single channel current at a fixed Ca^{2+} concentration; however, deviations from pure single-site behavior were found when the dependence on Ca^{2+} concentrations was examined. For example, the data in FIGURES 12B and 13B show reasonable fits to equation 1 using $z\delta = -0.40$ for external Ca^{2+} (FIG. 10B) and $z\delta = 0.15$ for internal Ca^{2+}. Similar $z\delta$ values were also obtained for Co^{2+}, another divalent inorganic cation, as listed in TABLE 2.

When plots of i_0/i_B were constructed as a function of $CaCl_2$ concentration, severe downward curvature was observed with increasing concentration. Such behavior could have several explanations, the simplest of which could be a simple deviation from solution ideality at high $CaCl_2$ concentrations (100 mM) such as are necessary in this experiment. In an attempt to correct for nonideal behavior, we plotted i_0/i_B as a function of Ca^{2+} activity, as calculated using published values for the mean activity of $CaCl_2$ solutions in this range.[61,62] This manipulation resulted in fairly linear i_0/i_B behavior for block by external Ca^{2+} but not for internal Ca^{2+} (see inserts of FIGS. 12A and 13A). The simple Woodhull model can thus adequately account for our results on external Ca^{2+} block by use of an activity scale for Ca^{2+}, but only accounts for internal Ca^{2+} block in the low concentration limit.

One reasonable explanation for this deviation is a surface charge effect caused by Ca^{2+} adsorption to the surface of the membrane, or the channel, which sets up an electrostatic potential that repels Ca^{2+} entry to the blocking site(s). Such behavior could also result from repulsion among multiple sites of Ca^{2+} blocking that causes lower binding affinity for the second ion. We have not attempted to distinguish these possibilities. Regardless of this problem, it is interesting that external Ca^{2+} exhibits about a threefold greater voltage dependence than internal Ca^{2+}, which is practically the converse of the situation that was observed for organic cations. This may support the view that the lining of the internal mouth of the channel is fairly hydrophobic in its deepest regions or is otherwise unsuitable for stable binding of hydrated inorganic cations.

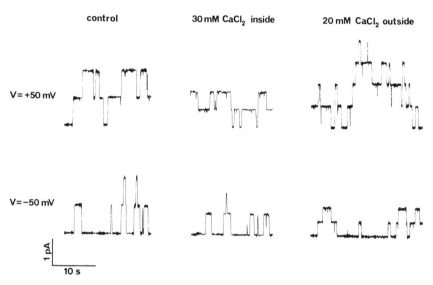

FIGURE 11. Effect of internal and external Ca^{2+} on batrachotoxin-activated Na channels. Current records from three different bilayers are compared at +50 mV (*top records*) and at −50 mV (*bottom records*). The control records on the left side were taken in the presence of 0.2 M symmetrical NaCl and 20 nM external decarbamoylsaxitoxin to induce discrete closing events. The middle pair of records is from a different bilayer in which 30 mM internal $CaCl_2$ was present, and the right pair of records is from a bilayer in which 20 mM external $CaCl_2$ was present. Channel opening is in the upward direction. In each experiment, all channels in the bilayer were oriented in the same direction.

SUMMARY AND CONCLUSIONS

Our results support the existence of three different Na-channel subtypes or isochannels. These isochannels can be readily distinguished as the predominant Na-channel types in mammalian brain, skeletal muscle, and cardiac muscle. The sensitivity to μ-conotoxin GIIIA and tetrodotoxin is sufficient to classify these channels. The skeletal muscle channel is very sensitive to both tetrodotoxin and μ-conotoxin, the brain channel is sensitive to tetrodotoxin but insensitive to μ-conotoxin, and the heart and denervated muscle channels are insensitive to both toxins.

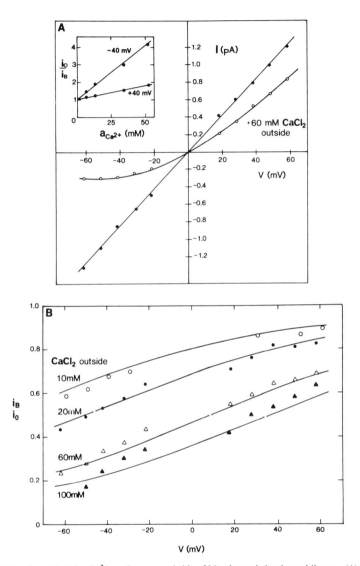

FIGURE 12. Fast block by Ca^{2+} on the external side of Na channels in planar bilayers. (**A**) Single channel current-voltage data is plotted in the presence of 200 mM symmetrical NaCl ($\bullet$, $g = 20.6$ pS) and after the addition of 60 mM $CaCl_2$ (O) to the external side. The *inset* shows the ratio, i_0/i_B, at $+40$ and -40 mV plotted as a function of Ca^{2+} activity. (**B**) The ratio of single channel current in the presence of external Ca^{2+}, i_B, to that in the absence of Ca^{2+}, i_0, is plotted at the indicated voltages and external $CaCl_2$ concentrations. The *solid lines* are fits of the data to equation **1** with best fit parameters given in TABLE 2.

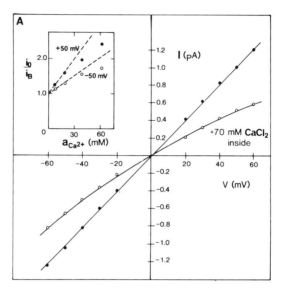

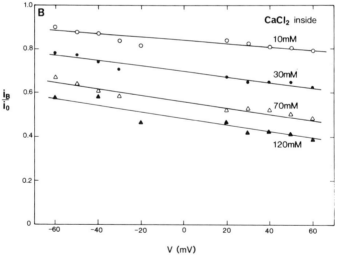

FIGURE 13. Fast block by Ca^{2+} on the internal side of Na channels in planar bilayers. (**A**) Single channel current-voltage data is plotted in the presence of 200 mM symmetrical NaCl ($\bullet$, $g = 20.6$ pS) and after the addition of 70 mM $CaCl_2$ (O) to the internal side. The inset shows the ratio i_0/i_B, at $+50$ and -50 mV plotted as a function of Ca^{2+} activity. (**B**) The ratio of single channel current in the presence of internal Ca^{2+}, i_B, to that in the absence of Ca^{2+}, i_0, is plotted at the indicated voltages and internal $CaCl_2$ concentrations. The *solid lines* are fits of the data to equation **1** using $z\delta = 0.15$ and $K_B(0) = 54$, 70, 89, and 113 mM at 10, 30, 70, and 120 mM external $CaCl_2$, respectively.

In addition to block at the external receptor site for guanidinium toxins, several other blocking modes can be generalized for batrachotoxin-activated Na channels. One mode is peculiar to certain hydrophobic molecules so far represented by our studies of benzocaine and procaine. These molecules induce discrete blocking events with dwell times that apparently increase with anesthetic concentration and a blocking frequency that increases with negative voltage. This mode is quite distinct from the fast internal block by charged organic molecules that increases with positive voltage. These results imply that it is not possible to ascribe the diverse effects of local anesthetics to a single site in the interior channel mouth, as previously proposed by Hille.[31] Our observations thus support the conclusions of other workers who used mixtures of two local anesthetics to show that the dose-response behavior does not fit single-site behavior, but requires at least two distinct sites.[63,64] Two additional blocking modes can be distinguished for the interactions of cations at the internal and external mouths of the channel. Organic molecules can apparently enter the electric field from the internal but not the external side of the channel. This result suggests a wide internal entryway to the field and an external constriction that prevents the entry of molecules with a single methyl group but permits entry of divalent inorganic cations such as Ca^{2+} and Co^{2+}.

REFERENCES

1. CAMPBELL, D. T. & B. HILLE. 1976. J. Gen. Physiol. **67:** 309–323.
2. PAPPONE, P. A. 1980. J. Physiol. **306:** 377–410.
3. BAER, M., P. M. BEST & H. REUTER. 1976. Nature **263:** 344–345.
4. COHEN, C. J., B. P. BEAN, T. J. COLATSKY & R. W. TSIEN. 1981. J. Gen. Physiol. **78:** 383–411.
5. BROWN, A. M., K. S. LEE & T. POWELL. 1981. J. Physiol. **318:** 479–500.
6. REDFERN, P. & S. THESLEFF. 1977. Acta Physiol. Scand. **82:** 70–78.
7. HARRIS, J. B. & S. THESLEFF. 1971. Acta Physiol. Scand. **83:** 382–388.
8. GONOI, T., S. J. SHERMAN & W. A. CATTERALL. 1985. J. Neurosci. **5:** 2559–2564.
9. CATTERALL, W. A. & J. COPPERSMITH. 1981. Molec. Pharmacol. **20:** 526–532.
10. CATTERALL, W. A. & J. COPPERSMITH. 1981. Molec. Pharmacol. **20:** 533–542.
11. FRELIN, C., P. VIGNE & M. LAZDUNSKI. 1983. J. Biol. Chem. **258:** 7256–7259.
12. FRELIN, C., P. VIGNE, H. SCHWEITZ & M. LAZDUNSKI. 1984. Mol. Pharmacol. **26:** 70–74.
13. FRELIN, C., H. P. M. VIJVERBERG, G. ROMEY, P. VIGNE & M. LAZDUNSKI. 1984. Pfluegers Arch. **402:** 121–128.
14. LAWRENCE, J. C. & W. A. CATTERALL. 1981. J. Biol. Chem. **256:** 6213–6222.
15. LAWRENCE, J. C. & W. A. CATTERALL. 1981. J. Biol. Chem. **256:** 6223–6229.
16. LOMBET, A., C. FRELIN, J. F. RENAUD & M. LAZDUNSKI. 1982. Eur. J. Biochem. **124:** 199–203.
17. RENAUD, J. F., T. KAZAZOGLOU, A. LOMBET, R. CHICHEPORTICHE, E. JAIMOVICH, G. ROMEY & M. LAZDUNSKI. 1983. J. Biol. Chem. **258:** 8799–8805.
18. ROGART, R. B. & L. J. REGAN. 1985. Brain Res. **329:** 314–318.
19. ROGART, R. B., L. J. REGAN, L. C. DZIEKAN & J. B. GALPER. 1983. Proc. Natl. Acad. Sci. **80:** 1106–1110.
20. SHERMAN, S. J., J. C. LAWRENCE, D. J. MESSNER, K. JACOBY & W. A. CATTERALL. 1983. J. Biol. Chem. **258:** 2488–2495.
21. TANAKA, J. C., D. D. DOYLE & L. BARR. 1984. Biochim. Biophys. Acta **775:** 203–214.
22. WOODHULL, A. M. 1973. J. Gen. Physiol. **61:** 687–708.
23. BEGENISICH, T. & M. DANKO. 1983. J. Gen. Physiol. **82:** 599–618.
24. MOZHAYEVA, G. N., A. P. NAUMOV & Y. A. NEGULYAEV. 1981. Biochim. Biophys. Acta **643:** 251–255.
25. YAMAMOTO, D., J. Z. YEH & T. NARAHASHI. 1984. Biophys. J. **45:** 337–344.
26. STRICHARTZ, G. R. 1973. J. Gen. Physiol. **62:** 37–57.

27. CAHALAN, M. D. & W. ALMERS. 1979. Biophys. J. 27: 39–59.
28. HORN, R., J. PATLAK & C. F. STEVENS. 1981. Biophys. J. 36: 321–327.
29. OXFORD, G. S. & J. Z. YEH. 1985. J. Gen. Physiol. 85: 583–602.
30. COURTNEY, K. R. 1975. J. Pharmacol. Exp. Ther. 195: 225–236.
31. HILLE, B. 1977. J. Gen. Physiol. 69: 497–515.
32. KRUEGER, B. K., J. F. WORLEY & R. J. FRENCH. 1983. Nature 303: 172–175.
33. MOCZYDLOWSKI, E., S. S. GARBER & C. MILLER. 1984. J. Gen. Physiol. 84: 665–686.
34. MOCZYDLOWSKI, E., S. HALL, S. S. GARBER, G. R. STRICHARTZ & C. MILLER. 1984. J. Gen. Physiol. 84: 687–704.
35. GRAY, W. R., A. LUQUE, B. M. OLIVERA, J. BARRET & L. J. CRUZ. 1981. J. Biol. Chem. 256: 4734–4740.
36. OLIVERA, B. M., J. M. MCINTOSH, L. J. CRUZ, F. A. LUQUE & W. R. GRAY. 1984. Biochemistry 23: 5087–5090.
37. CRUZ, L. J., W. R. GRAY, B. M. OLIVERA, R. D. ZEIKUS, L. KERR, D. YOSHIKAMI & E. MOCZYDLOWSKI. 1985. J. Biol. Chem. 260: 9280–9288.
38. SATO, S., H. NAKAMURA, Y. OHIZUMI, J. KOBAYASHI & Y. HIRATA. 1983. FEBS Lett. 155: 277–280.
39. HILLE, B. & D. T. CAMPBELL. 1976. J. Gen. Physiol. 67: 265–293.
40. MUELLER, P. & D. O. RUDIN. 1968. Bimolecular lipid membranes: Techniques of formation, study of electrical properties and induction of ionic gating phenomena. In Laboratory Techniques in Membrane Biophysics. H. Passow & R. Stampfli, Eds.: 141–156. Springer-Verlag. Berlin.
41. GREEN, W. N., L. B. WEISS & O. S. ANDERSON. 1984. Ann. N. Y. Acad. Sci. 435: 548–550.
42. MOCZYDLOWSKI, E. G. 1986. Biophys. J. 47: 190a.
43. MOCZYDLOWSKI, E. G. & R. LATORRE. 1983. Biochim. Biophys. Acta 732: 412–420.
44. MOCZYDLOWSKI, E. Unpublished results.
45. BARCHI, R. L. & J. B. WEIGELE. 1979. J. Physiol. 295: 383–396.
46. HANSEN-BAY, C. M. & G. R. STRICHARTZ. 1980. J. Physiol. 300: 89–103.
47. JONES, L. R., H. R. BESCH, J. W. FLEMING, M. M. MCCONNAUGHEY & A. M. WATANABE. 1979. J. Biol. Chem. 254: 530–539.
48. FRENCH, R. J., J. F. WORLEY, III & B. K. KRUEGER. 1984. Biophys. J. 45: 301–310.
49. GUO, X., S. H. BRYANT & E. G. MOCZYDLOWSKI. 1986. Biophys. J. 49: 380a.
50. NODA, M., S. SHIMIZU, T. TANABE, T. TAKAI, T. KAYANO, T. IKEDA, H. TAKAHASHI, H. NAKAYAMA, Y. KANAOKA, N. MINAMINO, K. KANGAWA, H. MATSUO, M. A. RAFTERY, T. HIROSE, S. INAYAMA, H. HAYASHIDA, T. MAYATA & S. NUMA. 1984. Nature 312: 121–127.
51. UEHARA, A. & E. MOCZYDLOWSKI. 1986. Membr. Biochem. 6: 111–147.
52. MOCZYDLOWSKI, E., A. UEHARA & S. HALL. 1986. Blocking pharmacology of batrachotoxin-activated Na-channels from rat skeletal muscle. In Reconstitution of Ion Channel Proteins. C. Miller, Ed.: 405–428. Plenum. New York.
53. HILLE, B. 1977. J. Gen. Physiol. 69: 475–496.
54. POSTMA, S. W. & W. A. CATTERALL. 1984. Molec. Pharmacol. 25: 219–227.
55. HILLE, B. 1971. J. Gen. Physiol. 58: 599–619.
56. HILLE, B. 1984. Ionic Channels of Excitable Membranes. Sinauer Associates. Sunderland, Mass.
57. HILLE, B. 1975. J. Gen. Physiol. 66: 535–560.
58. BEGENISICH, T. B. & M. D. CAHALAN. 1980. J. Physiol. 307: 217–242.
59. FRENCH, R. J. & J. J. SHOUKIMAS. 1985. J. Gen. Physiol. 85: 669–698.
60. VERGARA, C., E. MOCZYDLOWSKI & R. LATORRE. 1984. Biophys. J. 45: 73–76.
61. ROBINSON, R. A. & R. H. STOKES. 1959. Electrolyte Solutions. 2d ed. Academic. New York.
62. ATKINS, P. W. 1978. Physical Chemistry. W. H. Freeman. San Francisco.
63. MROSE, H. E. & J. M. RITCHIE. 1978. J. Gen. Physiol. 71: 223–225.
64. HUANG, L. M. & G. EHRENSTEIN. 1981. J. Gen. Physiol. 77: 137–153.

Functional Reconstitution of Purified Sodium Channels from Brain in Planar Lipid Bilayers[a]

ROBERT P. HARTSHORNE,[b,g] BERNARD U. KELLER,[b,c]
JANE A. TALVENHEIMO,[d,e] WILLIAM A. CATTERALL,[d]
AND MAURICIO MONTAL[b,f]

[b]Departments of Biology and Physics
University of California at San Diego
La Jolla, California 92093

[d]Department of Pharmacology
University of Washington
Seattle, Washington 98195

INTRODUCTION

The purified sodium channel from rat brain consists of three subunits: α, $\beta 1$, and $\beta 2$[1-3] (see Catterall *et al.*, this volume). It was followed through the purification process by its ability to bind ^{3}H-saxitoxin. Because the only functional properties of sodium channels that can be measured in detergent solution are the binding of saxitoxin, tetrodotoxin, and *Tityus* γ toxin,[4,5] it is necessary to reconstitute the purified protein into a lipid bilayer membrane and characterize its functional properties to establish that the entire sodium channel protein has been purified and to determine if it is functionally intact. The first stage of this process is reconstitution of purified sodium channels into proteoliposomes. In this system the competency of the purified sodium channels is assayed by the measurement of ^{22}Na$^+$ flux that has been stimulated by the sodium channel activating neurotoxins veratridine and batrachotoxin. It has been shown by using this approach that reconstituted sodium channels contain a functional sodium selective ion conduction pathway that can be opened by veratridine and batrachotoxin and blocked by saxitoxin and tetrodotoxin.[6-10] The concentration dependence of the effects of these toxins is very similar with reconstituted and native sodium channels. It has additionally been shown with purified reconstituted sodium channels from rat brain that there is a functional ion channel associated with at least 30% to 70% of the saxitoxin binding sites.[7]

[a]This research was supported by grants from the National Institutes of Health (EY-02084) and the Department of Army Medical Research (17–82–C-2221). RPH was a postdoctoral fellow of the National Multiple Sclerosis Society.
[c]Present address: Max Plank Institut für Biophysikalische Chemie, Göttingen, West Germany.
[e]Present address: Department of Pharmacology, University of Miami School of Medicine, Miami, Fla. 33101.
[f]Present address: Department of Neurosciences, Roche Institute of Molecular Biology, Nutley, N.J. 07110.
[g]Present address: Department of Pharmacology, Oregon Health Sciences University, Portland, Oreg. 97201.

293

Although $^{22}Na^+$ flux measurements in proteoliposomes demonstrate that many of the functional moieties of the sodium channel have survived the purification intact, this assay lacks the voltage control and time resolution needed to do the detailed analysis of the voltage dependence and kinetic and conductance properties of the purified sodium channel necessary to establish its functional integrity. Electrical measurement of these properties under voltage clamp conditions that allow direct comparison with electrophysiological data on native sodium channels is the best way to determine these parameters.[11,12] We have performed such experiments with purified sodium channels that have been incorporated into planar lipid bilayers by fusing sodium channel containing proteoliposomes with preformed bilayers.[11,13] The results of these experiments indicate that the α, $\beta 1$, and the $\beta 2$ subunits of the purified protein are sufficient to account for the entire structure of the rat brain sodium channel.

MATERIALS AND METHODS

Purification and Reconstitution into Proteoliposomes

Sodium channels were purified from rat brain to a specific activity of 2000–2900 pmol of ^{3}H-saxitoxin binding sites per milligram of protein as described by Hartshorne and Catterall.[2] To each milliliter of purified sodium channels 0.2 ml of a solution of 10% Triton X-100, 1.19% bovine brain phosphatidylcholine (Sigma), and 0.74% bovine brain phosphatidylethanolamine (Sigma) were added and the detergent was removed by adsorption on porous polystyrene beads (0.25–0.4 ml of BioBeads SM-2 per ml of reconstitution mixture) to form proteoliposomes.[6,7,14] The resulting proteoliposomes are composed of 2 mg/ml phosphatidylcholine, 1.05 mg/ml phosphatidylethanolamine, and 5–15 pmol/ml saxitoxin receptor in 50 mM NaCl, 10 mM Hepes/Tris pH 7.4, 0.5 mM $MgSO_4$, and ~400 mM sucrose.

Experimental Setup

A 25 μ thick Teflon sheet containing an aperture 40-220 μ in diameter is mounted with silicone grease over a hole in a partition separating two 450 μl chambers, labeled cis and trans, that have been milled from a block of teflon. The teflon block rests on a platform above a battery-powered magnetic stirrer that is enclosed in a Faraday cage on a vibration-free table. The cis chamber contains 1–5 μl of proteoliposomes and 0.5 M NaCl in medium A (10 mM Hepes/Na^+ pH 7.4, 0.15 mM $CaCl_2$, 0.1 mM $MgCl_2$, and 0.05 mM EGTA). The trans chamber initially contains 0.2–0.4 M NaCl in medium A plus 1 μM batrachotoxin. The chambers are connected by Ag/AgCl pellet electrodes (In Vivo Metric Systems, Healdsburg, Ca.) to a List Medical Electronics EPC-7 patch clamp amplifier in voltage clamp mode. The trans electrode is set to the command voltage relative to the cis electrode which is held at ground. The EPC-7 output is filtered at 3 kHz, monitored on an oscilloscope and recorded on a RACAL 4DS FM tape recorder. All experiments are performed at 21°C ± 2°C.

Bilayer Formation

We have used two different lipid mixtures to form bilayers: a solution of 40 mg/ml 1-palmitoyl-2-oleoyl phosphatidylethanolamine (POPE) with 10 mg/ml 1-palmitoyl-

2-oleoyl phosphatidylcholine (POPC, Avanti Polar Lipids) in *n*-decane (Sigma), as suggested by Weiss,[15] and nonoxidizable lipid, diphytanoylphosphatidylcholine (Avanti Polar Lipids), in a 50 mg/ml solution in *n*-decane.[16] In order to form stable bilayers the area of Teflon around the aperture is first thoroughly cleaned in hexane, then precoated on both sides with a thin film of 5% lipid in *n*-decane and dried for 3–5 minutes under a gentle stream of nitrogen. After the chambers are filled with their aqueous solutions, a small amount of the 5% lipid solution is spread across the cis side of the aperture of a no. 2 brush from which most of the bristles have been removed. Voltage steps 0.1–1 mV in amplitude and of 5 ms duration are applied to monitor bilayer formation by capacitance change.[17] A clean brush is then used to wipe away the excess lipid solution repeatedly until a large increase in capacitance signals bilayer formation. The specific capacitance of the bilayer and torus is 0.25–0.35 $\mu F/cm^2$. Bilayers made from either of the lipid solutions typically have high resistances (>300 $G\Omega$), are electrically stable between -150 mV and $+150$ mV, and can last several hours.

Channel Incorporation into Lipid Bilayers

Purified sodium channels are incorporated into the planar lipid bilayer by fusing proteoliposomes with it in a process that requires an osmotic gradient across the bilayer (cis osmolarity > trans osmolarity).[18–21] Following bilayer formation, proteoliposomes are added to the cis chamber and the solutions in the cis and trans chambers are gently stirred for three minutes while maintaining an applied voltage (V) of 70 mV across the bilayer. The current through the bilayer is then examined at $V = 70$ mV and -70 mV to determine if any channels have been incorporated. If not, the bilayer capacitance is rechecked and the stirring step repeated until one or more channels are seen.[11] Channel incorporation is stopped by eliminating the osmotic gradient across the bilayer with the addition of 4 M NaCl to the trans chamber to yield a final concentration of 0.5 M.

Voltage Convention

Because sodium channels are oriented randomly in the proteoliposomes,[7] their orientation in the bilayer is also random. When comparing a voltage-dependent property of channels oriented in opposite directions, this could cause confusion. In order to avoid this ambiguity, the voltage sensed by the channel is defined according to the electrophysiological convention ($V = V_{\text{"intracellular" side}} - V_{\text{"extracelluar" side}}$). The "extracellular" side of a sodium channel can be readily determined by the sidedness of tetrodotoxin block at the end of an experiment.[22] Alternatively, the polarity of the applied voltage sensed as a hyperpolarization that closes a channel will also indicate its orientation. When both methods have been employed to determine the orientation of a channel the results have always agreed ($n = 25$).

RESULTS AND DISCUSSION

Tetrodotoxin Sensitivity

The most specific test of whether an ion channel in a planar lipid bilayer is a sodium channel is its susceptibility to block by tetrodotoxin or saxitoxin. FIGURE 1 demonstrates that the ionic current through purified sodium channels is reversibly blocked by

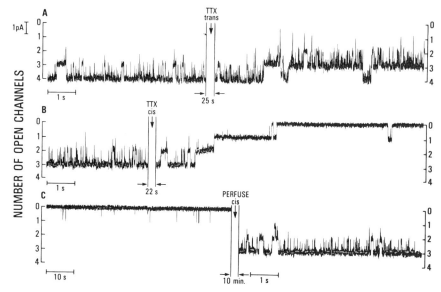

FIGURE 1. TTX block of reconstituted sodium channels in planar lipid bilayers. This bilayer contained one trans-facing and three cis-facing sodium channels in symmetric 0.5 M NaCl medium A with 1 μM BTX trans. The applied voltage was -50 mV for the cis-facing channels and $+50$ mV for the trans-facing channel. The current records were low-pass filtered at 500 Hz. **(A)** Orientation dependence of TTX block. The initial current record shows four open channels interrupted by occasional brief closures. At the *arrow*, 40 μM TTX (final concentration) was added to the trans chamber. The 25-s delay between the addition of TTX and channel block was the result of slow mixing of TTX with the solution. This was intentionally done to allow the channel blocking to be recorded. **(B)** Continuation of current record in A three minutes later following complete mixing of the trans chamber. Addition of 2 μM TTX to the cis chamber blocks the remaining channels. **(C)** Reversibility of TTX block. With TTX on both sides, all channels remain blocked with occasional brief openings. Upon removal of TTX from the cis chamber by perfusion (exchange of 14 volumes with stirring), the membrane current from the three cis-facing channels returns to the pre-TTX value, whereas the one trans-facing channel remains blocked.

tetrodotoxin in an orientation-dependent manner.[11] The bilayer in FIGURE 1 contains four active channels. Prior examination of the polarity of the voltage that closes the channels by hyperpolarization indicated that there are three cis-facing channels and one trans-facing channel. Following addition of tetrodotoxin to the trans chamber in FIGURE 1A, the one trans-facing sodium channel is blocked and remains blocked for the rest of the experiment whereas the three cis-facing channels are unaffected. Addition of tetrodotoxin to the cis side of the bilayer in FIGURE 1B reduces the current in three discrete steps to the value it had prior to channel incorporation as the three cis-facing channels are blocked. The initial segment of FIGURE 1C, on a tenfold slower time scale, shows that the channels remain blocked as long as tetrodotoxin is present. Following perfusion of the cis chamber to remove tetrodotoxin, the three cis-facing channels reappear, demonstrating that tetrodotoxin block is reversible. The tetrodotoxin sensitivity of these single-channel events is unequivocal evidence that they are mediated by the sodium channel protein.

Tetrodotoxin Block Is Voltage Dependent

The concentration and voltage dependence of tetrodotoxin block of purified batrachotoxin-activated sodium channels are shown in FIGURE 2. The concentration dependence of block is well described by a simple one-to-one binding curve at both voltages. At -50 mV the K_i for tetrodotoxin block is 8.3 nM, at 70 mV the K_i is 135 nM.[11] The voltage dependence of this shift in K_i corresponds to an *e*-fold increase in K_i for each 43 mV depolarization. These values are in close agreement with the K_i of tetrodotoxin block of 7–16 nM at -50 mV and its voltage dependence of 35–41 mV/*e*-fold change in K_i found with rat brain synaptosomal sodium channels incorporated into planar bilayers by French *et al.*[23]

Channel Opening Is Voltage Dependent

One of the major objectives of this research is to determine if purified sodium channels retain a voltage-sensing mechanism. This was examined by measuring the voltage dependence of channel opening in the presence of batrachotoxin. Batracho-toxin should shift the voltage dependence of sodium channel activation in the

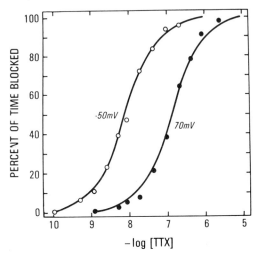

FIGURE 2. The concentration dependence of tetrodotoxin block of purified sodium channels at -50 mV (O) and 70 mV (●). Current records from a bilayer containing four cis-facing sodium channels in symmetric 0.5 M NaCl medium A were examined to determine the percentage of time the channels are blocked as a function of tetrodotoxin concentration in the cis chamber. In the absence of tetrodotoxin at these voltage closures longer than 1 s are rare ($\tau_c < 30$ ms). Hence only closures lasting longer than 1 s are attributed to tetrodotoxin block. In order to insure that representative samples of data were examined, 45 min current records were analyzed for each tetrodotoxin concentration less than 4 nM, 30 min current records were analyzed for tetrodotoxin concentrations between 4 and 20 nM, and 10 min current records were analyzed for all other tetrodotoxin concentrations. The smooth curves are the theoretical curves for one-to-one block by tetrodotoxin given by plotting $100[\text{TTX}]/K_i + [\text{TTX}]$ vs. log [TTX] for $K_i = 8.3$ nM at -50 mV and $K_i = 135$ nM at 70 mV.

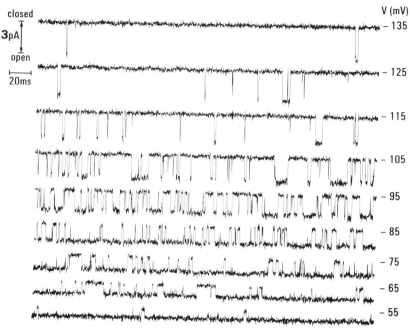

FIGURE 3. Single sodium channel current records. A trans-facing sodium channel was incorporated into a diphytanoyl phosphatidylcholine bilayer in a 70-μm aperture bathed by 0.5 M NaCl medium A cis and 0.2 M NaCl medium A plus 1 μM BTX trans. Representative current records, low-pass filtered at 1 kHz, are shown for the voltages indicated.

hyperpolarized direction and eliminate inactivation.[24-26] FIGURE 3 shows the single channel current through a batrachotoxin-modified sodium channel at the indicated holding potentials. In the first current record at -135 mV the channel is closed nearly all of the time except for the few brief openings indicated by downward deflections. At more positive voltages the channel spends an increasing fraction of time open. The channel is open 50% of the time at -95 mV (V_{50}). At -55 mV and more positive voltages the channel is open most of the time with occasional closures. As expected for a batrachotoxin-modified sodium channel, it does not inactivate.

For purified sodium channels the average value of V_{50} is -92 mV $\pm$ 17 mV (SEM, $n = 22$).[11] This agrees well with the V_{50} of -93 mV for batrachotoxin-modified rat brain synaptosomal sodium channels in planar bilayers,[21] -94 mV for batrachotoxin-modified rat sarcolemmal sodium channels in planar bilayers,[27] and -85 mV for batrachotoxin-modified sodium channels in NG-108-15 neuroblastoma cells.[26] The V_{50} of purified sodium channels varies from channel to channel. For most of the 22 channels V_{50} is between -80 mV and -105 mV. The extreme values were -130 mV and -64 mV. The voltage dependence of channel opening obtained by integration of conductance histograms at each voltage[11] is shown in FIGURE 4 for three different channels selected because of their widely differing V_{50} values. Channel opening is steeply voltage dependent over a limited voltage range for each channel. The curves are parallel to each other and shifted along the voltage axis. This indicates that the variation of V_{50} is not due to channels incorporated into the bilayer in such a way that they sense only a fraction of the applied electric field. The variability of V_{50} is not caused by an uncompensated electrode offset potential because the reversal potential for the Na^+ current is always within a few millivolts of the calculated Nernst potential for Na^+. Lipid surface charge effects are an unlikely cause because these experiments are conducted with symmetric bilayers of uncharged lipids in solutions with symmetric ionic composition. Is the variability due to alteration of the channel protein during its purification? Probably not, because similar results have been obtained with batracho-toxin-modified sodium channels incorporated into planar bilayers from native membranes[15,27] and variations, although smaller ones, in the voltage dependence of opening of batrachotoxin-modified sodium channels in patch clamped neuroblastoma cells have also been observed.[28] Two possibilities for the variation in V_{50} that we cannot presently rule out are variations in bilayer thickness and a naturally occurring heterogeneity in the sodium channel population, perhaps arising from variations in fixed charge on or near the voltage-sensing mechanism.

Gating Charge

The apparent gating charge of purified sodium channels was determined by fitting the voltage dependence data to a Boltzmann function.[23] Despite large differences in V_{50}, there is little difference in the apparent gating charge from channel to channel. The average value is 3.8 ± 0.3 (SEM, $n = 5$). This value agrees well with the apparent gating charge determined for batrachotoxin-modified native sodium channels from rat brain (4–6),[23] NG-108-15 neuroblastoma cells (4–5),[26] and frog node of Ranvier (3.5).[25]

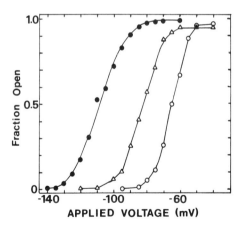

FIGURE 4. Voltage dependence of sodium channel opening. The fraction of time a channel was open was determined by integrating conductance histograms derived from 25 s of current record at each voltage. The voltage dependence for three different channels, selected because of their widely differing V_{50} values, are illustrated. The channels are in 80% 1-palmitoyl-2-oleoyl-phosphatidylethanolamine/20% 1-palmitoyl-2-oleoyl-phosphatidylcholine bilayers bathed in symmetric 0.5 M NaCl medium A plus 1 mM BTX trans.

Analysis of Channel Gating Kinetics

The opening and closing rates of purified sodium channels in the presence of 1 μM batrachotoxin were determined from closed and open dwell time histograms over the voltage ranges of -120 mV to -50 mV and 50 mV to 120 mV as described by Keller *et al.*[13] At a voltage of -80 mV or more negative, the closed dwell time distributions are well fit by single exponentials, indicating the presence of a single closed state, c_1. At

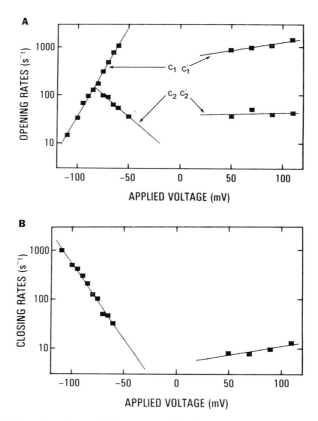

FIGURE 5. Voltage dependence of (**A**) opening and (**B**) closing rates. (**A**) Current records similar to those in FIGURE 4 lasting 30 to 60 s at each voltage were digitized and the opening rates at each applied voltage were determined by probability density analysis of the closed dwell time. In order to prevent noise from interfering with the determination of rapid channel transitions, only records for applied voltages $V < -50$ mV or $V > 50$ mV were analyzed. For applied voltages $V < -80$ mV the data were well fit by a single opening rate from c_1. For more positive applied voltages, the hypothesis of a single opening rate was rejected at a $p = 0.05$ significance level (chi-square-test). For all voltages more positive than -80 mV the data were well fit with two opening rates. For negative applied voltages both opening rates were found to be exponentially voltage dependent, whereas for positive applied voltages they were practically voltage independent. *Straight lines* were obtained by fitting different exponential functions to the four opening rates according to a least-square fit. (**B**) Closing rates were determined from probability density analysis of the open dwell time. For negative applied voltages the rate was exponentially voltage dependent, whereas for positive applied voltages the rate was almost voltage independent.

TABLE 1. Transition Rates and Their Voltage Dependence for the C-C-O Model of Native and Reconstituted Na$^+$ Channel

	Transition Rate (s^{-1})		Voltage Dependence (mV/*e*-fold Change)	
	Purified	Native	Purified	Native
α	477 ± 118 ($n = 5$)	73 ± 16 ($n = 4$)	13.5 ± 1	11 ± 1.5
β	63 ± 14 ($n = 5$)	96 ± 44 ($n = 5$)	−13.6 ± 1	−19 ± 1.6
γ	139 ± 44 ($n = 5$)	81 ± 10 ($n = 2$)	−20.2 ± 2.3	−25.8 ± 4.5
δ	40 ± 13 ($n = 5$)	4 ($n = 1$)	18.6 ± 3.5	9.5

Transition rates at −70 V and their voltage dependence for the C-C-O model of batrachotoxin-activated sodium channels are compared for purified rat brain sodium channels in planar bilayers and patch-clamped mouse neuroblastoma sodium channels (native) measured by Huang *et al.*[26]

voltages more positive than −80 mV, however, two exponential components are required to fit the closed dwell time distributions, indicating that an additional closed state, c_2, is also significantly populated in this voltage range. The mean closed dwell times in c_1 and c_2 are voltage dependent but in opposite direction. Depolarization decreases the mean dwell time in c_1 from 25 ms ± 6.2 (SEM, $n = 5$) at −100 mV to 1.8 ms ± 1.1 ($n = 5$) at −60 mV, whereas the mean dwell time in c_2 increases from 5.6 ms ± 2.6 ($n = 5$) at −75 mV to 12 ms ± 2.8 ($n = 5$) at −60 mV.[13] The opening rates from c_1 and c_2 (1/mean closed dwell times) are plotted semilogarithmically as a function of voltage in FIGURE 5a. These rates are exponentially voltage dependent in the negative voltage range with the opening rate from c_1 having a slope of 13.5 ± 0.9 mV/*e*-fold change, and the opening rate from c_2 having a slope of −20.2 ± 2.3 mV/*e*-fold change.

Over the positive voltage range the sum of two exponentials is also required to fit the closed dwell time histograms. The mean closed dwell times at 100 mV are 0.79 ± 0.9 ms ($n = 3$) for c'_1 and 27 ± 3.1 ms ($n = 3$) for c'_2. In contrast to the results in the negative voltage range, the corresponding opening rates in the positive voltage range shown in FIGURE 5 are essentially independent of voltage.

The open dwell time histograms are well fit by a single exponential over the entire voltage range investigated. This is consistent with there being a single open state. Depolarization prolongs the mean open dwell time from 1.4 ± 0.3 ms at −100 mV to 28 ± 4.5 ms at −60 mV. For the negative voltage range studied, the closing rate (1/mean open dwell time) is exponentially voltage dependent with a slope of 13.6 ± 0.6 mV/*e*-fold change as shown in FIGURE 5b. For the positive voltage range, the closing rate is only moderately voltage dependent with a slope of 71 ± 26 mV/*e*-fold change (FIGURE 5b).[13]

For negative applied voltages the data can be well fit by a linear kinetic scheme with two closed states, one open state, and exponentially voltage dependent rate constants:

$$c_2 \underset{\delta}{\overset{\gamma}{\rightleftharpoons}} c_1 \underset{\beta}{\overset{\alpha}{\rightleftharpoons}} o.$$

These results are in agreement with the kinetic scheme proposed for batrachotoxin-modified native sodium channels in patch-clamped mouse neuroblastoma cells by Huang *et al.*,[28] who examined the voltage range of −100 mV to −40 mV. The transition rate constants at −70 mV and their channel dependence for both purified rat brain sodium channels and mouse neuroblastoma sodium channels are given in TABLE

1 for comparison. The voltage dependence of the transition rates agrees quite well. However, the transition rates at -70 mV for leaving state c_1, α, and δ, are higher for the purified channel indicating that the energy barriers for leaving c_1 are lower. Although the values for these rate constants differ, the fact that the kinetics of purified rat brain sodium channels and native sodium channels in mouse neuroblastoma cells can be well described by the same C-C-O model is further evidence that the purified sodium channel is essentially intact.

The voltage-independent opening and closing rate constants seen in the positive voltage range could be due to the appearance of new voltage independent states of the sodium channel. At present, however, we favor a simpler alternative hypothesis. Rather than invoking three new states to account for this data, these rate constants can be attributed to the states of the sodium channel seen at negative voltages for which the voltage-dependent changes of the rate constants have saturated. More data will be required to resolve this question.

Batrachotoxin Is Required for Channel Incorporation

Sodium channel activity in the absence of batrachotoxin or veratridine has not yet been observed. Does this mean that channels that are nonfunctional in the absence of batrachotoxin are being incorporated into the bilayer, or, alternatively, is batracho-toxin required for channel incorporation into the bilayer under the conditions used? The following experiment favors the second possibility. Under conditions chosen to promote fusion (5 μl of proteoliposomes, a 0.5 M_{cis}–0.2 M_{trans} NaCl gradient and a diphytanoyl PC bilayer in a 220 μm aperture), we attempted to incorporate sodium channels into the bilayer using the procedure described in MATERIALS AND METHODS in the absence of batrachotoxin for 1 hour. At this time, to stop any further fusion, the osmotic gradient across the planar bilayer was eliminated by adding 4 M NaCl to the trans chamber to yield a final concentration of 0.5 M NaCl. In order to determine if any sodium channels had been incorporated during the one-hour incubation, batracho-toxin (1 μM final trans) was added and the current through the bilayer was monitored for 30 minutes. No sodium channels were observed, demonstrating that during the one-hour incubation in the absence of batrachotoxin no channels were incorporated into the bilayer. The osmotic gradient across the planar bilayer was then reestablished by diluting the contents of the trans chamber with distilled water to reduce the concentration of NaCl to 0.3 M. In each of four separate experiments batrachotoxin-activated sodium channels (1 to 3) were then seen within ten minutes. These results clearly indicate that batrachotoxin is required for proteoliposome fusion under these conditions. Whether batrachotoxin promotes fusion by increasing the osmotic gradient across the proteoliposome bilayer by increasing its sodium permeability, or by causing a hydrophobic surface on the sodium channel to become exposed is not known. We are currently examining other methods of promoting channel incorporation into the bilayer to allow us to study the voltage-dependent activation and inactivation of purified sodium channels in the absence of batrachotoxin.

Single Channel Conductance and Ionic Selectivity

The single channel current-voltage curves for Na$^+$, K$^+$, and Rb$^+$ in FIGURE 6 show that purified sodium channels are selectively permeable to Na$^+$. The average single channel conductance (γ) in 0.5 M solutions of these ions is $\gamma_{Na^+} = 25.2$ pS $\pm$ 0.5 pS (SEM, $n = 10$), $\gamma_{K^+} = 3.5$ pS $\pm$ 0.2 pS (SEM, $n = 3$), and $\gamma_{Rb^+} = 1.2$ pS $\pm$ 0.1 pS

(SEM, n = 3).[11] The single channel conductance for Na^+ of 25.2 pS is a little lower than the 30 pS found by Krueger *et al.*,[21] and slightly higher than the 24 pS found by Moczydlowski *et al.*[27] for native rat brain sodium channels incorporated into planar bilayers and activated by batrachotoxin. The permeability ratios of K^+ and Rb^+ relative to NA^+ are 0.14 ± 0.02 and 0.05 ± 0.01, respectively. These permeability ratios agree well with the permeability ratios directly measured from ion flux determinations with batrachotoxin-activated sodium channels in N18 neuroblastoma

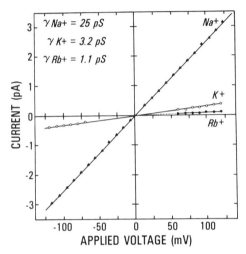

FIGURE 6. Current-voltage relationship of single sodium channels for Na^+, K^+, and Rb^+. The amplitude of single channel currents was determined in 0.5 M symmetric solutions of NaCl (△), KCl (○), and RbCl (●) in 10 mM Hepes/Tris pH 7.4, 0.15 mM $CaCl_2$, 0.1 mM $MgCl_2$, and 0.05 mM EGTA with 1 μM BTX trans. In order to accurately determine the small single channel current in RbCl accurately, 200 nM TTX was added to the cis chamber to produce long closed periods and the current records were low-pass filtered at 50 Hz to resolve the open and blocked channels from the noise. For this reason, only the positive branch of the curve for Rb^+ is shown. The continuous lines are the least-square fits to the data points. The slope of a line is the single channel conductance for the ion: γ_{Na^+} = 25 pS, γ_{K^+} = 3.2 pS, and γ_{Rb^+} = 1.1 pS in this experiment. The uncorrected zero-current potentials were 1.4 mV and 1.5 mV for Na^+ and K^+, respectively.

cells (P_{K^+} = 0.17 and P_{Rb^+} = 0.08),[29] and sodium channels purified from rat muscle (P_{K^+} = 0.14 and P_{Rb^+} = 0.02).[9] The agreement is not as good with the relative permeability of K^+ (0.07) determined from reversal potential measurements on batrachotoxin-activated rat brain sodium channels in planar bilayers. Because the relative permeability of ions through sodium channels calculated from reversal potential measurements varies with the ionic composition of the medium,[30] only a qualitative agreement is expected.

CONCLUSIONS

Studies on the properties of the purified sodium channel protein from rat brain reconstituted into proteoliposomes and planar lipid bilayers have demonstrated the existence of the following moieties that function in the same manner as in intact sodium channels: an ion-conducting pore, a sodium-selective ion selectivity filter, a voltage-sensing mechanism, a batrachotoxin-veratridine receptor, a gating mechanism that is appropriately connected to the voltage sensor and the batrachotoxin binding site, a Leiurus scorpion binding site,[31] and a receptor site for tetrodotoxin and saxitoxin. It is therefore probable that the α, $\beta1$, and $\beta2$ subunits are sufficient to account for the entire structure of the sodium channel from rat brain.

The initial goal of reconstitution, to establish whether all the functional elements of the sodium channel are in the purified protein, has nearly been achieved. The next objectives are to determine which subunits and domains of subunits are involved in opening and closing the channel, forming its structure, and governing its voltage regulation.

ACKNOWLEDGMENT

We are indebted to Dr. John W. Daly for generously providing the batrachotoxin used in these experiments.

REFERENCES

1. HARTSHORNE, R. P. & W. A. CATTERALL. 1981. Purification of the saxitoxin receptor of the sodium channel from rat brain. Proc. Natl. Acad. Sci. U.S.A. **78:** 4620–4624.
2. HARTSHORNE, R. P. & W. A. CATTERALL. 1984. The sodium channel from rat brain: Purification and subunit composition. J. Biol. Chem. **259:** 1667–1675.
3. HARTSHORNE, R. P., D. J. MESSNER, J. C. COPPERSMITH & W. A. CATTERALL. 1982. The saxitoxin receptor of the sodium channel from rat brain: Evidence for two nonidentical β subunits. J. Biol. Chem. **257:** 13888–13891.
4. CATTERALL, W. A., C. S. MORROW & R. P. HARTSHORNE. 1979. Neurotoxin binding to receptor sites associated with voltage-sensitive sodium channels in intact, lysed and detergent solubilized brain membranes. J. Biol. Chem. **254:** 11379–11387.
5. BARHANIN, J., D. PAURON, A. LOMBET, R. NORMAN, H. VIJVERBERG, J. R. GIGLIO & M. LAZDUNSKI. 1983. Electrophysiological characterization, solubilization and purification of the Tityus γ toxin receptor receptor associated with the gating component of the Na$^+$ channel from rat brain. EMBO J. **2:** 915–920.
6. TALVENHEIMO, J. A., M. M. TAMKUN & W. A. CATTERALL. 1982. Reconstitution of neurotoxin-stimulated sodium transport by the voltage-sensitive sodium channel purified from rat brain. J. Biol. Chem. **257:** 11868–11871.
7. TAMKUN, M. M., J. A. TALVENHEIMO & W. A. CATTERALL. 1984. The sodium channel from rat brain: Reconstitution of neurotoxin-activated ion flux and scorpion toxin binding from purified components. J. Biol. Chem. **259:** 1676–1688.
8. WEIGELE, J. B. & R. L. BARCHI. 1982. Functional reconstitution of the purified sodium channel protein from rat sarcolemma. Proc. Natl. Acad. Sci. U.S.A. **79:** 3651–3655.
9. TANAKA, J. C., J. F. ECCELSTON & R. L. BARCHI. 1983. Cation selectivity characteristics of the reconstituted voltage-dependent sodium channel purified rat skeletal muscle sarcolemma. J. Biol. Chem. **258:** 7519–7526.
10. ROSENBERG, R. L., S. A. TOMIKO & W. S. AGNEW. 1984. Reconstitution of neurotoxin-modulated ion transport by the voltage-regulated sodium channel isolated from the electroplax of *Electrophorus electricus*. Proc. Natl. Acad. Sci. U.S.A. **81:** 1239–1243.
11. HARTSHORNE, R. P., B. U. KELLER, J. A. TALVENHEIMO, W. A. CATTERALL & M. MONTAL. 1985. Functional reconstitution of the purified brain sodium channel in planar lipid bilayers. Proc. Natl. Acad. Sci. U.S.A. **82:** 240–244.
12. ROSENBERG, R. L., S. A. TOMIKO & W. S. AGNEW. 1984. Single channel properties of the reconstituted voltage-regulated Na$^+$ channel isolated from the electroplax of *Electrophorus electricus*. Proc. Natl. Acad. Sci. U.S.A. **81:** 5594–5598.
13. KELLER, B. U., R. P. HARTSHORNE, J. A. TALVENHEIMO, W. A. CATTERALL & M.

MONTAL. 1986. Sodium channels in planar lipid bilayers: Channel gating kinetics of purified sodium channels modified by batrachotoxin. J. Gen. Physiol. **88**: 1–23.

14. HOLLOWAY, P. W. 1973. A simple procedure for removal of Triton X-100 from protein samples. Anal. Biochem. **53**: 304–308.

15. WEISS, L. B., W. N. GREEN & O. S. ANDERSEN. 1984. Single channel studies on the gating of batrachotoxin modified sodium channels in lipid bilayers. Biophys. J. **45**: 67. Abstract.

16. REDWOOD, W. R., F. R. PFEIFFER, J. A. WEISBACH & T. E. THOMPSON. 1971. Physical properties of bilayer membranes formed from a synthetic saturated phospholipid in n-decane. Biochim. Biophys. Acta **233**: 1–6.

17. MUELLER, P. & D. O. RUDIN. 1969. Bimolecular lipid membranes: Techniques of formation, study of electrical properties and induction of gating phenomenon. *In* Laboratory Techniques of Membrane Biophysics. M. Passow & R. Stampfli, Eds.: 141–156. Springer-Verlag. Berlin.

18. MILLER, C. & E. RACKER. 1976. Ca^{2+} induced fusion of fragmented sarcoplasmic reticulum with artificial bilayers. J. Membr. Biol. **30**: 283–300.

19. COHEN, F. S., M. H. AKABAS & A. FINKELSTEIN. 1982. Osmotic swelling of phospholipid vesicles causes them to fuse with a planar phospholipid bilayer membrane. Science **217**: 458–460.

20. COHEN, F. S., M. H. AKABAS, J. ZIMMERBERG & A. FINKELSTEIN. 1984. Parameters affecting the fusion of unilamellar phospholipid vesicles with planar bilayer membranes. J. Cell Biol. **98**: 1054–1062.

21. KRUEGER, B. K., J. F. WORLEY & R. J. FRENCH. 1983. Single sodium channels from rat brain incorporated into planar lipid bilayer membranes. Nature **303**: 172–175.

22. NARAHASHI, T., N. C. ANDERSON & J. W. MOORE. 1966. Tetrodotoxin does not block excitation from inside the nerve membrane. Science **153**: 765–767.

23. FRENCH, R. J., J. F. WORLEY & B. K. KRUEGER. 1984. Voltage-dependent block by saxitoxin of sodium channels incorporated into planar lipid bilayers. Biophys. J. **45**: 301–310.

24. ALBUQUERQUE, E. X., J. W. DALY & B. WITKOP. 1971. Batrachotoxin: Chemistry and pharmacology. Science **172**: 995–1002.

25. KHODOROV, B. I. & S. V. REVENKO. 1979. Further analysis of the mechanisms of action of batrachotoxin of the membrane of myelinated nerve. Neuroscience **4**: 1315–1330.

26. HUANG, L. M., N. MORAN & G. EHRENSTEIN. 1982. Batrachotoxin modifies the gating kinetics of sodium channels in internally perfused neuroblastoma cells. Proc. Natl. Acad. Sci. U.S.A. **79**: 2082–2085.

27. MOCZYDLOWSKI, E., S. S. GARBER & C. MILLER. 1984. Batrachotoxin-activated Na^+ channels in planar lipid bilayers: Competition of tetrodotoxin block by Na^+. J. Gen. Physiol. **84**: 687–704.

28. HUANG, L. M., N. MORAN & G. EHRENSTEIN. 1984. Gating kinetics of batrachotoxin modified sodium channels in neuroblastoma cells determined from single channel measurements. Biophys. J. **45**: 313–322.

29. HUANG, L. M., W. A. CATTERALL & G. EHRENSTEIN. 1979. Comparison of ionic selectivity of batrachotoxin-activated channels with different tetrodotoxin dissociation constants. J. Gen. Physiol. **73**: 839–854.

30. CAHALAN, M. & T. BEGENISICH. 1976. Sodium channel selectivity: Dependence on internal permeant ion concentration. J. Gen. Physiol. **68**: 111–125.

31. FELLER, D. J., J. A. TALVENHEIMO & W. A. CATTERALL. 1985. The sodium channel from rat brain: Reconstitution of scorpion toxin binding site in vesicles of defined lipid composition. J. Biol. Chem. **260**: 11542–11547.

Surface Charges near the Guanidinium Neurotoxin Binding Site[a]

WILLIAM N. GREEN[b] AND OLAF S. ANDERSEN

Department of Physiology and Biophysics
Cornell University Medical College
New York, New York 10021

INTRODUCTION

The guanidinium neurotoxins saxitoxin (STX) and tetrodotoxin (TTX) have been used to identify, classify, and purify voltage-dependent sodium channels in excitable membranes, as discussed in many papers in this volume. STX and TTX can also be used to probe the surface characteristics of sodium channels, *e.g.*, whether there are fixed surface charges in the vicinity of the toxin binding site.[1,2]

Addition of alkali metal cation salts to the extracellular solution bathing sodium channels decreases the binding of STX and TTX to the channels. This effect of the alkali metal cations on toxin binding can formally be described as a one-to-one competitive inhibition.[3-6] Other studies have shown that increases in extracellular Ca^{2+} concentration inhibit the binding of the divalent STX more than the binding of the monovalent TTX.[1,2] The results of the latter studies suggest that there are fixed negative surface charges near the toxin binding site. If this were the case, the interaction between alkali metal cations and the neurotoxins could result from a combination of a competitive displacement and a reduction in the local toxin concentration due to screening of surface charges and the associated reduction in surface potential.

We report here the results of experiments designed to test whether sodium channels possess a net surface charge density near the neurotoxin binding site. This question can be studied using sodium channels that have been incorporated into planar lipid bilayers,[7] because one has control over the lipid composition of the host bilayer.

EXPERIMENTAL APPROACH

In order to examine whether there are fixed negative surface charges near the toxin binding site, we compared the sodium channel block induced by the monovalent TTX and the divalent STX over a wide range of $[Na^+]$ ($0.02 \ M \leq [Na^+] \leq 1.0 \ M$). Batrachotoxin-modified sodium channels from canine forebrain were incorporated into planar lipid bilayers formed from a 4:1 mixture of 1-palmitoyl-2-oleoyl-phosphatidyl-ethanolamine and 1-palmitoyl-2-oleoyl-phosphatidylcholine in *n*-decane as described elsewhere.[8] The experiments were done at room temperature (21°–25°C), pH 7.4, with Na^+ as the only cation in the (symmetrical) aqueous solutions bathing the membrane; changes in $[Na^+]$ are thus associated with changes in ionic strength.

[a]This work was supported by NIH grant GM 21342.
[b]WNG was supported by the Cornell Departmental Associates Program.

A net surface charge density at the toxin binding site will give rise to a potential difference between the bulk aqueous phase and the site, the surface potential, V_s (e.g., refs. 9 and 10). The local toxin and Na^+ concentrations will generally differ from their bulk concentrations because

$$c = C \exp \{-zeV_s/kT\}, \qquad (1)$$

where c and C denote the local and the bulk concentration, respectively, of the charged species, z is the valency, e is the elementary charge, k is Boltzmann's constant, and T is temperature in Kelvin. The sign and magnitude of V_s is determined by the charge distribution and geometry in the vicinity of the binding site and the bulk phase ionic strength. This relation can, to a first approximation, be expressed from the Gouy-Chapman equation[9]:

$$V_s = (2kT/e) \text{ arc sinh } \{\sigma/(8N[Na^+]\epsilon_o\epsilon_r kT)\}, \qquad (2)$$

where σ is an apparent surface charge density, N is Avogadro's number, ϵ_o is the permittivity of free space, and ϵ_r is the relative dielectric constant of H_2O.

The valencies of the active forms of STX and TTX are different: $+2$ for STX and $+1$ for TTX (e.g., ref. 11). A differential displacement of the toxins by extracellular Na^+ can thus be used as an assay for surface charges in the vicinity of the toxin binding site. In the presence of a net surface charge density, STX block should be affected more than TTX block by changes in $[Na^+]$. V_s will vary as a function of Na^+ concentration (equation 2) to produce larger changes in the local STX concentration than in TTX concentration (equation 1). Further, since the channels were incorporated into lipid bilayers that carry no net charge, a detectable negative surface charge density can be ascribed to fixed negative charges on the extracellular surface of the channel protein.

We used a two-state model to quantify the toxin block. The channel may be in an unblocked (open) or a blocked (closed) state, and the toxins bind reversibly to the same physical site on the channel; toxin binding and channel block are indistinguishable. We have the following scheme:

$$\text{unblocked} \underset{k_{off}}{\overset{k_{on} \cdot [TX]}{\longleftrightarrow}} \text{blocked},$$

where $[TX]$ is the toxin concentration, and k_{on} is the association and k_{off} the dissociation rate constant for toxin binding. The dissociation constant for toxin binding, K_d, was evaluated from the fractional closed time based on channel closures lasting longer than 0.6 s (see ref. 12 for details). Estimates for k_{on} and k_{off} were obtained from the average duration of toxin-induced channel closures, τ_c, and the average duration of the interval between toxin-induced closures, τ_o:

$$k_{on} = 1/([TX] \cdot \tau_o), \qquad (3)$$

and

$$k_{off} = 1/\tau_c. \qquad (4)$$

Both k_{on} and k_{off} vary as functions of the membrane potential difference,[13-15] with a voltage dependence that is approximately independent of $[Na^+]$.[12,15] The k_{on} and k_{off} vs. $[Na^+]$ relations will therefore be based on 0 mV estimates of the rate constants. The data for TTX are illustrated in FIGURE 1. These data are well described by a simple competitive model where the relation between k_{on} and $[Na^+]$ is

$$k_{on} = k'_{on}/(1 + [Na^+]/K_{Na}), \tag{5}$$

and k_{off} is independent of $[Na^+]$. K_{Na} is the dissociation constant between Na^+ and the toxin binding site; k'_{on} is the TTX association rate constant for the hypothetical situation where $V_s = 0$ and $[Na^+] = 0$. The small variation in k_{off} with $[Na^+]$ is ignored for the present. We estimate k'_{on}, k_{off}, and K_{Na} to be about 3×10^7 $M^{-1}s^{-1}$, 6×10^{-2} s^{-1}, and 0.04 M, respectively, and $K_d \simeq 2$ nM. These estimates are similar to those obtained for sodium channels from rat skeletal muscle.[15]

The interaction between TTX and Na^+ could well be a simple competition, but similar data for STX block as a function of $[Na^+]$ cannot be described this way. This is illustrated in a log-log plot of k_{on} (and k_{off}) vs. $[Na^+]$, see FIGURE 2. The TTX data cluster around a line with a slope $\simeq -0.85$, whereas the STX data cluster around a line with a slope $\simeq -1.6$. The k_{on} values for STX decrease much more than the corresponding values for TTX as $[Na^+]$ is increased. Inspection of equation 5 shows that the data at high $[Na^+]$ should cluster around a straight line with a slope of -1.0. It is not possible to have a steeper Na^+ dependence within the framework of a simple one-to-one competition. A similar steep Na^+ dependence of STX binding has been observed by other workers.[6]

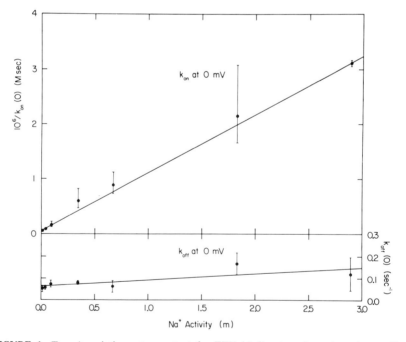

FIGURE 1. *Top:* Association rate constant for TTX binding to voltage-dependent sodium channels as a function of $[Na^+]$. The plot, $1/k_{on}$ vs. $[Na^+]$, emphasizes that $1/k_{on}$, according to a one-to-one competitive model, should be a linear function of $[Na^+]$. The straight line represents a nonlinear least-squares fit of equation 5 to the untransformed data. $K_{Na} = 0.038$ M, $k'_{on} = 2.5$ $M^{-1}s^{-1}$. *Bottom:* Dissociation rate constant for TTX as a function of Na^+ activity; k_{off} is almost independent of Na^+ activity. The straight line was drawn by eye (slope ~ 0.3).

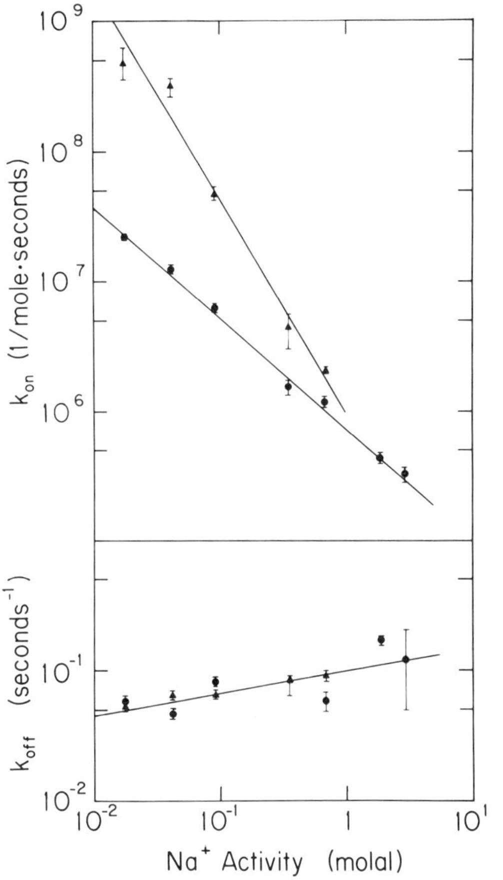

FIGURE 2. *Top:* Association rate constants for TTX (●) and STX (▲) binding to voltage-dependent sodium channels as a function of $[Na^+]$. The straight lines denote least-squares fits to the log-log transformed data. The slopes are -0.85 for TTX and -1.62 for STX. *Bottom:* Dissociation rate constants for TTX (●) and STX (▲). The *straight line* denotes a least-squares fit to the log-log transformed combined data set; the slope is 0.17.

The steep Na^+ dependence of the STX binding could result because two Na^+ ions compete with one STX at a neutral binding site. It could also result from a one-to-one competition at a charged binding site. (We will disregard the many intermediate cases between these fairly extreme alternatives.) For several reasons, the former mechanism is unlikely to be correct. First, there is no evidence for a two-to-one competition between Na^+ and TTX. Second, competitive displacements done at a constant ionic strength, where the surface potential should be independent of variations in $[Na^+]$, is consistent with a one-to-one competition between Na^+ and STX.[5] Third, at low $[Na^+]$, k_{on} approaches 10^9 $M^{-1}s^{-1}$, which is uncomfortably close to the diffusion-controlled rate of ligand binding to a neutral binding site.[16,17]

One can, however, account for the Na^+ dependence of not only the STX block but also the TTX block if one extends the one-to-one competitive mechanisms to incorporate a fixed surface charge density at the toxin binding site. One finds in this situation that k_{on}, and K_d, varies as function of $[Na^+]$ and V_s, where the latter again is a function of Na^+ concentration (see equation 2). When equation 5 is extended to include the surface charge effects, we obtain[12]:

$$k_{on} = k'_{on} \exp\left(-V_s z e/kT\right)/[1 + [Na^+]\exp\left(-V_s e/kT\right)/K_{Na}], \qquad (6)$$

where z is the valency of the active form of the toxin. The variation in K_d, equal to k_{off}/k_{on}, can be similarly described:

$$K_d = K'_d \exp (V_s ze/kT)\{1 + [Na^+] \exp [-V_s e/kT]/K_{Na}\}, \qquad (7)$$

where K'_d denotes the (local) toxin dissociation constant at $[Na^+] = 0$. FIGURE 3 depicts our (0 mV) estimates of K_d for STX and TTX as a function of $[Na^+]$; the curves represent fits of equation 7 to the data. The surface charge density was estimated to be $-1/300\ e\text{Å}^{-2}$, K_{Na} was 0.3 M, and K'_d was 20 nM for both STX and

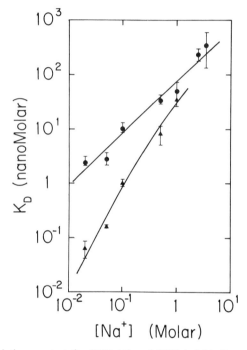

FIGURE 3. Dissociation constant for TTX ($\bullet$) and STX ($\blacktriangle$) binding to voltage-dependent sodium channels as a function of $[Na^+]$. The curves denote fits of equation 7 to the data for the monovalent TTX and the divalent STX. $K'_d = 20$ nM for both STX and TTX, $K_{Na} = 0.3$ M, and $\sigma = -1/300\ e\text{Å}^{-2}$.

TTX (k'_{on} was 3×10^{-7} M^{-1}s^{-1} for both toxins). Both the STX and TTX data are well described by the predictions of the one-to-one competitive model extended to include surface charges in the vicinity of the binding site.

It is of interest to compare these estimates for K_{Na} and K'_d for TTX with those obtained by fitting equation 5 to the TTX data (FIG. 1). The estimates obtained after including surface charges differ by an order of magnitude from the estimates obtained assuming one-to-one competition and no net surface charge in the vicinity of the binding site.

DISCUSSION

Changes in Na^+ concentration alter STX binding to a greater extent than TTX binding. The different behavior observed with the monovalent TTX and the divalent STX can be described by a model that incorporates competitive interactions between one Na^+ and one toxin molecule, as well as a negative surface charge density near the toxin binding site. The steeper Na^+ dependence of the STX binding could, in principle, also result from a two-to-one competition. But this is unlikely for the reasons outlined above, and because we find that addition of supposedly inert cations to the "extracellular" solution affect STX binding much more than TTX binding.[12] Our results on batrachotoxin-modified sodium channels thus confirm and extend earlier studies suggesting that there are fixed negative surface charges in the vicinity of the guanidinium binding site.[1,2]

A net surface charge density at the toxin binding site has implications for attempts to obtain estimates for the binding parameters for Na^+ (or other cations) and the toxins. It will also have implications for the interpretation of H^+-toxin interactions (e.g., refs. 18 and 19), as they may arise from direct competitive interactions, from titration of the toxin itself, as well as from titration of (positive and negative) surface charges in the vicinity of the binding site. The surface charge density, $-1/300\ e\text{Å}^{-2}$, is similar to what we estimate from the data of Hille et al.[2] In addition, Moczydlowski et al.[20] obtained suggestive evidence for a surface potential of about -40 mV at an ionic strength of 0.2 M, corresponding to a surface charge density of about $-1/300\ e\text{Å}^{-2}$. The similar estimates for the apparent surface charge density obtained on sodium channels from a variety of sources further support the notion that the structural features of the guanidium neurotoxin binding site and its environment are remarkably conserved (e.g., ref. 21). The evolutionary stability of the toxin binding site suggests that it somehow is important for the normal function of sodium channels. If the neurotoxin binding site is spatially separate from the permeation path,[12,22,23] the question arises: What role does the toxin binding site play in sodium channel development and function?

ACKNOWLEDGMENTS

We thank Dr. J. W. Daly, Laboratory of Bioorganic Chemistry, National Institutes of Health, for the generous gifts of batrachotoxin that made these studies possible. We also wish to thank Dr. L. B. Weiss for help with some of the experiments, and Dr. L. D. Chabala for critically reading the manuscript.

REFERENCES

1. HENDERSON, R., J. M. RITCHIE & G. R. STRICHARTZ. 1974. Evidence that tetrodotoxin and saxitoxin act at a metal cation binding site in the sodium channels of nerve membrane. Proc. Natl. Acad. Sci. (U.S.A.) 71: 3936–3940.
2. HILLE, B., J. M. RITCHIE & G. R. STRICHARTZ. 1975. The effect of surface charge on the nerve membrane on the action of tetrodotoxin and saxitoxin in frog myelinated nerve. J. Physiol. 250: 34–35P.
3. HENDERSON, R., J. M. RITCHIE & G. R. STRICHARTZ. 1973. The binding of labelled saxitoxin to the sodium channels in nerve membrane. J. Physiol. 235: 783–804.
4. REED, J. & M. RAFTERY. 1976. Properties of the tetrodotoxin binding component in plasma membranes isolated from Electrophorus electricus. Biochemistry 15: 944–953.

5. WEIGELE, J. B. & R. L. BARCHI. 1978. Saxitoxin binding to the mammalian sodium channel. Competition by monovalent and divalent cations. FEBS Lett. **95:** 49–53.
6. RHODEN, V. A. & S. M. GOLDIN. 1979. The binding of saxitoxin to axolemma of mammalian brain. J. Biol. Chem. **254:** 11199–11201.
7. KRUEGER, B. K., J. F. WORLEY & R. J. FRENCH. 1983. Single sodium channels from rat brain incorporated into planar lipid bilayer membranes. Nature **303:** 172–175.
8. GREEN, W. N., L. B. WEISS & O. S. ANDERSEN. 1986. Batrachotoxin-modified sodium channels in planar lipid bilayers: Ionic permeation and block. Submitted to J. Gen. Physiol.
9. AVEYARD, R. & D. A. HAYDON. 1973. An Introduction to the Principles of Surface Chemistry. Cambridge University Press. London.
10. MCLAUGHLIN, S. 1977. Electrostatic potentials at membrane-solution interphases. Curr. Top. Membr. Transp. **9:** 71–144.
11. RITCHIE, J. M. & R. B. ROGART. 1977. The binding of saxitoxin and tetrodotoxin to excitable tissue. Rev. Physiol. Biochem. Pharmacol. **79:** 1–50.
12. GREEN, W. N., L. B. WEISS & O. S. ANDERSEN. 1986. Batrachotoxin-modified sodium channels in planar lipid bilayers: Characterization of the saxitoxin and tetrodotoxin block. Submitted to J. Gen. Physiol.
13. FRENCH, R. J., J. F. WORLEY & B. K. KRUEGER. 1984. Voltage-dependent block by saxitoxin of sodium channels incorporated into lipid bilayers. Biophys. J. **45:** 301–310.
14. GREEN, W. N., L. B. WEISS & O. S. ANDERSEN. 1984. Batrachotoxin-modified sodium channels in lipid bilayers. Ann. N.Y. Acad. Sci. **435:** 548–550.
15. MOCZYDLOWSKI, E., S. S. GARBER & C. MILLER. 1984. Batrachotoxin-activated Na$^+$ channels in planar lipid bilayers. Competition of tetrodotoxin block by Na$^+$. J. Gen. Physiol. **84:** 665–686.
16. BURGEN, A. S. V. 1966. The drug-receptor complex. J. Pharm. Pharmacol. **18:** 137–149.
17. EIGEN, M. 1974. Diffusion control in biochemical reactions. *In* Quantum Statistical Mechanics in the Natural Sciences. S. L. Mintz & S. M. Widmayer, Eds. Plenum. New York.
18. STRICHARTZ, G. 1984. Structural determinants of the affinity of saxitoxin for neuronal sodium channels. J. Gen. Physiol. **84:** 281–305.
19. HU, S. L. & C. Y. KAO. 1985. The pH dependence of the tetrodotoxin-blockade of the sodium channel and implications for toxin binding. Toxin. In press.
20. MOCZYDLOWSKI, E., A. UEHARA & S. HALL. 1986. Blocking pharmacology of batrachotoxin-activated sodium channels from rat skeletal muscle. *In* Reconstitution of Ion Channels. C. Miller, Ed. Plenum. New York. In press.
21. HILLE, B. 1984. Ionic Channels of Excitable Membranes. Sinauer Associates. Sunderland, Mass.
22. CHABALA, L. D., W. N. GREEN, O. S. ANDERSEN & C. L. BORDERS, JR. 1986. Covalent modification of external carboxyl groups of batrachotoxin-modified canine forebrain sodium channels. Biophys. J. **49:** 40a.
23. GREEN, W. N., L. B. WEISS & O. S. ANDERSEN. 1986. The tetrodotoxin and saxitoxin binding site of voltage-dependent sodium channels is negatively charged and distant from the permeation pathway. Biophys. J. **49:** 40a.

Genetic Variants of Voltage-Sensitive Sodium Channels

LINDA M. HALL

Department of Genetics
Albert Einstein College of Medicine
Bronx, New York 10461

A genetic approach provides a powerful new dimension to the study of voltage-sensitive sodium channels. By saturating the genome for mutations that affect sodium channel function it should be possible to determine the number of gene products required to produce a functional sodium channel and keep it stably inserted in its membrane environment. Some mutants will define genes coding for structural components of the channel. These mutants, originally isolated because of their effects on the behavior and/or survival of the organism, will act like very specific chemical probes to identify physiologically important domains in the sodium channels.

For a molecule as large as the α subunit of the sodium channel, these mutations will provide powerful tools for dissecting structure-function relationships. A genetic approach to the study of sodium channels can also provide information about the molecular basis for distinct sodium channel subtypes. Such an approach can be used to determine whether pharmacologically or electrophysiologically distinguishable subtypes are due to different gene products or to posttranslational modifications of a single gene product. Finally, a genetic approach is very versatile because it does not restrict the investigator to studies of structural components alone. By identifying mutant interactions in which second site mutations can be shown to either enhance or suppress the phenotype of known channel mutants, it should be possible to identify new gene products that either interact with sodium channels physiologically or are involved in regulation of their expression.

The fruitfly *Drosophila melanogaster* is an ideal experimental organism for such genetic studies because it has a short life cycle of only 10 to 14 days depending on the culture temperature. In addition, large numbers can be readily grown in the laboratory to facilitate isolation of rare mutations.[1] It can also be readily mass cultured to provide large amounts of material required for biochemical studies of the nervous system.[2] Indeed, 50 g of adults can be easily produced daily for biochemical studies of ion channels. Although muscles in this insect do not have sodium-based action potentials, *Drosophila* neurons (like those of other organisms) use voltage-sensitive sodium channels in the propagation of action potentials. Pharmacologically, these sodium channels in *Drosophila* resemble those from other species in that they are activated by veratridine[3] and blocked by tetrodotoxin[4] and saxitoxin.[5] Both [³H]saxitoxin and [³H]tetrodotoxin have been used in binding studies to characterize voltage-sensitive sodium channels from *Drosophila*.[5,6] These channels have toxin-binding properties similar to those from other species. Therefore, it appears that this important ion channel has been phylogenetically conserved throughout evolution.

The first step in a genetic analysis of sodium channels is to screen systematically for mutations that affect the structure, function, or regulation of these channels. At first, this might seem to be an impossible task because nerve function is crucial for survival. Mutants which disrupt that function by changing the properties of the voltage-sensitive sodium channel would be expected to be lethal. Fortunately, we can bypass that difficulty by screening for conditional mutations that are temperature sensitive with respect to mutant expression. These mutants behave normally at one temperature (the permissive temperature) and express the defect at another, usually higher, temperature (the nonpermissive temperature).[7] Because inactivation of neuronal function would be expected to result in locomotor paralysis, a number of laboratories have screened for temperature-sensitive mutants that are paralyzed at high temperature (29°–39°C) but show normal locomotor activity at low temperature (22°C).[1,4,8–10]

This type of temperature-sensitive mutant is expected to be much rarer than nonconditional mutants, and therefore mutagenesis must be used to increase their frequency. Alkylating agents such as ethylmethane sulfonate[11] are commonly used as mutagens because they often cause single base changes leading to an alteration in the amino acid sequence of the protein product. Mutagenized males are put through a mating scheme to generate homozygous autosomal mutations[12] or hemizygous X-linked mutations.[1]

Even following mutagenesis, the frequency of temperature-sensitive paralytic mutations is very low and it is necessary to screen through thousands of normal sibs in order to find the rare new mutant. This screening is facilitated through the use of a large plexiglass box with a shelf on one side.[1] As illustrated in FIGURE 1, all adult flies are placed in the preheated (38°C) plastic box (2,000 to 4,000 flies per test) and are tested for paralysis within 10 minutes. Separation of immobile flies from the rest of the population is accomplished by entrapment of paralyzed flies on a ledge while their mobile sibs are drowned in a solution of vinegar and detergent. Individual paralyzed flies that recover and are fertile are used to establish lines and true breeding new paralytic mutations may then be characterized genetically, biochemically, behaviorally, and electrophysiologically.

Temperature-induced paralysis may be due to a variety of defects. In order to identify those that affect voltage-sensitive sodium channels, additional characterization is required. Some laboratories have used electrophysiological characterization to identify mutants (*nap* and *para*) that show temperature-induced loss of action potentials.[4,13] Our approach has been to test for alterations in [³H]saxitoxin binding parameters such as the dissociation constant (K_d), the total number of saturable binding sites (B_{max}), and the pH sensitivity of toxin binding. To date we have tested 11 different temperature-sensitive paralytic strains and have identified four strains

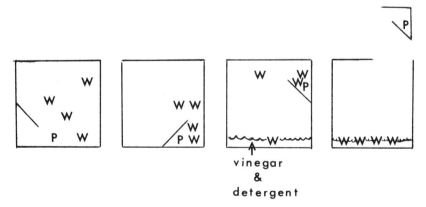

FIGURE 1. Selection of temperature-sensitive paralytic mutations (*P*) from a large population of normal sibs (*W*).

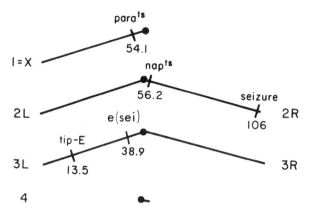

FIGURE 2. Chromosomal locations of temperature-sensitive paralytic mutations that affect the voltage-sensitive sodium channel or interact with such mutations.

(corresponding to three different genetic loci) that affect saxitoxin binding. The chromosome locations of these genes (*nap, sei,* and *tip-E*) are shown in FIGURE 2. The biochemical and electrophysiological properties of these mutants are summarized in TABLE 1; their genetic properties are summarized in TABLE 2. A comparison of the properties of the different mutants reveals that each is phenotypically distinct.

The *para*[ts] (paralytic temperature sensitive) mutation on the X chromosome was the first temperature-sensitive paralytic locus to be described.[8] It exhibits a very rapid paralysis and a sharp cut-off for the nonpermissive temperature.[4,8,15] When shifted down to the permissive temperature, this mutant shows instantaneous recovery that is independent of the length of exposure to the nonpermissive temperature. The locus appears to be readily mutable to a temperature-sensitive phenotype because three alleles were reported by Grigliatti *et al.,*[1] and an additional three alleles were described by Siddiqi and Benzer.[15] Several lines of evidence suggest that this locus may affect the voltage-sensitive sodium channel. Mutants cause a temperature-induced blockade of action potentials[13,15,16] in larvae and adults. In addition, primary cultures of *para*[tsl] neurons show a resistance to veratridine that becomes more pronounced at restrictive temperatures.[17] All *para* alleles are unconditionally lethal[18] when homozygous with another mutant (*nap*[ts]), which also blocks action potentials[4] and reduces the number of saxitoxin-binding sites.[6,19] These observations have led to the suggestion that the products of the *nap* and *para* loci interact either as sodium channel subunits or as enzyme and substrate in the posttranscriptional modification of sodium channel polypeptides.[18]

There are, however, several additional observations that should be considered in building a model for the *para*[ts] gene product. First, our laboratory has been unable to find any consistent differences in [³H]saxitoxin binding to *para*[ts] extracts over a range of assay temperatures from 0° to 38°C. Secondly, the temperature that causes paralysis in *para*[ts] mutants depends on the preconditioning temperature. For example, *para*[tsl] flies raised at 17°C will paralyze at least transiently when shifted to 21°C, whereas flies raised at 21°C require higher temperatures for paralysis. When *para*[tsl] flies raised at 21°C are shifted to 29°C, they initially show a very rapid paralysis. However, if they are held at 29°C for a period of time (on the order of 5–30 minutes), paralyzed flies will recover and then are resistant to further paralysis at that temperature. Finally, electrophysiological analysis of the flight muscles of *para*[ts] flies has suggested that

TABLE 1. Summary of Biochemical and Electrophysiological Characteristics of Mutants

	para	nap	sei	tip-E	e(sei)
Behavioral phenotype	rapid paralysis followed by recovery; temperature of paralysis depends on growth temperature.	rapid paralysis	hyperactive → paralysis	rapid paralysis	sluggish
STX binding phenotype[19,21,23,24]	none, regardless of assay temperature (0°C–38°C)	$\downarrow B_{max}$	ts-1: $\downarrow B_{max}$ → ts-2: ts $\uparrow K_d$	labile binding $\downarrow B_{max}$	not done
pH Sensitivity of STX binding[19,24]	not done	no change	differs from wild-type	no significant change	not done
Electrophysiological phenotype Larvae[4,13,25]	temperature-induced block of action potentials	temperature-induced block of action potentials prolonged refractory period sensitive to TTX	?	no effect	not done
Adult giant fiber pathway[14,25]	not blocked	not blocked blocked at 35°C	not blocked	blocked at 40°C	not done
Pharmacological phenotype[17,24]					
TTX	normal	sensitive	not done	slightly sensitive	sensitive to all drugs tested due to behavioral defect
Veratridine	resistant (resistance enhanced at high temperatures)	resistant	not done	slightly resistant	
Pyrethroids	not done	resistant	normal	normal	not done

TABLE 2. Summary of Genetic Characteristics of Mutants

	para	*nap*	*sei*	*tip-E*	*e(sei)*
Chromosome map position[1,4,8,9,19]	X-53.9-54.1	II-56.2	II-106	III-13.5	III-39.1
Dominance[23,24]					
Behaviorally	some alleles partial dominant, others recessive; dominant in combination with nap^{ts}	recessive	*ts-1* recessive *ts-2* partial dominant	recessive	recessive
Biochemically	no phenotype known	recessive	*ts-1* recessive *ts-2* partial dominant	recessive	not done
Interactions[13,18,25]					
Enhances	*nap*				
Suppresses	no effect on Sh	*para* *sei, Sh, bss*		*nap, para* *sei, Sh*	*sei*
Mutability of locus, alleles generated by:					
EMS or point mutagens	six independent isolates by two different groups	1	5	1	not done
Transposable element mutagenesis	1	0	0/238,000	not done	69/11,680 (may be a transposable element hot spot)
X- or γ-induced alleles	numerous deletions available which are lethal as heterozygotes in a nap^{ts} background	1/17,440	unknown	1/34,660	not done
Model	A. gene product interacts functionally with STX binding component B. gene product is a minor class of sodium channels C. gene product affects membrane environment	regulates level of STX binding site; catalytic interaction with sodium channel	STX binding site altered; stoichiometric interaction with sodium channel	affects stability of STX binding site	interacts with *sei* gene product.

various neurons are affected differently by $para^{ts1}$ gene expression[20] so that there are heterogeneous temperature effects on excitation in different neuronal elements.

To explain these observations, one must postulate that if $para^{ts1}$ affects the voltage-sensitive sodium channel directly, it must do so at a site distinct from the saxitoxin-binding region. This effect cannot result in thermolability of the channel because no temperature-induced changes on saxitoxin-binding were observed even at high assay temperatures. (It should be noted, however, that binding studies were done only on the $ts1$ allele. Some of the other alleles, especially those which act like deletions for the $para$ locus, might show more dramatic effects.) Another possibility is that the $para$ locus affects a genetically distinct subset of sodium channels that represents a minor fraction (20% or less) of the total saxitoxin binding component. Effects on such a small fraction would be within the noise level of the binding assay and would not be detected. A third possibility is that the $para^{ts}$ mutation affects the membrane environment of the channel rather than affecting the channel directly. The effects of the "preconditioning temperature" on the temperature of paralysis and the subsequent accommodation to the nonpermissive temperature by the $para^{ts}$ mutant may indicate that the $para$ gene product is extremely sensitive to changes in membrane lipids that may occur as the organism adapts to different temperatures.

The nap^{ts} (no action potential temperature sensitive) mutation on the second chromosome resembles the $para^{ts}$ mutation in that it shows a very rapid paralysis when shifted to the nonpermissive temperature. When shifted to the permissive temperature nap^{ts} also shows instantaneous recovery that is independent of the length of paralysis. Although the original nap^{ts} stock did not show accommodation at the nonpermissive temperature, as the mutant has been maintained in culture, the stock has apparently built up modifiers that cause an accommodation similar to that exhibited by $para^{ts}$. The nap locus is not readily mutable and only one allele induced by point mutagens has been reported despite numerous attempts to isolate new alleles. The locus does appear to be readily mutable by γ-radiation (see TABLE 2). If the nap locus were the structural gene for a large molecule such as the α subunit of the sodium channel, it would be expected to be a large target for chemical mutagenesis. Lethal alleles should be readily isolable. The apparent low mutation frequency at this locus argues against its being a large structural gene.

In contrast to the $para^{ts}$ mutation, nap^{ts} does have a dramatic effect on [³H]saxitox-in[19,21] and [³H]tetrodotoxin binding.[6] The total number of saturable binding sites (B_{max}) is 30%–50% lower in the nap^{ts} mutant compared with the wild-type regardless of assay temperature. There is no effect of the mutant on the dissociation constant or the pH dependence of toxin binding.[19] This reduction in number of binding sites is not due to a generalized reduction in neuronal tissue because levels of α-bungarotoxin binding[21] and (Na^+-K^+) ATPase[19] are the same in this mutant as in the wild-type.

These binding studies on the nap^{ts} mutant that show a decrease in number of saxitoxin-binding sites even at low assay temperature complement previous electro-physiological studies[13] which had demonstrated that nap^{ts} causes an increased sensitivity to tetrodotoxin and prolongs the refractory period of the compound action potential even at permissive temperatures. Thus, there appears to be a biochemical correlate to the physiological alterations seen at permissive temperatures.

Can the reduction in sodium channel levels also account for the temperature-induced paralysis? To test this suggestion we fed wild-type flies a sublethal dose of tetrodotoxin and compared them with buffer-fed control flies with respect to temperature-induced paralysis. We found that wild-type flies fed tetrodotoxin show rapid paralysis at 38°C, whereas their buffer-fed sibs show normal locomotor activity at this temperature.[19] These observations have led us to suggest that the nap locus may not affect sodium channel structure directly but rather may code for a gene product that interacts with the sodium channel to affect the number of binding sites inserted into the membrane.

As a further test of this model we have compared the behavioral and biochemical properties of *nap* heterozygotes with those of homozygous *nap* mutants and homozygous wild-type. As summarized in TABLE 2, we have found both the behavioral and the biochemical phenotypes of *nap^ts* to be completely recessive.[19] This recessive phenotype indicates that one copy of the normal gene is sufficient to give a completely wild-type phenotype.

One possible model for a recessive phenotype is indicated in FIGURE 3. If the nap gene product interacts with or regulates the production of the voltage-sensitive sodium channel in a catalytic rather than stoichiometric fashion, a 50% reduction in the *nap^+* gene product could still result in a completely wild-type phenotype as long as there is still enough *nap^+* product to carry the normal "reaction" to completion. For illustrative purposes in FIGURE 3, the *nap^+* product is shown to be involved in a posttranslational modification of the sodium channel, although other possibilities are equally likely. In this model, failure of posttranslational modification might partially destabilize the channel, resulting in fewer membrane-bound channels. This process might be similar to the glycosylation required for maintenance of functional sodium channels in neuroblastoma cells.[22]

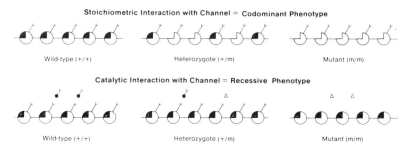

FIGURE 3. A codominant phenotype indicates a gene product that interacts stoichiometrically with the sodium channel whereas a completely recessive phenotype indicates a gene product that interacts catalytically with the sodium channel.

An alternative model would be that the *nap^+* gene product is involved in the transcriptional regulation of one genetically distinct sodium channel subtype. Once sodium channel genes have been cloned in *Drosophila,* these models will be distinguishable by comparing transcriptional activity in *nap* versus wild-type flies.

The *nap^ts* mutation may be viewed as a sodium channel "underproducer." Although this mutation may define a locus that directly regulates sodium channel production, it might also affect channel insertion into membranes or might affect channel stability. It would be interesting to identify genetic loci directly involved in sodium channel regulation because this is one way in which neurons might control their general level of excitability. Although there might be many genetic defects that would lead to a net decrease in sodium channel number, it is likely that screening for mutants that cause channel "overproduction" would be a more effective way to identify interesting regulatory loci. The pharmacological phenotype of *nap^ts,* an underproducer mutant, suggests a strategy for screening for such overproducers. As shown in FIGURE 4, when *nap^ts* is fed a dose of tetrodotoxin which would kill ~50% of wild-type, fewer *nap^ts* flies survive indicating that this mutant strain is sensitive to channel antagonists.

In contrast, when fed veratridine, the *nap^{ts}* mutant is much more resistant than wild-type to this channel agonist. Because an underproducer is sensitive to antagonists and resistant to agonists, it should be possible to enrich for regulatory mutants that cause channel overproduction by screening for the reciprocal phenotype, that is, by screening for sensitivity to agonists and resistance to antagonists. Screening for changes in sensitivity in opposite directions using drugs with very different structures should help to eliminate mutants in which sensitivity changes are due to alterations in drug permeability or metabolism and should enrich for interesting regulatory mutants.

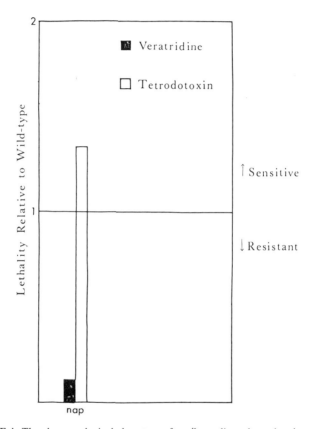

FIGURE 4. The pharmacological phenotype of *nap^{ts}*, a sodium channel underproducer.

The *sei^{ts}* (seizure, temperature sensitive) locus is on the second chromosome and has been defined by two alleles (*ts1* and *ts2*).[19,23] As shown in FIGURE 2, *sei^{ts}* maps to a much more distal region of the right arm of chromosome 2 than the *nap* locus. The *sei^{ts}* alleles are also behaviorally quite distinct from *nap^{ts}*. When *sei* flies are shifted to the nonpermissive temperature, they first go through a phase of hyperactivity and convulsions before they become paralyzed. Their behavior resembles that of veratridine-poisoned flies, whereas the behavior of *nap* more closely resembles that of tetrodotoxin-poisoned flies. For both *sei* alleles the time required for recovery is dependent on the length of time that the flies are paralyzed at the nonpermissive temperature. This behavior is very different from that of both *nap* and *para* flies and suggests that some important component is being depleted during paralysis that must be replenished before recovery can occur. [³H]Saxitoxin-binding studies have shown that *sei*^{ts2} extracts show an altered pH dependence for toxin binding and a temperature-sensitive increase in the dissociation constant for toxin-receptor binding. There is no change in the number of saturable binding sites.[19] As summarized in TABLE 2, the *sei*^{ts2} allele has partially dominant and dose-dependent effects on paralytic behavior and on saxitoxin binding.[23] As shown in the models in FIGURE 3, the codominant phenotype of *sei*^{ts2} suggests that in mutant heterozygotes both mutant and normal channels coexist, giving heterozygotes a phenotype intermediate between that of homozygous mutant and homozygous wild type. In general terms these results suggest that the *sei* gene product interacts with the sodium channel in a stoichiometric fashion. One interpretation would be that the *sei* locus may alter saxitoxin binding sites structurally.

This interpretation is complicated by the finding that the *sei*^{ts1} allele shows a reduced number of saxitoxin binding sites relative to wild-type, but no alteration in the dissociation constant. Furthermore, the *ts-1* allele is completely recessive with respect to both behavioral and biochemical phenotypes. The different effects of these two alleles on behavior and on saxitoxin binding may result because they affect different structural domains of the sodium channel. To explain the lack of codominant effect with the *sei*^{ts1} allele, we postulate that the *sei*^{ts1} mutation makes the mutant product less able to compete with the wild-type product so that in the heterozygote only the wild-type product remains and is functional. In a case such as this where different alleles give different phenotypes it will be interesting to characterize the phenotypic variability among new alleles. Eventually molecular analysis of many *sei* alleles will aid in the structure-function analysis of the *sei*⁺ gene product.

The *tip-E* (temperature-induced paralysis, locus E) mutant on the third chromosome (see FIG. 2) resembles *nap*^{ts} because it paralyzes rapidly at 38°C and recovers almost immediately when shifted back to the permissive temperature.[9] As in *nap*^{ts} the recovery time is completely independent of the duration of paralysis at the nonpermissive temperature. As summarized in TABLE 1, the *tip-E* mutant also resembles *nap* in [³H]saxitoxin binding studies because *tip-E* extracts show a 30%–40% decrease in the number of saxitoxin-binding sites per mg protein and have a K_d similar to wild-type for the remaining sites.[24] Again, this decrease seen in *tip-E* extracts is not due to general hypotrophy of the nervous system because the density of α-bungarotoxin binding sites is normal in *tip-E*.[24] In some *tip-E* extracts, an almost normal density of saxitoxin-binding sites was seen at low assay temperatures. In these "normal" extracts, the B_{max} decreased at high assay temperatures to 30%–40% less than wild-type controls. Both the ligand binding phenotype and the behavioral phenotype were completely recessive in *tip-E* mutants. One interpretation of this data is that the *tip-E* gene product is a labile component required for a fraction of saxitoxin binding. This component may be lost during extract preparation, but if it is not lost, then it is destroyed during incubation at high assay temperatures.

Because *nap* and *tip-E* both reduce saxitoxin binding sites by approximately the same amount, we were interested in determining whether they affect the same or different populations of sodium channels. Therefore, we constructed *nap, tip-E* double mutants and examined their behavioral phenotype and the saxitoxin-binding properties of extracts. We found that behaviorally 50% of the double mutants paralyzed after 40 s at 28°C, whereas 50% of *nap* homozygotes paralyzed after 40 s at 32.5°C and the *tip-E* homozygotes required 40 s at 39.2°C for 50% to become paralyzed. This increased behavioral sensitivity to temperature-induced paralysis was paralleled by decreases in longevity and also by decreases in the number of [³H]saxitoxin binding sites. The double mutant showed fewer binding sites than either single mutant alone.[24]

This suggested that *tip-E* and *nap* affect different sodium channel populations in an additive fashion. In view of the recently reported genetic heterogeneity in sodium channels in rat,[26] it will be interesting to use molecular biological approaches to determine whether *tip-E* and *nap* affect genetically distinct sodium channels.

The mutants described up to this point were all identified on the basis of a temperature-induced paralysis phenotype coupled with alterations in saxitoxin-binding properties or in electrophysiological properties. Another approach to identifying genes affecting membrane excitability is to look for second site mutations that act to enhance or suppress the behavioral phenotype of existing mutants. This approach has been used to categorize relationships among existing mutations.[13,18,25] We have recently used this approach to identify a new genetic locus called enhancer of seizure [*e(sei)*]. This locus maps to the third chromosome at a site distinct from *tip-E* and causes both seizure alleles to paralyze at lower temperatures than usual. This interaction is specific because this enhancer does not affect the behavioral phenotype of other temperature-sensitive paralytic mutations including *nap*, *tip-E*, *para*, and shibire[1,27] (D.P. Kasbekar and L.M. Hall, unpublished observations). This enhancer locus may code for a product that interacts specifically with the seizure gene product. This enhancer gene has been cytogenetically localized to a six-band region on the left arm of chromosome 3, and appears to be a hot spot for transposable element mutagenesis (D.P. Kasbekar and L.M. Hall, in preparation). Therefore, it may be cloned by the approach of transposon tagging. Then antibodies produced against the cloned gene product will be a useful first approach to studying the nature of this product and its interaction with seizure. This approach provides a general strategy to identify gene products of interest based on their involvement in a common physiological pathway.

This report has described a number of different genes that affect sodium channel structure, function, or regulation, but the genetic, biochemical, and electrophysiological approaches discussed do not provide conclusive information about which, if any, of these genes actually code for structural components of the voltage-sensitive sodium channel. In order to identify the structural gene (or genes) in *Drosophila* homologous to the α subunit of the voltage-sensitive sodium channel, we have made oligonucleotide probes from regions of the sodium channel that are highly conserved between the electric eel (*Electrophorus*) and the rat,[26] and we have used these probes to identify positive clones from a *Drosophila* library. Further characterization of these clones by sequence analysis will identify those that are homologous to vertebrate sodium channel cDNA. These clones will then be hybridized to *Drosophila* salivary gland chromosomes to determine the location of the homologous gene. By this cytogenetic localization we will be able to determine if the homologous gene corresponds to any that we have identified to date or alternatively, if it corresponds to a new genetic locus. Mutants that affect this structural locus will be useful for structure-function analysis. The remaining mutants will be even more interesting because they will help to identify additional aspects of channel regulation. Such processes might be difficult to identify by classical biochemical approaches.

Even though the gene product has not been identified for the mutants summarized in this article, these mutants are still useful for defining the role of cell excitability in various biological processes. For example, the *nap*[ts] mutant has recently been used to demonstrate that cell excitability is required for the biological clock involved in the *Drosophila* male courtship song oscillation.[28] This song has an oscillatory rhythm that continues even when the male is not courting. Kyriacou and Hall[28] used temperature-shift studies to block action potentials and demonstrated that when action potentials stopped, the clock governing this oscillatory rhythm also stopped.

This experiment demonstrates the advantage of using mutants as pharmacological agents. In this case the nap^{ts} mutant acts like immediately reversible tetrodotoxin or saxitoxin because the mutant effects can be rapidly turned on or off by shifting the temperature. The mutant approach has an additional advantage. Since every cell in the organism carries the mutant gene, there is no problem with accessibility of different cell populations to the "reagent." This same approach may be readily extended to the dissection of other complex behavioral processes such as learning and memory. In terms of future directions, conditional mutants such as those described in this paper are potentially very versatile pharmacological agents that may serve as the tetrodotoxins and saxitoxins of the future.

REFERENCES

1. GRIGLIATTI, T. A., L. HALL, R. ROSENBLUTH & D. T. SUZUKI. 1973. Temperature-sensitive mutations in *Drosophila melanogaster*. XIV. A selection of immobile adults. Mol. Gen. Genet. **120**: 107–114.
2. FAN, C. L., L. M. HALL, A. J. SKRINSKA & G. M. BROWN. 1976. Correlation of guanosine triphosphate cyclohydrolase activity and the synthesis of pterins in *Drosophila melanogaster*. Biochem. Genet. **14**: 271–280.
3. WU, C.-F., N. SUZUKI & M.-M. POO. 1983. Dissociated neurons from normal and mutant *Drosophila* larval central nervous system in cell culture. J. Neurosci. **3**: 1888–1899.
4. WU, C.-F., B. GANETZKY, L. Y. JAN, Y.-N. JAN & S. BENZER. 1978. A Drosophila mutant with a temperature-sensitive block in nerve conduction. Proc. Natl. Acad. Sci. U.S.A. **75**: 4047–4051.
5. GITSCHIER, J., G. R. STRICHARTZ & L. M. HALL. 1980. Saxitoxin binding to sodium channels in head extracts from wild-type and tetrodotoxin-sensitive strains of *Drosophila melanogaster*. Biochim. Biophys. Acta **595**: 291–303.
6. KAUVAR, L. M. 1982. Reduced [^{3}H]-tetrodotoxin binding in the nap^{ts} paralytic mutant of *Drosophila*. Mol. Gen. Genet. **187**: 172–173.
7. SUZUKI, D. T. 1970. Temperature-sensitive mutations in *Drosophila melanogaster*. Science **170**: 695–706.
8. SUZUKI, D. T., T. GRIGLIATTI & R. WILLIAMSON. 1971. Temperature-sensitive mutations in *Drosophila melanogaster* VII. A mutation ($para^{ts}$) causing reversible adult paralysis. Proc. Natl. Acad. Sci. U.S.A. **68**: 890–893.
9. KULKARNI, S. J. & A. PADHYE. 1982. Temperature-sensitive paralytic mutations on the second and third chromosomes of *Drosophila melanogaster*. Genet. Res. **40**: 191–199.
10. SHYNGLE, J. & R. P. SHARMA. 1985. Studies on paralysis and development of second chromosome temperature sensitive paralytic mutants of *Drosophila melanogaster*. Indian J. Exp. Biol. **23**: 235–240.
11. LEWIS, E. B. & F. BACHER. 1968. Method of feeding ethyl-methanesulphonate (EMS) to *Drosophila* males. Drosophila Information Service **43**: 193.
12. GETHMAN, R. C. 1974. Meiosis in male *Drosophila melanogaster* I. Isolation and characterization of meiotic mutants affecting second chromosome disjunction. Genetics **78**: 1127–1142.
13. WU, C.-F. & B. GANETZKY. 1980 Genetic alteration of nerve membrane excitability in temperature-sensitive paralytic mutants of *Drosophila melanogaster*. Nature **286**: 814–816.
14. NELSON, J. C. & D. H. BAIRD. 1985. Action potentials persist at restrictive temperatures in temperature sensitive paralytic mutants of adult *Drosophila*. Soc. Neurosci. Abstr. **11**: 213.
15. SIDDIQI, O. & S. BENZER. 1976. Neurophysiological defects in temperature-sensitive paralytic mutants of *Drosophila melanogaster*. Proc. Natl. Acad. Sci. U.S.A. **73**: 3253–3257.
16. SIDDIQI, O. 1975. Genetic blocks in the elements of neural network in *Drosophila*. *In* Regulation of Growth and Differentiated Function in Eukaryotic Cells. G. P. Talwar, Ed.: 541–549. Raven Press. New York.

17. SUZUKI, N. & C.-F. WU. 1984. Altered sensitivity to sodium channel-specific neurotoxins in cultured neurons from temperature-sensitive paralytic mutants of *Drosophila*. J. Neurogenet. **1:** 225–238.
18. GANETZKY, B. 1984. Genetic studies of membrane excitability in Drosophila: Lethal interaction between two temperature-sensitive paralytic mutations. Genetics **108:** 897–911.
19. JACKSON, F. R., S. D. WILSON, G. R. STRICHARTZ & L. M. HALL. 1984. Two types of mutants affecting voltage-sensitive sodium channels in *Drosophila melanogaster*. Nature **308:** 189–191.
20. BENSHALOM, G. & D. DAGAN. 1981. Electrophysiological analysis of the temperature-sensitive paralytic *Drosophila* mutant, *para*ts. J. Comp. Physiol. A. **144:** 409–417.
21. HALL, L. M., S. D. WILSON, J. GITSCHIER, N. MARTINEZ & G. R. STRICHARTZ. 1982. Identification of a *Drosophila melanogaster* mutant that affects the saxitoxin receptor of the voltage-sensitive sodium channel. Ciba Found. Symp. **88:** 207–220.
22. WAECHTER, C. J., J. W. SCHMIDT & W. A. CATTERALL. 1983. Glycosylation is required for maintenance of functional sodium channels in neuroblastoma cells. J. Biol. Chem. **258:** 5117–5123.
23. JACKSON, F. R., J. GITSCHIER, G. R. STRICHARTZ & L. M. HALL. 1985. Genetic modifications of voltage-sensitive sodium channels in *Drosophila*: Gene dosage studies of the *seizure* locus. J. Neurosci. **5:** 1144–1151.
24. JACKSON, F. R., S. D. WILSON & L. M. HALL. 1986. The *tip-E* mutation of *Drosophila* decreases saxitoxin binding and interacts with other mutations affecting nerve membrane excitability. J. Neurogenet. **3:** 1–17.
25. GANETZKY, B. 1986. Neurogenetic analysis of *Drosophila* mutations affecting sodium channels: Synergistic effects on viability and nerve conduction in double mutants involving *tip-E*. J. Neurogenet. **3:** 19–31.
26. NODA, M., T. IKEDA, T. KAYANO, H. SUZUKI, H. TAKESHIMA, M. KURASAKI, H. TAKAHASHI & S. NUMA. 1986. Existence of distinct sodium channel messenger RNAs in rat brain. Nature **320:** 188–192.
27. POODRY, C. A., L. HALL & D. T. SUZUKI. 1973. Developmental properties of *shibire*ts: A pleiotropic mutation affecting larval and adult locomotion and development. Dev. Biol. **32:** 373–386.
28. KYRIACOU, C. P. & J. C. HALL. 1985. Action potential mutations stop a biological clock in *Drosophila*. Nature **314:** 171–173.

Analysis of Mutations Affecting Sodium Channels in *Drosophila*[a]

BARRY GANETZKY,[b] KATE LOUGHNEY,[b] AND
CHUN-FANG WU[c]

[b]*Laboratory of Genetics*
University of Wisconsin
Madison, Wisconsin 53706

[c]*Department of Biology*
University of Iowa
Iowa City, Iowa 52242

INTRODUCTION

The appeal of saxitoxin (STX) and tetrodotoxin (TTX) as research tools lies in their remarkable affinity and specificity in binding to sodium channels. These toxins have been incomparably useful as ligands that enable the purification of sodium channel polypeptides and as pharmacological agents that permit the precise reduction or elimination of Na^+ current in excitable cells. In a genetically tractable organism such as *Drosophila melanogaster*, mutations that affect the function of ion channels have much the same appeal. Mutations provide specific molecular handles that make possible the identification and characterization of the relevant gene products. In addition, they provide specific tools that allow membrane excitability to be manipulated in defined ways for a variety of experimental purposes.

The cloning and sequencing of a sodium channel polypeptide in other organisms[1] have provided the crucial information for beginning to understand the function of sodium channels in molecular terms. Still, many questions remain to be answered before a complete and detailed picture of the structure and function of sodium channels is achieved. In addition, the synthesis, assembly, and membrane distribution of sodium channels appear to be precisely regulated.[2,3] The basis of this regulation at the molecular level is unclear at present.

Among a collection of mutations in *Drosophila* that affect sodium channels, we expect to identify both the genes that encode sodium channels and those involved in their regulation. Methodology exists in *Drosophila* to clone genes identified by mutation and to reintroduce these genes following *in vitro* mutagenesis into an intact organism with a complete nervous system. Thus, analysis of mutations in *Drosophila* can help elucidate questions concerning the structure and regulation of sodium channels. Two mutations that we have been particularly concerned with are *nap*[ts] (no action potential, temperature sensitive) and *para*[ts] (paralytic, temperature sensitive). Here we review the electrophysiological, pharmacological, and genetic properties of these mutants. In addition, we will describe the molecular cloning of the *para* gene.

[a]This work was supported by the National Institutes of Health (grants NS1539, GM35099, and a Research Career Developmental Award NS00719 to B. G., and grants NS00675 and NS18500 to C.-F. W.) and a postdoctoral fellowship from the American Heart Association of Wisconsin to K. L. This is paper no. 2863 from the Laboratory of Genetics, University of Wisconsin, Madison.

THE *nap^ts* MUTATION

The first mutation clearly shown to affect sodium channels in *Drosophila* in some way was *nap^ts*.[4] It is a recessive mutation on the second chromosome and was originally isolated because of its behavioral phenotype. At 25°C *nap^ts* flies behave normally but when they are shifted to 37°C they undergo complete paralysis within seconds and remain immobilized. If they are returned to 25°C they recover completely from paralysis, also within seconds.

By recording compound action potentials extracellularly from larval nerve bundles,

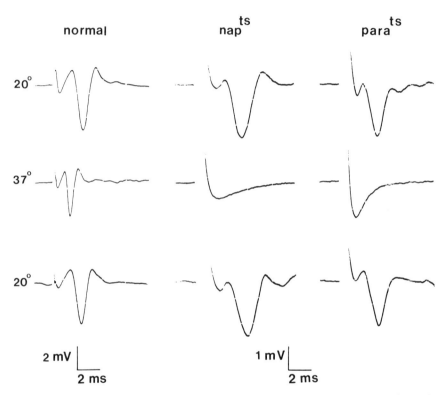

FIGURE 1. Temperature dependence of action potential propagation in normal, *nap^ts*, *para^ts* nerves. Larval segmental nerves were cut near the ganglion and stimulated at that end. The compound action potential was recorded en passant by a suction electrode at some distance from the stimulation site. The exact waveform depends on the length of the nerve loop drawn up in the suction electrode. At 20°C, the compound action potential in the mutants is similar to that in normal flies. In these records, the amplitude of the mutant action potentials is smaller than normal at 20° (notice the difference in scale), but more detailed studies are required to determine whether this difference is reproducible. At 37°C the compound action potential is still prominent in normal nerves. In *nap^ts*, action potentials are completely absent at this temperature and only the stimulus artifact is recorded. In *para^ts*, action potentials are almost completely abolished at 37°C, although a very small remaining active response may be superimposed on the stimulus artifact. Upon lowering the temperature again to 20°C the active response in the mutants recovers rapidly.

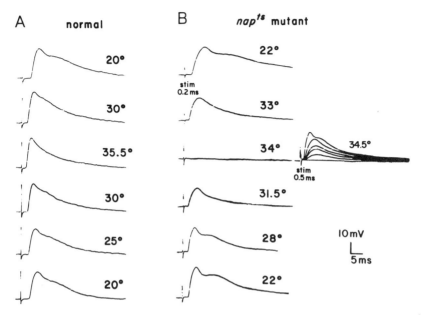

FIGURE 2. Intracellular recording from ventrolateral longitudinal muscles in normal and *nap^{ts}* larvae at various temperatures, showing ejps in response to nerve stimulation (0.2 ms duration). (A) Normal larva. The ejp persisted as the temperature was raised to 35°C and lowered again. (B) *nap^{ts}* larva. As the temperature was raised to 34°C, the ejp disappeared; it reappeared as the temperature was lowered. *Inset,* At 34°C, when the response failed, a graded potential could still be induced by passive electrotonic depolarization of the nerve terminal by applying stronger stimuli (0.5 ms duration) of varied intensity. Therefore, transmitter release and postsynaptic response in *nap^{ts}* remain functional even at 37°C. The bath solution contains 2 mM Ca^{2+} for all traces. (From Wu *et al.*[4])

we showed that the paralytic behavior was paralleled by a defect in nerve conduction.[4] As the temperature is raised from 20°C to 37°C there is an abrupt loss of the action potential in *nap^{ts}* but not in normal larvae (FIG. 1). Nerve conduction returns within seconds after lowering the temperature back to 20°C.

The postsynaptic excitatory junctional potentials (ejps) recorded from muscle fibers in response to nerve stimulation are alike in *nap^{ts}* and normal larvae at 20°C. At elevated temperatures the ejp abruptly disappears in mutant but not normal larvae (FIG. 2). Loss of the ejp can be entirely accounted for by the failure in nerve conduction because synaptic transmission, evoked by passive electrotonic depolarization of the nerve terminal, is unimpaired even at the restrictive temperature.[4]

This specific block in nerve conduction suggests an effect on sodium channels. Direct examination of sodium current has not yet been achieved, but a variety of indirect evidence supports this interpretation. Even at nominally permissive temperatures (23°C), *nap^{ts}* manifests defects in nerve membrane properties. The refractory period of the nerve action potential is more than twice as long in *nap^{ts}* as in normal larvae.[5] In addition, TTX blocks nerve conduction in *nap^{ts}* larvae at concentrations four to five times lower than required to effect a similar block in normal larvae (FIG. 3).[5] Finally, *nap^{ts}* neurons cultured *in vitro* are significantly more resistant than normal to veratridine (FIG. 4), which is cytotoxic to neurons because it persistently activates

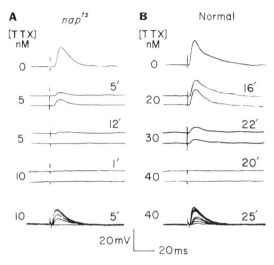

FIGURE 3. Continuous recordings (23°C) from ventrolateral longitudinal muscles in *nap^{ts}* and normal larvae showing ejps at the TTX concentration indicated at the left of each trace. TTX was added to the bath solution to change concentrations in increments of 5–10 nM. Traces were made at different times after change of TTX concentration as indicated at the right of each trace. (**A**) *nap^{ts}* larva. At 5 nM TTX, the ejp is almost entirely blocked within 12 min. After active conduction is blocked by TTX, graded potentials can still be evoked electrotonically showing that synaptic transmission is not affected. For 11 *nap^{ts}* larvae examined, the TTX concentration at which nerve conduction was blocked was 9.8 ± 4.4 nM (x ± SD). (**B**) Normal larva. Failure occurs only after 20 min in 40 nM TTX. Graded responses can be evoked electrotonically at this point. For 9 normal larvae examined, the critical dose of TTX was 40.3 ± 11.1 nM. The bath solution contains 0.8 mM Ca^{2+} for all traces. (From Wu and Ganetzky.[5] Reprinted by permission from *Nature*.)

sodium channels.[6] These results, together with the reduced saxitoxin binding in membrane preparations from *nap^{ts}* heads reported by Hall and her colleagues,[7,8] support the conclusion that *nap^{ts}* alters the function and/or the stability of sodium channels. The consequences of this defect are most striking near 37°C, but can be detected by appropriate assays, even at 23°C.

This notion receives additional support from results of a different kind of experiment involving the *Sh* (Shaker) mutation. In contrast with normal flies, when anesthetized with ether, *Sh* flies manifest vigorous leg-shaking behavior (FIG. 5).[9] It has been shown that *Sh* abolishes a particular potassium outward current (I_A) resulting in a delay in nerve membrane repolarization.[10–13] At the larval neuromuscular junction, *Sh* causes a very prolonged ejp, which is associated with anomalous repetitive firing of motor axons in response to a single stimulus (FIG. 6).[10]

If double mutants are constructed between *nap^{ts}* and *Sh,* the behavioral defect of *Sh* is suppressed by *nap^{ts}* (FIG. 5) even at 23°C.[14] Furthermore, the repetitive nerve activity and prolonged ejp associated with *Sh* are also suppressed by *nap^{ts}* (FIG. 6) in double mutants.[13] This suppression is not limited to *Sh*. The *eag* (ether a go-go)[16,17] and *Hk* (hyperkinetic)[18] mutations affect other classes of potassium channels, again leading to enhanced membrane excitability. The effects of these mutations are also suppressed by *nap^{ts}* in double mutants.[14] The basis of this suppression is apparently the reduction in membrane excitability caused by *nap^{ts}*, which is sufficient even at 23°C to counterbalance the enhanced excitability produced by the other mutants. Since *Sh*, *eag*, and *Hk* are all known to affect potassium channels, the counterbalancing effect of *nap^{ts}* points to a defect in sodium channels.

THE *para^{ts}* MUTATION

The results with *nap^{ts}* raised the question of whether other mutations with similar properties could be found among temperature-sensitive paralytic mutants. Attention focused on *para^{ts1}* because out of a number of paralytic mutants examined, behaviorally it was most similar to *nap^{ts}*. It is an X-linked mutation isolated by Suzuki and co-workers and was the first temperature-sensitive paralytic mutation to be discovered. Like *nap^{ts}*, *para^{ts1}* causes flies to become paralyzed within seconds after they are exposed to the restrictive temperature (29°C for adults, 35°C for larvae). Recovery from paralysis at permissive temperatures is equally rapid.

The behavioral similarity of *nap^{ts}* and *para^{ts1}* is paralleled by similarities in their

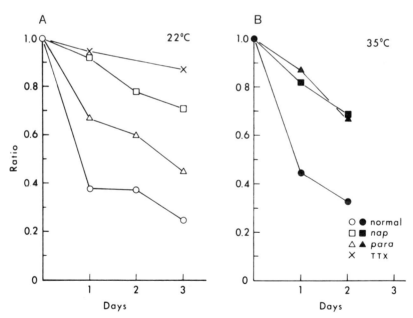

FIGURE 4. Relative sensitivity to veratridine of normal (*circles*), *para^{ts1}* (*triangles*), *nap^{ts}* (*squares*), and TTX-pretreated (1 μM) normal (*crosses*) neurons. The fractions of viable neurons at 22°C and 35°C in veratridine-treated (500 μM) and control cultures were determined by time lapse study over three consecutive days. The ratio of the neuronal density in veratridine-treated cultures to control cultures is shown. For each data point, 150–550 neurons in 6 to 14 different veratridine-treated and control cultures were examined. (A) 22°C. (B) 35°C. Data for the third day at 35°C are excluded because of the extensive premature cell death that occurs when cultures are maintained at this temperature. (From Suzuki and Wu.[6] Reprinted by permission from the *Journal of Neurogenetics*.)

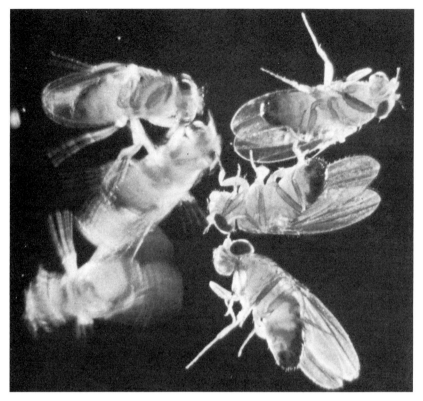

FIGURE 5. Long exposure time (ten seconds) photograph of flies after ether anesthesia. Sh^{KS133} mutants (*left*) display rapid and vigorous leg shaking and wing scissoring. The *Sh* phenotype is suppressed by nap^{ts} since Sh^{KS133}, nap^{ts} double mutants (*right*) appear like normal flies and remain immobile after anesthetization. $T = 23°C$. (From Ganetzky and Wu.[14] Reprinted by permission from *Genetics*.)

electrophysiological defect as well: the compound action potential recorded extracellularly from $para^{ts1}$ larval nerve bundles is blocked at elevated temperatures (FIG. 1).[5] Other phenotypes associated with nap^{ts} such as the enhanced sensitivity to TTX and the altered binding to STX were not found in $para^{ts1}$. In general, it appears that whereas defects in nap^{ts} are apparent at 23°C, the defects in $para^{ts1}$ are less evident until the temperature is raised.

This is demonstrated by the veratridine resistance of $para^{ts1}$ neurons *in vitro*. At 23°C, $para^{ts1}$ neurons are more resistant than normal to the cytotoxic effects of veratridine, but less so than nap^{ts}. However, at 35°C the resistance of $para^{ts1}$ neurons increases to the level displayed by nap^{ts} (FIG. 4).[6]

The $para^{ts1}$ allele also does not suppress the *Sh* phenotype at 23°C. However, we recently discovered new temperature-sensitive alleles of the *para* gene that do suppress the behavioral defect in *Sh* at permissive temperatures. (M. Stern and B. Ganetzky, unpublished). It will be of interest to characterize the physiological and pharmacological properties of these new alleles.

INTERACTION OF *nap^{ts}* AND *para^{ts}* MUTANTS

The similarities in phenotype between *nap^{ts}* and *para^{ts}* are not fortuitous but reflect an important underlying relationship between the products of these two genes. This conclusion is based on the finding that double mutants for *para^{ts1}* and *nap^{ts}* are lethal and the lethality occurs regardless of temperature.[5,20] The usual genetic interpretation of synergistic interactions of this kind is that there is a functional overlap between the two gene products. We think this interpretation applies in this instance as well. For example, disruption of the *nap$^+$* or *para$^+$* function results in a temperature-dependent failure to propagate action potentials, but simultaneous interference with both could lead to such severe defects in the function or stability of sodium channels that the ability to propagate action potentials is lost at all temperatures.

Direct evidence for this interpretation is provided by the observation that doubly mutant sensory axons, which can be produced as small tissue patches in viable genetic mosaics, are unable to relay signals in response to tactile stimuli regardless of the temperature.[21] It is tempting to think in terms of physical interactions between polypeptides in order to explain the synergism between *nap^{ts}* and *para^{ts}* mutants, but direct evidence for this is not available.

From a genetic point of view, one of the important aspects of the interaction between *nap^{ts}* and *para^{ts}* is that it readily suggests a basis for isolating additional

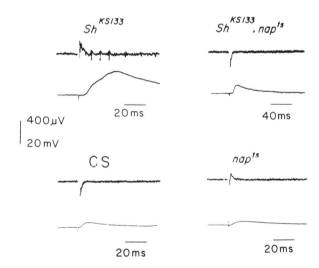

FIGURE 6. Simultaneous intracellular recordings of ejps (*lower traces*) from larval ventrolateral longitudinal muscles and extracellular recordings of action potentials from nerve (*upper traces*) innervating the muscle. In a normal (CS) larva, the nerve response to a stimulus consists of a single compound action potential and the ejp has a small amplitude at the Ca^{2+} concentration used (0.2 mM). In *Sh^{KS133}*, a single stimulus applied to the nerve elicits multiple nerve action potentials and an ejp of greater amplitude and duration than normal. Note the stepwise increase in amplitude of the ejp correlated with the occurrence of the extra nerve action potentials. In the *Sh^{KS133}*, *nap^{ts}* double mutant the repetitive firing and prolonged ejp are suppressed. The nerve and muscle responses of *nap^{ts}* are similar to those of normal larvae under these conditions. Voltage calibration: 400 μV for nerve traces, 20 mV for muscle traces. Note the different time scale for the *Sh^{KS133}*, *nap^{ts}* traces. $T = 23°C$. (From Ganetzky and Wu.[14] Reprinted by permission from *Genetics*.)

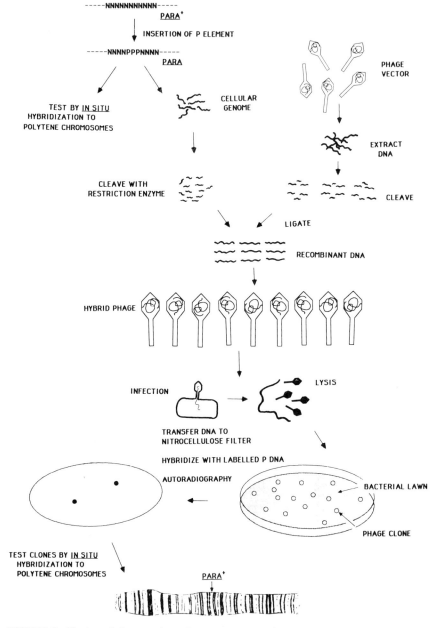

FIGURE 7. Cloning of the *para* locus by transposon tagging. Insertion of a transposable P element in the *para⁺* gene disrupts its function to produce a *para* mutation. After confirming the presence of a P element at the *para* locus by *in situ* hybridization (see FIG. 8), a recombinant DNA library is made using DNA from the mutant strain. To identify clones that contain P DNA sequences, DNA from all the clones is blotted onto nitrocellulose filters, denatured, and probed with ³²P-labeled P element DNA. Since the P element resides in multiple chromosomal locations as well as in the *para* locus, several different clones are recovered. After *in situ* hybridization of each clone to polytene chromosomes (which completely lack any P elements), the clones from the *para* locus are identifiable because they are the only ones that label the chromosome region containing *para*. (Based on a figure in Weinberg.[32])

mutations affecting sodium channels. For example, screening for new mutations that interact synergistically with *nap^ts* and/or *para^ts* may help identify other mutations affecting every step of sodium channel expression, assembly, and function. Two specific examples will suffice to illustrate this point. The *tip-E* (temperature-induced paralysis) mutation, discovered by Kulkarni,[22] was found to reduce viability in synergistic fashion when combined in double mutants with either *nap^ts* or *para^ts*.[23] The results of both STX binding experiments[24] and electrophysiological studies[23] indicate that *tip-E* affects sodium channels.

We have not yet exhausted all the mutations affecting functionally relevant components of this system. Recently, we found a new temperature-sensitive paralytic mutation that displays synergistic interactions with *para^ts*, *nap^ts*, and *tip-E* (B. Ganetzky, R. Kreber, and C. F.-Wu, unpublished). In addition, this mutation is dominant, suggesting that the product may serve a structural role. Analysis of this mutation is still underway, but like the mutations it interacts with, we expect it will turn out to affect sodium channels in some way.

CLONING OF *para* BY TRANSPOSON TAGGING

The mutations described here may be in genes that encode sodium channel subunits or they may be in genes affecting some other aspect of sodium channel production. Because we are interested in dissecting all the steps involved in the expression and assembly of sodium channels as well as their structure and function, we wish to identify and to characterize the protein products of the mutated genes. *Drosophila* is uniquely suited for such studies because it is possible to clone genes identified by mutations even in the absence of *a priori* information about the gene product and because the cloned genes can be reintroduced into flies after *in vitro* mutagenesis. We have concentrated on the cloning of *para* and *nap* to initiate molecular studies. Thus far, the cloning of *para* has progressed more rapidly and will serve to exemplify the approach.

Our protocol took advantage of the technique called transposon tagging (FIG. 7), which has been used successfully in a number of *Drosophila* laboratories to clone genes of interest.[25] Transposons are pieces of DNA of unknown function inhabiting the genomes of most organisms.[26] They occupy no fixed chromosomal location and are capable of transposing from one site to another, often at high frequencies. Should a transposon happen to insert itself into the normal allele of a gene of interest, the gene is interrupted to cause a mutant phenotype and a molecular tag for the gene is produced. A particularly useful transposon for this purpose in *Drosophila* is the P element because it can either be mobilized or made inert by a simple genetic cross.[27] When mobilized, it transposes at high frequency and inserts essentially randomly. The P element itself has been cloned so that it can be used to retrieve from a recombinant DNA library any gene in which it has inserted itself.[28]

From a cross in which the P element was mobilized, we recovered a new mutant *para* allele named *para^hd2*. To confirm that the new mutation was caused by the insertion of a P element at the *para* gene, we performed *in situ* hybridization to the giant polytene chromosomes (FIG. 8). Purified P element DNA was radioactively labeled and hybridized to polytene chromosomes from the *para^hd2* strain. Autoradiographic exposure revealed many different labeled chromosomal sites in the *para^hd2* strain. This was not surprising because the P element was present in the genome in multiple copies. What was critical was that one of the labeled sites corresponded exactly to the chromosomal position of the *para* gene, which we had determined previously by cytogenetic techniques. Thus, it seemed likely that the insertion of the P element at this site was the cause of the *para* mutation.[29] Conclusive evidence for this came from an experiment in which the P element was remobilized and revertants back to *para*[+] were recovered. Reversion to *para*[+] was correlated with loss of P element DNA from this chromosomal site.

Most of the extraneous P elements were removed by genetic crosses and a phage library was constructed using DNA from the resultant strain. The library was screened by using radioactively labeled P DNA as a probe and all phage plaques that hybridized to this probe were recovered. Because P elements were still inserted in at least three chromosome sites besides the *para* gene, we recovered clones deriving from each of these sites. Each of these clones was tested by *in situ* hybridization using chromosomes that lacked any P elements to identify those from the *para* region. Using DNA from a *para*[hd2] clone as a probe, we screened another phage library to recover the corresponding region from *para*[+] flies. We have now isolated approximately 50 kb of DNA from the *para*[+] region and mapped this region using restriction enzymes.

To determine what portion of this region actually corresponds to the *para* gene, we have located on the molecular map lesions associated with various mutant *para* alleles, including two associated with small insertions and two associated with the breakpoints of chromosomal inversions. These lesions are spread out over a distance of about 20 kb (FIG. 9). This gives us a minimum estimate of the size of the region involved in the

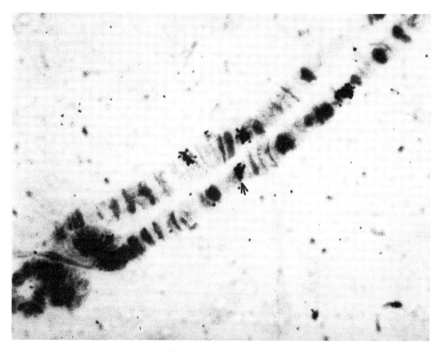

FIGURE 8. *In situ* hybridization of ^{32}P-labeled P element DNA to polytene chromosomes in the *para*[hd2] strain. Several sites of insertion of P elements are seen. One corresponds to the exact cytological location of the *para* locus (*arrow*). Thus the origin of the *para*[hd2] mutation as an insertion of the P element in the *para*[+] gene is confirmed.

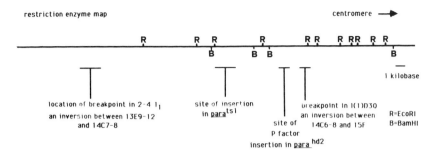

FIGURE 9. Molecular map of the DNA cloned from the *para* region. The site of insertion of the P element in the *para^hd2* strain and the location of chromosome breakpoint associated with other *para* mutations are indicated.

normal function of the *para⁺* gene. Still, we do not know what portion of this segment is transcribed into mRNA and translated into a polypeptide sequence.Thus, we are trying to identify the relevant transcripts from this region by RNA (Northern) blot analysis.

Once the transcript has been found the cDNA corresponding to this transcript can be sequenced to determine the amino acid sequence of the *para* gene product. Large amounts of this polypeptide can be produced in bacterial expression systems and used to generate specific antibodies. These antibodies can be used to identify the cellular location of *para⁺* gene product (cf. ref. 30). Mutations can be systematically created *in vitro* and the modified genes reintroduced into flies[31] to assess the effect of specific mutations on sodium channel function. In this way, the structure, function, and expression of this product will be elucidated at the molecular level. By application of similar techniques, other mutations affecting sodium channels such as *nap^ts* can also be characterized in molecular terms. These studies are currently underway.

CONCLUSIONS

Among higher organisms, *Drosophila* is perhaps unique in lending itself to detailed studies using genetic, electrophysiological, and molecular approaches. Using this combination of techniques to address the structure and function of sodium channels, we have been able to identify several genes that play prominent roles and to initiate the molecular analysis of these genes. Ultimately, we expect that the unique attributes of *Drosophila* will enable us to contribute to the understanding of sodium channels in novel ways.

ACKNOWLEDGMENTS

We gratefully acknowledge the expert technical assistance of Robert Kreber and James Berneking.

REFERENCES

1. NODA, M., S. SHIMAZU, T. TANABE, T. TAKAI, T. KAYANO, T. IKEDA, H. TAKAHASHI, H. NAKAYAMA, Y. KANAOKA, N. MINAMINO, K. KENGAWA, H. MATSUO, M. A. RAFTERY, T. HIROSE, S. INAYAMA, H. HAYASHIDA, T. MIYATA & S. NUMA. 1984. Primary structure of *Electrophorus electricus* sodium channel deduced from cDNA sequence. Nature **312**: 121–127.

2. SHERMAN, S. J. & W. A. CATTERALL. 1984. Electrical activity and cytosolic calcium regulate levels of tetrodotoxin-sensitive sodium channels in cultured rat muscle cells, Proc. Natl. Acad. Sci. U.S.A. **81**: 262–266.

3. WAXMAN, S. G. & J. M. RITCHIE. 1985. Organization of ion channels in the myelinated nerve fiber. Science **228**: 1502–1507.

4. WU, C.-F., B. GANETZKY, L. Y. JAN, Y. N. JAN & S. BENZER. 1978. A *Drosophila* mutant with a temperature-sensitive block in nerve conduction. Proc. Natl. Acad. Sci. U.S.A. **75**: 4047–4051.

5. WU, C.-F. & B. GANETZKY. 1980. Genetic alteration of nerve membrane excitability in temperature-sensitive paralytic mutants of *Drosophila melanogaster*. Nature **286**: 814–816.

6. SUZUKI, N. & C.-F. WU. 1984. Altered sensitivity to sodium channel-specific neurotoxins in cultured neurons from temperature-sensitive paralytic mutants of *Drosophila*. J. Neurogenet. **1**: 225–238.

7. JACKSON, F. R., S. D. WILSON, G. R. STRICHARTZ & L. M. HALL. 1984. Two types of mutants affecting voltage-sensitive sodium channels in *Drosophila melanogaster*. Nature **308**: 189–191.

8. KAUVAR, L. 1982. Reduced [³H]tetrodotoxin binding in the *nap^{ts}* paralytic mutant of *Drosophila*. Mol. Gen. Genet. **187**: 172–173.

9. KAPLAN, W. D. & W. E. TROUT. 1969. The behavior of four neurological mutants of *Drosophila*. Genetics **61**: 399–409.

10. JAN, Y. N., L. Y. JAN & M. J. DENNIS. 1977. Two mutations of synaptic transmission in *Drosophila*. Proc. R. Soc. (London) Ser. B. **198**: 87–108.

11. SALKOFF, L. & R. WYMAN. 1981. Genetic modification of potassium channels in *Drosophila Shaker* mutants. Nature **293**: 228–230.

12. TANOUYE, M., A. FERRUS & S. FUJITA. 1981. Abnormal action potentials associated with the *Shaker* complex locus of *Drosophila*. Proc. Natl. Acad. Sci. U.S.A. **78**: 6548–6552.

13. WU, C.-F. & F. J. HAUGLAND. 1985. Voltage clamp analysis of membrane currents in larval muscle fibers of *Drosophila:* Alteration of potassium currents in *Shaker* mutants. J. Neurosci. **5**: 2626–2640.

14. GANETZKY, B. & C.-F. WU. 1982. Indirect suppression involving behavioral mutants with altered nerve excitability in *Drosophila melanogaster*. Genetics **100**: 597–614.

15. GANETZKY, B. & C.-F. WU. 1982. *Drosophila* mutants with opposing effects on nerve excitability: Genetic and spatial interactions in repetitive firing. J. Neurophysiol. **47**: 501–514.

16. WU, C.-F., B. GANETZKY, F. N. HAUGLAND & A. X. LIU. 1983. Potassium currents in *Drosophila:* Different components affected by mutations of two genes. Science **220**: 1076–1078.

17. GANETZKY, B. & C.-F. WU. 1983. Neurogenetic analysis of potassium currents in *Drosophila:* Synergistic effects on neuromuscular transmission in double mutants. J. Neurogenet. **1**: 17–28.

18. SUN, Y.-A. & C.-F. WU. 1985. Genetic alteration of single-channel currents in dissociated CNS neurons of *Drosophila*. Soc. Neurosci. Abstr. **11**: 787.

19. SUZUKI, D. T., T. GRIGLIATTI & R. WILLIAMSON. 1971. Temperature-sensitive mutants in *Drosophila melanogaster* VII. A mutation (*para^{ts}*) causing reversible adult paralysis. Proc. Natl. Acad. Sci. U.S.A. **68**: 890–893.

20. GANETZKY, B. 1984. Genetic studies of membrane excitability in Drosophila: Lethal interaction between two temperature-sensitive paralytic mutations. Genetics **108**: 897–911.

21. BURG, M. G. & C.-F. WU. 1984. Blockage of a reflex response in genetic mosaics by

temperature-sensitive mutations: Effects on sensory cells derived from imaginal discs of *Drosophila*. Soc. Neurosci. Abstr. **11:** 917.
22. KULKARNI, S. & A. PADHYE. 1982. Temperature-sensitive paralytic mutations on the second and third chromosomes of *Drosophila melanogaster*. Genetic Res. **40:** 191–199.
23. GANETZKY, B. 1986. Neurogenetic analysis of *Drosophila* mutations affecting sodium channels: Synergistic effects on viability and nerve conduction in double mutants involving *tip-E*. J. Neurogenet. **3:** 19–31.
24. JACKSON, F. R., S. D. WILSON & L. M. HALL. 1986. The *tip-E* mutation of *Drosophila* decreases saxitoxin binding and interacts with other mutations affecting nerve membrane excitability. J. Neurogenet. **3:** 1–17.
25. BINGHAM, P. M., R. LEVIS & G. M. RUBIN. 1981. Cloning of DNA sequences from the *white* locus of *D. melanogaster* by a novel and general method. Cell **25:** 693–704.
26. CALOS, M. P. & J. H. MILLER. 1980. Transposable elements. Cell **20:** 579–595.
27. ENGELS, W. R. 1983. The P family of transposable elements in *Drosophila*. Ann. Rev. Genet. **17:** 315–344.
28. SEARLES, L. L., R. S. JOKERST, P. M. BINGHAM, R. A. VOELKER & A. L. GREENLEAF. 1983. Molecular cloning of sequences from a Drosophila RNA polymerase locus by P element transposon tagging. Cell **31:** 585–592.
29. LOUGHNEY, K. & B. GANETZKY. 1985. Cloning of a gene affecting sodium channels in *Drosophila*. Soc. Neurosci. Abstr. **11:** 782.
30. WHITE, R. A. H. & M. WILCOX. 1984. Protein products of the bithorax complex in Drosophila. Cell **39:** 163–171.
31. RUBIN, G. M. & A. C. SPRADLING. 1982. Genetic transformation of Drosophila with transposable element vectors. Science **218:** 348–353.
32. WEINBERG, R. A. 1983. A molecular basis of cancer. Sci. American **249:** 126–142.

Molecular Structure of Sodium Channels

SHOSAKU NUMA AND MASAHARU NODA

Departments of Medical Chemistry and Molecular Genetics
Kyoto University Faculty of Medicine
Kyoto 606, Japan

INTRODUCTION

The sodium channel is a transmembrane protein that mediates the voltage-dependent modulation of the sodium ion permeability of electrically excitable membranes.[1-3] Biochemical evidence has indicated that the sodium channels purified from the electric organ of the eel *Electrophorus electricus*[4,5] and from chick cardiac muscle[6] consist of a single polypeptide of relative molecular mass (M_r) ~260,000, whereas those purified from rat brain[7] and skeletal muscle[8] contain, in addition to the corresponding large polypeptide, two or three smaller polypeptides of M_r 37,000–45,000. The purified *Electrophorus* and rat sodium channel preparations have been shown to be functional when reconstituted into phospholipid vesicles.[9-13]

Very little was known, however, about the molecular basis for the selective ion transport and voltage-dependent gating operated by the sodium channel. Furthermore, several types of tetrodotoxin (or saxitoxin) binding sites or sodium currents have been observed in many excitable membranes,[14-23] despite the apparent homogeneity of the purified sodium channel preparations. It has not been determined whether these distinguishable populations of sodium channels are due to different states of the same channel protein or to different channel proteins. A promising approach to these issues has been provided by the use of recombinant DNA techniques. The complete amino acid sequences of the *Electrophorus electricus* electroplax sodium channel as well as two distinct sodium channel large polypeptides (designated as sodium channels I and II) from rat brain have been elucidated by these techniques. A partial amino acid sequence of a third rat brain protein homologous to the sodium channel large polypeptides has also been deduced. Structural features characteristic of the sodium channel proteins are discussed in terms of the function of the voltage-gated ionic channel.

PRIMARY STRUCTURE

The isolation of cDNA clones encoding the *Electrophorus* electroplax and rat brain sodium channels has been described.[24,25] FIGURES 1–3 show the nucleotide sequences of the cloned cDNAs encoding the *Electrophorus* sodium channel and rat sodium channels I and II, respectively, together with the respective amino acid sequences deduced from the cDNA sequences. The three sodium channels consist of 1,820, 2,009 (or 1,998, see legend to FIG. 2), and 2,005 amino acid residues (including the initiating methionine), with calculated M_r 208,321, 228,758 (or 227,576), and 227,840, respectively; at positions where amino acid differences are predicted by the nucleotide differences found among the individual clones, the amino acids given in FIGURE 4 have been taken for the calculation of M_r. These values agree with the reported M_r of the protein moiety of the sodium channels.[5,27] Nucleotide sequence

338

analysis of a rat brain cDNA clone of the third type revealed that it encodes a sequence of 573 amino acids highly homologous with the carboxy-terminal sequences of sodium channels I and II.[25]

FIGURE 4 shows the alignment of the amino acid sequences of rat sodium channels I and II and the *Electrophorus* sodium channel. The degree of sequence homology is 87%, 62%, and 62% for the rat I: rat II, rat I: *Electrophorus* and rat II: *Electrophorus* pairs, respectively. Homology matrix comparison[28] of the amino acid sequences revealed the presence of four internal repeats with homologous sequences, referred to as repeats I, II, III, and IV. The amino acid sequences of the four repeats are aligned in FIGURE 5. This observation strongly suggests that the four repeated homology units evolved from a single common ancestor by internal duplications. The regions corresponding to these repeats are highly conserved among the three sodium channels, whereas the remaining regions, all of which are assigned to the cytoplasmic side of the membrane (see below), are less well conserved, except the region between repeats III and IV. A large insertion of 166–178 amino acids occurs in the region between repeats I and II of the rat sodium channels, as compared with the *Electrophorus* counterpart. The inserted segment contains several potential sites of phosphorylation by cyclic AMP-dependent protein kinase,[29] which are conserved in the two rat sodium channels.

FUNCTIONAL IMPLICATIONS

FIGURE 6 shows the hydropathy profiles[30] of the three sodium channel molecules. Each internal repeat has five hydrophobic segments (S1, S2, S3, S5, and S6) and one positively charged segment (S4), all of which exhibit predicted secondary structure.[31] Segments S1, S2, and S3 generally contain a few charged residues. S3 has a few negative charges, and S2 a few negative and positive charges, whereas S1 is not uniform in charge. Segment S4 contains four to eight arginine or lysine residues located at every third position with mostly nonpolar residues intervening between the basic residues. Segments S5 and S6 are highly hydrophobic regions without any charged residues (except S6 in repeat II of sodium channel I).

It seems reasonable to assume that the four repeated homology units of the sodium channel are oriented in a pseudosymmetric fashion across the membrane. This implies the presence of an even number of transmembrane segments in each repeat because no additional hydrophobic segments are predicted outside the repeats (FIG. 6). Segments S1–S6 in each repeat presumably traverse the membrane, forming α-helical structures.[24,25] Furthermore, the sodium channels have no hydrophobic prepeptide,[32] and may, like some transmembrane proteins devoid of a cleavable prepeptide, have their amino terminus on the cytoplasmic side of the membrane. The transmembrane topology of the sodium channel molecule has therefore been described as shown in FIGURE 7A. The proposed transmembrane topology is consistent with six of the seven potential N-glycosylation sites[33] that are conserved in all the three sodium channels as well as with all the potential cyclic AMP-dependent phosphorylation sites.[29]

The ion selectivity of the sodium channel makes it unlikely that segment S4 with many positive charges constitutes the inner wall of the channel. It seems more reasonable to locate this segment within clusters of other segments (FIG. 7B). The formation of ion pairs between many of the positive charges in segment S4 and the negative charges in other segments such as S3 and S1 would stabilize the intramembranous location of the charged segments. The voltage-dependent gating of the sodium channel implies the presence of a voltage sensor, which is thought to be a collection of

```
                                          5'-----ACCGTGATGACGCTTTAGTGTGCAGTTCTGCTGGGTGTCGTATACCAGAAATCGAATCTTGTTACCTCACTGCAGTGACTCTCT   -301
AGATGCTGTTCTTAGATTAATATATAATTAGAAGTAATCCTGTGTCTTTAAGCTTGAATACAAGTACTTTTCTTTATTTTATAGTGTAAATCCATTTTTTTTTACACTTTTTTAGAGGAAGCAAAAAAAACCAAAAACCCAAAAACTTAG  -151
CATTGAGTTTGCAATACTAATGCTCTCTACTGGTTGTGGAGTATTGCTATTCTATCTCTGGGCTATTGCTAGTCTGCAACATTGATCTTCTGCATCTTGAGCTTCGGATAGAGATTCCACTCTGAGGTGATATCTTTCCGCGATGCGAAG    -1
  1         10        20        30        40        50
MetAlaArgLysPheSerSerAlaArgProGluMetPheArgArgPheThrProAspSerLeuGluGluIleGluAlaPheThrGluLeuLysLysSerCysThrLeuGluLysLysGluProGluSerThrProArgIleAspLeuAla
ATGGCTCGCAAGTTCTCTTCCGCACGCCCCGAAATGTTTCGCCGCTTCACCCCAGATTCACTGGAGGAGATTGAGGCGTTCACTGAGCTGAAGAAAAGTTGTACGTTAGAGAAGAAGGAGCCGGAGTCAACACCTAGAATTGACCTGGAG    150
  60        70        80        90        100
AlaGlyLysProLeuProMetIleTyrGlyAspProProGluAspLeuAsnIleProLeuGluGluAspLeuAspProPheTyrLysThrGlnLysThrPheIleValIleSerLysGlyAsnIleIleAsnArgPheAsnAlaGluArg
GCGGGGAAACCTCTGCCCATGATATATGGAGACCCACCAGAGGACCTGCTCAACATCCCACTGGAGGATCTTGACCCCTTCTACAAAACTCAGAAAACATTTATTGTGATTAGCAAGGGAAACATAATCAACAGATTCAATGCAGAACGA    300
  110       120       130       140       150
AlaLeuTyrIlePheSerProPheAsnProIleArgArgGlyAlaIleArgValPheValAsnSerAlaPheAsnPhePheIleMetPheThrIlePheSerAsnCysIlePheMetThrIleSerAsnProProAlaTrpSerLysIle
GCTTTGTACATCTTCAGTCCGTTTAACCCTATCAGAAGAGGAGCCATTCGGGTTTTTGTAAACTCGGCATTTAATTTTTTCATCATGTTCACCATCTTCTCTAACTGCATATTCATGACTATAAGCAACCCTCCTGCCTGGAGTAAAATT    450
  160       170       180       190       200
ValGluTyrThrPheThrGlyIleTyrThrPheGluValIleValLysValLeuSerArgGlyPheCysIleGlyHisPheThrPheLeuArgAspProThrrpAsnTrpLeuAspPheSerValValThrPheMetThrTyrIleThrGluPhe
GTGGAATATACTTTTACAGGTATATATACCTTTGAAGTAATAGTCAAAGTCCTATCCAGAGGCTTCTGTATTGGACATTTTACATTCCTTCGTGATCCATGGAACTGGCTGGATTTTCTGGTGGTCACCATGACGTATATCACAGAGTTT    600
  210       220       230       240       250
IleAspLeuArgAsnValSerAlaLeuArgThrPheArgValLeuArgAlaLeuLysThrIleThrIlePheProGlyLeuLysThrIleValArgAlaLeuIleGlnSerMetLysGlnMetGlyAspValValAllIleLeuThrValPhe
ATTGACCTTAGAAACGTGTCAGCACTTAGGACATTCCGTGTGCTCCGAGCTCTCAAGACAATCACTATTTTTCCTGGACTGAAAACTATTGTCAGAGCTTTGATCGAGTCGATGAAGCAGATGGGTGACGTGGTGATCCTGACCGTCTTC    750
  260       270       280       290       300
SerLeuAlaValPheThrLeuAlaGlyMetGlnLeuPheMetGlyAsnLeuArgHisLysCysIleArgTrpProIleSerAsnValThrLeuAspTyrGluSerAlaTyrAsnThrPheAspAsnPheAlaTyrIleGluAsnGlu
TCTCTGGCTGTGTTCACCCTCGCCGGGATGCAGCTGTTCATGGGGAACCTACGACACAAGTGCATTCGCTGGCCCATCTCTAACGTTACCCTCGATTATGAATCTGCCTACAACACCACTTTTGACTTTACAGCCTACATTGAAAATGAA    900
  310       320       330       340       350
GluAsnGlnTyrPheLeuAspGlyValAspAspAlaLeuLeuCysGlyAsnAsnSerAspAlaGlyLysCysProGluGlyTyrThrCysMetLysAlaGlyArgAsnProAsnTyrGlyTyrThrAsnTyrAspAsnPheAlaTrpThr
GAAAATCAGTACTTTCTCGATGGTGCTTGATGCCTTACTATGTGGCAACAATTCTGATGCTGGAAAGTGTCCAGAAGGCTATACGTGTATGAAGGCTGGGCGGAACCCAAACTACGGCTACACAAACTATGACAACTTTGCCTGGACT    1050
  360       370       380       390       400
PheLeuCysLeuPheArgLeuMetLeuGlnAspTyrTrpGluAsnLeuTyrGlnMetThrLeuArgAlaAlaGlyLysSerTyrMetValPhePheMetValIlePheLeuGlySerPheTyrLeuIleAsnLeuIleLeuAlaValAval
TTCCTGTGCCTCTTTAGGCTCATGCTTCAAGACTACTGGGAGAACCTCTATCAGATGACCTCTCCGTGCTGCTGGGAAAGGCTACATGGTGTTCTTCATCATGGTCATATTCCTGGGTTCCTTCTATCTTATCAACCTAATCCTGGCTGTA    1200
  410       420       430       440       450
ValAlaMetAlaTyrGluGluGlnAsnGlnAlaThrLeuAlaGluAlaGlnGluLysGluGlnAlaGluPheGlnAsnMetLeuGluGlnLeuLysLysGlnGlnGluGluIleGlnGlnGluLeuAsnAspGluArgLysAlaSerLeuAlaSerGlnLeuThr
GTTGCTATGGCATATGAGGAGCAGAATCAGGCAACACTGGCTGAGGCTCAAGAGAAAGAAGCTGAGTTCCAGAACATGCTAGAACAGCTCAAGAAGCAGCAGGAAGAGATCCAGCAGGAGCTCAATGATGAGAGGAAGGCATCTTTAGCCAGTCAGTTAACT    1350
```

(sequence continues)

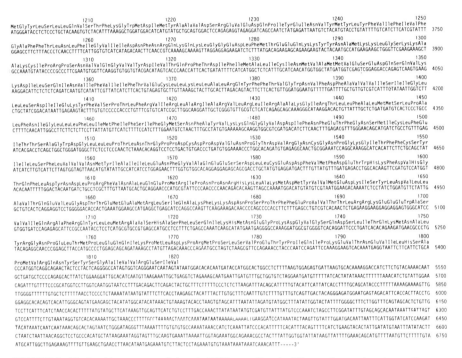

FIGURE 1. Nucleotide sequence of cloned cDNA encoding the *Electrophorus electricus* sodium channel. Nucleotide residues are numbered in the 5' to 3' direction, beginning with the first residue of the ATG triplet encoding the initiating methionine, and the nucleotides on the 5' side of residue 1 are indicated by negative numbers; the number of the nucleotide residue at the right end of each line is given. The deduced amino acid sequence of the sodium channel is shown above the nucleotide sequence, and amino acid residues are numbered beginning with the initiating methionine. (From Noda *et al.*[24] Reprinted from *Nature*, Copyright 1984 Macmillan Journals Limited.)

```
                          5'-----TACTGCAGAGGTCTCTGGTGCATGTGTATGTGTGTGCGTGTGTTTGTGTACGTATGTTCTGCCCCTGTCAGGCTGCAGCCCTTGTGAAACACTTGGTCACC  -151
TTTTGCAAGAAGGAAATCTCTGAATCGTTGCAACTGAAGGTGCGGACTCGGCTCGGGAGATGTTGTTCCTTACTGCAGATAGATAATTTTCCTTTTTATCAGGAATCTCACATGAAGAGTAAAGAGTAATTAAAATGTGCAGGATGACAAG  -1
  1                  10                 20                 30                 40                 50
ATGGAGCAAACAGTGCTTGTACCACCAGGACCTGACAGCTTCAACTTCTTCACCAGAGAATCTCTTGCAGCTATTGAAAGGCGCATTGCAGAAGAAAAAGCTAAGAATCCCAAGCCAGACAAAAAGATGATGATGAAAATGGCCTCAAAG  150
MetGluGlnThrValLeuValProProGlyProAspSerPheAsnPheTheThrArgGluSerLeuAlaAlaIleGluArgArgIleAlaGluGluLysAlaLysAsnProLysProAspLysLysAspAspAspAspLysAsnGlyProLys
 60                 70                 80                 90                100
CCGAACAGTGACTTGGAAGCTGGGAAGAACCTTCCATTTATCTATGGAGACATTCCTCCAGAGATGGTGTCGGAGCCTGGAGGACCTGGACCCCTACTATATCAATAAGAAAACTTTTATAGTATTGAATAAAGGGAAGGCCATCTTC  300
ProAsnSerAspLeuGluAlaGlyLysAsnLeuProPheIleTyrGlyAspIleProProGluMetValSerGluProGlyGlyProGlyProLeuLeuTyrIleAsnLysLysThrPheIleValLeuAsnLysGlyLysAlaIlePhe
 110                120                130  .             140                150
CGGTTCAGTGCCACTTCTGCCCTGTACATTTTAACTCCCTTCAATCCTCTTAGGAAAATAGCTATTAAGATTTTGGTACACTCATTATTCAGCATGTTAATTATGTGCACTATTTTGACGAACTGTGTATTTATGACAATGAGTAACCCT  450
ArgPheSerAlaThrSerAlaLeuTyrIleLeuThrProPheAsnProLeuArgLysIleAlaIleLysIleLeuValHisSerLeuPheSerMetLeuIleMetCysThrIleLeuThrAsnCysValPheMetThrMetSerAsnPro
 160                170                180                190                200
CCTGACTGGACAAAGAATGTAGAGTACACCTTCACAGGAATATATACCTTTGAATCACTAATAAAAATTATTGCAAGGGGCTTCTGTTTAGAAGATTTTACTTTCCTTCGTGACCCATGGAACTGGCTGGACTTCACTGTCATTACATTC  600
ProAspTrpThrLysAsnValGluTyrThrPheThrGlyIleTyrThrPheGluSerLeuIleLysIleIleAlaArgGlyPheCysLeuGluAspPheThrPheLeuArgAspProTrpAsnTrpLeuAspPheThrValIleThrPhe
 210                220                230                240                250
GCATATGTGACGGAGTTTGTGGACCTGGGCAATGTCTCAGCGTTGAGAACATTCAGAGTTCTTCGAGCATTGAAAACAATATCAGTCATTCCAGGCCTGAAGACCATCGTGGGGGCCCTGATCCAGTCTGTGAAGAAGCTCTCTGACGTC  750
AlaTyrValThrGluPheValAspLeuGlyAsnValSerAlaLeuArgThrPheArgValLeuArgAlaLeuLysThrIleSerValIleProGlyLeuLysThrIleValGlyAlaLeuIleGlnSerValLysLysLeuSerAspVal
 260                270                280                290                300
ATGATCCTCACCGTGTTCTGTCTCAGTGTGTTTGCTCTAATCGGGTTGCAGCTTTTCATGGGCAACCTGAGGAATAAGTGTGTACAGTGGCCCCCAACCACCCTTGAGGAACATAGCATAGAGAAGAATGTAACTACGGATTAC  900
MetIleLeuThrValPheCysLeuSerValPheAlaLeuIleGlyLeuGlnLeuPheMetGlyAsnLeuArgAsnLysCysValGlnTrpProProThrThrLeuGluHisSerIleGluLysAsnValThrThrAspTyr
 310                320                330                340                350
AACGGCACACTTGTAAATGAAACCGTGTTTGAATTTGACTGGAAATCATACATTCAAGACTCAAGATATCATTATTTCCTGGAGGGTGTTTTAGATGCACTACTGTGTGGAAATAGCTCTGATGCAGGCCAATGTCCAGAAGGTTACATG  1050
AsnGlyThrLeuValAsnGluThrValPheGluPheAspTrpLysSerTyrIleGlnAspSerArgTyrHisTyrPheLeuGluGlyValLeuAspAlaLeuLeuCysGlyAsnSerSerAspAlaGlyGlnCysProGluGlyTyrMet
 360                370                380                390                400
TGTGTAAAAGCTGGCAGAAACCCTAACTATGGTTACACAAGCTTTGACACCTTCAGCTGGGCATTTCTGTCCCTGTTTCGACTGATGACTCAGGACTTCTGTGGGAAAATCTTTACCAACTGACATTGCGTGCTGCCGGGAAAACATACATG  1200
CysValLysAlaGlyArgAsnProAsnTyrGlyTyrThrSerPheAspThrPheSerTrpAlaPheLeuSerLeuPheArgLeuMetThrGlnAspPheCysGlyLysIlePheThrAsnCysValValAlaGlyProGluGlyTyrMet
 410                420                430                440                450
ATATTTTTGTGCTGGTCATTTTCTTGGGCTCATTCTACCTGATAAACTTGATCCTGGCTGTGGTGGCCATGGCCTATGAGGAACAGAACCAGGCCACATTGGAGGAGGCTGAACAGAAGGAGGCAGAGTTTCAGCAGATGCTGGAGCAA  1350
IlePhePheValLeuValIleSerPheTyrLeuIleAsnLeuIleLeuAlaValValAlaMetAlaTyrGluGluGlnAsnGlnAlaThrLeuGluGluAlaGluGlnLysGluAlaGluPheGlnGlnMetLeuGluGln
 460                470                480   Asn          490                500
CTGAAGAAGCAGCAGGAGGCCGCACAGCAGGCGGCGGCGGCAACAGCATCAGACATCCAGGGACCCCAGTGCAGCGGGAGGCTCTCAAGTTGAGTTCAAAGAGCGCTAAAGAAAGGCGGAATCGG  1500
LeuLysLysGlnGlnGluAlaAlaGlnGlnAlaAlaAlaAlaThrAlaSerGluHisSerArgGluProSerAlaAlaGlyArgLeuSerAspSerSerSerGluAlaSerLysLeuSerSerLysSerAlaLysGluArgArgAsnArg
 510                520   A            530                540                550
AGGAAAAAAGAAAACAGAAAGAGCAGTCTGGAGGGGAAGAGAAAGATGATGATGAATTCCACAAATCCGAGTCCGAAGATACATCAGGAGAGGAAGGGCTTCCGCTTCTCCCATAGAAGGGACAGACTGACTATGAAAAGAGGTACTCT  1650
ArgLysLysArgLysGlnLysGlnGluGlyGlyGluGluLysAspAspAspGluPheHisLysSerGluSerGluAspTheSerGlyGluGluGlyLeuProPheLeuProPheArgArgLysIleLeuGlnSerLysGlnGluArgTyrSer
 560                570                580                590   Lys          600
TCCCCACATCAGTCTCTGTTGAGCATTCGCGGCTCACTGTTTTCCCCGAGACGCAATAGCAGAACAAGTCTTTTCAGCTTCAGAGGGCGAGCGAAGGACGTGGGGTCTGAGATTGGATTTGGCAGCATGAGCACACGACACCTTCGAGGAC  1800
SerProHisGlnSerLeuLeuSerIleArgGlySerLeuPheSerProGluArgAsnSerArgThrSerLeuPheSerPheArgGlyArgAlaLysAspValGlySerAsnSerSerThrPheGlyAsp
 610                620                630   A            650
AATGAAGCAGGAGAACTCTCTGTTTGTTCCCCGAAGACATTGAAGACGCAACAGTAACCTCAGCCAAACCAGCAGATCCTCCCGAATGCTGGCGGGGCTTCCAGCAAACGGGAAGATGCACAGCACAGTGGATTGGTGTG  1950
AsnGluSerArgArgAspSerLeuProValProArgArgIleGlyAlaGlnArgThrSerSerLeuSerGlnThrSerArgSerSerArgMetLeuAlaGlyLeuProAlaAsnGlyLysMetHisSerThrValAspCysAsnGlyVal
 660                670                680                690                700
GTTTCCTTGGTGGGCGGACCCTCGGTTCCGACATCGCCAGTTGGACAGCTTCTGCCAGAGGTGATAATAGATAAGCCAGCTACTGATGACAATGGACAACTACTGAACTGAGATGAGAAAGAGGAGGTCAAGTTCTTTCCCATGTTTCC  2100
ValSerLeuValGlyGlyProSerValProThrSerProValGlyGlnLeuLeuProGluValIleIleAspLysProAlaThrAspAspAsnGlyGlnLeuLeuAsnLeuArgMetArgLysArgArgGlnValLysLysSerGlnValPheAla
 710                720                730                740                750
ATGGACTTTCTTGAGGATCCTTCCCAGAGGCAAAGGGCAATGAGCATTGCCAGCATCTTAACAAATACAGTAGAAGAACTAGAAGAATCCAGCAGAAATGTCCACCCTGTTGGTATAAATTTTCCAACATATTTTTTAAATTTGGGACTGT  2250
MetAspPheLeuGluAspProSerGlnArgGlnArgAlaMetSerIleAlaSerIleLeuThrAsnThrValGluGluLeuGluGluSerSerArgAsnValHisProValGlyIleAsnPheProThrProTyrLysPheSerAsnIlePheTrpAspCys
 760                770                780                790                800
TCTCCATATTGGCTAAAAGTTAAACATATTGTCAACCTGGTTGTGATGGACCCATTTGTTGACCTGGCAATTACTATCTGTATTGTGTTAAATACCCTTTTCATGGCCATGGAGCACTACCCCATGACTGAACATTTCAATCATGTACTT  2400
SerProTyrTrpLeuLysValLysHisIleValAsnLeuValValMetAspProPheValAspLeuAlaIleThrIleCysIleValLeuAsnThrLeuPheMetAlaMetGluHisTyrProMetThrGluHisPheAsnHisValLeu
 810                820   Asn          830                840                850
ACAGTAGGAAACTTGGTTTTCACTGGGATCTTCACAGCAGAAATGTTCCTGAAAATCATTGCCATGGACCCTTACTATTATTTCCAAGAGGGCTGGAATATCTTTGATGGTTTCATTGTGACACTCAGCCTGGTAGAACTTGGCCTT  2550
ThrValGlyAsnLeuValPheThrGlyIlePheThrAlaGluMetPheLeuLysIleIleAlaMetAspProTyrTyrTyrPheGlnGluGlyTrpAsnIlePheAspGlyPheIleValThrLeuSerLeuValGluLeuGlyLeuAla
 860                870   A            880                890                900
AATGTGAAGGGTTATCAGTTCTCCGTTCATTCCGGATCTTCCAAGTTGGCAAAGTCCTGGCCCACACTGAACATGCTCATTAAGATCATCGGCAACTCGGTGGGCGCACTGGGGCAACCTGACCCTGGTGCTGGCCATCATC  2700
AsnValGluSerValLeuArgTyrSerPheHisSerGlySerSerLysLeuAlaLysSerTrpProThrLeuAsnMetLeuIleLysIleIleGlyAsnSerValGlyAlaLeuGlyAsnLeuThrLeuValLeuAlaIleIle
 910                920                930                940                950
GTCTTCATTTTTGCCGTGGTCGGCATGCAGCTGTTCGGCAAAAGTTACAAAGATTGTGTCTGCAAAATTGCCACTGACTGCAAACTCCCGCGGCTGGCACATGAACGACTCTTTCCCACTCCTTCCTGATCGTGTTCGTCGTGTTCGGG  2850
ValPheIlePheAlaValValGlyMetGlnLeuPheGlyLysSerTyrLysAspCysValCysLysIleAlaThrAspCysLysLeuProArgTrpHisMetAsnAspPheHisHisSerPheLeuIleValPheArgValLeuCysGly
 960                970                980                990               1000
GAGTGGATAGAGACCATGTGGGACTGCATGGAGGTCGCGGGTCAGGCCATGTGCCTTACTGTCTTCATGATGGTCATGGTGATTGGGAACCTGGTGGTCCTCAACCTT  3000
GluTrpIleGluThrMetTrpAspCysMetGluValAlaGlyGlnAlaMetCysLeuThrValPheMetMetValMetValIleGlyAsnLeuValValLeuAsnLeuPheLeuAlaLeuLeuLeuSerSerPheSerAlaAspAsnLeu
1010               1020               1030               1040               1050
GCAGCCACTGCGATGACAACGAAATGAACAACCTTCAAATTGCTGTGGACAGGATGCACAAAGGAGTAGCTTATGTAAAAGAAAAATATATGAGTTTATTCAACAGTCCTTGTTAGGAAACAGAAGATCCTAGATGAAATTAAGCCA  3150
AlaAlaThrAlaMetThrThrLysMetAsnAsnLeuGlnIleAlaValAspArgMetHisLysGlyValAlaTyrValLysLysLysTyrGluPheIleGlnSerProValLeuGlyGlyLysLeuLeuAspGluIleLysPro
1060               1070               1080               1090               1100
CTTGATGATCTAAACAACAAGAAAGACAATTGTACATCTAACCACACGACAGAGATTGGGAAAGATCTGGACTGTCTGGAAGGAGAGATCGACAGGTGCACAAGGACCGGCAGAGGGTGGAAAAGTACATCATTGATGAGAGT  3300
LeuAspAspLeuAsnAsnLysLysAspAsnCysIleSerAsnHisThrThrGluIleGlyLysAspLeuAspCysLeuLysAspAlaAsnGlyThrThrSerGlyIleGlyThrGlySerSerValGluLysTyrIleIleAspGluSer
1110               1120               1130               1140               1150
GACTACATGTCATTCATAAACAACCCCAGCCTCACCGTGACTGTGCCCATTGCTGTGGGAGAGTCTGACTTTGAAAACTTAAACACAGAGGATTTTAGCAGTGAATCAGATCTAGAAGAAAGCAAAGAAAAGCTCAACGAAAGCAGTAGT  3450
AspTyrMetSerPheIleAsnAsnProSerLeuThrValThrValProIleAlaValGlyGluSerAspPheGluAsnLeuAsnThrGluAspPheSerSerGluSerAspLeuGluGluSerLysGluLysLeuAsnGluSerSerSer
1160               1170               1180               1190               1200
TCCTCAGAAGGAAGCACAGTAGACATCGGGGCGCCTGCGGAGGAACAGCCTGTCGTGGAACCAGAAGAAACCTTGAGCCCCGAAGCTTGCTTCACTGAAGGCTGTGTCCAAAATCAGTGTGGAAAGAAGGAAGA  3600
SerSerGluGlySerThrValAspIleGlyAlaProAlaGluGluGlnProValValGluProGluGluThrLeuSerProGluAlaCysPheThrGluGlyCysValGlnAsnGlnCysGlyLysLysPheProSerArgPro
1210               1220               1230               1240               1250
GGAAAACAGTGGTGAACCTTCGGAGAACCTGTCTTCCCGAATAGTTGAGCACATCATCGATCAGCAAGAGAACAATCAAGACC  3750
GlyLysGlnTrpTrpAsnLeuArgArgThrCysPheArgIleValGluHisAsnTrpPheGluThrPheIleValPheMetIleLeuLeuSerSerGlyAlaLeuAlaPheGluAspIleTyrIleGluAspArgLysThrIleLysThr
1260               1270               1280               1290               1300
ATGCTGGAGTATGCAGACAAGGTTTTCACTTACATTTTTATCCTGGAGATGCTCCTCAAATGGGTAGCCTACGGCTATCAAACGTATTTCACCAATGCCTGGTGTTGGCTGGACTTCTTAATTGTTGATGTTTCATTGGTCAGTTTAACA  3900
MetLeuGluTyrAlaAspLysValPheThrTyrIlePheIleLeuGluMetLeuLeuLysTrpValAlaTyrGlyTyrGlnThrTyrPheThrAsnAlaTrpCysTrpLeuAspPheLeuIleValAspValSerLeuValSerLeuThr
1310               1320               1330               1340               1350
GCAAATGCCTTGGGTTACTCGGAACTTGGGGCCATCAAGTCCCTCAGGACACTAAGAGCTCTCGAGACCCCTAAGAGCCTTTATCACGATTTGAAGGGATGAGGGTGGTTGTGAGACGCCGTGTTAGGAGCAATTCCATCCATCATGAATGTG  4050
AlaAsnAlaLeuGlyTyrSerGluLeuGlyAlaIleLysSerLeuArgThrLeuArgAlaLeuArgProLeuArgAlaLeuSerArgGlnGlyMetArgValValValValAsnAlaLeuLeuGlyAlaIleProSerIleMetAsnVal
```

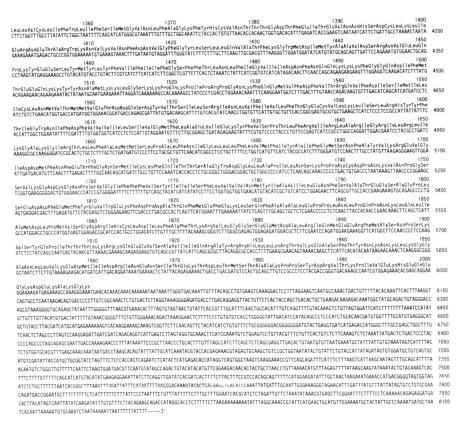

FIGURE 2. Nucleotide sequence of cloned cDNA encoding rat sodium channel I (see legend to FIG. 1). The nucleotide differences observed among the individual clones analyzed, together with the resulting amino acid substitutions, are given. Deletion of nucleotide residues 2,011–2,043 (amino acid residues 671–681, underlined) occurs in some of the clones. S_1 nuclease mapping of rat brain poly(A)$^+$ RNA indicated the presense of the mRNA both with and without this deletion. (From Noda et al.[25] Reprinted from Nature, Copyright 1986 Macmillan Journals Limited.)

```
                                            5'-----ACCCCCTGTCTTTGCTTTTCCTCTTTAGTAAGGATATTATTGCACATGTGAGATTTTTAC  -151
TTCCTACTGTAGGCTGAATTCTAGAAACCTGCACTGGAGACTGCTACATTCAACACGCACATGGATTCTGTGCTATGATTACCATTCCTTTTATTTCAGCACTTTCTTACGCGAGGAGCTAAACAGTGACTAAAGAAGCAGGATGAAAAG   -1

 1                 10                  20                  30                  40                  50
MetAlaArgSerValLeuValProProGlyProAspSerPheArgPhePheThrArgGluSerLeuAlaAlaIleGlnGlnArgIleAlaGluGluLysAlaLysArgProLysGlnGluArgLysAspGluAspGluAsnGlyPro
ATGGCACGGTCAGTGCTGGTACCTCCAGGACCTGACAGCTTCCGCTTCTTTACCAGGGAATCCCTTGCTGCTATCGAACAGCGCATTGCAGAAGAGAAAGCTAAGAGACCCAAACAGGAACGCAAGGACGAAGACGATGAAAATGGCCCA   150

 60                 70                  80                  90                 100
LysProAsnSerAspLeuGluValAlaGlyLysSerLeuProPheIleTyrGlyAspIleProProGluMetValSerGluProLeuGluAspLeuAspAspProTyrTyrIleAsnLysLysThrPheIleValLeuAsnLysGlyLysAlaIle
AAGCCAAATAGTGACTTGGAAGCAGGAAAATCCCTTCCTTTTATTTATGGAGACATTCCTCCAGAGATGGTGTCAGAACCACTGGAGGACCTGGACCCCTACTATATCAATAAGAAAACCTTCATAGTATTGAATAAGGGGAAAGCAATC   300

110                120                 130                 140                 150
SerArgPheSerAlaThrSerArgAlaLeuTyrIleLeuThrProThrPheAsnProIleLeuArgLysAlaLeuAlaIleLysIleLeuValHisSerLeuPheAsnValLeuIleMetCysThrIleLeuThrAsnCysValPheMetThrMetSerAsn
TCGCGGTTCAGCGCCACCTCTGCCCTGTACATTTTAACTCCCTTCAACCCCATTAGAAAATTAGCTATTAAGATTTTGGTACATTCTTTATTCAATGTGCTTATCATGTGCACAATTCTTACCAACTGTGTGTTTATGACCATGAGTAAC   450

160                170                 180                 190                 200
ProProAspTrpThrLysAsnValGluTyrThrPheThrGlyIleTyrThrPheGluSerLeuIleLysIleLeuAlaArgGlyPheCysLeuGluAspPheThrPheLeuArgAspAsnProTrpAsnTrpLeuAspPheThrValIleThr
CCTCCAGACTGGACAAAGAATGTGGAGTATACTTTTACAGGAATTTATACTTTTGAATCACTTATTAAAATCCTTGCAAGGGGCTTTTGTCTAGAAGATTTCACATTTCTACGGGAATCCCTGGAATTGGATTTCACAGTCATTACT   600

210                220                 230                 240                 250
PheAlaTyrValThrGluPheValAsnLeuGlyAsnValSerAlaLeuArgThrPheArgValLeuArgAlaLeuLysThrIleSerProLeuLysThrIleGlyAlaLeuGlnIleSerValLysLysLeuSerAsp
TTTGCGTATGTAACAGAATTTGTAAACCTAGGCAATGTTTCAGCTCTTCGAACTTTCAGAGTCTTGAGAGCTTTGAAAACTATTTCTCCAGGCCTGAAGACTATCGTGGGGGCCCTGATCCAGTCAGTGAAGAAGCTCTCTGAC   750

260                270                 280                 290                 300
ValMetIleLeuThrValPheCysLeuSerValPheAlaLeuIleGlyLeuGlnLeuPheMetGlyAsnLeuArgAsnLysCysLeuGlnTrpProProAspAsnSerThrPheGluIleAsnIleThrSerPhePheAsnAsnSerLeu
GTCATGATCCTCACCGTGTTCTGTCTCAGTGTCTTTGCTCTAATCGGGCTGCAGCTCTTCATGGGCAACCTGAGGAATAAAGTCTTGCAGTGGCCCCCAGACAATTCTACCTTTGAAATAAATATCACTTCCTTCTTTAATAACTCATTG   900

310                320                 330                 340                 350
AspTrpAsnGlyThrAlaPheAsnArgThrValAsnMetPheAsnArgThrAspGluTyrIleGluAspLysSerHisPheTyrPheLeuGluGlyGlnAsnAspAlaLeuLeuCysGlyAsnSerSerAspAlaGlyGlnCysProGluGly
GATTGGAATGGTACTGCCTTCAATAGGACGGTGAACATGTTTAACCGGACGGAATATATTGAAGATAAAAGTCACTTTTATTTTTTGGAAGGACAAAACGATGCTCTGCTTTGTGGGAACAGCTCAGATGCTGGACAGTGTCCAGAAGGA  1050

360                370                 380                 390                 400
TyrIleCysValLysAlaGlyArgAsnTyrGlyTyrThrSerPheAspThrPheSerTrpAlaPheLeuSerLeuPheArgLeuMetThrGlnAspPheTrpGluAsnLeuTyrGlnLeuThrLeuArgAlaAlaGlyLysThr
TACATCTGTGTGAAGGCTGGGAGAAACCCCAACTACGGCTACACAAGTTTTGACACCTTCAGCTGGGCCTTCTTGTCCTTATTTCGTCTCATGACTCAAGACTTCTGGGAAAACCTTTATCAGCTGACCTTGCGTGCTGCCGGGAAAACA  1200

410                420                 430                 440                 450
TyrMetIlePhePheValLeuValIlePheLeuGlySerPheTyrLeuIleAsnLeuIleLeuAlaValValAlaMetAlaTyrGluGlnGlnAsnAlaThrLeuGluGluAlaGluGlnLysGluAlaGluPheGlnGlnMetLeu
TACATGATATTTTTTGTGCTGGTCATTCTACCTGGTAAATTTGATCCTGGCTGGTGGGCCATGGCTTACGAGCAGCAGAATGCCACACTGGAGGAGGCTGAACAGAAGGAGGCAGAGTTTCAGCAGATGCTG  1350

460                470                 480                 490                 500
GluGlnLeuLysLysGlnGlnGluGluAlaGlnAlaAlaAlaAlaAlaSerAlaGluSerArgAspPheSerGlyAlaGlyGlyIleGlyValPheSerGluSerSerSerValAlaSerLysLysSerGlyGlnGlu
GAGCAACTGAAGAAGCAGCAGGAGGAAGCTCAGGCAGCAGCTGCAGCAGCGTCCGCAGAATCCAGAGACTTCAGCGGGGCAGGCGGGATAGGTGTTTCTCGGAGAGTTCGTCAGTAGCCTCAAAGTTAAGTTCCAAAAGTGAAAAGGAG  1500

Lys                510                 520                 530                 540                550
LeuLysAsnArgArgLysLysLysLysLysGlnLysGluGlnuAlaGlyIleArgLysSerArgSerGluAspSerIleLysArgLysSerLysGlyPheGlnPheSerLeuGluGlySerArgLeuThrTyrGluLys
TTGAAAAACAGAAGAAGAAGAAAAACAAGAGAAACAGGCTGGGGAGGAAGAGAAGGAGCAGCGGCGGGAAATCTGCCTCTGAGGACAGCATACGAAAGAAAGGCTTCCAGTTTTCCCTGGAAGGAAGTAGATTGACCTATGAAAAG  1650

A                  560                 570                 580                 590                600
ArgPheSerSerProHisIleGlnSerLeuLeuSerIleArgGlySerLeuPheSerProArgArgAsnSerArgAlaSerPheAsnPheLeuGlyValLysAspGlnValAlaArgGluLeuHisSerThr
AGATTTTCCTCTCCGCACCAGTCTCTCTTGAGCATCCGAGGCTCCCTATTTTCTCCAAGACGCAACAGTAGAGCAAGCCTTTTCAACTTCAAAGGTCGAGTGAAGGATATTGGTTCCGAAAATGACTTTGCAGACGATGAACACAGCACA  1800

610                620                 630                 640                650
PheGluAspAsnGluSerArgArgAspSerLeuPheValProArgArgHisGlyGluArgArgAsnSerAsnValSerGlnAlaSerArgSerSerArgMetLeuAlaValPheProMetGluAsnGlyGlyLysMetHisSerAlaValAspCys
TTTGAGGACAACGACAGCAGAAGAGACTCTCTATTTGTACCACACAGACATGGAGAAAGGCGTCCTAGCAATGTCAGCCAGGCCAGCCGTGCCTCCCGGGGGATACCCACTCTACCCATGAATGGGAAGATGCACAGTGCAGTGGACTGC  1950

660                670                 680                 690                700
AsnGlyValValSerLeuValGlyGlyProSerAlaLeuThrHisSerProValGlyGlnLeuLeuProGluGlyThrThrThrGluThrGluIleArgLysArgArgSerSerSerTyrHisValSerMetAspLeuGluAspGluProSer
AACGGTGTGGTGTCCCTGGTTGGAGGCCCCTCTGCGCTCACATCGCCTGTGGGGCAGCTGCTGCCGGAGGGCACAACTACTGAGACAGAAATAAGGAAGAGGAGATCCAGTTCTTACCACGTCTCTATGGACTTGTTGGAAGACCCTTCA  2100

710                720                 730                 740                750
ArgGlnArgAlaMetSerMetAlaSerIleLeuThrAsnThrValGluGluLeuGluGluSerArgGlnLysCysProProCysTrpTyrCysProSerProTrpLeuLysValLysHis
AGGCAAAGGGCAATGAGTATGGCCAGTATTTTGACGAACACTATGGAAGAACTTGAAGAGAATCCAGACAGAAATGCCCACCCTGCTGGTATAAATTTGCTAATATGTGCCTGATTTGGGACTGTTGTAAGCCATGGCTAAAGGTAAAACAC  2250

760                770                 780                 790                800
ValValAsnValValMetAlaSerProProPheValAspLeuAlaIleThrIleCysIleValLeuAsnThrLeuPheMetAlaMetGluHisTyrProMetThrGluGlnPheSerSerValLeuSerValGlyAsnLeuValPheThrGly
GTTGTCAATCTGGTAGTGATGGATCCATTTGTTGACCTGGCCATCACCATCTGCATTGTGCTGAATACGCTCTTCATGGCCATGGAGCATTACCCCATGACTGAGCAGTTCAGCAGTGTGCTGTCTGTTGGTAATCTTGTCTTCACTGGG  2400

810                820                 830                 840                850
IlePheThrAlaGluMetPheLeuLysIleIleAlaMetAspProTyrTyrPheGlnGluGlyTrpAsnIlePheAspSerPheIleValThrLeuSerLeuMetGluLeuGlyLeuAlaAsnValGluGlyLeuSerValLeuArg
ATCTTCACGGCAGAAATGTTTCTCAAGATAATAGCCATGGATCCATATTATTACTTCCAAGAAGGCTGGAATATCTTTGATAGCTTTATTGTGACCCTTAGTTTAATGGAACTCGGCCTTGCCGAATGTGGAAGGATTGTCAGTTCTCCGA  2550

860                870                 880                 890                900
SerPheArgGluLeuArgValPheLysLeuAlaLysSerTrpProThrLeuAsnMetLeuIleLysIleIleGlyAsnLeuEuLysAlaLeuIleGlyAlaLeuIleGlnSerValLysGlyLeuSerAspValMetSerPheAspAsnProSer
TCATTCCGGCTGCTTAGAGTCTTCAAGTTGGCAAAGTCCTGGCCCACACTGAACATGCTCATTAAGATCATCGGCAACCTGGTGAAGGCACTGATCGGTGCGCTCATTCAGTCTGTAAAAGGGCTATCTGATGTCATGTCTTCAGATAACCCCTCA  2700

910                920                 930                940                950
GlnLeuPheGlyLysTyrLysGluCysValCysLysIleSerAsnAspCysGluLeuProArgTrpHisMetHisAspPhePheHisSerPheLeuIleValPheArgValLeuCysGlyGluTrpIleGluThrMetTrpAspCys
CAGCTGTTTGGAAAGAGCTACAAGGAGTGTGTCTGTAAGATTTCCAATGATTGTGAGCTCCCGCGCTGGCACATGCACGACTTCTTCCACTCTTTCCTGATCGTGTTTCGAGTGCTGTGTGGGGAGTGGATTGAGACCATGTGGGACTGC  2850

960                970                 980                 990                1000
MetGluValAlaGlyGlnThrMetCysLeuThrValPheMetMetValMetValIleGlyAsnLeuValAlaLeuGluSerLeuArgSerSerSerAlaThrAspAlaAspAsnGluAsnGlu
ATGGAGGTCGCGGGCCAGACCATGTGCCTTACTGTCTTCATGATGGTCATGGTGATTGGGAACCTTGTTGCTCTGGAAAGTCTTCGTAGCTCCTCGGCTACTGATGCAGACAATGAGAATGAGAATG  3000

1010               1020    His        1030                1040                1050
AsnAsnLeuGlnIleAlaValGlyArgMetGlnLysGlyIleAspPheValLysAlaGluIleGlnPheIleGlnLysAlaMetGluValLysLysGlnuAlaGluLeuLysProLeuGluAspLeuAsnAsnLysAspAsp
AACAACCTCCAGATAGCCGTGGGAAGGATGCAGAAGGGATCGATTTTGTTAAAGCAGAAATACAGTTCATTCAGAAGGCCTTTGAAGTGAAATCAAAGCCTGGAGGTGAAGTTAAAAAGCAAGAGGCTGAACTCAAGAAACCCCTGGATGAGCTCAATAAT   3150

1060               1070     A          1080                1090                1100
SerCysIleSerAsnHisThrThrIleGluIleGlyLysAspLeuAsnTyrLeuLysAspGlyAsnGlyThrThrSerGlyIleGlySerSerValGluTyrValAspAspGluSerAspTyrMetTyrPheAsnAsnProSer
AGTTGTATCTCCAACCACACGACCATAGAAATAGGGAAGGACCTCAATTACTTAAAGATGGAAACGGGCAGACAGTGGCATCAGGCACGTGGAGAAGTATGTGGTAGATGAGAGTGATTACATGTACTTCAATAACCCCAGC   3300

Met                1110                1120                1130                1140                1150
LeuThrValThrProIleLeuAlaUGlyLysSerAspPheGluAlaAsnLeuAsnThrGlyGluPheSerGlnSerAspAlaTyrLysLysGluLeuAsnAlaThrSerSerSerGluGlyTyrSerThrValAspIleGlyAla
CTCACCGTGACTGTGCCCATCGCCCTTGGAGAGTCTGACTTTGAAAACTTAAACACGGGAGAATTCAGTAGTAGTCAGATATGGAAGAAACAAGGAGGAATTTGAATGCAACTAGCTCATCTGAGGGCTATAGCACTGTTGATATAGGGGCT   3450

A                  1160                 A          1170                1180                1190                1200
ProAlaGluGlyGlnInProGluGluSerLeuGluProGluAlaCysGlyPheThrGlyAspCysValArgLysLysAlaGlyLeuGlnGlnLeuLysGluGluLeuTrpTrpAsnGlu
CCGGCAGAGGGGAGCAGCAGGCCGAACCCGGGAAGAATCGCTTGAACCGGAAGGCGTGTTTCACAGAGATGATGTTGTCAGAAGTATCTGTCATAAGCATAGAACAGGGCAAAGCCAAGCTCTGGTGGAACTTGAGGGAAAACG   3600

1210               1220    Gly        1230                1240
CysTyrIleValGlyValHisAsnTrpPheGluGlyThrPheIleValPheMetIleLeuLeuSerSerGlyAlaLeuAlaPheGluAspIleTyrIleGluGlnArgThrIleLysThrMetGluGluTyrAlaAspLysValPheThr
TGCTACAAGATAGTAGGCGTACAATGGTTTGAAACCTTCATCGTTTTTATGATTCTGCTCAGCAGTGGTGCTCTTGCCTTTGAAGACATTTATATTGAGCAGCGAAAGACCATCAAGACCATGCTGGAGTATGCTGACAAAGTTTTCACT   3750
```

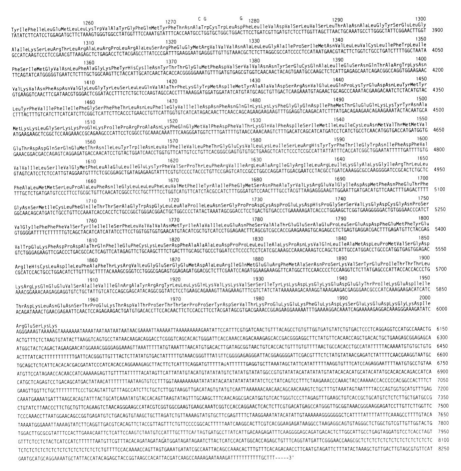

FIGURE 3. Nucleotide sequence of cloned cDNA encoding rat sodium channel II (see legend to FIG. 1). The nucleotide (and amino acid) differences observed among the individual clones analyzed are shown. (From Noda et al.[25] Reprinted from *Nature*, Copyright 1986 Macmillan Journals Limited.)

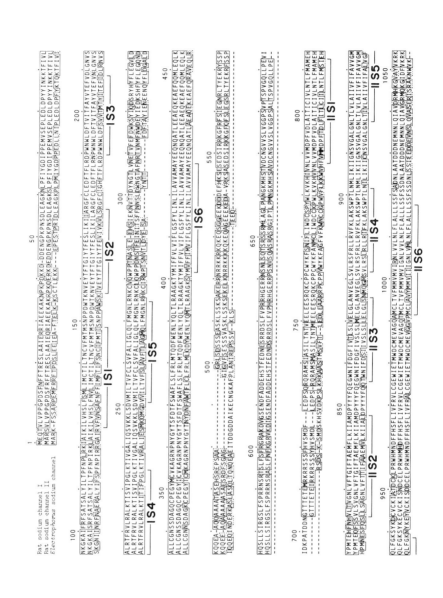

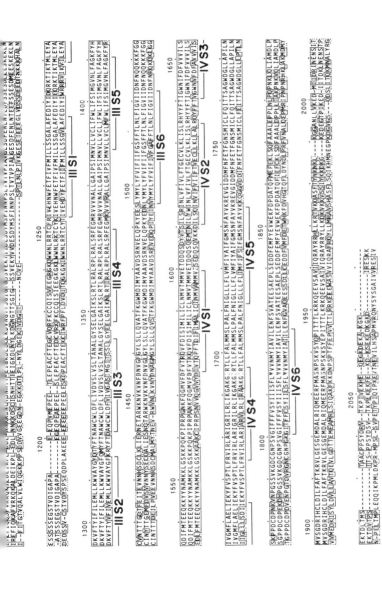

FIGURE 4. Alignment of the amino acid sequences of rat sodium channels I (*top*) and II (*middle*) and the *Electrophorus electricus* sodium channel (*bottom*). The one-letter amino acid notation is used. At positions where amino acid differences occur (FIGS. 2 and 3), the residue given below has been adopted. Sets of identical residues are enclosed with *solid lines*, and sets of conservative residues by *dotted lines*. Conservative amino acid substitutions are defined as pairs of residues belonging to one of the following groups: S, T, P, A, and G; N, D, E, and Q; H, R, and K; M, I, L, and V; F, Y, and W (ref. 26). Gaps (---) have been inserted to achieve maximum homology. In order to evaluate homology (see text), gaps have been counted as one substitution regardless of their length. Positions in the aligned sequences including gaps are numbered beginning with that of the initiating methionine. The putative transmembrane segments S1–S6 in each of repeats I–IV are indicated; the termini of these segments have been tentatively assigned. (From Noda *et al.*[25] Reprinted from *Nature*, Copyright 1986 Macmillan Journals Limited.)

```
                                  1                                                50
Repeat I   Rat I          ILTPFNPLRKIA-IKÏLVHSLFSMLÏM--CTÏLTNCVFMÏMSNPPDWTK-----NVVEYT---FTGÏYTFESLÏKÏÏARGFCLEDF   110- 183
           Rat II         ILTPFNPIRKLA-IKÏLVHSLFNVLÏM--CTÏLTNCVFMÏMSNPPDWTK-----NVVEYT---FTGIYTFESLIKILARGFCLEDF   111- 184
           Electrophorus  IFSPFNPIRRGA--NLVVLKKHIV-FTÏFSNCIFMTÏSNPPAWSK---IWEYT---FTGIVKVLSRGFCIGHF                104- 177
Repeat II  Rat I          CSPYWLKVKHIV-NLVVMDPFVDLAÏT--ICÏVLNTLFMAMEHYPMTEH---FNHVLTVGNLVFTGÏFTAEMFLKIÏA-MDPYYYF   750- 828
           Rat II         CCKPWLKVKHVV-NLVVMDPFVDLAÏT--ICÏVLNTLFMAMEHYPMTEQ---FSSVVLSVGNLVFTGÏFTAEMFLKIÏA-LDPYYYF   741- 819
           Electrophorus  CCGPWVFLKKWV-HFVMMDPFTDLFIÏT--LCÏÏLNTLFMSÏEHHPMNES---FQSLLLSAGNLVFTÏFAAEMVLKIÏA-LDPYYF    548- 626
Repeat III Rat I          RGKQWWNLRRTCFRIVEHNWF-ETFÏV--FMÏLLSSGALAFEDIYIDQRKTIKTMLEYADKVFTYÏFILEMLLKWVAYGYQT-YF   1200-1280
           Rat II         KGKLWWNLRKTCYIVEHNWF-ETFÏV--FMÏLLSSGALAFEDIYIEQRKTIKTMLEYADKVFTYÏFILEMLLKWVAYGFOM-YF    1190-1270
           Electrophorus  IPRPGNKFQGMVFDFV-TRQVFDISÏÏMLÏCLNMVT--MMVETDDQSDY--VTSILSRINLVFIVLFTGECVLKLÏS-LRHY-YF    982-1062
Repeat IV  Rat I          IPRPANKFQGMVFDFV-TKQVFDISÏMILÏCLNMVT--MMVETDDQSOE--MTNILYWINLVFIVLETGECVLKLÏS-LRHY-YF   1523-1600
           Rat II         IPRPSNVVQGVVYDIYJ-TQPFTDIFÏMALICÏNMVA--MMVESEDQSOV--KKDIÏLSQINVÏFVÏÏFYVECLLKLÏL_S-LRQY-FF 1513-1590
           Electrophorus                                                                                          1304-1381

                           |___S1___|                                          |___S2___|
```

```
                       100                              150
TFLRDPÏMNWLDFTVÏTFAYVVT-EFVD----------LGNVSALÏTFRVLRALKTISVIPGLKTIVGALÏQSVKKLSDVMÏLTVFCLSVFALÏGLQLFMGNLRN-KCVQW   184- 280
TFLRNPÏMNWLDFTVIITFAYVVT-EFVN----------LGNVSALÏTFRVLRALKTISVIPGLKTIVGALIQSVKKLSDVMÏLTVFCLSVFALIGLQLFMGNLRN-KCLQW  185- 281
TFLRDPÏMNWLDFSVVTMTYIÏT-EFID----------LRNVSALÏTFRVLRALKTITFPGLKTÏVRALIESMKQMGDVVIÏTVFSLAVFTLAGMQLFMGNLRIH-KCIRW   178- 274
Q---EGWNIFDGFIVTLSILVELGLAN-----------VEGLISVLRSFRLLRVFKLRVFKLAKSWPTLNMLIKIIIGNSVGALGNLTÏLVLAIIVFIVLAIIVFIFAVVGMQLFGKSYKDCVC---  829- 921
Q---EGWNIFDGFIVSLSILMEL GLAN----------VEGLISVLRSFRLLRVFKLRVFKLAKSWPTLNMLÏKIIIGNSVGALGNLTÏLVLAIIVFIFAVVGMQLFGKSYKECVC---           820- 912
Q---QTWNIFDSIÏVSLSLLELGLSN-------------MQGMSVLRSVLRSLRTLRALRPLRALSRFEGMRVVVNALLGAÏPSÏMNVLLVCLIFWLIFSIMGVNLFAG--KFYHCV---            627- 719
T---NAWCWLDFLIVDVSILVSLT-ANAL---------GYSELGAIKSLRTLRALRPLRALSRFEGMRVVVNALLGAÏPSÏMNVLLVCLFWLIFSIMGVNLFAG--KFYHCI---              1281-1377
T---NAWCWLDFLIVDVSILVSLT-ANAL---------GYSELGAIKSLRTLRALRPLRALSRFEGMKVVVRALLGAÏPSÏMNVLLVCLMFWLIFSÏMGVNLFAG--KFYRCI---              1271-1367
T---DAWCWLDFVIVGASIMGIT-SSLL----------GYEELGAIKNLRTIRALRGRÏLRLIKGAKGIRTL----LFALMMSLPALFNIGLLLFLVMFIYAÏFGMSNFAYVKRE---            1063-1159
T---IGWNIFDFVVVILSIIVGMFLAELIEKYFVSPTLFRVLRLARÏGRÏLRLIKGAKGIRTL----LFALMMSLPALFNIGLLLFLVMFIYAÏFGMSNFAYVKRE---                     1601-1698
T---IGWNIFDFVVVILSIIVGMFLAELIEKYFVSPTLFRVIRLARÏGRÏLRLÏKGAKGIRTL----LFALMMSLPALFNIGLLLFLVMFIYAÏFGMSNFAYVKRE---                     1591-1688
T---VGMNVFDFÏAVVVISÏÏJGLLLSDIIEKYFVSPTLFRVÏRLARÏARÏVLRLÏRJAAKGIRTLJ---LFALMMSLPALFNIGLLLFLIMFIYSJFGMSNFAYVKKQ-----                1382-1479

   |___S3___|                              |___S4___|                   |___S5___|
```

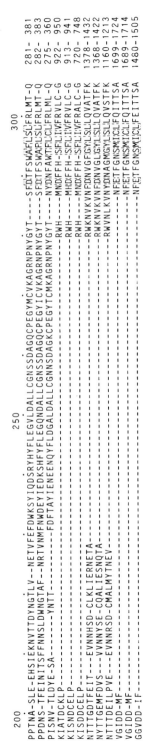
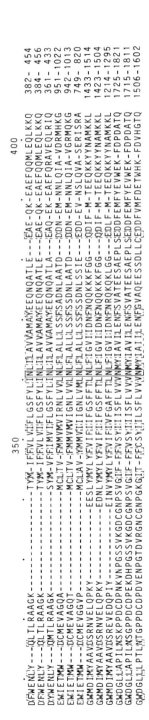

— S6 —

FIGURE 5. Alignment of the amino acid sequences of the four internal homology units of rat sodium channels I and II and the *Electrophorus electricus* sodium channel. The sequences of repeats I (rows 1–3), II (rows 4–6), III (rows 7–9), and IV (rows 10–12) are aligned. The numbers of the residues (see FIGS. 1–3) on each line are given on the right side. Sets of twelve identical residues at one aligned position are enclosed in *solid boxes*, and sets of twelve identical or conservative residues at one aligned position with *dashed boxes*. Positions in the aligned sequences including gaps (---) are numbered beginning with the amino terminus of the repeats. Segments S1–S6 are indicated; the termini of these segments are tentative and may vary with the individual segments (see FIG. 4).

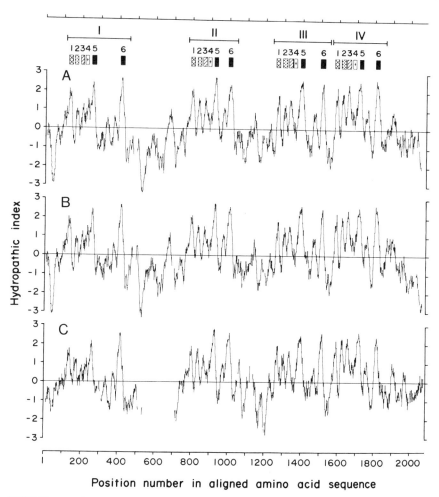

FIGURE 6. Hydropathy profiles of **(A)** rat sodium channel I, **(B)** rat sodium channel II, and **(C)** the *Electrophorus electricus* sodium channel. The averaged hydropathic index[30] of a nonadeca-peptide composed of amino acids $i - 9$ to $i + 9$ is plotted against i, where i represents the position number in the aligned sequences in FIGURE 4; no plots are given for the positions corresponding to gaps. The locations of repeats I–IV are shown by *bars*. The positions of segments S1–S6 in each repeat are indicated. The hydropathy profile in C is based on data from Noda *et al.*[24]

charges or equivalent dipoles moving under the influence of the membrane electric field;[1,34] in fact, this movement can be measured as a gating current.[35,36] The finding that the equivalent of four to six charges must move fully across the membrane to open one sodium channel[1,34] suggests the intramembranous location of many dipoles that move by smaller distances.

The unique structure of segment S4 in all repeats is strikingly well conserved among the three sodium channels (FIG. 5). It seems most likely that the positive charges present in this segment, many of which presumably form dipoles, represent the voltage sensor. They would move outward in response to depolarization, causing conformational changes and possible rearrangement of ion pairs. Segment S4 in repeats I, II, III, and IV contain four, five, six, and eight positive charges, respectively. This may underlie the proposal that the successive transitions among several closed states are fast and involve less charge movement than does the slow transition from the last closed state to the open state.[37] The presence of four homologous repeats in a single sodium channel molecule is consistent with the sigmoid activation kinetics characteristic of this channel.[1]

As the minimum cross section of the sodium channel is thought to be 3×5 Å (refs. 38 and 39), at least one helical segment from each repeat would take part in forming the inner wall of the channel at the narrowest point. Remarkably, segment S2 in every repeat contains, at equivalent positions, a glutamic acid residue (position 70 in the aligned sequences in FIG. 5) and a lysine residue (position 74), which are conserved in all the three sodium channels. These acidic and basic residues are located on one side of the α-helix. In addition, segment S2 in repeats I and III contains a conserved glutamic acid (position 57) or aspartic acid residue (position 60) located ten residues apart from the above-mentioned glutamic acid on nearly the same side of the α-helix (note gaps at positions 60–62 in repeat I); segment S2 in repeat III has two more conserved charged residues (glutamic acid at position 57 and lysine at position 61), which face another side of the α-helix. In view of the high degree of conservation of the charged residues in segment S2, it is tempting to hypothesize that this segment forms the inner wall of the channel (FIG. 7B).

Segment S3 in every repeat also contains a conserved aspartic acid residue (position 96) at an equivalent position. It is an intriguing speculation that this aspartic

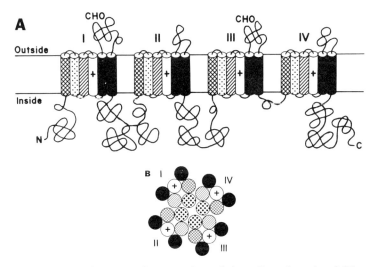

FIGURE 7. (A) Proposed transmembrane topology of the sodium channel and (B) proposed arrangement of the transmembrane segments viewed in cross section. In A, the four homology units spanning the membrane are displayed linearly. Segments S1–S6 in each repeat (I–IV) are shown by cylinders marked as follows: S1, *cross-hatched;* S2, *stippled;* S3, *hatched;* S4, *plus signs;* S5 and S6, *filled.* Putative sites of N-glycosylation (CHO) are indicated. In B, the ionic channel is represented as a central pore surrounded by the four homology units. Segments S1–S6 in each repeat (I–IV) are shown by circles marked as in A. (From Noda *et al.*[25] Reprinted from *Nature,* Copyright 1986 Macmillan Journals Limited.)

acid, which may be paired with a basic residue in segment S4 in the closed state of the channel, may be shifted by depolarization to interact with the lysine (position 74) present in segment S2 of every repeat. This would cause a conformational change of the putative channel wall and simultaneously mask the positive charge on the channel lining to allow sodium ions to pass through the central pore. Clusters of positively charged residues (predominantly lysine) and of negatively charged residues are conserved in the regions preceding segment S1 and following segment S6 of repeat IV,

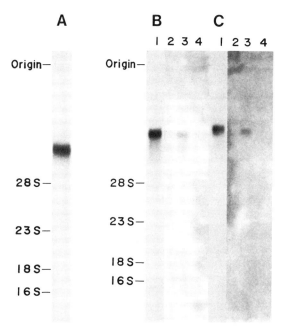

FIGURE 8. Autoradiograms of RNA blot hybridization analysis. The RNA samples used were as follows: (A) 20 μg of total RNA from *Electrophorus electricus* electric organ; (B), (C) 20 μg of poly (A)$^+$ RNA from whole brain (lane 1), skeletal muscle (lane 2), cardiac muscle (lane 3), and liver (lane 4) of male adult rats. The probes were excised from (A) *Electrophorus electricus* sodium channel cDNA, (B) rat sodium channel I cDNA or (C) rat sodium channel II cDNA. The autoradiograms in B and C were derived from the same electrophoresis experiment; the duration of autoradiography was about seven times shorter for lane 1 than for lanes 2–4. The size markers were *E. coli* rRNA and calf (A) or rat (B and C) RNA. (From Noda *et al.*[24,25] Reprinted from *Nature*, Copyright 1984, 1986 Macmillan Journals Limited.)

respectively. It is conceivable that these segments, which are assigned to the cytoplasmic side of the membrane, are involved in the inactivation of the sodium channel.[37]

RNA BLOT HYBRIDIZATION ANALYSIS

RNA preparations from *Electrophorus* electric organ and from rat brain, skeletal muscle, and cardiac muscle were subjected to blot hybridization analysis with respective sodium channel cDNA probes (FIG. 8). The *Electrophorus* electroplax contained a hybridizable RNA species of ~8,000 nucleotides (FIG. 8A). The rat brain contained RNA species of ~9,000 and ~9,500 nucleotides hybridizable with the sodium channel I and II cDNA probes, respectively, in comparable amounts (FIG. 8B and 8C, lane 1). The cardiac muscle also contained two RNA species that were hybridizable with the sodium channel I and II cDNA probes and indistinguishable in size from the brain mRNAs, although the hybridization signals were much weaker (lane 3); note the difference in the duration of autoradiography (see legend to FIG. 8). No hybridizable RNA species were detected with the skeletal muscle RNA (lane 2) or with the liver RNA used as a control (lane 4). The weak or undetectable hybridization observed with the cardiac muscle and skeletal muscle RNAs may be accounted for by the low content of the sodium channel mRNAs or by the presence of different sodium channel mRNAs in these tissues. It has been reported that adult rat cardiac muscle contains a sodium channel species with a low affinity for tetrodotoxin, in addition to a sodium channel species that, like the brain counterpart, has a high affinity for the toxin, and that the content of the high-affinity sodium channel is much lower than that of the low-affinity sodium channel.[14,15] The structurally distinct sodium channels encoded by the mRNAs we have found may be responsible for the different types of sodium currents observed in excitable tissues.[18-23]

STRUCTURAL COMPARISON WITH NICOTINIC ACETYLCHOLINE RECEPTOR

It is of interest to compare the molecular structure of the sodium channel with that of the nicotinic acetylcholine receptor (AChR). Both have a transmembrane ionic channel. The AChR is a pentameric protein complex consisting of homologus subunits,[40,41] whereas the sodium channel is a single large polypeptide with a molecular size comparable to that of the whole AChR complex and contains four homologous internal repeats. The structural repeats of the sodium channel may correspond functionally to the AChR subunits in that both contain about an equal number of transmembrane segments and are oriented presumably in a pseudosymmetric fashion across the membrane, forming an ionic channel. Thus the two channel proteins, though their gating is effected in different ways, may be similar in basic structural organization. Moreover, the AChR and the sodium channel share common evolutionary features. The AChR subunits are encoded by separate genes that apparently have been generated from a single common ancestor by gene duplications, whereas the four repetitive units of the sodium channel are encoded by a single gene that presumably evolved from a primordial gene by internal duplications.

CONCLUDING REMARKS

The complete amino acid sequences of the *Electrophorus* electroplax sodium channel and two distinct sodium channels from rat brain have been elucidated by cloning and sequencing the cDNAs. The deduced primary structure suggests putative functional regions involved in the operation of this voltage-gated ionic channel. Future studies will be directed towards expression of the cloned cDNAs and to functional analysis of the wild-type channels as well as of mutant channels produced by site-specific mutagenesis of the cDNAs.

ACKNOWLEDGMENTS

We thank Dr. Takashi Miyata and Mr. Hidenori Hayashida for computer analysis.

REFERENCES

1. HODGKIN, A. L. & A. F. HUXLEY. 1952. J. Physiol. **117:** 500–544.
2. AGNEW, W. S. 1984. Ann. Rev. Physiol. **46:** 517–530.
3. CATTERALL, W. A. 1984. Science **223:** 653–661.
4. AGNEW, W. S., S. R. LEVINSON, J. S. BRABSON & M. A. RAFTERY. 1978. Proc. Natl. Acad. Sci. U.S.A. **75:** 2606–2610.
5. MILLER, J. A., W. S. AGNEW & S. R. LEVINSON. 1983. Biochemistry **22:** 462–470.
6. LOMBET, A. & M. LAZDUNSKI. 1984. Eur. J. Biochem. **141:** 651–660.
7. HARTSHORNE, R. P. & W. A. CATTERALL. 1981. Proc. Natl. Acad. Sci. U.S.A. **78:** 4620–4624.
8. BARCHI, R. L. 1983. J. Neurochem. **40:** 1377–1385.
9. WEIGELE, J. B. & R. L. BARCHI. 1982. Proc. Natl. Acad. Sci. U.S.A. **79:** 3651–3655.
10. TAMKUN, M. M., J. A. TALVENHEIMO & W. A. CATTERALL. 1984. J. Biol. Chem. **259:** 1676–1688.
11. ROSENBERG, R. L., S. A. TOMIKO & W. S. AGNEW. 1984. Proc. Natl. Acad. Sci. U.S.A. **81:** 1239–1243.
12. HANKE, W., G. BOHEIM, J. BARHANIN, D. PAURON & M. LAZDUNSKI. 1984. EMBO J. **3:** 509–515.
13. HARTSHORNE, R. P., B. U. KELLER, J. A. TALVENHEIMO, W. A. CATTERALL & M. MONTAL. 1985. Proc. Natl. Acad. Sci. U.S.A. **82:** 240–244.
14. LOMBET, A., J. -F. RENAUD, R. CHICHEPORTICHE & M. LAZDUNSKI. 1981. Biochemistry **20:** 1279–1285.
15. LOMBET, A., T. KAZAZOGLOU, E. DELPONT, J. -F. RENAUD & M. LAZDUNSKI. 1983. Biochem. Biophys. Res. Commun. **110:** 894–901.
16. RENAUD, J. -F., T. KAZAZOGLOU, A. LOMBET, R. CHICHEPORTICHE, E. JAIMOVICH, G. ROMEY & M. LAZDUNSKI. 1983. J. Biol. Chem. **258:** 8799–8805.
17. SHERMAN, S. J. & W. A. CATTERALL. 1985. *In* Regulation and Development of Membrane Transport Processes. J. S. Graves, Ed. 237–263. Wiley. New York.
18. BARRETT, J. N. & W. E. CRILL. 1980. J. Physiol. **304:** 231–249.
19. GUNDERSEN, C. B., R. MILEDI & I. PARKER. 1983. Proc. R. Soc. London Ser. B. **220:** 131–140.
20. JAIMOVICH, E., R. CHICHEPORTICHE, A. LOMBET, M. LAZDUNSKI, M. ILDEFONSE & O. ROUGIER. 1983. Eur. J. Physiol. **397:** 1–5.
21. EICK, R. T., J. YEH & N. MATSUKI. 1984. Biophys. J. **45:** 70–73.
22. GILLY, W. F. & C. M. ARMSTRONG. 1984. Nature **309:** 448–450.
23. BENOIT, E., A. CORBIER & J. -M. DUBOIS. 1985. J. Physiol. **361:** 339–360.
24. NODA, M., S. SHIMIZU, T. TANABE, T. TAKAI, T. KAYANO, T. IKEDA, H. TAKAHASHI, H. NAKAYAMA, Y. KANAOKA, N. MINAMINO, K. KANGAWA, H. MATSUO, M. A. RAFTERY, T. HIROSE, S. INAYAMA, H. HAYASHIDA, T. MIYATA & S. NUMA. 1984. Nature **312:** 121–127.
25. NODA, M., T. IKEDA, T. KAYANO, H. SUZUKI, H. TAKESHIMA, M. KURASAKI, H. TAKAHASHI & S. NUMA. 1986. Nature. **320:** 188–192.
26. DAYHOFF, M. O., R. M. SCHWARTZ & B. C. ORCUTT. 1978. *In* Atlas of Protein Sequence and Structure, vol. 5. suppl. 3. M. O. Dayhoff, Ed.: 345–352. National Biomedical Research Foundation. Silver Spring, Md.
27. MESSNER, D. J. & W. A. CATTERALL. 1985. J. Biol. Chem. **260:** 10597–10604.
28. TOH, H., H. HAYASHIDA & T. MIYATA. 1983. Nature **305:** 827–829.
29. KREBS, E. G. & J. A. BEAVO. 1979. Ann. Rev. Biochem. **48:** 923–959.
30. KYTE, J. & R. F. DOOLITTLE. 1982. J. Mol. Biol. **157:** 105–132.
31. CHOU, P. Y. & G. D. FASMAN. 1978. Ann. Rev. Biochem. **47:** 251–276.

32. BLOBEL, G. & B. DOBBERSTEIN. 1975. J. Cell Biol. **67:** 852–862.
33. BAUSE, E. 1983. Biochem. J. **209:** 331–336.
34. HILLE, B. 1984. Ionic Channels of Excitable Membranes. Sinauer Associates. Sunderland, Mass.
35. ARMSTRONG, C. M. & F. BEZANILLA. 1973. Nature **242:** 459–461.
36. KEYNES, R. D. & E. ROJAS. 1974. J. Physiol. **239:** 393–434.
37. ARMSTRONG, C. M. 1981. Physiol. Rev. **61:** 644–683.
38. HILLE, B. 1971. J. Gen. Physiol. **58:** 599–619.
39. HILLE, B. 1972. J. Gen. Physiol. **59:** 637–658.
40. NUMA, S., M. NODA, H. TAKAHASHI, T. TANABE, M. TOYOSATO, Y. FURUTANI & S. KIKYOTANI. 1983. Cold Spring Harb. Symp. Quant. Biol. **48:** 57–69.
41. NUMA, S. 1986. Chemica Scripta. **26B.** In press.

Biosynthesis of Electroplax Sodium Channels[a]

WILLIAM B. THORNHILL AND S. ROCK LEVINSON

Department of Physiology
University of Colorado, School of Medicine
Denver, Colorado 80262

INTRODUCTION

Electrically excitable cells, such as nerve and muscle tissue, possess voltage-regulated ion channels that are responsible for the initiation and propagation of the action potential.[1] Over the past thirty-five years, the voltage-regulated sodium channel has been extensively studied using biophysical and pharmacological techniques in an attempt to understand its complex operation.[2,3] Although a wealth of function information has been accumulated on sodium channel operation it has been only relatively recently that attention has been focused on the isolation and physiochemical characterization of this important membrane protein.[4-6] This biochemical approach is expected to result eventually in further insights into how the channel operates on a molecular level through structural-functional correlations.

The successful isolation of the sodium channel was achieved by using the binding of tritiated neurotoxins, tetrodotoxin (TTX) or saxitoxin (STX) as affinity markers for the channel in lipid-detergent solutions.[7] Miller *et al.*[8] have shown that the TTX-binding component from electroplax membranes of *Electrophorus electricus* is a single, large, heavily glycosylated protein (M_r approximately 260,000 daltons). The polypeptide is about 30% carbohydrate by weight with sialic acids representing 40% of the total sugar moieties.

In this report, we describe the cell-free biosynthesis of the electroplax sodium channel and we contrast some physiochemical properties of this core polypeptide with those of the mature, native molecule. We also present preliminary studies on the biosnythesis and posttranslational processing of eel sodium channels in frog oocytes.

THE EEL SODIUM CHANNEL BINDS LARGE AMOUNTS OF SDS

When analyzed by a Ferguson plot,[9] in which the porosity of the separating polyacrylamide gel is varied to estimate the mobility of a protein in free solution, the eel sodium channel has been shown to have a fourfold greater electrophoretic free mobility compared to standard proteins.[8] This unusual characteristic has been inferred to be the result of binding of large amounts of sodium dodecyl sulfate (SDS) to hydrophobic domains on the native channel, an inference well supported by the

[a]This work was supported in part by grants from the National Institutes of Health (NS–15879), the Muscular Dystrophy Association of America, and a Research Career Development Award to SRL.

extensive literature on SDS-protein interactions and their affects on SDS-PAGE behavior.[10–13]

Recent studies from our laboratory have confirmed the eel sodium channel does indeed bind unusually high amounts of SDS compared to bovine serum albumin (BSA), a well-characterized protein. We have directly measured the binding of ^{35}S-SDS to the sodium channel by equilibrium dialysis at both high and low ionic strengths (FIGURE 1). Under both conditions the channel polypeptide bound much more SDS than BSA, which has been shown to bind 1.4 and 0.4 grams of SDS per gram protein at low and high ionic strengths, respectively.[10] In addition, most of this elevated binding of SDS occurred well above the critical micelle concentration (CMC) for the detergent. This is also in contrast to standard proteins, like BSA, which mainly

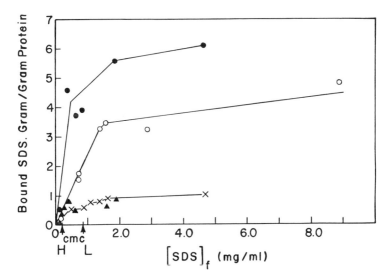

FIGURE 1. Binding of [^{35}S]SDS to the biochemically isolated sodium channel and bovine serum albumin; ● = binding of SDS to sodium channel glycopeptide at high ionic strength; O = sodium channel in low ionic strength; ▲ = binding of detergent to BSA at high ionic strength; × = BSA at low ionic strength. H and L show the critical micelle concentrations (cmc) for SDS at the respective ionic strengths.

interact with detergent monomers and bind saturating amounts of SDS just below the CMC,[10] and suggest the sodium channel is binding detergent micelles around very hydrophobic domains on the molecule.

The extensive binding of micelles to the channel polypeptide is also supported by our observations that at high ionic strengths the amount of SDS bound to the molecule is greater than at low ionic strengths (FIGURE 1). For standard proteins, such as BSA, the amount of detergent bound actually decreases with increasing ionic strength.[10] The most likely explanation for the behavior of the sodium channel polypeptide is that increased detergent binding at high ionic strength is a result of increased size of the SDS micelles which are bound or organized by the polypeptide in high salt.[14] This increased binding of SDS to the channel should be sufficient to explain its unusually high electrophoretic free mobility on polyacrylamide gels.

HYDROPHOBIC DOMAINS ARE ADDED POSTTRANSLATIONALLY TO THE SODIUM CHANNEL

The above results suggest, therefore, that extensive hydrophobic domains must exist on the mature, native channel. Although the amino acid composition of the channel is not unusually hydrophobic,[8] extensive sequences of hydrophobic amino acids are present[15] that may be responsible for the binding of large amounts of SDS. Alternatively, the hydrophobic domains may be added posttranslationally in the form of covalently attached fatty acids or phospholipids. In order to distinguish between these two possibilities, we have used a cell-lysate system to synthesize the sodium channel core polypeptide, in the absence of posttranslational processing, to determine whether the unmodified polypeptide exhibits the unusually high electrophoretic free mobility characteristic of the native channel. Total electroplax RNA was isolated by standard methods[16] and used to direct protein synthesis in a rabbit reticulocyte lysate system.[17] The ^{35}S-methionine-labeled proteins that were synthesized ranged in apparent molecular mass from 12,000 to 200,000 daltons when analyzed by SDS-PAGE (FIGURE 2, lane 2). Antisera raised against the highly purified sodium channel specifically precipitated a polypeptide with a M_r of 230,000 daltons from the translation mixture (FIGURE 2, lane 3). This polypeptide accounted for approximately 0.1% of the total proteins synthesized from the addition of electroplax RNA, as estimated by comparing the radioactivity precipitated with channel antisera with the total radioactivity precipitated by trichloroacetic acid. Ferguson analysis of the core

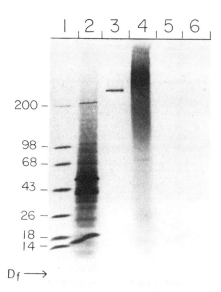

FIGURE 2. Autoradiograph of the ^{35}S-methionine-labeled proteins synthesized as a result of the addition of electroplax RNA to an *in vitro* translation system. The total proteins synthesized are shown in lane 2; the polypeptide precipitated by anti-eel sodium channel antibody is shown in lane 3. Controls: lane 6, antibody preblocked with biochemically purified unlabeled sodium channel; lane 5, proteins synthesized by the reticulocyte lysate system in the absence of eel RNA. Lane 1, ^{14}C-labeled protein standards; lane 4, the ^{125}I-labeled native sodium channel (note the characteristic spreading of the band). Samples were run on a 5%–30% gradient SDS-polyacrylamide gel with low cross-linking.

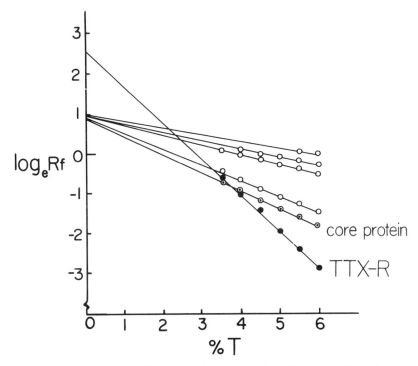

FIGURE 3. Ferguson analysis of the electrophoretic behavior of the native sodium channel and the core polypeptide synthesized *in vitro*, compared with that of standard proteins. This is a plot of the natural logarithm of the relative electrophoretic mobility (Rf) vs. the acrylamide concentration used to cast the separating SDS gel ($\%T$).[14]C-labeled protein standards (O) from top to bottom were ovalbumin, bovine serum albumin, phosphorylase B, and myosin; ⊙ = migration of the ^{35}S-labeled core polypeptide synthesized *in vitro;* ● = migration of the peak (middle) of the ^{125}I-labeled native sodium channel band.

polypeptide was then performed to determine if it had a high electrophoretic free mobility. The core polypeptide actually exhibited a slightly lower free solution mobility than the standard proteins, as is shown in FIGURE 3.

We therefore conclude that posttranslational processing of the core polypeptide to the native form is necessary before the mature channel exhibits it unusual electrophoretic behavior. A slight correction for the lowered free mobility of the core polypeptide allows us to estimate its molecular mass as approximately 200,000 daltons. This is in close agreement with both the value derived from electronmicroscopy[18] and primary amino acid sequence data derived from cDNA clones of the channel gene.[15]

LIPIDS ARE TIGHTLY ASSOCIATED WITH THE SODIUM CHANNEL

The most likely posttranslational modification that would be consistent with the binding of micellar SDS to the sodium channel is the covalent attachment of fatty acids or phospholipids. Further compositional analysis of the highly purified channel has recently detected significant amounts of hydrocarbon chains tightly associated with the molecule through both hydrophobic and presumably covalent interactions (see Levinson *et al.*,[36] this volume). For example, of the total lipids tightly associated with the channel, one fraction can be extracted with organic solvents whereas another fraction is resistant. The lipids that interact hydrophobically with the native molecule are probably doing so with posttranslationally attached fatty acids and not hydrophobic amino acid sequences, because the core polypeptide exhibited near normal electrophoretic behavior on SDS gels, which is indicative of the binding of normal amounts of SDS and not suggestive of any unusual hydrophobic characteristics. Recently a number of integral membrane proteins have been reported to be fatty acid acylated and to contain 1–2 hydrocarbon chains per polypeptide.[19,20] These polypeptides appear to be fairly well behaved on SDS-PAGE, although a full investigation of their interaction with detergents and electrophoretic properties has not usually been conducted. In contrast, the eel sodium channel contains a total of approximately 6%–8% fatty acid by weight, even after SDS-gel filtration on Sepharose 4B followed by extensive dialysis. It can be estimated that there are approximately 50–65 fatty acid chains tightly associated with the channel molecule; this is an unprecedented amount, even taking into consideration the large size of the polypeptide and the probability that most of the hydrophobically associated lipids are actually phospholipids. After extensive extractions with organic solvents, the channel still contains about 3.0% fatty acid by weight, or about 25 hydrocarbon chains per molecule. Thus the hydrophobic characteristics of the sodium channel are apparently due to this close association of posttranslationally acquired lipids.

POSTTRANSLATIONAL PROCESSING OF SODIUM CHANNELS

The eel sodium channel has been shown to contain N-linked sugars, which is indicative of processing in the rough endoplasmic reticulum (RER), sialic acids, and presumably covalently attached fatty acids, suggestive of extensive processing in the Golgi apparatus.[21] An intact cell system is needed to follow the complete posttranslational processing of sodium channels because the RER to Golgi export requires specific cell machinery.

We have chosen the frog oocyte system to analzye the posttranslational processing of eel sodium channels for a number of reasons. *Xenopus laevis* stage VI oocytes are actively engaged in the synthesis of endogeneous proteins and their large size (up to 1.5 mm in diameter) makes them easy to inject with exogeneous mRNA.[22] To date, a number of tissue specific mRNAs, coding for secretory or membrane proteins, have been injected in this system and shown to be translated and the polypeptides properly posttranslationally processed.[23] In addition, Miledi and collaborators have injected mRNA from electrically excitable tissue into oocytes and have detected the presence of a number of voltage-sensitive ion channels via the two-electrode voltage clamp (see Yellen[24] for a short review). In particular, the injection of rat brain mRNA,[25] or size-fractionated mRNA,[26] resulted in the appearance of voltage-dependent, TTX-blockable sodium currents, suggesting the mammalian sodium channel is faithfully processed to a functional form. The oocyte therefore appears to be an ideal system in which to analyze the production of eel sodium channels both biochemically and electrophysiologically.

Preliminary studies with oocytes injected with electroplax RNA have begun to determine whether eel sodium channels will be expressed in this system. After injection with electroplax total RNA, the oocytes were incubated in a medium containing ^{35}S-methionine for different periods of time. Specific eel sodium channel antisera then was used to precipitate the channel molecules from whole oocyte homogenates as a function of time (FIGURE 4). At the earliest time point (10 hours), only a 230,000 dalton polypeptide, indistinguishable in molecular mass from the core polypeptide synthesized in the cell-free system, is visible. This band increases in intensity with time.

T
10
20
30
40
60
N
C1
C2
200-
98-
68-
43-
26-
18-
14-

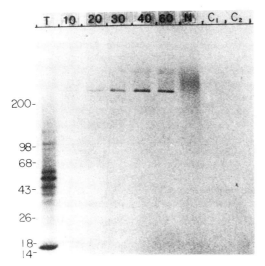

FIGURE 4. Autoradiograph of the ^{35}S-methionine-labeled eel sodium channels synthesized as a result of the injection of electroplax RNA into *Xenopus* oocytes. The medium with fresh ^{35}S-methionine was changed every 20 hours. The total proteins synthesized are shown in lane T. Batches of oocytes were homogenized and eel sodium channels immunoprecipitated with specific channel antisera at 10, 20, 30, 40, and 60 h, indicated above the lanes. Controls (at 60 h): C_1, antisera preblocked with unlabeled native sodium channel; C_2, immunoprecipitation of homogenates of noninjected oocytes with channel antisera; lane N is the ^{125}I-labeled native sodium channel.

Processing of the channel also apparently occurs, with the increasing appearance of polypeptide bands of higher molecular mass than the core polypeptide, similar to the native molecule. In our hands, different oocyte batches were found to vary greatly with the speed and degree of posttranslational processing of eel sodium channels. Further studies will be necessary to elucidate the modifications occurring and to discern whether channels are being inserted into the oocyte's cell surface in a functional state.

200-
98-
68-
43-
26-
18-
14-
Df

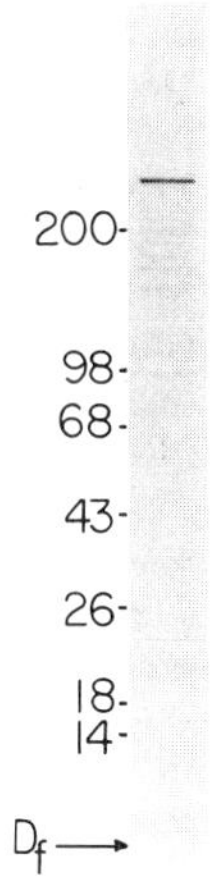

FIGURE 5. Autogradiograph of the ^{35}S-labeled sodium channel polypeptide synthesized in the rabbit reticulocyte lysate system. A ladder of polypeptides is visible below the completed core polypeptide.

Finally, in the course of the cell-free biosynthetic studies, we observed the sodium channel antisera variably precipitated a "ladder" of polypeptides below the 230,000 dalton polypeptide (FIGURE 5). We postulate these polypeptides are incomplete translation products of the 230,000 dalton polypeptide and result from ribosomes, containing the partially completed radiolabeled peptide, prematurely dissociating from the channel mRNA at specific preterminal codons. The following observations lend support to this hypothesis (1) the ladder polypeptides are part of the sodium channel because they are blocked with unlabeled native channel, (2) the sodium channel mRNA is probably not degraded during its isolation because in the oocyte system the ladder has not been detected, (3) the ladder still occurs with a RNase inhibitor and five protease inhibitors in the translation mixture, (4) the ladder's intensity increases with time of incubation of the translation mixture and chasing with unlabeled methionine does not diminsh its intensity, and (5) although the ladder is variable in intensity compared to the completed core polypeptide, when the ladder is present its pattern is invariable. Although the rabbit reticulocyte lysate system has not often been described as producing partial translation products, another cell-free system, the wheat germ lysate, is widely known to be an "early quitter" and is not recommended for translation of large mRNAs coding for polypeptides larger than 70–100 kilodaltons.[27]

CONCLUSION

The cell-free biosynthesis of the sodium channel core polypeptide has been described along with preliminary studies on the posttranslational processing of eel sodium channels in frog oocytes. The cell-free biosynthetic studies suggest that the unusual properties exhibited by the mature, native sodium channel on SDS gels are due to posttranslational modifications of the core polypeptide. Although the diffuse banding pattern on SDS gels has been inferred to result from differing degrees of glycosylation of the polypeptide,[8,28] we have presented evidence here that the high binding of SDS to the native channel and its high electrophoretic free mobility on polyacrylamide gels are due to a posttranslationally acquired property and not the intrinsic hydrophobicity of the core polypeptide. In this volume (Levinson et al.[36]) we have presented evidence that highly hydrophobic domains, in the form of large amounts of lipids, are tightly associated with the native sodium channel and are apparently the posttranslationally acquired domains responsible for the channel's unusual hydrophobic characteristics.

In recent years, a number of cytosolic and membrane-associated proteins have been shown to contain covalently attached hydrocarbon chains.[19,20,29] Integral membrane proteins that are fatty acid acylated include the transferrin receptor,[30] the α and β subunits of the nicotinic acetylcholine receptor from a mouse cell line,[31] and sialoglyco-proteins from murine erythrocytes.[32] The membrane-associated form of the variant surface coat glycoprotein from Trypanosoma brucei has recently been reported to be released from the membrane by phospholipases.[33] Therefore, a phosphodiester linkage between a phospholipid in the outer leaflet of the plasma membrane and the glycoprotein has been postulated.

The precise role played by the covalent attachment of hydrocarbon chains to either cytosolic or membrane proteins is still speculative. In the case of membrane proteins, a number of roles have been postulated, including the anchoring of the protein in the lipid bilayer, a signal for protein sorting within membranes, and a signal for subunit assembly of some receptors in the Golgi apparatus and their cell surface expression.[31,34] In the case of the sodium channel, the lipid association may play a role in gating mechanisms, because it is believed the voltage-sensitive gates partially reside in a hydrophobic lipid environment.[35]

It seems probable these modifications are required for normal channel operation, because the sodium channel is very heavily posttranslationally processed. If this is the case, then biosynthetic studies of sodium channel maturation will be an essential approach to the understanding of how the channel operates on a molecular level.

REFERENCES

1. HILLE, B. 1984. Ionic Channels of Excitable Membranes. Sinauer Associates. Sunderland, Mass.
2. HODGKIN, A., A. HUXLEY & B. KATZ. 1952. J. Physiol. (London) 116: 424–448.
3. AIDLEY, A. R. 1978. The Physiology of Excitable Cells. Cambridge University Press. Cambridge.
4. LEVINSON, S. R. 1981. In Molecular Basis of Drug Action. T. Singer & T. Ondazara, Eds.: 315–331. Elsevier/North Holland. New York.
5. AGNEW, W. S. 1984. Ann. Rev. Physiol. 46: 517–530.
6. CATTERALL, W. A. 1984. Science 223: 653–666.
7. AGNEW, W. A., S. R. LEVINSON, J. S. BRABSON & M. A. RAFTERY. 1978. Proc. Natl. Acad. Sci. U.S.A. 75: 2606–2610.
8. MILLER, J. A., W. S. AGNEW & S. R. LEVINSON. 1983. Biochemistry 12: 462–470.
9. FERGUSON, K. A. & A. L. C. WALLACE. 1961. Nature (London) 190: 629.
10. REYNOLDS, J. A. & C. TANFORD. 1970. Proc. Natl. Acad. Sci. U.S.A. 66: 1002–1007.
11. REYNOLDS, J. A. & C. TANFORD. J. Biol. Chem. 245: 5161–5165.
12. GREFRATH, S. P. & J. A. REYNOLDS. 1974. Proc. Natl. Acad. Sci. U.S.A. 71: 3913–3916.
13. PITT-RIVERS, R. & F. S. A. IMPIOMBATO. 1968. Biochem. J. 409: 825–830.
14. TANFORD, C. 1980. The Hydrophobic Effect: Formation of Micelles and Biological Membranes. 2d ed., chap. 7. Wiley. New York.
15. NODA, M., S. SHIMIZU, T. TANABE, T. TAKAI, T. KAYAMA, T. IKEDA, H. TAKAHASHI, H. NAKAYAMA, Y. KANAOKA, N. MINAMINO, K. KANGAWA, H. MATSUO, M. A. RAFTERY, T. HIROSE, S. INAYAMA, H. HAYASHIDA, T. MIYATA & S. NUMA. 1984. Nature 312: 121–127.
16. CHIRGWIN, J. M., A. D. PRZUBYLA, R. J. MACDONALD & W. J. RUTTER. 1979. Biochemistry 18: 5294–5299.
17. PELHAM, H. R. B. & R. J. JACKSON. 1976. Eur. J. Biochem. 67: 247–256.
18. ELLISMAN, M. H. & S. R. LEVINSON. 1982. Proc. Natl. Acad. Sci. U.S.A. 79: 6707–6711.
19. SCHMIDT, M. F. G. 1983. Curr. Top. Microbiol. Immunol. 102: 101–129.
20. MAGEE, A. I. & M. J. SCHLESINGER. 1982. Biochim. Biophys. Acta 694: 279–289.
21. STRUCK, D. K. & W. J. LENNARZ. 1980. The Biochemistry of Glycoproteins and Proteoglycans. W. J. Leenarz, Ed.: 35–83. Plenum. New York.
22. GURDON, J. B., C. D. LANE, H. R. WOODLAND & G. MARBAIX. 1971. Nature 223: 177.
23. COLMAN, A. 1984. Transcription and Translation: A Practical Approach, chap. 10. B. D. Hames & S. J. Higgens, Eds. IRL Press. Oxford.
24. YELLEN, G. 1984. Trends Neurosci. Dec., pp. 457–458.
25. GUNDERSON, C. B., R. MILEDI & I. PARKER. 1984. Nature 308: 421–424.
26. SUMIKAWA, K., I PARKER & R. MILEDI 1984. Proc. Natl. Acad. Sci. 81: 7994–7998.
27. CLEMENS, M. J. 1984. Transcription and Translation: A Practical Approach, chap. 9. B. D. Hames & S. J. Higgins, Eds. IRL Press. Oxford.
28. AGNEW, W. S., J. A. MILLER, M. H. ELLISMAN, R. L. ROSENBERG, S. A. TOMIKO & S. R. LEVINSON. 1983. Cold Spring Harbor Symp. Quant. Biol. XLVIII: 165–179.
29. MAGEE, I. M. & S. A. COURTNEIDGE. 1985. EMBO J. 4: 1137–1144.
30. OMARY, M. B. & I. S. TROWBRIDGE. 1981. J. Biol. Chem. 256: 4715–4718.
31. OLSON, E. N., L. GLASER & J. P. MERLIE. 1984. J. Biol. Chem. 259: 5364–5367.
32. DOLCI, E. D. & G. E. PALADE. 1985. J. Biol. Chem. 260: 10728–10735.
33. JACKSON, D. G. & H. P. VOORHEIS. 1985. J. Biol. Chem. 260: 5179–5183.
34. SCHLESINGER, M. J. & C. MALFER. 1982. J. Biol. Chem. 257: 9887–9890.
35. HILLE, B. 1984. Ionic Channels of Excitable Membranes, chaps. 13 and 14. Sinauer Associates. Sunderland, Mass.
36. LEVINSON, S. R., D. S. DUCH, B. W. URBAN & E. RECIO-PINTO. 1986. The Sodium Channel from Electrophorus electricus. This volume.

Distribution of Sodium Channels in Muscle[a]

J. H. CALDWELL

Department of Molecular and Cellular Biology
National Jewish Center for Immunology and Respiratory Medicine
Denver, Colorado 80206
and
Department of Physiology
University of Colorado Medical Center
Denver, Colorado 80262

INTRODUCTION

It seems true, no matter what cell we consider, that a morphological specialization or polarity will have associated with it a specific distribution of membrane proteins. The distribution of ion channels in excitable cells such as neurons or muscle is an excellent case in point. Neurons segregate voltage-gated sodium channels, concentrating them at the axon hillock and node of Ranvier and excluding them from the internodal regions of myelinated axons. It has recently become clear that sodium channels in skeletal muscle also have a well-defined distribution. The sodium channel distribution along the length of a muscle fiber, from end plate to tendon, has been studied with the loose patch voltage clamp and is described here.

Several experiments provided the incentive for making the loose patch clamp measurements. The first suggestion of a nonuniform sodium channel distribution along the length of the fiber was a report by Nastuk and Alexander[1] that in frog sartorius the rate of rise of the action potential (recorded with an intracellular electrode) was greater near the end plate than in extrajunctional regions far from the end plate. Shortly thereafter, Thesleff *et al.*[2] performed similar experiments in rat muscle. Thesleff *et al.* suggested that sodium channels are concentrated near the end plate and also proposed that these channels in the end plate region might be tetrodotoxin insensitive. Several years later Betz *et al.*[3] reinvestigated this for two reasons. First, we had discovered that rat muscle has a reduced chloride conductance near the end plate[4] and this nonuniform leak conductance could, by itself, cause the increased rate of rise of the action potential near the end plate. Second, using a vibrating microelectrode[5,6] to measure extracellular current, we found that veratridine (bath applied) induced an inward current focused at the end plate. We studied both the rate of rise of the action potential (FIG. 1A) and the veratridine-induced inward current (FIG. 1B) in both normal saline and in chloride-free saline. The nonuniform chloride conductance accounted for some but not all of the difference in rate of rise of the action potential. We concluded that sodium conductance is increased near the rat end plate and that this increase is confined to membrane within 200 μm of the end plate.

These earlier experiments suffered from several disadvantages, most notable being the lack of spatial resolution and the indirect measure of sodium current. The loose

[a]This work was supported by the National Science Foundation and the Muscular Dystrophy Association.

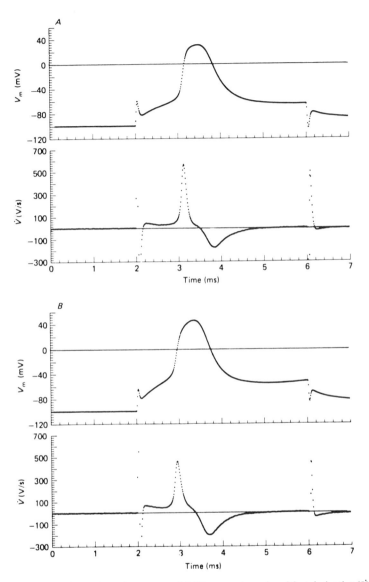

FIGURE 1A. Recordings of membrane potential (V_m, upper traces) and first derivative ($\dot{V}$, lower traces) recorded from end-plate (A) and extrajunctional (B) regions in low-chloride Krebs solution (chloride replaced by isethionate). Action potentials were elicited from a holding potential of -100 mV by a depolarizing pulse of 4 ms duration. The peak of the differentiated action potential gives the maximum rate of rise ($\dot{V}_{max}$) of the action potential. Note that $\dot{V}_{max}$ is greater at the end-plate than in the extrajunctional region.

366   ANNALS NEW YORK ACADEMY OF SCIENCES

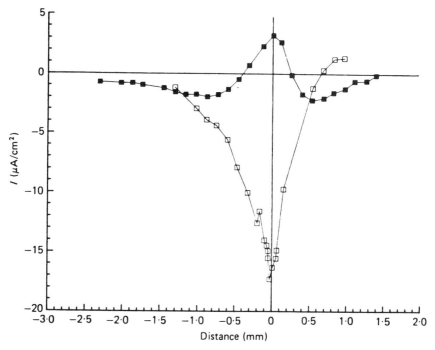

FIGURE 1B. Spatial maps of steady electrical current, measured with a vibrating microelectrode, before (■) and during (□) veratridine (500 μM) treatment. The electrode was vibrated perpendicular to the muscle edge and measured current entering or leaving the muscle. Muscle was pretreated with α-bungarotoxin (4 μg/ml) to block synaptic currents. The x-axis represents distance along the edge of the muscle, with zero being the point of maximum outward current in normal Krebs solution (end-plate region). The y-axis represents current density, positive corresponding to outward current. Note that the point of maximum outward current in normal Krebs solution corresponds to the maximum inward current in veratridine. (From Betz et al.[4] Reprinted by permission from the *Journal of General Physiology*.)

patch voltage clamp obviates these problems. Small patches of membrane (2–20 μm in diameter) can be voltage clamped and sodium current directly measured. Both Beam, Caldwell, and Campbell[7] and Roberts and Almers[8] have used this technique to show that sodium channels are concentrated near the end plate. We have now mapped sodium current density in all regions of the fiber and can give a more complete description of the distribution of sodium channels.

METHODS

The muscle preparations were chosen for their visibility, which allowed us to position the electrode with respect to defined features of the muscle fiber. We used intact muscles from the garter snake and both intact and enzymatically dissociated fibers from the rat flexor digitorum brevis (FDB) and omohyoid. The enzymatic dissociation was similar to that of Bekoff and Betz.[9] The muscles and recording electrode were viewed at 400× magnification with Hoffman modulation contrast optics.

The loose patch clamp, as described originally by Strickholm[10] and more recently by Stühmer and Almers,[11] was used for mapping. We used the single electrode rather than the concentric barrels developed by Roberts and Almers.[12] The details of our methods have been described earlier.[7] Two problems not mentioned previously were encountered in doing these experiments. First, when recording from the enzymatically dissociated fibers, the application of suction to improve the seal resistance sometimes caused the formation of large membrane "bubbles" in the pipette. One of these is illustrated in FIGURE 2. This increased the effective membrane area of recording and could increase the sodium current recorded. A more preliminary description of this phenomenon and its effect on currents has been made.[13] These membrane bubbles could arise with very little suction (20 mm Hg), and thus it was important to watch for them during the recording.

The second problem is that large membrane currents through the patch will change the potential across the patch. For a muscle cell this is normally not of any concern. When recording from the end plate, however, even a pipette of moderate size (e.g., 10 μm) can record a peak sodium current of 200 nA. If an intracellular electrode is inserted adjacent to the patch electrode, a depolarization of 30–40 mV is recorded; the loose patch clamp has become only a loose patch, not a clamp. By using small pipettes and thus keeping the peak current less than 20 nA, the membrane potential remains under voltage control when recording at the end plate. When the small pipettes (2–4 μm in diameter) were used, the pipette tip diameter was measured at 1000× magnification. Current densities are expressed relative to the pipette tip diameter rather than the effective membrane area in the patch (see DISCUSSION).

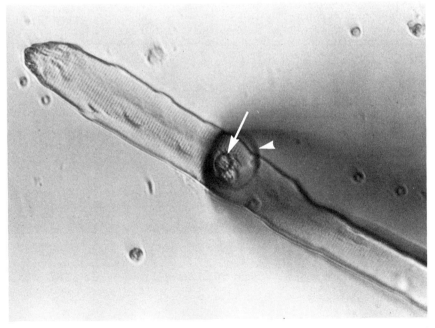

FIGURE 2. A "bubble" of membrane created by application of suction to the patch. The end of this single, dissociated FDB fiber is at the upper left. The pipette tip was 13 μm in diameter (arrow) and the "bubble" was 50 μm in diameter (arrowhead).

RESULTS

The fiber has been divided into four regions for convenience in presenting the data. These are (1) the end-plate region, (2) perijunctional or near end plate, (3) extrajunctional, far from both end plate and tendon, and (4) near the tendon. The extent of the end plate is defined by the outermost branches of the nerve terminal. In both the rat and snake this is an oval-shaped area. Not all of this area is covered by nerve terminals and thus this region includes both subsynaptic membrane and nonsynaptic membrane (without the high density of acetylcholine receptors). The perijunctional membrane is outside the nerve branches and extends several hundred micrometers away from the end plate.

End-Plate Region

These recordings have all been made from rat fibers whose nerve terminals were removed by enzymatic treatment. The largest current densities of any region of the fiber occur when the pipette is on the end plate. Current density as large as 400 mA/cm^2 has been recorded, although 100–200 mA/cm^2 is more typical. The average current density recorded with 2.5 μm pipettes was 169 ± 90 mA/cm^2 (mean ± SD, $n = 14$). Sodium current recorded from the end plate is shown in FIGURE 3. We assume that the pipette records simultaneously from subsynaptic membrane and from the nonsynaptic membrane that lies between nerve terminals. This can be appreciated from FIGURE 4, which shows the end plate region of a rat FDB fiber. The insets show the same end plate with Hoffman optics and labeled with FITC-α bungarotoxin. The dark ring on the end plate shows the location of one recording position.

Another feature of recording from the end plate is significant. When small pipettes (2.5 μm diameter) were used, large variations in current were found within an individual end plate. The same pipette at one position recorded very little current (less than 10 mA/cm^2), and yet at another position several hundred mA/cm^2. Variation in

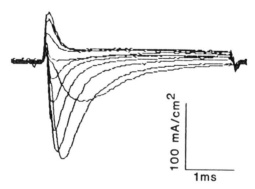

100 mA/cm^2

1ms

FIGURE 3. Sodium currents recorded directly from the end-plate membrane of a dissociated rat flexor digitorum brevis muscle fiber. In this fiber the enzymatic treatment resulted in complete removal of the nerve terminal. In addition, the fiber was situated in the dish such that the exposed end plate was accessible to the pipette. Sodium currents measured with the pipette on the end plate. Voltage steps were from −52 to +83 mV in 15 mV increments. The holding potential was −112 mV. Pipette diameter was 4 μm. Pipette resistance was 600 kΩ. Shunt resistance was 3.6 MΩ.

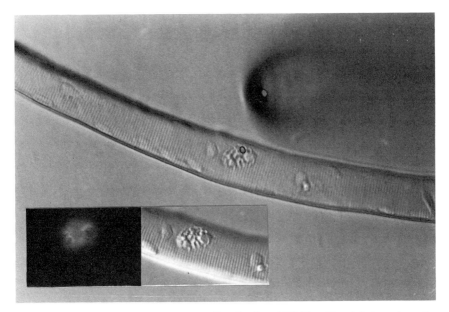

FIGURE 4. The end-plate region of a single dissociated rat FDB fiber. The *right inset* shows the end plate with Hoffman modulation contrast optics and the *left inset* shows the fluorescence from FITC-α bungarotoxin (4 μg/ml) which was bound to the fiber prior to recording. The recording position is indicated by the black oval and contains both subsynaptic and nonsynaptic membrane.

peak sodium current within one end plate is illustrated in FIGURE 5. This may be an artifact arising from incomplete removal of nerve and Schwann cell from the muscle, the small currents being measured when the pipette was over the debris. There did not appear to be obvious debris during these recordings, but we cannot rule this out. If the variations are real, they imply a nonuniform distribution within the end plate.

Near End Plate

Sodium current recorded adjacent to the end plate was four-to-five times lower than that recorded from the end plate. In dissociated rat FDB muscle the average current density was about 30 mA/cm^2 and in the snake it was 25 mA/cm^2. Some of the difference between end plate and perijunctional current density may be a consequence of the additional membrane folding in the end plate (see DISCUSSION).

In addition to the abrupt decrease from end plate to perijunctional membrane, current density decreases with distance from the end plate in both snake[7,8] and rat.[7] Peak sodium currents recorded at different positions from a rat FDB fiber are shown in FIGURE 6. The largest of these currents is found near the end plate (recording from the end plate membrane is not shown here). Peak current versus distance from the end plate for the snake fiber is plotted in FIGURE 7. In both rat and snake the current density fell smoothly with distance from the end plate and reached far-extrajunctional levels (see below) when the electrode was 100–200 μm from the end plate. Thus sodium channels are concentrated not only within the end plate but also near the end plate.

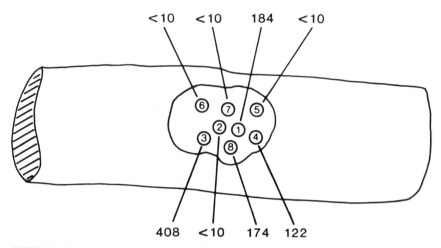

FIGURE 5. Sodium current recorded at eight positions within a single end plate of a dissociated FDB fiber. The numbers within the circles indicate the sequence of recording. The numbers above and below the fiber indicate the current density (mA/cm^2) at each spot. The pipette diameter was 2.5 μm (pipette resistance = 680 kΩ). Seal resistances were between 1 MΩ–1.9 MΩ and there was no correlation between the magnitude of the seal and the large or small currents. The membrane potential was held at -132 mV (-80 mV hold with resting membrane potential estimated to be -52 mV).

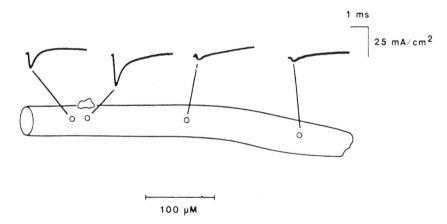

FIGURE 6. Representative Na currents recorded at different positions along a rat muscle fiber. Circles indicate the recording positions. Na currents, elicited by a test pulse to a potential estimated to be -7 mV, from four sites on an isolated rat fiber. The test currents were measured 2–4 min after the establishment of a holding potential, estimated to be -97 mV. The pipette had a tip diameter of 5 μm and a resistance of 400 kΩ. The seal resistance varied from 600–900 kΩ. (From Beam, et al.[7] Reprinted from Nature **313**: 588–590, Copyright 1985 Macmillan Journals Limited.)

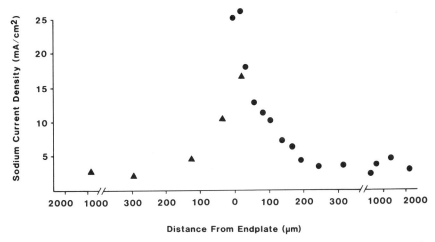

FIGURE 7. Variation of sodium current density with distance from the end plate in a snake muscle fiber. The abscissa gives the distance from the recording site to the closest portion of the end plate. Note the change in horizontal scale for points at distances greater than 350 μm from the end plate. The points plotted as circles were measured sequentially at sites from left to right along the fiber and the points plotted as triangles were measured sequentially at sites from right to left along the fiber. (From Beam *et al.*[7] Reprinted from Nature **313**: 588–590, Copyright 1985 Macmillan Journals Limited.)

These recordings in FIGURES 6 and 7 show current density versus longitudinal distance. How does current density vary with circumferential distance from the end plate?

An example of a snake fiber whose end plate was on the side is illustrated in FIGURE 8. The fiber was 80 μm in diameter, which allowed us to map circumferentially from the end plate to the antipode. It is evident that current density fell rapidly in any direction from the end plate. We conclude that the end plate itself is the focal point of the increased density.

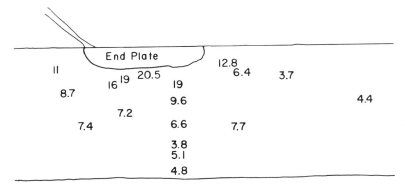

FIGURE 8. Circumferential decrease in Na current density. Snake external abdominal oblique muscle. Current density (mA/cm^2) is indicated at each recording position. No holding potential was applied. The estimated resting potential was -90 mV. Pipette diameter was 10 μm, fiber diameter 80 μm, pipette resistance 210 kΩ; seal resistance varied from 210–310 kΩ.

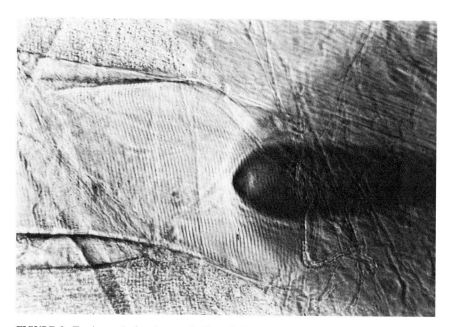

FIGURE 9. Tendon end of a short scale fiber of the garter snake. The shadow of the pipette extends over the connective tissue sheet in which the muscle terminates. Pipette tip diameter was 10 μm.

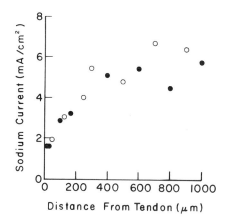

Distance From Tendon (μm)

FIGURE 10. Decrease of sodium current near the end of a short scale fiber of the snake. Pipette diameter was 12.5 μm and resistance 150 kΩ. Estimated resting potential was 94 mV. No hold was applied. The shunt resistance varied from 250–410 kΩ. Recordings were first made moving the electrode toward the tendon (●) and then away from the tendon (○).

Extrajunctional

For most muscles this region which is far from both the end plate and tendon constitutes the majority of the fiber. Almers et al.[14] found that sodium current density in frog sartorius varied severalfold over a few micrometers. We made similar measurements in snake external abdominal oblique muscle, although not as closely spaced as were those of Almers et al. Current density also varied by a factor of 2–3 over 10–20 μm in the snake; these fluctuations were never as large as those at the end plate nor were they associated with any obvious morphological feature.

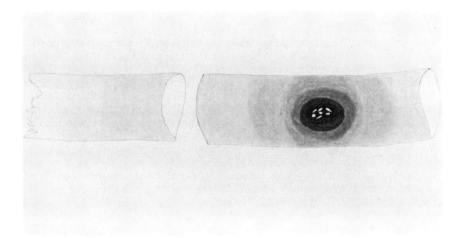

FIGURE 11. Sketch of a single muscle fiber illustrating the distribution of sodium channels. The darkest area (oval-shaped) is the end-plate region where the largest current densities were recorded. Within the end plate are light patches to indicate that the current density is not uniform. The current density decreases in all directions from the end plate. The gap in the fiber represents the extrajunctional region where the current density fluctuates without any correlation to external morphology. The lightest area near the tendon indicates the low current density at the end of the fiber.

Near Tendon

As the electrode comes within 200–500 μm of the end of the fiber, the current density progressively decreases. FIGURE 9 shows the end of a short scale fiber of the snake. Sodium current density from one of these fibers is shown in FIGURE 10. This decrease also occurs in the rat FDB and soleus.

These measurements of sodium current in all regions of the fiber are summarized schematically in FIGURE 11. The highest concentration of sodium channels occurs at and near the end plate. Channel density may be extremely nonuniform within the end plate. Channel density decreases with both circumferential and longitudinal distance from the end plate. At distances greater than about 200 μm from the end plate, the density fluctuates about a low level (5–10 mA/cm^2 in the rat and 4 mA/cm^2 in the snake) for many millimeters. The density begins to decrease further when the electrode is 200–500 μm from the tendinous end. When the electrode is within 25 μm of the end, current density is only ~1mA/cm^2.

Are sodium channels at the end plate different from those far from the end plate? We have tested the TTX sensitivity of channels at end plate and extrajunctional regions in both rat and snake muscle. There was no evidence for any TTX-resistant channels in normal muscle.

DISCUSSION

The pattern of Na channel distribution in skeletal muscle described here is probably true for most, or perhaps all, vertebrates. The original observation by Nastuk and Alexander[1] suggests that it is correct for frog muscle, and it has been found in all of the various snake and rat muscles that we have studied. One would still like to know the absolute density of Na channels. Estimating channel density requires several assumptions. First, one needs to know the membrane area being voltage clamped. We have calculated current density based on the area of the tip of the pipette. This is valid if all the current we measure is generated by surface membrane and if the surface is not heavily infolded. We have begun to measure the capacitance of the patch as Roberts and Almers[8] did in the snake, and we also find that the pipette records from both surface membrane and transverse-tubular membrane. There is, however, evidence that Na channel density is low in the transverse tubular membrane[15] and therefore it is not clear how much, if any, of this should be included in the current density calculation. The question of membrane area is especially important at the end-plate region, because the synaptic folds cause a 4–5 fold increase in surface area and the currents we record are also increased by a similar amount. On the other hand, sodium channels are probably not uniformly distributed in the end-plate region. If we therefore take the maximum current densities as expressed here and assume a single channel current of 1 pA, the sodium channel density at the end plate is several thousand per μm^2, a value close to that at the node of Ranvier.

Is the nonuniform distribution reasonable from a functional viewpoint? The end plate and perijunctional membrane could be considered analogous to the axon hillock of a neuron. The increased channel density would improve the safety factor for neuromuscular transmission and ensure that an action potential is initiated. The additional channels would compensate for the shunt caused by open AchRs during the end plate potential[16] and for the fact that both halves of the fiber need to be brought to threshold. What would explain the decrease in channel density at the tendon? One might posit a biological conservation of energy, stating that the channels are not at the end because they are not needed there. Current for continued propagation of the action potential is not required at the end and current supplied from regions near the tendon would be sufficient to bring the membrane to threshold for contraction. This logic may be comforting, but it is not especially compelling. It may be worthwhile to consider the possibility that having sodium channels at the tendon would be detrimental. Membrane at the extreme end of frog fibers is increased 50-fold[17]; this would alter the shape of the action potential in this region and sodium channels in this membrane might lead to a reflected action potential propagating back toward the end plate.

It is not hard to rationalize the sodium channel distribution that we find, but this does not help us to understand how the fiber achieves this distribution or what controls the distribution. The best studied ion channel distribution is that of the acetylcholine receptor (AChR). A variety of mechanisms have been proposed but the basis of the distribution remains unexplained. We should be aware that it is unlikely that the control of channel distribution will be identical for all channels, especialy since their distributions are not the same. Sodium channels and AChRs are both concentrated at the end plate, but given the large variation in Na current density described earlier, it is conceivable that AChR and Na channels are in separate areas within the end plate. In soleus muscle, AChR density is increased at the tendon whereas sodium channel denisty is decreased. Finally, chloride channels have a distribution very different from both AChR and Na channels; they are reduced in the end-plate region.[4]

The focal increase in sodium channel density at the end plate implicates the nerve in inducing and/or maintaining the high concentration of sodium channels. The reduced density at the tendon would be predicted to be linked to muscle activity and thus only indirectly dependent on the presence of the nerve. Denervation of the muscle could be expected to affect Na channel distribution. However, in preliminary experiments denervation had no effect on the nonuniform distribution in either rat or snake muscle.

The persistence of the increased density near the endplate in denervated muscle may help to explain why fibrillation potentials (spontaneous action potentials) tend to originate at the denervated end plate.[18,19] Apparently, once the mechanism for Na channel localization is established, it no longer requires the nerve.

ACKNOWLEDGMENTS

The unpublished experiments described here were done in collaboration with Drs. Kurt Beam, Donald Campbell, and Richard Milton. FIGURE 11 was drawn by Diane Nicholl.

REFERENCES

1. NASTUK, W. L. & J. T. ALEXANDER. 1973. Nonhomogeneous electrical activity in single muscle fibers. Fed. Proc. 32: 333.
2. THESLEFF, S., F. VYSKOCIL & M. R. WARD. 1974. The action potential in end-plate and extrajunctional regions of rat skeletal muscle. Acta Physiol. Scand. 91: 196–202.
3. BETZ, W. J., J. H. CALDWELL & S. C. KINNAMON. 1984. Increased sodium conductance in the synaptic region of rat skeletal muscle fibers. J. Physiol. 352: 189–202.
4. BETZ, W. J., J. H. CALDWELL & S. C. KINNAMON. 1984. Physiological basis of a steady endogenous current in rat lumbrical muscle. J. Gen. Physiol. 83: 175–192.
5. JAFFE, L. F. & R. NUCCITELLI. 1974. An ultrasensitive vibrating probe for measuring steady extracellular current. J. Cell Biol. 63: 614–628.
6. BETZ, W. J. & J. H. CALDWELL. 1984. Mapping electric currents around skeletal muscle with a vibrating probe. J. Gen. Physiol. 83: 143–156.
7. BEAM, K. G., J. H. CALDWELL & D. T. CAMPBELL. 1985. Na channels in skeletal muscle concentrated near the neuromuscular junction. Nature 313: 588–590.
8. ROBERTS, W. M. & W. ALMERS. 1985. Increased Na$^+$ current density near endplates in snake skeletal muscle. Biophys. J. 47: 189a.
9. BEKOFF, A. & W. J. BETZ. 1977. Physiological properties of dissociated muscle fibers obtained from innervated and denervated adult rat muscle. J. Physiol. 271: 25–40.
10. STRICKHOLM, A. 1961. Impedance of a small electrically isolated area of the muscle cell surface. J. Gen. Physiol. 44: 1073–1088.
11. STÜHMER, W. & W. ALMERS. 1982. Photobleaching through glass micropipettes: Sodium channels without lateral mobility in the sarcolemma of frog skeletal muscle. Proc. Natl. Acad. Sci. U.S.A. 79: 946–950.
12. ROBERTS, W. M. & W. ALMERS. 1984. An improved loose patch voltage clamp method using concentric pipettes. Pflügers Arch. 402: 190–196.
13. MILTON, R. L. & J. H. CALDWELL. 1986. Vesicles extracted from skeletal muscle fibers via suction: Possible implications for loose and tight patch voltage clamping. Biophys. J. 49: 172a.

14. ALMERS, W., P. R. STANFIELD & W. STÜHMER. 1983. Lateral distribution of sodium and potassium channels in frog skeletal muscle: Measurements with a patch clamp technique. J. Physiol. **336:** 261–284.
15. HILLE, B. & D. T. CAMPBELL. 1976. An improved vaseline gap voltage clamp for skeletal muscle fibers. J. Gen. Physiol. **67:** 265–293.
16. FATT, P. & B. KATZ. 1951. An analysis of the end-plate potential recorded with an intra-cellular electrode. J. Physiol. **115:** 320–370.
17. MILTON, R. L., R. T. MATHIAS & R. S. EISENBERG. 1985. Electrical properties of the myotendon region of frog twitch muscle fibers measured in the frequncy domain. Biophys. J. **48:** 253–267.
18. BELMAR, J. & C. EYZAGUIRRE. 1966. Pacemaker site of fibrillation potentials in denervated mammalian muscle. J. Neurophysiol. **29:** 425–441.
19. PURVES, D. & B. SAKMANN. 1974. Membrane properties underlying spontaneous activity of denervated muscle fibres. J. Physiol. **239:** 125–153.

Distribution and Mobility of Voltage-gated Ion Channels in Skeletal Muscle[a]

W. M. ROBERTS,[b] W. STÜHMER,[c] R. E. WEISS,[d]
P. R. STANFIELD,[e] AND W. ALMERS

Department of Physiology and Biophysics
University of Washington
Seattle, Washington 98195

INTRODUCTION

Cell membranes are widely held to be fluid lipid bilayers wherein membrane proteins may diffuse freely. As a consequence of their mobility, membrane proteins are expected to distribute themselves uniformly over the cell membrane. In embryonic or transformed cells grown in tissue culture, uniform distribution and mobility have indeed been found for many membrane proteins (for a review, see ref. 1). When cells differentiate to form adult tissues, however, cell membrane proteins often segregate and become regionalized; this is especially true for membrane proteins that mediate transport of salts or water-soluble nutrients across cell membranes (for a review see ref. 2). In skeletal muscle, a widely known and striking example of regionalization is the congregation of acetylcholine receptors beneath the innervating nerve terminal at the neuromuscular junction. The mobility of these receptors is so low (diffusion coefficient $D < 10^{-12}$ cm^2/s) that it cannot be detected with present methods.

While voltage-gated Na and K channels are found everywhere on the sarcolemma, they too are nonuniformly distributed over the cell membrane. Both Na and K channels[3,4] are present in the sarcolemma at higher density than in the membranes of the transverse tubules, a system of cell membrane invagination that serves to conduct the action potential from the sarcolemma to the fiber interior. The distribution of channels between sarcolemma and tubules seems to be carefully optimized.[5] Conduction of action potentials down the tubules requires at least some Na channels there; however, too many Na channels could result in escape of the tubule membrane potential from control by the sarcolemma, and jeopardize the tight control of skeletal muscle by the motor nerve. With too many K channels in the tubules, an action potential would lead to excessive K accumulation there, and this in turn can cause the repetitive after-discharges observed in congenital myotonia.[6]

The uneven distribution of K and Na channels could be explained if, like AChR at

[a]This work was supported by a National Institutes of Health (Department of Health and Human Services) grant (AM17803) and by a grant-in-aid from the Muscular Dystrophy Association.
[b]Present address: Department of Physiology S-762, University of California Medical School, San Francisco, Calif. 94143.
[c]Present address: Max Planck Institute for Biophysical Chemistry, P.O. Box 1841, 3400 Göttingen, Federal Republic of Germany.
[d]Present address: Physiology Dept., University of California Medical School, Los Angeles, Calif. 90024.
[e]Present address: Dept. of Physiology, University of Leicester, Leicester LE1 7RH, United Kingdom.

the end plate, the two channels are immobile, or at least severely restricted in their mobility. This paper reviews our recent work on this and related topics.

METHODS

We used a method for electrical recording now known as the loose patch voltage clamp.[7,8] The tip of a fire-polished micropipette is pushed against a muscle fiber, electrically isolating a 10–15 μm patch of sarcolemma. Potential steps are applied to the pipette, and the resulting current measured. We wished to record from muscle fibers that retained their normal basal lamina, a 20 to 150 nm thick extracellular layer of collagen, glycoproteins, and other constituents. Hence we had to accept inferior electric seals between pipette tip and sarcolemma and develop electronic methods to cancel them out. We also developed a version of this method employing concentric pipettes. Such pipettes may be used to divide the patch into a central and a peripheral, annular region. By keeping center and periphery isopotential by electronic feedback, one can simulate an operationally infinite seal resistance for the inner pipette, even though the actual seal resistance may be quite low.[9] In the present work, however, only simple, single-barreled micropipettes were used.

Besides electrical recording, we also performed measurements of "fluorescence recovery after photobleaching" (FRAP) in order to measure the mobility of wheat germ agglutinin (WGA) receptors. Our method follws that of previous workers[10–13] and is described elsewhere.[14]

RESULTS AND DISCUSSION

Distribution of Na and K Channels over the Sarcolemma

When depolarizing potential steps are applied to patch pipettes pressed against the sarcolemma of a frog sartorius or snake costocutaneous muscle, one readily records transient inward currents through voltage- and tetrodotoxin-sensitive Na channels. These currents are followed by outward currents through voltage-activated K channels of the "delayed rectifier" type. Similar membrane currents were observed by earlier investigators who used other methods to record from large portions of muscle cells.[15] With local recording, however, one finds that the amplitudes of Na and K currents vary from position to position on a fiber. The amplitudes do not vary in parallel, hence the variations in current amplitude cannot be the result of, for example, variable amounts of membrane infolding, or of a variable thickness of the basal lamina. We interpret it to represent a variation of ion channel density with positon.

We have recorded peak I_{Na} at over 60 positions within a 20×90 μm strip of sarcolemma crossing the fiber. From the results we have constructed a contour map of I_{Na} and hence, of Na channel density. The area contained two "hot spots" where I_{Na} was three times larger than elsewhere in that area. The gradient of Na channel density was fairly steep, with density falling e-fold within 10–15 μm. If Na channels survive as long as AChR, such gradients could be maintained only if Na channels were immobile, or diffused with a diffusion coefficient less than 2×10^{-12} cm^2/s. This is 1000 times smaller than the diffusion coefficient of AChR,[16] a protein of similar size, after AChRs have been released from cytoskeletal constraints. One may conclude that the Na channels within "hot spots" are anchored in the cell membrane. A detailed description of this work has been published.[7]

The costocutaneous muscle of the garter snake forms a single layer of parallel muscle fibers. The motor end plates are clearly visible, and the surface of the muscle fibers may be visualized under differential interference contrast. Hot spots have been detected by scanning along a muscle fiber, but the largest I_{Na} densities are found at the motor end plate.[17,18] I_{Na} amplitude declines steeply as one moves away from the end plate, falling e-fold within 20 to 30 μm. The membrane capacity, measured with small potential steps at the same locations where I_{Na} was recorded, shows little variation from its average value (4 μF/cm^2). This demonstrates that the increased Na channel density near the end plate is not due to membrane infoldings that may increase the membrane area from which current is recorded. Evidently the increased I_{Na} near the end plate reflects a genuinely increased density of Na channels. K currents do not increase as one moves towards the end-plate region. Apparently the end plate concentrates Na channels and ACh receptors but not voltage-dependent K channels.

It seemed possible that increased Na channel density is a result of proximity to muscle fiber nuclei, which are known to congregate beneath the end plate. The dye Hoechst 33342, a membrane-permeant fluorescent stain selective for DNA, was used to visualize nuclei in living muscle fibers. The fluroescence of nuclei was visible under epifluorescence illumination, so that pipettes could be placed onto patches of sarcolemma that covered a nucleus and others that did not. The mean ratio of I_{Na} in patches that were located above nuclei to patches that were not was 0.98 ± 0.08 SEM ($n = 16$); this is not significantly different from unity. It appeared that nuclei were absent beneath those portions of sarcolemma where a nerve or capillary crossed the fiber. I_{Na} density in such regions was not significantly different from other extrajunctional regions. Evidently the proximity to muscle cell nuclei has no significant influence on the local density of Na channels.

The findings reported so far may be summarized thus: Na and K channels are unevenly distributed not only between tubular membranes and sarcolemma, but also on the sarcolemma itself. For Na channels the observed gradients in Na channel density are steep, suggesting that Na channels are immobile or greatly restricted in their mobility.

Mobility of Lectin Receptors in the Sarcolemma

It seemed possible that immobility is a general property of membrane proteins in a highly stable and differentiated cell such as an adult skeletal muscle fiber. In order to test this, we stained single fibers dissected from frog semitendinosus muscles with fluorescently labeled wheat germ agglutinin (WGA). WGA binds to a wide variety of integral membrane proteins, so that the mobility of WGA receptors may be taken as representing an average for many sarcolemmal membrane proteins.

Mobility of WGA receptors was measured by FRAP. A spot of dim light 5.0 to 7.2 μm in diameter was imaged onto the sarcolemma, and the fluorescence excited by the light was monitored with a photomultiplier. Chromophores in the spot were then bleached by intensifying, for a short period, the beam of light 10 to 100 times, so that fluorescence was greatly diminished. Over the next 20 to 40 min fluorescence gradually recovered. We attribute the recovery of fluorescence to appearance in the spot of new WGA receptors that, carrying with them their unbleached chromophore, reach the spot by diffusion within the plane of the membrane, a conclusion reached by other workers who have done similar experiments on other tissues. An example is shown in FIGURE 1 (top). The continuous curve drawn through the data points describes diffusion into a disk; it is a least-squares fit and was calculated with a diffusion coefficient for WGA receptors of 2.5 $\times$ 10^{-11} cm^2/s, and on the assumption

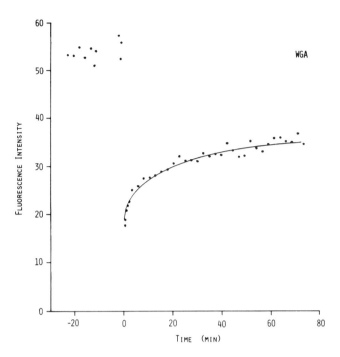

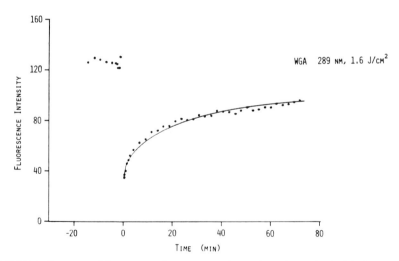

FIGURE 1. Recovery of fluorescence from two sarcolemmal patches stained with fluorescein-conjugated WGA. Two experiments were carried out on the same fiber, one without irradiation (*top*) and another after preirradiation with UV light at the indicated energy density and wavelength (*bottom*). The curves are least-squares fits describing diffusion into a disk, assuming that only a fraction of all WGA receptors are mobile. Diffusion coefficients were 2.5×10^{-11} cm^2/s (*top*) and 2.4×10^{-11} cm^2/s (*bottom*); mobile fractions were 49% (*top*) and 72% (*bottom*). Irradiation, bleaching, and fluorescence measurements were all carried out through a $72\times$ reflecting objective.

that 49% of all WGA receptors were mobile. Average values from experiments on eleven fibers were 6.4×10^{-11} cm^2/s ($\pm 0.8 \times 10^{-11}$ cm^2/s) for the diffusion coefficient and 0.53 ± 0.02 for the mobile fraction. These results are very similar to results with WGA receptors on human embryo fibroblasts.[12] One must remember, however, that an adult muscle fiber is surrounded by a basal lamina; at least some of the apparently immobile WGA receptors are undoubtedly attributable to that structure. Receptors for succinyl concanavalin A (Con A), another divalent lectin, appeared to be entirely immobile in our measurements. Concanavalin A is known to be avidly bound by the basal lamina (see, for example, ref. 19), and we suppose that the overwhelming majority of Con A receptors from which we collected fluorescence were constituents of the basal lamina.

The conclusion from our results with WGA receptors is that the sarcolemma of adult skeletal muscle contains immobile as well as many mobile membrane proteins. There appears to be nothing special about the cell membrane fluidity of an adult skeletal muscle fiber.

K and Na Channels Have Little or No Mobility

We have developed a method for measuring the mobility of voltage-gated Na and K channels. The method takes advantage of the finding that both Na and K channels may be destroyed by irradiation with weak ultraviolet light.[20,21] Destruction is thought to be due to a direct, one-hit, one-photon event. The effect has an action spectrum with a maximum at 280 to 290 nm, suggesting that UV attacks aromatic amino acids in the channel proteins.

The experimental strategy was to use through-the-pipette irradiation with UV light in order to destroy ion channels locally in the patch of membrane from which current is recorded. If these channels are mobile in the plane of the membrane, fresh Na and K channels from neighboring, unirradiated membrane areas should reach the irradiated patch by diffusion, causing recovery of Na and K current there. UV light was directed into the back end of the pipette via a quartz fiber functioning as a light guide. The light traveled down the pipette and was found to emerge from the pipette tip as a well-defined beam of the same diameter as the pipette tip orifice. Hence UV will reach only the patch of membrane beneath the pipette tip orifice, and destruction of channels is expected to be confined to that area only. This was verified by mapping the patch current amplitude as a function of distance from the center of the irradiated patch.

When Na and K channels were locally destroyed by through-the-pipette irradiation with UV light, both I_{Na} and I_K were found to diminish, as expected. With I_{Na}, however, no recovery was observed within 100 min after irradiation. Comparison with theoretical curves (see ref. 22) indicates that diffusion with $D = 10^{-12}$ cm^2/s would have been just detectable with our method, hence we conclude that Na channels are immobile, or have a diffusion coefficient less than 10^{-12} cm^2/s.[23]

In other experiments it was found that Na channels are unable to move under large electric fields in the plane of the membrane. Not even the "surface charge" of Na channels has lateral mobility, as judged by the failure of membrane-parallel electric fields to influence the gating of Na channels.[24]

Our results on Na channels may be compared with those of Angelides,[25] who measured Na channel mobility with FRAP using a scorpion toxin as a fluorescent ligand. In mammalian myotubes cocultured with spinal cord neurons, he found Na channels to be immobile at the nerve-muscle synapse, whereas a minority of extrajunctional Na channels had some mobility.

In similar experiments with K channels, a small fraction of I_K was seen to recover after irradiation. The effect was small, but appeared consistently. When both K and Na currents were recorded in the same patch, recovery was seen only with I_K, and not I_{Na}. Averaged results with K channels were best fit by assuming that about 25% of all K channels had a mobility similar to that of WGA receptors, with the rest being immobile (FIG. 2).

These results may be summarized by saying that all Na and most K channels are immobile or have a mobility less than 10^{-12} cm^2/s, the limit of detection in our experiments. Evidently Na channels are anchored in the cell membrane. The same may apply also to most K channels.

It seemed possible that the restricted mobility of ion channels is a result of UV irradiation. To test this point, the mobility of WGA receptors was measured in a patch

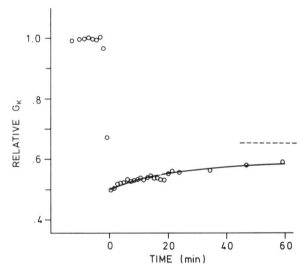

FIGURE 2. Recovery of K current after photodestruction of K channels by 289 nm light. Averaged results from four fibers are shown. The average UV energy density required to cause destruction of half of the K channels is estimated to be 0.8 to 0.9 J/cm^2 from action spectrum measurements (not shown). The curve is predicted if both photodestruction and the efficiency of current collection fall with distance from the center of the patch along a Gaussian curve.[22] The diffusion coefficient is 5×10^{-11} cm^2/s, the mobile fraction 25%.

that had been preirradiated with 289 nm UV at an energy density 2–4 times larger than we used in our electrical measurements. The result is shown in FIGURE 1 (bottom), along with results from an unirradiated patch from the same fiber (FIG. 1, top). The rates at which fluorescence recovers, and hence the diffusion coefficients for WGA, are identical within experimental error. Evidently UV light of the wavelength and energy densities used here does not significantly diminish mobility.

One may conclude that mobile and immobile membrane proteins coexist in the sarcolemma of adult skeletal muscle. Na and K channels are among the membrane proteins that are singled out for immobilization. The immobility of Na channels and of most K channels may explain how these channels remain at specific places through the life of a muscle cell.

REFERENCES

1. PETERS, R. 1981. Translational diffusion in the plasma membrane of single cells as studied by fluorescence microphotolysis. Cell Biol. Intl. Rep. **5:** 733–760.
2. ALMERS, W. & C. E. STIRLING. 1984. Distribution of transport proteins over animal cell membranes. J. Membr. Biol. **77:** 169–186.
3. JAIMOVITCH, E., R. A. VENOSA, P. SHRAGER & P. HOROWICZ. 1976. Density and distribution of tetrodotoxin receptors in normal and detubulated frog sartorius muscle. J. Gen. Physiol. **67:** 399–416.
4. KIRSCH, G. E., R. A. NICHOLS & S. NAKAJIMA. 1977. Delayed rectification in the transverse tubules. Origin of the late after-potential in frog skeletal muscles. J. Gen. Physiol. **70:** 1–21.
5. ALMERS, W. 1980. Potassium concentration changes in the transverse tubules of vertebrate skeletal muscle. Fed. Proc. **39:** 1527–1532.
6. ADRIAN, R. H. & S. H. BRYANT. 1974. On the repetitive discharge in myotonic muscle fibers. J. Physiol. (London) **240:** 505–515.
7. ALMERS, W., P. R. STANFIELD & W. STÜHMER. 1983. Lateral distribution of sodium and potassium channels in frog skeletal muscle: measurements with a patch-clamp technique. J. Physiol. (London) **336:** 261–284.
8. STÜHMER, W., W. M. ROBERTS & W. ALMERS. 1983. The loose patch clamp. *In* Single Channel Recording. B. Sakmann & E. Neher, Eds.: 123–132. Plenum. New York.
9. ROBERTS, W. M. & W. ALMERS. 1984. An improved loose patch voltage clamp method using concentric pipettes. Pflügers Arch. **402:** 190–196.
10. PETERS, R., J. PETERS, K. H. TEWS & W. BÄR. 1974. A microfluorimetric study of translational diffusion in erythrocyte membranes. Biochim. Biophys. Acta **367:** 282–294.
11. EDIDIN, M., Y. ZAGYANSKI & T. J. LARDNER. 1976. Measurement of membrane lateral diffusion in single cells. Science **191:** 466–468.
12. JACOBSON, K., Z. DERZKO, E.-S. WU, Y. HOU & G. POSTE. 1976. Measurement of the lateral mobility of cell surface components in single, living cells by fluorescence recovery after photobleaching. J. Supramol. Struct. **5:** 565–576.
13. AXELROD, D., P. RAVDIN, D. E. KOPPEL, J. SCHLESSINGER, W. W. WEBB, E. L. ELSON & T. R. PODLESKI. 1976. Lateral motion of fluorescently labeled acetylcholine receptors in membranes of developing muscle fibers. Proc. Natl. Acad. Sci. U.S.A. **73:** 4594–4598.
14. WEISS, R. E., W. M. ROBERTS, W. STÜHMER & W. ALMERS. Mobility of voltage-dependent ion channels and lectin receptors in the sarcolemma of frog skeletal muscle. J. Gen. Physiol. **87:** 955–983.
15. ADRIAN, R. H., W. K. CHANDLER & A. L. HODGKIN. 1970. Voltage clamp experiments in striated muscle fibres. J. Physiol. (London) **208:** 607–644.
16. TANK, D. W., E. S. WU & W. W. WEBB. 1982. Enhanced molecular diffusibility in muscle membrane blebs: Release of lateral constraints. J. Cell Biol. **92:** 207–212.
17. BEAM, K. G., J. H. CALDWELL & D. T. CAMPBELL. 1985. Na channels in skeletal muscle concentrated near the neuromuscular junction. Nature **313:** 588–590.
18. ROBERTS, W. M. & W. ALMERS. 1985. Increased Na^+ current density near endplates in snake skeletal muscle. Biophys. J. **47:** 189a.
19. WAKAYAMA, Y., E. BONILLA & D. L. SCHOTLAND. 1980. Ultrastructural localization of concanavalin A-binding sites in satellite cells of human skeletal muscle. Cell Tissue Res. **210:** 79–84.
20. FOX, J. M. & R. STÄMPFLI. 1971. Modification of ionic membrane currents of Ranvier nodes by UV-radiation under voltage clamp conditions. Experientia **27:** 1289–1290.
21. OXFORD, G. S. & J. P. POOLER. 1975. Ultraviolet photoalteration of ion channels in voltage-clamped lobster giant axons. J. Membr. Biol. **20:** 13–30.
22. AXELROD, D., D. E. KOPPEL, J. SCHLESSINGER, E. ELSON & W. W. WEBB. 1976. Mobility measurement by analysis of fluorescence photobleaching recovery kinetics. Biophys. J. **16:** 1055–1069.
23. STÜHMER, W. & W. ALMERS. 1982. Photobleaching through glass micropipettes: sodium

channels without lateral mobility in the sarcolemma of frog skeletal muscle. Proc. Natl. Acad. Sci. U. S. A. **79:** 946–950.

24. ALMERS, W., P. R. STANFIELD & W. STÜHMER. 1983. Slow changes in currents through sodium channels in frog muscle membrane. J. Physiol. (London) **339:** 253–271.

25. ANGELIDES, K., T. NUTTER, H. DARBON, S. TERAKAWA & G. B. BROWN. 1986. Spatial relations of the neurotoxin binding sites on the sodium channel. This volume.

Distribution of Saxitoxin-binding Sites in Mammalian Neural Tissue

J. MURDOCH RITCHIE

Department of Pharmacology
Yale University School of Medicine
New Haven, Connecticut 06510

Since the initial demonstration by Moore *et al.*[1] that tetrodotoxin could be used as a chemical marker for sodium channels in excitable tissue, and the subsequent development of radiolabeled tetrodotoxin by Hafemann[2] and of saxitoxin by Ritchie *et al.,*[3] both tetrodotoxin and saxitoxin have been widely used to determine the density and distribution of sodium channels in the excitable membranes of a variety of muscles and of nonmyelinated and myelinated nerves.[4-6] For example, amphibian and mammalian muscle fibers are found to have a channel density of about 200–400 μm^{-2} (given the assumption that channels are uniformly distributed over the sarcolemma). Nonmyelinated fibers have a greater range of densities, probably because of the greater range of diameter size. The density determined with labeled saxitoxin is thus 35 μm^{-2} in garfish olfactory fibers ($d = 0.24$ μm),[3] 100 μm^{-2} in nonmyelinated fibers of the rabbit vagus ($d = 0.7$ μm),[3] and 200 μm^{-2} in the nonmyelinated fibers of the rat cervical sympathetic ($d = 1$ μm),[7] whereas for the much larger giant axons of the squid *Loligo pealii* ($d = 450$ μm)[8] and of the squid *Loligo forbesi* ($d = 660$ μm)[9] it is 170 μm^{-2} and 290 μm^{-2}, respectively. In experiments using labeled tetrodotoxin, an even higher density of 550 μm^{-2} has been reported for *Loligo forbesi.*[10]

It is interesting that these experimentally determined values for nonmyelinated axons are smaller (considerably smaller for the very smallest fibers) than the theoretical estimate of the density of sodium channels that is optimal for maximal conduction velocity,[11,12] which is between 500 and 1,000 μm^{-2}. This deviation from optimum may well represent an evolutionary adaptation to reduce the energetic cost of conduction. Because smaller fibers have a larger surface-to-volume ratio, their ionic fluxes would be larger (per unit weight of tissue) if they had the same channel density as in the squid, which comes nearest to the optimal value, and they would require a correspondingly larger expenditure of energy both to maintain this resting condition and to restore the ionic balance after each impulse.

This paper focuses on the use of saxitoxin and tetrodotoxin, in conjunction with electrophysiological techniques, to determine the distribution of sodium channels in mammalian myelinated nerve,[4-6,13-18] and on the presence of extraneuronal voltage-dependent sodium channels.[15,19-23]

THE COMPLEMENTARY DISTRIBUTION OF SODIUM AND POTASSIUM CHANNELS IN MAMMALIAN MYELINATED NERVE

Sodium Channels

Saxitoxin-binding experiments on nerve fiber were first carried out in nonmyelinated axons[1,3] because the small diameter of these fibers means there is a large area of axonal membrane per unit weight of tissue. Initially, myelinated fibers were not

studied because they suffer two disadvantages that apparently made them unsuitable
for binding experiments. First, their diameter is much larger than in the nonmyelinated fibers of the lobster and rabbit, so that myelinated nerve has a relatively small
area of axonal membrane per gram of tissue. Secondly, in a myelinated fiber there is
relatively little active membrane, most of the axolemma being under the myelin sheath.
These disadvantages are compensated for, however, by the membrane conductance of
nodes of Ranvier being considerably higher than that of other tissues.[24] Hence these
nodes of Ranvier are expected to have a higher density of sodium channels. Indeed, in
all mammalian species studied (cat, guinea pig, rabbit, and rat) experiments on
desheathed sciatic nerves, which consist mainly of myelinated fibers, reveal a distinct
saturable component of saxitoxin binding.[4,6,15]

 This saturable uptake of saxitoxin by myelinated peripheral nerve does not involve
the internodal axolemma. Thus, as shown in FIGURE 1 (upper panel), the saturable
component of binding, determined by the difference between the total binding curve
and the nonspecific linear binding curve obtained in the presence of a high concentration of unlabeled tetrodotoxin, is about 40 fmol/mg wet tissue. Under these experimental conditions, saxitoxin in the bathing medium gains ready access to the nodal
axolemma but not to the internodal axolemma, which is protected by the myelin. When
this protection is removed by homogenization, however (FIG. 1, lower panel), there is

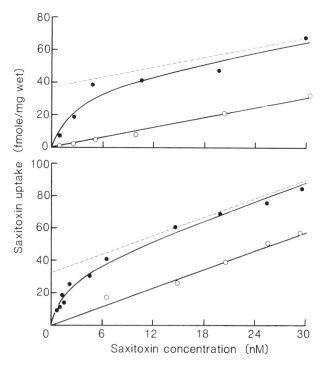

FIGURE 1. Uptake of labeled saxitoxin by the myelinated fibers of cat desheathed sciatic nerve,
showing the total (●) and linear (○) components of binding. The *dashed line* shows the asymptote
to the total binding curve. The *upper panel* shows the binding to desheathed but otherwise intact
nerve trunks. The *lower panel* shows the corresponding binding to homogenized nerve trunks.

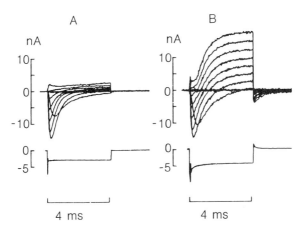

FIGURE 2. Ionic currents in a rabbit node of Ranvier (**A**) before and (**B**) after acute treatment disrupt the myelin. The families of currents in both **A** and **B** (*upper records*) were generated by the same series of depolarizations from an initial holding value of -80 mV to various test potentials in the range -72.5 mV to $+62.5$ mV in 15 mV increments. The current response associated with a hyperpolarization to -125 mV is shown in the *lower pair* of records.

virtually no change in the size of the saturable saxitoxin-binding component, suggesting that the internodal axolemma, even though its membrane area is two-to-three orders of magnitude greater than that of the nodal axolemma, is virtually devoid of sodium channels.[4]

Potassium Channels

Voltage-dependent potassium channels seem to be distributed in a fashion complementary to sodium channels. Compared to other excitable tissue, such as frog myelinated fibers or the squid giant axon, the nodal membrane of mammalian myelinated fibers contains relatively few voltage-dependent potassium channels.[25,26] As FIGURE 2A shows, rabbit single myelinated axons exhibit very little delayed outward current under voltage clamp. But if voltage-dependent channels are absent from the node, they are present in large numbers in the internodal axolemma. This can be seen by recording from the internodal axolemma. As FIGURE 2B shows, when paranodal demyelination is produced by any of a variety of experimental procedures there is an abrupt appearance of outward potassium current.[28] When this occurs there is no consistent increase in the inward sodium current (FIG. 2B), confirming the conclusion of the saxitoxin binding experiments that there are few, if any, sodium channels in the internodal axolemma.

Function of the Complementary Distribution of Na+ and K+ Channels

The experiments in FIGURES 1 and 2 clearly demonstrated a complementary distribution of sodium and potassium channels in mammalian myelinated nerve fibers. Virtually all the sodium channels are concentrated in the node of Ranvier with few if any in the internodal region. On the other hand, there are few potassium channels in the mammalian node of Ranvier, but there is a large number of them in the internodal axolemma of both frog[29] and mammalian[28] nerves. This is a major example of the high degree of regional specialization that is found in mammalian myelinated axons.[30] The presence of sodium channels in the nodal membrane (where they are absolutely necessary for conduction) and their absence from the internodal axolemma (where they would be inactive physiologically) need little comment. But why are the potassium channels distributed in the way they are?

The absence of potassium channels from the node seems to have at least two physiological advantages. The first is a consequence of the fact that any persistence of an increased voltage-dependent potassium conductance following an impulse (as in the squid giant axon) necessarily produces a period of refractoriness following the impulse during which time it is difficult to elicit, or conduct, another impulse. The lack of this persisting increase in potassium conductance in mammalian fibers, together with a speeding up of the inactivation kinetics of the sodium channel,[26] means that a mammalian fiber of a given size and at a given temperature can pass impulses at a higher frequency than the corresponding fiber in the frog,[28] which may confer some evolutionary advantage.

A second advantage stems from the fact that an absence of nodal voltage-dependent potassium channels has a favorable effect on the metabolic cost of conduction[31] because the presence of a voltage-sensitive potassium conductance leads to a faster repolarization of the membrane[32] so that, during the later stages of the action potential, the inward currents that flow through the still incompletely inactivated sodium channels must be larger. A greater number of sodium ions must therefore be pumped out during the recovery process, requiring a correspondingly greater expenditure of energy by the sodium pump. The absence of potassium channels from the mammalian node of Ranvier thus confers the advantage of an improved economy of conduction in addition to an improved ability to carry impulses at a higher rate.

These advantages of removing voltage-dependent potassium channels from the nodal membrane cannot apply to the internodal axolemma, which is not actively involved in conduction. Indeed, there are reasons to believe that as far as the internodal axolemma is concerned it is advantageous to retain potassium channels. One reason, discussed by Chiu and Ritchie,[28] is that potassium channels in the paranodal axolemma may prevent spurious nodal reexcitation. Generation of ectopic impulses might occur because the sodium channels in the mammalian node recover so rapidly from inactivation (as a result of the faster inactivation kinetics) that they are at risk of being reexcited by any local persisting depolarization. Such a depolarization might occur in the ring of axolemmal tissue at the node-paranode junction, which may not be entirely devoid of sodium channels. The activation of these channels, and their subsequent recovery, may be delayed because of the high access resistance along the paranodal seal between the myelin and axon. The function of the potassium channels in the paranodal region would be to prevent a delayed persisting depolarization of the paranode from occurring. The more the membrane in this region is depolarized, the more the depolarization will be opposed by the delayed turning on of the conductance of the voltage-dependent potassium channel.

Perhaps a more critical function of the voltage-dependent potassium channels in the internodal axolemma is their support of the generation of an internodal resting potential. This factor is important because the internodal axolemma, although it does not participate actively in the generation of the impulse, is, however, connected electrotonically to the nodal axolemma. Calculation shows[33,34] that if there were no such internodal resting potential, the resulting electrotonic loading of the node would lead to a nodal depolarization of about 10 mV for a 20 μm diameter fiber and about 22 mV for a 1 μm diameter fiber. In the latter case, the value of h-infinity would be reduced to about 0.1, which would almost certainly prevent generation of the impulse and the fiber would be permanently inactive.

Early experimental evidence for the presence and importance of this normally hidden internodal resting potential had already been obtained by Bohm and Straub[35] to explain their curious experimental finding that after frog nodes of Ranvier are briefly exposed to a high-potassium solution, TEA produces a partial repolarization which, however, only occurs if the potassium channel blocking agent is applied immediately; with prolonged exposure to the high-potassium solution the repolarization effect of TEA decreased to zero. They suggested that with the increase in nodal membrane resistance as a result of the blocking of the nodal potassium channels by TEA the still-polarized internode can repolarize the node partially. However, with prolonged exposure to potassium, the internodal axolemma would also be depolarized (because there would be time for the applied potassium ions to diffuse into the periaxonal space) so that the internodal axolemma can now no longer repolarize the nodal membrane.

It is unfortunate that there is at present no generally available high-affinity ligand for potassium channels. This means it is not possible to carry out binding experiments (similar to those involving saxitoxin binding to sodium channels) to determine the densities of potassium channels in nodal and internodal membranes. It is, however, clear that the number of potassium channels in the mammalian nodal axolemma is relatively small and that their density is low both compared with the potassium channel density in other excitable membranes (such as the frog nodal membrane) and compared with the nodal sodium channel density. Furthermore, it is clear that both the density and number of potassium channels in the internodal region is high compared with the density and number of sodium channels in the internodal region. The overall effect in a peripheral nerve fiber, therefore, is that sodium currents predominate in the nodal membrane, whereas potassium currents predominate in the internodal axolemma. The large number of potassium channels in the internodal axolemma generating the large potassium current (which is the product of the area of membrane and channel density) might reflect, however, the very much larger membrane of the area recorded from rather than an actual high density of potassium channels. Indeed, in both internodal and nodal membrane the same low density of potassium channels might prevail.

EXTRANEURONAL SODIUM CHANNELS

Although both the saxitoxin-binding experiments and the electrophysiological experiments (FIGS. 1 and 2) demonstrated that sodium channels are absent from the internodal axolemma of mammalian myelinated axons, a major difficulty arose when all the saxitoxin binding sites in the nodal region were assumed to be present in the nodal axolemma. Thus, gating-current measurements in rabbit myelinated nerve[13,14] suggested a value of 1200 sodium channels μm^{-2} on the assumption of a nodal area of 66 μm^2 for a 20 μm diameter fiber. Even with the somewhat lower nodal area obtained for a mammalian fiber of this size by Rydmark and Berthold[36] of about 40 μm^2, the sodium channel density would be about 2000 μm^{-2}. This value compares favorably with the value of 1200–1300 μm^{-2} obtained from counting particles in freeze-fracture studies on the rabbit node of Ranvier[37] as well as independent estimates of the channel density in frog nodes obtained electrophysiologically from noise measurements and from gating-current measurements,[13,24,38] all of which give values of 1300–5000 μm^{-2}.

The difficulty arises because these values for the sodium channel density obtained electrophysiologically are considerably smaller than the calculated density of saxitoxin-binding sites based on the assumption that all the binding sites are in the nodal axolemma; this latter value[4,39] is 10,000–12,000 μm^{-2}. This discrepancy is now seemingly resolved by the demonstration that, at least in certain preparations, there is an abundance of extraneuronal voltage-sensitive sodium channels. These channels, which are missed in conventional electrophysiological recordings from excitable tissue, make an important contribution to saxitoxin binding.

Saxitoxin Binding to Degenerated Nerve Trunks

The fact that saxitoxin-binding sites exist in nonneuronal tissue was established both in tissue culture experiments in a variety of fibroblasts and normal human glia-like cells[39-41] and in electrophysiological experiments on the Schwann cell membrane of squid giant axon.[43] In these tissues, veratridine produces a depolarization (squid Schwann cells) or an increased ^{22}Na influx (glia and fibroblasts) that is blocked by tetrodotoxin, suggesting the presence of sodium channels.[43] That such nonneuronal

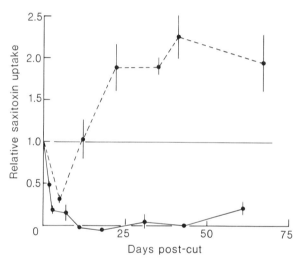

FIGURE 3. The binding of saxitoxin to rat (——) and rabbit (-------) desheathed sciatic nerve trunks. The curves show the saxitoxin uptake in the nerve trunks distal to nerve section. The uptakes are expressed as fractions of the uptake in the control contralateral sciatic nerves.

sodium channels might not just be present but actually abundant was first suggested by the experiment illustrated in FIGURE 3. The assumption that voltage-sensitive sodium channels are confined to excitable membranes requires that when the excitable membrane in a tissue disappears so also must the saxitoxin binding sites. In order to test this hypothesis mammalian sciatic nerves were sectioned, allowed to degenerate, and the saxitoxin-binding capacity of the degenerated distal stump was examined. In the cat,[44] as well as the guinea pig and rat,[15] axonal degeneration leads to the expected substantial loss of saxitoxin binding, although it was noted that in the cat the loss is not complete with about 20% of the saxitoxin-binding capacity remaining. In the rat, nerve section does lead to the virtual complete disappearance of saxitoxin-binding capacity (FIG. 3). In the rabbit, however, after an initial fall, the saxitoxin-binding capacity of the degenerated nerve trunk not only ceases to decrease after a few days but it then becomes two-to-three times larger than in the original intact trunk. In this axon-free preparation the Schwann cells that have proliferated to fill the space vacated by the degenerating axons exhibit a marked saxitoxin-binding capacity. This immediately raises the question of whether a saxitoxin-binding capacity is indeed tantamount to the presence of voltage-dependent sodium channels or whether saxitoxin binding is less specific and binds to sites other than sodium channels. If the former pertains, the intriguing question of the function of these extraneuronal sodium channels immediately arises. But if the latter is the case, there arises the disturbing question of the validity of the use of saxitoxin (or tetrodotoxin) in biochemical experiments as a marker for voltage-dependent sodium channels.

VOLTAGE-DEPENDENT SODIUM AND POTASSIUM CHANNELS IN MAMMALIAN SATELLITE CELLS

The experiments of FIGURE 3 prompted an examination of the satellite cells of both the central and peripheral nervous systems, and electrophysiological experiments have been carried out with the patch-clamp method of recording to search for voltage-dependent channels in rabbit cultured Schwann cells[19,20] and in rat cultured astrocytes.[21] In parallel with these electrophysiological experiments, saxitoxin-binding experiments have also been carried out.[20,21] In summary, both Schwann cells and astrocytes express voltage-dependent Hodgkin-Huxley–type sodium and potassium channels, and both bind labeled saxitoxin. Furthermore, astrocytes, but not Schwann cells, express plasmalemmal voltage-dependent chloride channels.

Hodgkin-Huxley Sodium and Potassium Channels

FIGURE 4A shows a typical record of the currents from a patch-clamped rat astrocyte using the whole-cell configuration. Because of the large surface area (the cell capacity being on average about 60 pF) the clamping conditions are not optimal. Nevertheless, it is clear that there is an early inward current followed by a late outward current. FIGURE 4B shows a similar pattern in a rabbit Schwann cell. In both kinds of satellite cells the relative sizes of the sodium and potassium currents are found to be extremely variable. The Schwann cell in FIGURE 4B had a relatively large outward current and a smaller inward current; it is used to show the complete abolition of the outward current by 4-aminopyridine, which is part of the evidence that this outward current is a potassium current.[19,20] The outward current is also abolished by TEA and by cesium (in the pipette) as shown in FIGURE 4C, taken from a Schwann cell, which shows that the inward current is largely blocked by tetrodotoxin.

FIGURE 5 shows the h-infinity curve (upper panel) and peak current-voltage curve (lower panel) obtained from a rat astrocyte.[21] Similar curves were obtained from the rat Schwann cell.[19,20] In both kinds of satellite cells, the h-infinity curve is in much the same position as it is in the mammalian nodal axolemma.[26] The peak current-voltage curve, however, is shifted by about 30 mV in the depolarizing direction.

Extraneuronal Saxitoxin Binding to Satellite Cells

As might be expected from the presence of voltage-dependent sodium channels both astrocytes and Schwann cells bind saxitoxin (FIG. 6). The binding capacity for astrocytes[21] and Schwann cells[20] (150–200 fmol/mg protein corresponds with an

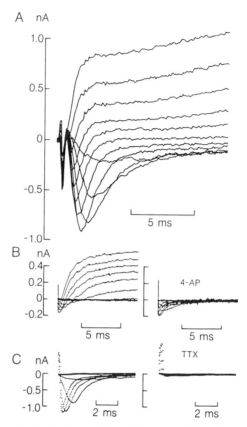

FIGURE 4. Ionic currents (leak-subtracted) in whole-cell recordings from cultured satellite cells. (A) Rat astrocyte. The pipette solution contained 150 mM potassium gluconate. The cell was held at -70 mV, pulsed for 100 ms to -100 mV to remove sodium channel inactivation, and then taken in 10 mV steps to a series of final potentials between -50 and $+50$ mV. (B) Rabbit Schwann cells. The patch pipette contained (mainly) 140 mM KCl. The protocol was similar to that in **A**. The *right-hand record* was taken after adding 6 mM 4-AP externally. (C) Rabbit Schwann cell. The patch pipette was filled (mainly) with 140 mM cesium fluoride. The protocol was similar to that of **A** and **B**. The *right-hand record* was taken after addition of 60 nM tetrodotoxin externally.

uptake of about 40 fmol/mg wet tissue, which is comparable in size to the values obtained in intact nerve and brain. Shrager *et al.*[20] have estimated that the density of the channels on the rabbit Schwann cell plasmalemma is about 30 μm^{-2}. A corresponding estimate for rat astrocytes based on the findings of Bevan *et al.*[21] suggests a density on the astrocytic plasmalemma of about 10 μm^{-2}. Since the regular array of Schwann cell microvilli at the node may have a plasmalemmal area an order of magnitude larger than that of the nodal axolemma,[36] and furthermore since the external plasmalemma of the Schwann cell in the internodal region is about three orders of magnitude greater than the nodal axolemma, even such a relatively low density of sodium channels in the satellite cell could account for the apparent discrepancy previously noted between the number of saxitoxin binding sites and the number of sodium channels determined electrophysiologically. All these Schwann cell channels would be readily accessible from the bathing medium in experiments on desheathed nerve (such as in FIG. 1), and they could easily outnumber the true axolemmal sodium channels by an order of magnitude.

HIGH-AFFINITY AND LOW-AFFINITY BINDING SITES IN SATELLITE CELLS

Recent experiments in a variety of different tissues have made it clear that two quite different sites for binding saxitoxin and tetrodotoxin exist that can be distinguished on the basis of their differing affinities for the toxin.[45-49] This also seems to be the case for satellite cells—at least for those in the CNS. In experiments with rabbit Schwann cells[20] the equilibrium dissociation constants for the toxins determined electrophysiologically compare favorably with those obtained in saxitoxin binding experiments. In the rat astrocyte, however, two distinct populations exist.[21] Whereas the saxitoxin-binding experiments with both Schwann cells and astrocyte cells reveal the well-known high-affinity binding site with an equilibrium dissociation constant for saxitoxin (K_{STX}) and for tetrodotoxin (K_{TTX}) of 3.4 and 7.1 nM, respectively, electrophysiological experiments with astrocytes reveal another site with a much lower affinity.[21] FIGURE 7 shows the peak current-voltage curve in a rat cultured astrocyte. As can be seen, the peak current is reduced by application of tetrodotoxin. A concentration of 1 μM tetrodotoxin, however, is required to reduce the size of the response by slightly more than half. Indeed, the average values for K_{STX} and K_{TTX} found in these electrophysiological experiments are 30 and 500 nM, respectively.[21]

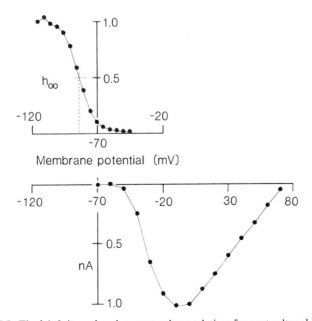

FIGURE 5. The *h*-infinity and peak current-voltage relations for a rat cultured astrocyte.

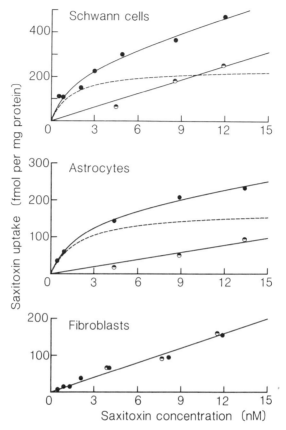

FIGURE 6. The uptake of [³H]saxitoxin by rabbit cultured Schwann cells (*top panel*), rat cultured astrocytes (*middle panel*), and rabbit cultured fibroblasts (*bottom panel*). In all panels the curves were taken in the absence (●) and presence (◓) of 4 μM tetrodotoxin. The *dashed lines* show the saturable component of binding.

In satellite cells of the CNS, therefore, there are two distinct populations binding saxitoxin (and tetrodotoxin). There is a high-affinity binding site revealed by the labelled saxitoxin experiments, and in addition there is a low-affinity site revealed in the electrophysiological experiments. Whether these represent two distinct populations of sites or whether they are two states of the same population remains unclear at the moment.

VOLTAGE-DEPENDENT CHLORIDE CHANNELS

As can be seen in FIGURES 5B and 5C, the delayed outward current in cultured Schwann cells is abolished by agents that block the voltage-dependent potassium channel (4-AP, cesium, TEA). In the rat astrocyte, however, these agents block only about 70% of the outward current. The remaining outward current (FIGURE 8, top panel) is, in fact, a voltage-gated chloride current.[21,22,50] This current (FIG. 8, middle and bottom panels) is immediately (and reversibly) abolished when the chloride in the bathing medium is replaced by a large organic anion such as gluconate. This voltage-dependent chloride current is similar to that described by Inoue[51] for the squid giant axon; like the squid current, the glial cell chloride current is blocked by the disulfonic stilbenes DIDS and SITS.[50]

These voltage-gated chloride channels could provide a useful adjunct to the potassium buffering mechanism often ascribed to astrocytes whereby potassium is taken up from a region of high concentration and is released remotely (the potassium movement being driven by the difference between the local and remote potassium equilibrium potentials).[21,22,50] When there is a substantial accumulation of potassium extracellularly, the resulting depolarization will open the astrocytic chloride channels. This will then permit chloride to enter the astrocytes with the potassium that has been released by the active neurons. The potassium can then be stored locally in the neighboring astrocyte rather than dumped remotely as is required by the hypothesis for potassium buffering that is generally proposed.[52,53] This, in turn, means that the potassium might be more readily available for recapture by the neuron during the recovery process. Such a mechanism, of course, would be complementary to the more classical mechanism.

THE NUMBER OF SAXITOXIN-BINDING SITES RELATIVE TO THE NUMBER OF NEURONAL SODIUM CHANNELS

The presence of nonneuronal sodium channels does complicate interpretation of saxitoxin-binding experiments. For example, Oaklander et al.[16] found that there was little difference in the binding of saxitoxin to various peripheral and central nervous

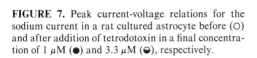

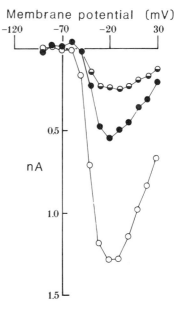

FIGURE 7. Peak current-voltage relations for the sodium current in a rat cultured astrocyte before (O) and after addition of tetrodotoxin in a final concentration of 1 μM (●) and 3.3 μM (◓), respectively.

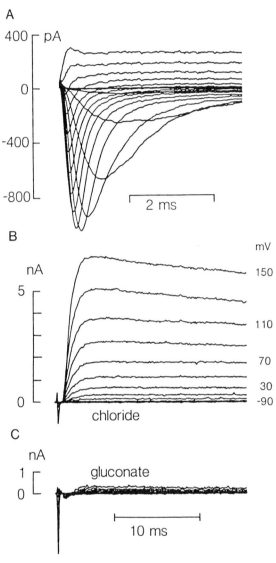

FIGURE 8. Ionic currents (leak-subtracted) in whole-cell recordings from rat cultured astro-cytes. The cells were held at -70 mV, pulsed for 100 ms to -100 mV to remove sodium channel inactivation, and then taken in 10 mV steps to a series of potentials between -70 and $+120$ mV (only some of which are shown). In **A** the pipette solution contained 150 mM cesium chloride. In **B** and **C**, the pipette solution was N-methyl-$(+)$-glucamine gluconate. Panel **C** shows the same family of records as in panel **B** obtained shortly after the sodium chloride of the bathing medium had been replaced by sodium gluconate.

tissues of myelin-deficient rats compared to their normal litter-mates. This was interpreted to mean that sodium channel insertion and maintenance within the axolemma is independent of myelination. This interpretation would become less secure, however, if the bulk of the saxitoxin binding in the brain were to glial cells. It should be pointed out that even in rat Schwann cells, sodium channels are not completely absent. Shrager et al.[20] in fact showed that rat cultured Schwann cells exhibited both electrophysiological sodium channels and saxitoxin binding, but only to about 7% of the corresponding values in the rabbit Schwann cells.

The earlier discrepancy between the number of saxitoxin-binding sites in myelinated nerve and the number of sodium channels found electrophysiologically can now be accounted for, at least in principle. The number of sodium channels in the axolemma of a single node of a 20 μm diameter myelinated rabbit fiber[13] is about 8×10^4 (Chiu, 1980) compared to the number of saxitoxin binding sites of about 50×10^4 (based on a nodal area[36] of 40 μm^2 and a binding site density[4,39] of 10^4 μm^{-2}. The discrepancy arose originally because all the saxitoxin-binding sites were believed to be on the axolemma. However, now that it is clear that Schwann cells can bind saxitoxin (and express sodium channels), the much larger area of Schwann cell membrane must be taken into account. The hexagonal nodal array of Schwann cell microvilli would contribute about 400 μm^2 plasmalemma at the node,[36] which would only contribute a relatively small number of sites if the membrane density of 30 μm^2 estimated by Shrager et al.[20] obtains. The external Schwann cell membrane in the 2 mm stretch of internode; however, would contribute about 12.5×10^4 μm^2. Thus the density of Schwann cell sodium channels could be as little as 4 μm^{-2} and yet account for the discrepancy. This calculation is based on the assumption that the channels are distributed evenly over the plasmalemma. It is possible, however, that a higher density might prevail in the paranodal region of the Schwann cell plasmalemma with few if any in the internode proper. In either case it is now possible to resolve the difference between the electrophysiological estimate, which pertains to the axolemma only, and the much larger estimate based on saxitoxin binding, which pertains both to axolemma and Schwann cell plasmalemma.

More serious is any discrepancy between the number of sodium channels and the number of saxitoxin-binding sites on the cultured Schwann cells themselves. The saturable binding capacity of the Schwann cells in FIGURE 3A is 240 fmol/mg protein. As the measured protein content of these cells is about 0.6×10^{-9} g protein per cell, this binding corresponds to about 86,000 binding sites per cell. However, even with the maximum sodium current recorded in these Schwann cells of (2100 pA), Shrager et al.[20] estimated that each cell contained only about 920 functional sodium channels, which is very much less than the number of binding sites. However, this estimate (based on the ratio of the peak whole-cell and the single channel conductances) implicitly assumes that all the channels are open simultaneously at the peak of the sodium current. Recent kinetic studies[54,55] indicate that this is not the case, at least not in neuroblastoma and some other cells.

A more general approach is to estimate the number of channels from the ratio of the charge carried by the whole-cell current during a depolarizing epoch to the charge carried by a single channel during a similar depolarizing epoch. During steps to -5 mV, in solutions giving an E_{Na} of $+42$ mV, the charge carried by whole-cell sodium currents[56] can be as large as 4 pC. The mean open lifetime of each channel[20] is about 0.3 ms and their conductance[20] is 20 pS. Therefore, if each channel opens on average only once during a depolarizing epoch (as assumed by Aldrich et al.,[54] and by Horn and Vandenburg[55]), the mean charge carried is 2.8×10^{-4} pC. On this basis, the number of electrophysiological sodium channels would be nearly 14,000 per cell, still leaving a large gap to be bridged between the electrophysiological and saxitoxin binding data.

Two factors, however, would operate to close this gap. First, Schwann cells have long, narrow processes which must largely be ignored by the recording system in the voltage-clamp experiment and so would not contribute to the peak current recorded. Secondly, not all Schwann cell sodium channels may be functional electrophysiologically. In astrocytes, for example, the electrophysiological sodium channels have a much smaller affinity for tetrodotoxin and saxitoxin than do those most readily studied in the binding experiments. The high-affinity sites in the astrocytes could be an inoperative or incomplete form of the channel, and there might be a similar type of inoperative binding site in Schwann cells.

CONCLUSION

The anomalous binding of saxitoxin to nonneuronal tissue has led directly to the discovery of a diverse set of voltage-dependent channels in Schwann cells in the PNS and glial cells in the CNS. It has been suggested above that the function of the voltage-gated chloride channels in astrocytes is to assist in the spatial buffering of potassium ions during activity. What could be the function, however, of the Hodgkin-Huxley–type sodium and potassium channels in both Schwann cells and astrocytes? The shift in the peak current-voltage curve of FIGURE 5 makes it unlikely that Schwann cells can generate or conduct an electrical impulse; before activation could occur, the sodium channels would be totally inactivated. One cannot exclude the possibility that these channels appear adventitiously under the abnormal conditions of cell culture and have no normal physiological role. One possible role for these channels,[20–22] however, is that the satellite cells may be acting as local factories for sodium channels that become incorporated in the nodal membrane. A long mammalian axon has to maintain a large area of membrane and a large number of channel proteins (perhaps as many as 10^8 sodium channels). Little is known, at present, about the turnover rate of such channels in the nodal membrane. A system in which the satellite cells act as local factories for some axonal proteins would clearly be advantageous. Circumstantial evidence exists that suggests that proteins synthesized by Schwann cells can indeed be incorporated into axons, and therefore such a hypothesis is not untenable.[21] Furthermore, the presence of saxitoxin binding to proliferating Schwann cells in degenerating nerve (FIG. 3) indicates that the presence of sodium channels on cultured Schwann cells cannot simply be an aberrant expression of these channels that occurs only in culture. Clearly, much more work needs to be done before speculation on the function of these glial channels can be proved or disproved. Further studies of the ion channels of Schwann cells promise to provide interesting insights into the function of the accessory cells of the peripheral and central nervous systems, and thus, of the nerve cells themselves.

REFERENCES

1. MOORE, J. W., T. NARAHASHI & T. I. SHAW. 1967. An upper limit to the number of sodium channels in nerve membrane? J. Physiol. (London) **188:** 99–105.
2. HAFEMANN, D. R. 1972. Binding of radioactive tetrodotoxin to nerve membrane preparations. Biochim. Biophys. Acta **266:** 548–556.
3. RITCHIE, J. M., R. B. ROGART & G. R. STRICHARTZ. 1976. A new method for labelling saxitoxin and its binding to non-myelinated fibres of the rabbit vagus, lobster walking leg, and garfish olfactory nerves. J. Physiol. (London) **261:** 477–494.
4. RITCHIE, J. M. & R. B. ROGART. 1977. The density of sodium channels in mammalian

myelinated nerve fibers and the nature of the axonal membrane under the myelin sheath. Proc. Natl. Acad. Sci. U.S.A. **74:** 211–215.

5. RITCHIE, J. M. & R. B. ROGART. 1977. The binding of saxitoxin and tetrodotoxin to excitable tissue. Rev. Physiol. Biochem. Pharmacol. **79:** 1–50.

6. RITCHIE, J. M. & S. Y. CHIU. 1981. Distribution of sodium and potassium channels in mammalian myelinated nerve. Adv. Neurol. **31:** 329–342.

7. PELLEGRINO, R. G., P. S. SPENCER & J. M. RITCHIE. 1984. Sodium channels in the axolemma of unmyelinated axons: A new estimate. Brain Res. **305:** 357–360.

8. STRICHATRZ, G. R., R. B. ROGART & J. M. RITCHIE. 1979. Binding of radioactively labelled saxitoxin to the squid giant axon. J. Membr. Biol. **48:** 357–364.

9. KEYNES, R. D. & J. M. RITCHIE. 1984. On the binding of labelled saxitoxin to the squid giant axon. Proc. R. Soc. London, Ser. B. **222:** 147–153.

10. LEVINSON, S. R. & H. MEVES. 1975. The binding of tritiated tetrodotoxin to squid giant axons. Phil. Trans. R. Soc. London, Ser. B. **270:** 349–352.

11. HODGKIN, A. L. 1975. The optimum density of sodium channels in an unmyelinated nerve. Phil. Trans. R. Soc. London, Ser. B. **270:** 297–300.

12. ADRIAN, R. H. 1975. Conduction velocity and gating current in the squid giant axon. Proc. R. Soc. London, Ser. B. **189:** 81–86.

13. CHIU, S. Y. 1980. Asymmetry currents in the mammalian myelinated nerve. J. Physiol. (London) **309:** 499–519.

14. CHIU, S. Y. & J. M. RITCHIE. 1981. Evidence for the presence of potassium channels in the internodal region of acutely demyelinated mammalian single nerve fibres. J. Physiol. (London) **313:** 415–437.

15. RITCHIE, J. M. & H. P. RANG. 1983. Extraneuronal saxitoxin binding sites in rabbit myelinated nerve. Proc. Natl. Acad. Sci. U.S.A. **80:** 2803–2807.

16. OAKLANDER, A. L., R. G. PELLEGRINO & J. M. RITCHIE. 1984. Saxitoxin binding to central and peripheral nervous tissue of the myelin deficiency (md) mutant rat. Brain Res. **307:** 393–397.

17. PELLEGRINO, R. G. & J. M. RITCHIE. 1984. Sodium channels in the axolemma of normal and degenerating rabbit optic nerve. Proc. R. Soc. London, Ser. B. **222:** 155–160.

18. RITCHIE, J. M. 1982. Sodium and potassium channels in regenerating and developing mammalian myelinated nerves. Proc. R. Soc. London, Ser. B. **215:** 273–287.

19. CHIU, S. Y., P. SHRAGER & J. M. RITCHIE. 1984. Neuronal-type Na^+ and K^+ channels in rabbit cultured Schwann cells. Nature **311:** 156–157.

20. SHRAGER, P., S. Y. CHIU & J. M. RITCHIE. 1984. Voltage-dependent sodium and potassium channels in mammalian cultured Schwann cells. Proc. Natl. Acad. Sci. U.S.A. **82:** 948–952.

21. BEVAN, S., S. Y. CHIU, P. T. A. GRAY & J. M. RITCHIE. 1985. The presence of voltage-gated sodium, potassium and chloride channels in rat cultured astrocytes. Proc. R. Soc. London Ser. B. **225:** 299–313.

22. GRAY, P. T. A. & J. M. RITCHIE. 1985. Ion channels in Schwann and glial cells. Trends Neurosci. **8:** 411–415.

23. GRAY, P. T. A., S. BEVAN, S. Y. CHIU & J. M. RITCHIE. 1985. Ion channels in rabbit cultured fibroblasts. Proc. R. Soc. London, Ser. B. **227:** 1–16.

24. NONNER, W., E. ROJAS & R. STÄMPFLI. 1975. Displacement currents in the node of Ranvier. Pflügers Arch. **354:** 1–18.

25. HORACKOVA, M., W. NONNER & R. STÄMPFLI. 1968. Action potentials and voltage-clamp currents of single rat Ranvier nodes. Proc. Int. Union Physiol. Sci. **7:** 198.

26. CHIU, S. Y., J. M. RITCHIE, R. B. ROGART & D. STAGG. 1979. A quantitative description of membrane currents in rabbit myelinated nerve. J. Physiol. (London) **292:** 149–166.

27. BRISMAR, T. 1980. Potential clamp analysis of membrane currents in rat myelinated nerve fibres. J. Physiol. (London) **198:** 171–184.

28. CHIU, S. Y. & J. M. RITCHIE. 1981. Ionic and gating currents in mammalian myelinated nerve. Adv. Neurol. **31:** 313–328.

29. CHIU, S. Y. & J. M. RITCHIE. 1982. Evidence for the presence of potassium channels in the internode of frog myelinated nerve fibres. J. Physiol. (London) **322:** 485–501.

30. WAXMAN, S. G. & J. M. RITCHIE. 1985. Organization of ion channels in the myelinated nerve fiber. Science **228:** 1502–1507.

31. RITCHIE, J. M. 1985. A note on the mechanism of resistance to anoxia and ischaemia in pathophysiological mammalian myelinated nerve. J. Neurol. Neurosurg. Psychiatry **48:** 274–277.

32. HODGKIN, A. L. & A. F. HUXLEY. 1952. A quantitative description of membrane current and its application to conduction and excitation in nerve. J. Physiol. (London) **119:** 500–544.

33. SELEKTOR, L. J. & B. I. KHODOROV. 1979. The nerve impulse propagation in a myelinated fibre under varying the parameters of internodes (English translation). Biofizika **24:** 910–916.

34. CHIU, S. Y. & J. M. RITCHIE. 1984. On the physiological role of internodal potassium channels and the security of conduction in myelinated nerve fibres. Proc. R. Soc. London, Ser. B. **220:** 415–422.

35. BOHM, H. W. & R. W. STRAUB. 1961. Der Effekt von Tetraethylammonium an Kalium-depolarisierten markhaltigen Nervenfasern. Pflügers Arch. Ges. Physiol. **274:** 528–29.

36. RYDMARK, M. & C.-H. BERTHOLD. 1983. Electron microscopic serial section analysis of nodes of Ranvier in lumbar spinal roots of the cat: Amorphometric study of nodal compartments in fibres of different sizes. J. Neurocytol. **12:** 537–565.

37. ROSENBLUTH, J. 1981. Freeze-fracture approaches to ionophore localization in normal and myelin-deficient nerves. Adv. Neurol. **31:** 391–418.

38. CONTI, F., B. HILLE, W. NONNER & R. STÄMPFLI. 1976. Conductance of the sodium channel in myelinated nerve fibres with modified sodium inactivation. J. Physiol. (London) **262:** 729–742.

39. RITCHIE, J. M. 1978. Sodium channel as a drug receptor. In Cell Membrane Receptors for Drugs and Hormones: A Multi-disciplinary Approach. R. Straub & L. Bolis, Eds.: 227–242. Raven. New York.

40. MUNSON, R., B. WESTERMARK & L. GLASER. 1979. Tetrodotoxin-sensitive sodium channels in normal human fibroblasts and normal human glia-like cells. Proc. Natl. Acad. Sci. U.S.A. **76:** 6425–6429.

41. ROMEY, G., Y. JACQUES, H. SCHWEITZ, M. FOSSET & M. LAZDUNSKI. 1979. The sodium channel in non-impulsive cells. Interaction with specific neurotoxins. Biochim. Biophys. Acta **556:** 344–353.

42. POUYSSEGUR, J., Y. JACQUES & M. LAZDUNSKI. 1980. Identification of a tetrodotoxin-sensitive Na^+ channel in a variety of fibroblast lines. Nature (London) **286:** 162–164.

43. VILLEGAS, J., C. SEVCIK, F. V. BARNOLA & R. VILLEGAS. 1976. Grayanotoxin, veratrine, and tetrodotoxin-sensitive sodium pathways in the Schwann cell membrane of squid nerve fiber. J. Gen. Physiol. **67:** 369–380.

44. PELLEGRINO, R. G., M. J. POLITIS, J. M. RITCHIE & P. S. SPENCER. 1986. Morphological and biochemical events in Schwann cells accompanying Wallerian degeneration in cat peripheral nerve. J. Neurocytol. **15:** 17–28.

45. STRICHARTZ, G. R. & C. M. H. BAY. 1981. Saxitoxin binding in nerves from walking legs of the lobster Homarus americanus. J. Gen. Physiol. **77:** 205–221.

46. LOMBET, A., C. FRELIN, J.-F. RENAUD & M. LAZDUNSKI. 1982. Na^+ channels with binding sites of high and low affinity for tetrodotoxin in different excitable and non-excitable cells. J. Biochem. **124:** 199–203.

47. ROGART, R. B. & L. J. REGAN. 1985. Two subtypes of sodium channel with tetrodotoxin-sensitivity and insensitivity detected in denervated mammalian skeletal muscle. Brain Res. **329:** 314–318.

48. ROGART, R. B., L. J. REGAN, L. C. DZIEKAN & J. B. GALPER. 1983. Identification of two sodium channel subtypes in chicken heart and brain. Proc. Natl. Acad. Sci. U.S.A. **80:** 1106–1110.

49. ROGART, R. B. 1986. "High" versus "low" STX-affinity Na^+ channel subtypes in nerve, heart, and skeletal muscle. This volume.

50. GRAY, P. T. A. & J. M. RITCHIE. 1986. A voltage-gated chloride conductance in rat cultured astrocytes. Proc. R. Soc. London, Ser. B. In press.

51. INOUE, I. 1985. Voltage-dependent chloride conductance of the squid giant axon membrane and its blockade by disulfonic stilbene derivatives. J. Gen. Physiol. **85:** 519–537.

52. COLES, J. A. & R. K. ORKAND. 1983. Chloride enters receptors and glia in response to light

or raised external potassium in the retina slices of the bee drone *Apis mellifera*. J. Physiol. (London) **357:** 11P.

53. GARDNER-MEDWIN, A. R. 1983. A study of the mechanisms by which potassium moves through brain in the rat tissue. J. Physiol. (London) **335:** 358–374.
54. ALDRICH, R. W., D. P. CORY & C. F. STEVENS. 1984. A re-interpretation of mammalian sodium channel gating based on single channel recording. Nature **306:** 436–441.
55. HORN, R. & C. A. VANDENBURG. 1984. Statistical properties of single sodium channels. J. Gen. Physiol. **84:** 505–534.
56. GRAY, P. T. A., S. BEVAN, S. Y. CHIU, P. SHRAGER & J. M. RITCHIE. 1986. Ionic conductances in mammalian Schwann cells. *In* Ionic Channels in Neural Tissue. J. M. Ritchie, R. D. Keynes & L. Bolis, Eds. Liss. New York.

High-STX-Affinity vs. Low-STX-Affinity Na$^+$ Channel Subtypes in Nerve, Heart, and Skeletal Muscle[a]

RICHARD B. ROGART

Department of Medicine
University of Chicago
Chicago, Illinois 60637

INTRODUCTION

Tetrodotoxin (TTX) and saxitoxin (STX), two small and highly potent neurotoxins, depend for their effect on a highly specific action of blocking Na$^+$ channels at extremely low concentrations. About ten years ago, Ritchie, Strichartz, and I[1] introduced a novel way of exchange-labeling saxitoxin ([^{3}H]STX) with ^{3}H$_2$O to high specific activity. This has provided a chemical probe that has been used with great success to characterize Na$^+$ channels with "high-affinity" receptors for STX in a large number of nerve and skeletal muscle preparations.[2,3] A second type of Na$^+$ channel with a "low-affinity" STX and TTX receptor has been hypothesized to account for a "TTX-insensitive" action potential (AP) found in a number of preparations. Despite the high specific activity of [^{3}H]STX, Na$^+$ channels with low-affinity STX receptors have eluded detection in many studies[4-12] of preparations where other measurements suggest that these channels seem to be present.

In preparations with high-affinity STX receptors, physiological block of the rapid permeability increase to Na$^+$ which underlies the rising phase of the action potential occurs in the nanomolar concentration range. This correlates well with the equilibrium dissociation constant (K_d value) for binding of ^{3}H-labeled STX and TTX to the Na$^+$ channel. This close correlation between physiological effects and pharmacological binding properties has allowed their use as pharmacologic markers to study the Na$^+$ channel protein. [^{3}H]STX and [^{3}H]TTX have been used successfully to estimate Na$^+$ channel density and distribution in excitable membranes,[2,3] to probe the chemical nature of the channel's toxin binding site,[2] and to allow purification of the Na$^+$ channel from eel electroplaque, rat skeletal muscle, and rat brain.[14,16]

In tissues[3] found to maintain Na$^+$-dependent toxin-insensitive APs, block of the AP by STX and TTX occurs at concentrations of toxin that are 2–4 orders of magnitude greater than in excitable membranes with "toxin-sensitive" APs, which are blocked by nanomolar concentrations of STX and TTX. These TTX-insensitive APs, first described by Redfern and Thesleff[13] in denervated mammalian skeletal muscle, have subsequently been found in widespread distribution in other mammalian tissues,[3] including newborn mammalian skeletal muscle, mammalian cardiac muscle, mouse dorsal root ganglion cells *in vivo* and in culture, cultured mammalian skeletal muscle, and L6 cells.

[a]Dr. Rogart was an Established Investigator (83–253) of the American Heart Association while this research was performed. This work was supported by grants from the NIH (NS–23360), the American Heart Association, and the Muscular Dystrophy Association.

The toxin-insensitive Na$^+$ channel, postulated to account for this toxin-insensitive AP, has been detected in numerous electrophysiological and Na$^+$ flux studies in these preparations. However, multiple earlier attempts[4-12] at pharmacologic identification of binding sites failed to demonstrate a corresponding low-affinity uptake of labeled toxin. The binding techniques used in these studies were too insensitive to detect the low-affinity component of labeled toxin uptake. Studies will be described here in which low-STX-affinity receptor sites on toxin-insensitive Na$^+$ channels have been characterized in a variety of preparations. From these studies, we suggest a simple classification scheme for Na$^+$ channels into two major subtype groups, those with "high-STX-affinity" and "low-STX-affinity" receptors.

Toxin-insensitive Na$^+$ channels have generally been assumed to be unique to mammalian excitable membranes. Electrophysiological studies in chick heart and denervated skeletal muscle have shown only Na$^+$ channels with high sensitivity to TTX, acting at concentrations in the 10 nM region.[17-18] Hence, Na$^+$ permeability in chick heart has been attributed to only a single class of Na$^+$ channels with high-affinity binding sites for TTX. We have demonstrated[19] that there are two subtypes of [^{3}H]STX binding sites in chicken as well: high-STX-affinity Na$^+$ channels are found in chick brain and low-STX-affinity Na$^+$ channels are found in chick heart. We have also demonstrated that the apparent discrepancy between electrophysiological findings and pharmacological data is due to differences between properties of STX and TTX, which have previously been used nearly interchangeably, and have been assumed to be virtually identical in their interaction with the Na$^+$ channel.[20]

The studies described here measure with high resolution the binding of exchange-labeled [^{3}H]STX to high-STX-affinity and low-STX-affinity receptors on the Na$^+$ channel. They should pave the way for elucidation of the pharmacological and biochemical properties of Na$^+$ channels with low-STX-affinity binding sites, and determine how they differ from those with high-STX-affinity binding sites. This information should be significant for eventual correlation with molecular biological studies determining the detailed structural differences between Na$^+$ channel subtypes.

MATERIALS AND METHODS

The binding of labeled saxitoxin ([^{3}H]STX) was measured to membrane homogenates of chick brain and cardiac membrane, rat brain and cardiac membrane, and rat skeletal muscle membrane prepared as described below. Membrane samples were incubated for 30 minutes in a series of concentrations of [^{3}H]STX, and the uptake of toxin by the preparation was determined and expressed in fmol/mg wet. Similar preparations were exposed to the same series of concentrations of labeled [^{3}H]STX solutions which also contained a large concentration of unlabeled TTX (10 μM) or STX (5–10 μM) sufficient to inhibit by simple competition more than 99% of the binding of [^{3}H]STX to the Na$^+$ channel. For chick brain and heart, TTX and STX could be used interchangeably as the unlabeled competitor. For experiments with mammalian tissues containing low-STX-affinity receptors, it was necessary to use unlabeled STX as the competitor, due to the substantially lower affinity of TTX for the toxin-insensitive Na$^+$ channel. All experiments were performed at 2°–4°C.

The choline-substituted Locke solution used for most experiments contained choline chloride (154 mM) and MOPS (10 mM), pH = 7.2. The standard wash solution used for the filtration step contained choline chloride (600 mM), KCl (2.5 mM), CaCl$_2$ (2 mM) and MOPS (10.0 mM), pH 7.2.

Tritiated STX

Purified STX provided by the NIH was exchange-labeled with tritium and purified by high-voltage electrophoresis as described by Ritchie, Rogart, and Strichartz.[1] The specific activity of the preparation, 70 dpm/fmol, was determined by comparing the biological activity of the toxin to a standard paralytic shellfish poison (PSP) obtained from the Food and Drug Administration. A radiochemical purity of 0.78 was determined from direct measurement of the fraction of radioactivity and biological activity removed from a solution in which a brain homogenate was incubated, as described previously.[19]

Membrane Preparations

Hearts, brains, and skeletal muscle were dissected from 250-g rats or from chicks sacrificed 10–20 days after hatching. Hearts were trimmed of fat, great vessels, and atria, and washed to remove blood. Tissue was homogenized with a Polytron homogenizer for two 5-15–s periods at half speed in ice-cold Locke solution. The material was centrifuged at 30,000 g for 20 min, the supernatant discarded, and the entire pellet resuspended in Locke solution with a glass homogenizer.

Rat distal leg muscles were denervated by removal of a 1–2 cm length segment of the sciatic nerve in the thigh. Four to five days after denervation, the gastrocnemius and anterior and posterior tibial muscles were removed and a crude membrane homogenate was prepared.

STX Uptake Determination

A new two-step ligand binding assay technique was introduced in these experiments. The first step performed was analogous to that used in a standard centrifugation assay. The second step was to resuspend, filter, and wash the pellet rapidly on a Whatman GFB or GFC filter. Resuspension of the pellet, filtration, and washing were easily accomplished in less than 10 seconds. Advantages of this centrifugation/filtration assay are discussed and demonstrated in the results below.

Extracellular Space Determination

One source of linear, nonspecific uptake in binding assays is the free ligand in the incubation media which is trapped in the pellet during a standard centrifugation assay or on the filter during a standard filtration assay. The volume of trapped media was estimated with [^{14}C]mannitol in each sample, providing a good approximation of the "extracellular space" (ECS) of the preparation. The ECS can be subtracted from the total [^{3}H]STX uptake in each sample.

Data Analysis of Binding Measurements

Binding uptake measurements were fitted to curves which were the sum of a saturable hyperbolic Langmuir component of binding representing a simple bimolecular reaction between [^{3}H]STX and the Na$^+$ channel plus a linear nonspecific component of toxin uptake:

$$\frac{M[\text{STX}]}{K_d + [\text{STX}]} + b[\text{STX}],$$

where b is the coefficient for linear uptake, [STX] is toxin concentration, M is maximum saturable binding capacity, and K_d is the equilibrium dissociation constant. For studies where two components of specific [³H]STX uptake are present, the binding curve used was determined as follows:

$$\text{uptake} = \frac{M_H[\text{STX}]}{K_H + [\text{STX}]} + \frac{M_L[\text{STX}]}{K_L + [\text{STX}]} + b[\text{STX}],$$

where M_H and M_L are the M values and K_H and K_L are the K_d values for high-STX-affinity and low-STX-affinity binding, respectively.

Measurements for the dissociation (or backward rate) and association (or forward rate) constant for toxin binding were fitted to

$$\text{uptake} = U_o \exp(-k_{-1} t)$$

and

$$\text{uptake} = U_o (1 - \exp -k_{+1} t),$$

where U_o represents uptake at $t = 0$ and k_{-1} and k_{+1} are the dissociation and association rate constants, respectively. A nonlinear least-squares curve-fitting program was used to estimate all parameters and their standard errors.

RESULTS

A New Ligand Binding Assay: Centrifugation/Filtration

Our initial experiments examined [³H]STX binding to chick cardiac Na⁺ channels, to determine whether there was any evidence that a low-STX-affinity Na⁺ channel was found in the chick heart, analogous to that found in mammalian heart. In FIGURE 1, we compare binding of [³H]STX to Na⁺ channels in chick brain and heart using an equilibrium centrifugation assay. The [³H]STX uptake by chick brain homogenates in FIGURE 1A is similar to that found for other nerve and skeletal muscle preparations, and demonstrates high-STX-affinity binding to the Na⁺ channel. The total binding is well fitted by the sum of a hyperbolic saturable and a linear nonspecific component of binding. In the presence of a huge excess of unlabeled STX or TTX (5–10 μM), the saturable component is completely inhibited, leaving only the linear component of [³H]STX uptake. FIGURE 1B shows uptake of [³H]STX to chick heart homogenate, under conditions identical to those (FIG. 1A) for brain homogenate. Although a specific component of binding, competitively inhibited by an excess of unlabeled toxin (5μM), is readily apparent, it is much smaller than the linear nonspecific component of binding. Whereas 85%–90% maximal uptake is reached by 5 nM in chick brain (FIG. 1A), no evidence for saturation in chick heart (FIG. 1B) occurs at this concentration. Experimental conditions, however, prevent further quantitative comparison, because in FIG. 1B the linear component becomes so large above 5 nM that neither saturation nor K_d value for specific uptake of [³H]STX can be accurately assessed.

To further characterize the saturable specific component of [^{3}H]STX binding to the cardiac Na$^+$ channel, it was necessary to decrease nonspecific STX uptake. One way of doing this was to change the conditions of the assay solution in a way that would enhance the toxin affinity for the Na$^+$ channel binding site. STX and TTX binding to

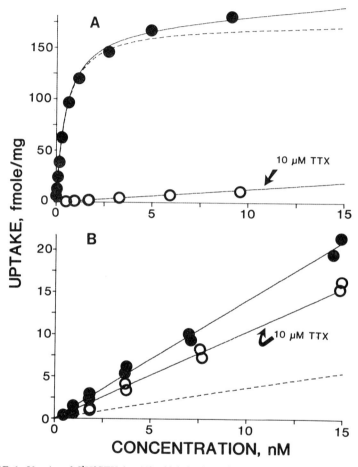

FIGURE 1. Uptake of [^{3}H]STX by **(A)** chick brain and **(B)** chick heart measured by the centrifugation assay; ● = total binding; ○ = linear component of binding; --- = saturable component of binding. The binding parameters for brain were M = 174.8 ± 3.0 fmol/mg (wet weight) of tissue, K_d = 0.5 ± 0.03 nM, and B_{max} = 1.37 ± 0.2 fmol/mg (wet weight) of tissue/nmol.

the Na$^+$ channel occurs at a cationic binding site, and is inhibited by simple competition with cations such as Na$^+$. Substituting choline for Na$^+$ in the assay solution should decrease competitive inhibition of [^{3}H]STX binding, and was found to increase [^{3}H]STX affinity by 2–4 fold, allowing the specific component of binding to saturate at a lower concentration range of [³H]STX, where the linear component of binding would be proportionately smaller.

We also developed a new two-step ligand binding assay technique,[21] our most significant improvement, which allows us to detect easily a variety of types of low-affinity [³H]STX binding sites. This new assay technique provides considerable enhancement of the resolution of specific [³H]STX binding. First, a centrifugation step is used to separate a membrane pellet from the bulk of free, unbound toxin in the supernatant. The pellet is then rapidly resuspended and washed on a filter (taking less than 10 seconds). This brief wash step eliminates the incubation medium trapped in the pellet (which can amount to 10–20 μl in a 10–15 mg pellet, and can specifically contain free [³H]STX 10 times the amount of that bound to the pellet.) The wash step also minimizes the toxin bound nonspecifically to the membrane preparation.

FIGURES 2A–2C show control binding curves for three ligand binding methods: centrifugation, filtration, and the new centrifugation/filtration method. The decrease in linear nonspecific [³H]STX uptake with the new centrifugation/filtration assay compared to filtration and centrifugation is 7.9-fold and 30-fold, respectively. The improved resolution of specific [³H]STX binding in FIGURE 2C is obvious. Other studies demonstrated that the saturable component of [³H]STX uptake was the same using the new centrifugation/filtration assay and conventional centrifugation and filtration assays. The new centrifugation/filtration assay is also generally applicable for study of binding of other radiolabeled ligands to low-affinity receptors.

Chick Brain and Heart Na⁺ Channels

Using the new centrifugation/filtration assay, we were easily able to resolve specific [³H]STX binding to Na⁺ channels in chick cardiac membrane.[19] FIGURE 3 compares the measured uptake of [³H]STX to Na⁺ channels in chick brain and heart membrane after 30 min incubation in Choline-Locke solution with [³H]STX, followed by separation of free from bound [³H]STX. The binding of [³H]STX to chick cardiac membrane, illustrated in FIGURE 3B, shows a substantial reduction in the linear [³H]STX uptake compared to FIGURE 1B. Clear resolution of the saturable specific [³H]STX uptake is obtained, accounting for 80%–90% of total [³H]STX uptake in FIGURE 3B. The observed lower affinity for [³H]STX and the decreased number of [³H]STX binding sites in chick cardiac membrane accounted for the previous difficulty in FIGURE 1B in resolving a specific component of uptake in heart. The specific component of [³H]STX binding in heart has a maximum saturable uptake of 6.7 fmol/mg wet, which is only 5% of that in brain, and an equilibrium dissociation constant (K_d) of 6.2 nM, 20 times greater than that in brain.

The [³H]STX affinity of chick heart and brain Na⁺ channels also differed at physiological Na⁺ concentrations. The saturable component of [³H]STX binding measured simultaneously at three Na⁺ concentrations (0, 154, and 300 mM) for the same membrane preparation as in FIGURE 2 is shown in FIGURE 3. Although [³H]STX uptake at 154 and 300 mM Na⁺ reached only 65%–75% maximum saturable uptake in chick heart (FIG. 3B), relative K_d values were easily determined because all three curves shared the same maximum specific uptake and the 0 mM Na⁺ curve more closely approached full saturation. The K_d increased from 0.3 to 0.6 to 1.0 nM in chick brain and from 6.2 to 9.2 to 11.8 nM in chick heart.

Mammalian Cardiac Na⁺ Channel

We next measured [³H]STX binding to rat cardiac membrane,[23] to see whether we could detect a low-affinity [³H]STX receptor site that corresponded to the electro-

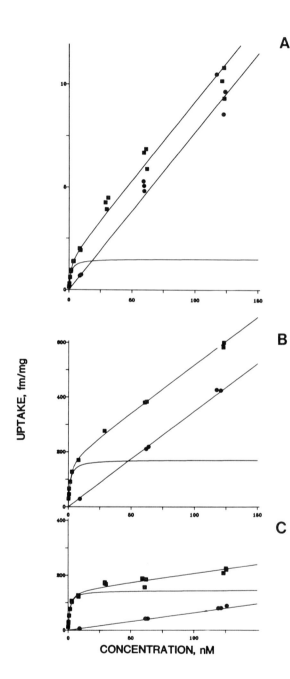

FIGURE 2. Ligand assay methods, no "ECS" correction. The uptake of labeled saxitoxin by chick brain measured by **(A)** filtration assay, **(B)** centrifugation assay, and **(C)** combined centrifugation-filtration assay. Results are before correction for [³H]STX in the mannitol-accessible space. Nonspecific [³H]STX update was measured in the presence of an excess of unlabeled STX (5–10 nM) and was the nondisplaceable linear portion (●) of the total uptake (■). The hyperbola is the saturable specific component of toxin binding, defined as the difference between the total and linear uptake components. The binding parameters were **(A)** $M = 151.0 \pm 25.0$ fmol/mg wet, $K_d = 1.39 \pm .03$ nM, and $B = 7.7 \pm 0.22$ fmol/mg wet; **(B)** $M = 171.5 \pm 4.0$ fmol/mg wet, $K_d = 1.4 \pm .02$ nM, and $B = 3.49 \pm 0.2$ fmol/mg wet; and **(C)** $M = 145.2 \pm 3.5$ fmol/mg wet, $K_d = 1.28 \pm .14$ nM, and $B = 0.63 \pm 0.03$ fmol/mg wet.

physiologically observed toxin-insensitive AP in mammalian heart. FIGURE 5 illustrates [³H]STX binding curves to a rat heart membrane homogenate preparation, using the centrifugation/filtration assay.

[³H]STX binding to rat heart membrane in FIGURE 5A differs from the other

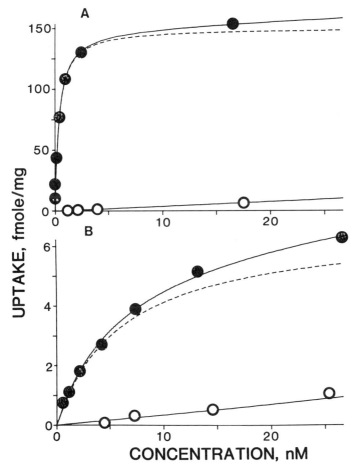

FIGURE 3. [³H]STX uptake to chick brain vs. heart. The uptake of [³H]STX by (A) chick brain and (B) chick heart, measured in isotonic Cs with new assay methods described in text. The *dashed line* is the saturable component of toxin binding. Each point is the mean of 3–5 determinations. The binding parameters were (A) $M = 149.3 \pm$ fmol/mg wet, $K_d = 0.3 \pm 0.004$ nM, $B = 0.4 \pm 0.09$ fmol/mg wet, and (B) $M = 6.7 \pm 0.4$ fmol/mg wet, $K_d = 6.2 \pm 0.8$ nM, and $B = 0.03 \pm 0.007$ fmol/mg wet.

binding curves presented thus far in that it consists of two populations of binding sites with high STX affinity and low STX affinity. The total [³H]STX uptake in FIGURE 5A consists of three components. The first saturable specific component of [³H]STX binding demonstrates high-STX-affinity sites with $K_H = 0.13$ nM and $M_H = 27.6$

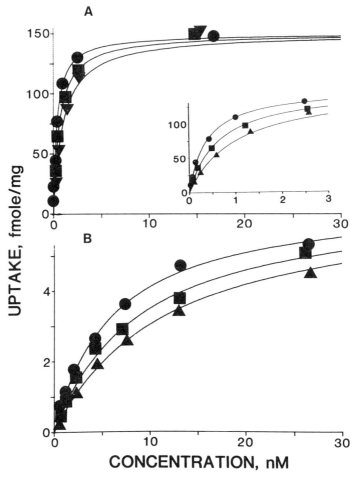

FIGURE 4. The saturable component of uptake of [³H]STX to chick (**A**) brain and (**B**) heart, obtained by subtracting the linear component from measured uptake points. *Inset:* Expanded view for brain at 0–3 nM, the range over which saturation occurs. Three solutions were used: isotonic Cs⁺ (●); 154 mM Na⁺ (■); 300 mM Na⁺ (▲). Each point is the mean of 3–5 determinations. The binding parameters for brain were M = 148.4 ± 0.6 fmol/mg (wet weight) of tissue and K_d = 0.3 ± 0.02 nM (isotonic Cs⁺), 0.6 ± 0.005 nM (154 nM Na⁺), and 1.0 ± 0.009 nM (300 mM Na⁺); those for heart were M = 6.7 ± 0.4 fmol/mg (wet weight) of tissue and K_d = 6.2 ± 0.8 nM (isotonic Cs⁺), 9.2 ± 0.6 nM (154 mM Na⁺), and 11.9 ± 0.9 nM (300 mM Na⁺).

fmol/mg wet (the [³H]STX affinity for this receptor is almost identical to that found in rat brain). A second saturable specific component demonstrates low-STX-affinity binding sites with K_L = 13.5 nM and M_L = 80.5 fmol/mg wet, and accounts for the remainder of the specific [³H]STX binding. A third component consists of linear nonspecific uptake of [³H]STX.

To resolve high-affinity and low-affinity components of ligand binding in a two-population binding curve, the concentration of ligand must be extended to 5–10 times the low-affinity K_L value. In FIGURE 5A, the specific [³H]STX binding is easily resolved at 100 nM [STX] by using the centrifugation/filtration assay in choline-substituted Locke solution; specific binding represents 85% and 35% of total binding at the K_L value and at 100 nM, respectively.

FIGURE 5 demonstrates the Scatchard plot for specific [³H]STX binding (determined by subtraction of linear nonspecific [³H]STX binding from total [³H]STX binding in FIG. 5A) to Na⁺ channels in the rat heart membrane preparation. The curved Scatchard plot for [³H]STX binding to rat heart membrane in FIGURE 5B

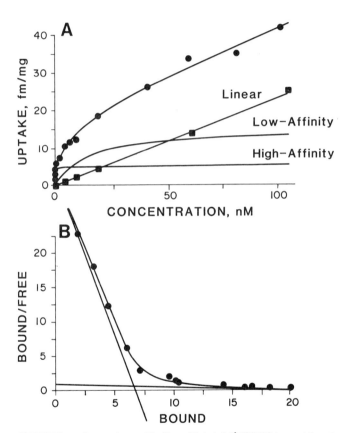

FIGURE 5. [³H]STX uptake: rat heart. Binding of labeled [³H]STX to a rat heart membrane homogenate, shown as (A) [³H]STX uptake, and (B) Scatchard plot. Nonspecific [³H]STX uptake was measured in the presence of an excess of unlabeled STX (5–10 nM) and was the nondisplaceable linear portion (■) of the total uptake (●). Specific saturable [³H]STX binding, defined as the difference between the total and linear uptake components, consists of low and high affinity components, as indicated. The Scatchard plots for specific [³H]STX uptake show the asymptotes corresponding to these two components. The binding parameters were (A) $M_H = 7.3$ fmol/mg wet, $K_H = 0.73$ nM, and $M_L = 16.4$ fmol/mg wet; (B) $K_L = 13.5$ nM, $B = 0.132 \pm 0.005$ fmol/mg wet nM.

indicates the presence of two populations of binding sites with high and low STX affinity (assuming the binding sites are noninteracting).

STX and TTX Differ in Distinguishing Mammalian and Chick Na⁺ Channel Subtypes

Our detection of low-STX-affinity Na^+ channels in mammalian heart is consistent with electrophysiological findings of toxin-insensitive APs in this preparation. Our finding of low-STX-affinity Na^+ channels in chick heart, however, is inconsistent with previous electrophysiological studies that have demonstrated only a single high-affinity site of TTX action in chick heart and nerve.

We hoped[20] that by comparing the affinity of TTX for chick heart and nerve Na^+ channels under identical conditions (measured from its ability to inhibit [³H]STX binding), we could shed some light on this discrepancy between electrophysiological and pharmacological results. As we will show, STX and TTX demonstrate differences in their ability to recognize Na^+ channel subtypes in chick excitable membranes, which resolves this issue.

FIGURE 6 shows the inhibition of [³H]STX binding to chick brain and heart membranes by unlabeled STX. The uptake (U) of a labeled ligand (L) by a competitive inhibitor (I) with affinity K_I can be expressed as

$$U = \frac{M - L}{L + K_d\,(1 + I/K_I)},$$

where M is the maximum saturable uptake. Normalizing by the uptake (U_0) at $I = 0$:

$$\frac{U}{U_0} = \frac{1}{1 + [K_d/(L + K_d)\,I]\,K_I}.$$

[³H]STX uptake was fitted to the second equation by nonlinear least-squares analysis. The K_I values for STX were determined by using the data for competition by unlabeled STX.

The uptake data were then plotted in FIGURES 6 and 7 with respect to a transformed inhibitor concentration, $I' = K_d/(L + K_d + I)$, as follows:

$$\frac{U}{U_0} = \frac{1}{1 + I'/K_I}.$$

This transformation is defined so that 50% inhibition of the normalized uptake ($U/U_0 = 0.5$) occurs at a transformed inhibitor concentration that equals the affinity constant for the inhibitor ($I' = K_I$). In this way we have eliminated the dependence of the competition curve upon the labeled ligand concentration (L), and ligand affinity (K_d), facilitating comparison between experiments carried out at different ligand concentrations. Analysis of the data in FIGURE 6 indicated K_d values for STX of 0.043 nM in chick brain, and 0.95 nM in chick heart (see TABLE 1). This is in agreement with the 20-fold difference in affinity between the chick cardiac and brain Na^+ channel subtypes observed in FIGURE 3 above and reported by Rogart et al.[19]

FIGURE 7 shows similar experiments in which [³H]STX binding was displaced by unlabeled TTX. The resulting K_d values for TTX were 0.24 nM in chick brain and 0.6 nM in chick heart (TABLE 1). Hence, the two Na^+ channel subtypes have only a 2.5-fold difference in affinity for TTX, as compared to a 20-fold difference in affinity

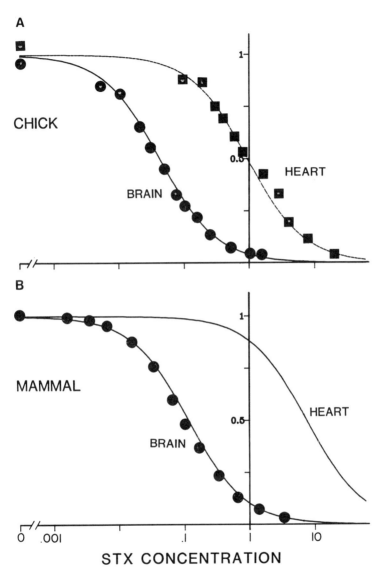

FIGURE 6. STX competition: chick and mammal brain and heart. Inhibition of specific [³H]STX binding (**A**) to chick heart and brain, and (**B**) to rat heart and brain, at 1 nM [³H]STX, by unlabeled STX ranging in concentration from 0 to 1000 nM. Membrane homogenates were exposed to labeled [³H]STX at 1 nM concentration, along with unlabeled STX ranging from 0 to 50 nM concentration, in 1.5 ml of an assay solution containing 154 mM choline chloride and 10 nM MOPS. Nonspecific [³H]STX uptake was measured in the presence of an excess of unlabeled STX (5–10 nM) and was the nondisplaceable linear portion of the total uptake. Points shown are the means of three samples. The abscissa used a transformed inhibitor concentration ($I' = [K_{d/L} + K_d] I$). The *solid line* shows the [³H]STX displacement curve, normalized to uptake at [³H]STX = 0, $U/U_0 = 1/ (1 + I'/K_I)$. The binding parameters determined were (**A**) chick heart, $K_d(STX) = 0.95$ nM; chick brain, $K_d(STX) = 0.043$ nM; (**B**) rat brain, $K_d(STX) = 0.114$ nM; rat heart, $K_d(STX) = 10$ nM.

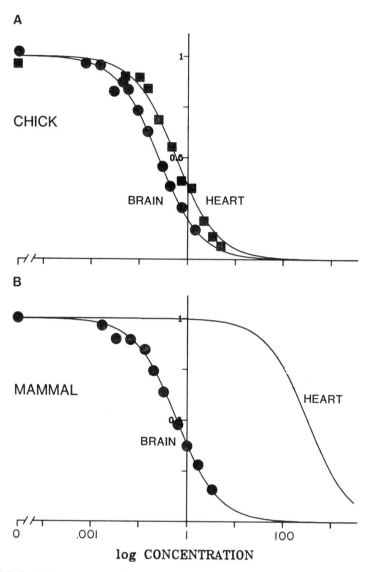

FIGURE 7. TTX competition: chick and mammal brain and heart. Inhibition of specific [³H]STX binding to (A) chick heart and brain and (B) mammal heart and brain at 1 nM [³H]STX by unlabeled TTX ranging in concentration from 0 to 500 nM. Conditions are those found in the legend to FIGURE 6. The binding parameters determined were (A) chick heart, K_d(TTX) = 0.60 nM and chick brain, K_d(TTX) = 0.24 nM; (B) rat heart, K_d(TTX) = 300 nM and rat brain, K_d(TTX) = 0.64 nM.

for STX. This small difference in TTX affinity could easily go undetected in electrophysiological studies designed to demonstrate a TTX-resistant Na^+ channel in chick (particularly when the anticipated affinity for TTX was around 1 μM).

Identical experiments were performed with rat brain and rat heart. Analysis of the data in FIGURE 6B indicated a K_d value for STX of 0.114 nM in rat brain, and 10 nM in rat heart. FIGURE 7B shows similar experiments in which [³H]STX was displaced by unlabeled TTX. K_d values for TTX were 0.64 nM in rat brain and 300 nM in rat heart. Hence both STX and TTX recognize significant differences in Na^+ channel subtypes in rat brain and rat heart. Recognition in chick of two Na^+ channel subtypes has eluded other previous studies not only because in chick TTX is not capable of adequately resolving differences in Na^+ channel subtypes, but also because both channel subtypes in chicken show a shift towards increasing absolute toxin affinity compared to those in mammal. As a result, the low-STX-affinity chick cardiac Na^+ channel (K_d = 0.6 nM for TTX) is shifted so that it nearly superimposes with the high-affinity TTX binding site in rat brain (K_d = 0.64 nM for TTX). Hence it is understandable that electrophysiological studies have found a TTX affinity at the chick cardiac Na^+ channel that is quite similar to that found at the high-affinity Na^+ channel in many mammalian nerve preparations. Although these data have been interpreted as consistent with only a single population of chick Na^+ channels with high affinity for TTX, examination of the affinity of STX clearly indicates two populations of Na^+ channels in chick brain and heart.

TABLE 1. Comparison of K_d Values (nM) for STX and TTX Binding to Chick and Rat Brain and Heart

	Heart	Brain	Ratio
Chick			
STX	0.95	0.043	22
TTX	0.60	0.24	2.5
Mammal			
STX	10.0	0.114	88
TTX	300.0	0.64	470

STX Kinetics at the Na^+ Channel Binding Site

Binding of STX to the Na^+ channel is an equilibrium process, with one toxin molecule binding to one receptor. For a simple bimolecular binding reaction of this sort, the equilibrium dissociation constant, K_d, is equal to k_{-1}/k_{+1}, where k_{+1} is the forward or association rate constant, and k_{-1} is the reverse or dissociation rate constant. FIGURE 8A illustrates the dissociation of [³H]STX from chick brain and cardiac homogenates. The dissociation rates were 0.31 min^{-1} and 0.61 min^{-1} respectively for brain and heart Na^+ channels at 2°–4° C.[19] Although the dissociation of [³H]STX from the cardiac Na^+ channel is about two times faster than in brain, this difference is far too small to explain the 20-30–fold decrease in [³H]STX affinity.

We have also measured[22] the association rate of STX to the Na^+ channel, and found an eightfold slower STX on-rate to chick heart than to chick brain Na^+ channel, as illustrated in FIGURE 8B. This confirms that the twentyfold lower STX affinity to Na^+ channel in chick heart compared to brain is due primarily to an association rate which is about tenfold slower in heart, whereas the dissociation rate is only twofold higher in heart.

STX binding to the chick cardiac and brain Na^+ channels is therefore a

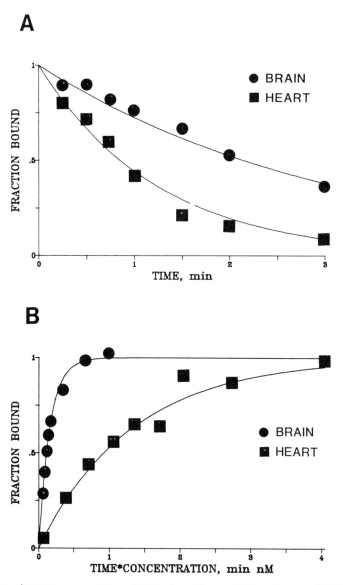

FIGURE 8. [³H]STX on-and off-time chick brain and heart. **(A)** Dissociation of [³H]STX from the Na⁺ channel of chick brain and chick heart after addition of an excess of unlabeled toxin. **(B)** Association of [³H]STX with the Na⁺ channel of chick brain and chick heart under same conditions. Observed uptakes have been normalized by maximum uptake. Fitted curves are **(A)** exponential; **(B)** 1-exponential with rate constants of $1.7 \times 10^7/M$ min and 3.2 min for chick brain, and $0.2 \times 10^7/M$ min and 1.6 min for chick heart.

bimolecular process, consistent with association and dissociation processes that follow first-order kinetics, as shown in FIGURE 8. We have hypothesized one mechanism consistent with these kinetic observations: some variable structural feature of the chick cardiac Na$^+$ channel slows STX association, while having little effect on dissociation. For instance, a hinged portion of the cardiac Na$^+$ channel opens and closes in a stochastic fashion, exposing and blocking the toxin binding sites. FIGURE 9 illustrates such a hypothetical model of the toxin binding site in the cardiac Na$^+$ channel, where an additional highest portion, not found on the nerve channel, slows STX association but has little effect on TTX dissociation.

Rat Denervated Muscle Na$^+$ Channels

We next went on[24] to measure [^{3}H]STX binding to rat denervated skeletal muscle, in order to determine whether we could detect low-STX-affinity receptor sites corresponding to the toxin-insensitive AP that has been observed in this preparation.

A   B

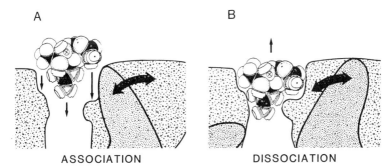

ASSOCIATION   DISSOCIATION

FIGURE 9. Hypothetical STX binding site in cardiac Na$^+$ channel. STX binding to a hypothetical cardiac Na$^+$ channel binding site, which contains a hinged "blocking particle" that moves rapidly back and forth across the toxin binding site. (A) STX association rate is slowed by the blocking particle when it is in the binding site. (B) Once STX has bound to its receptor site, STX dissociation rate is little affected by the blocking particle.

FIGURE 10 shows [^{3}H]STX uptake curves and Scatchard plots for normal and denervated rat skeletal muscle, respectively. For normal muscle, the Scatchard plot observations fall on a straight line, indicating a single population of receptor sites. For denervated muscle, the Scatchard plot is clearly nonlinear, indicating that there are two populations of channels present (assuming the [^{3}H]STX binding sites are noninteracting).

The untransformed data in FIGURE 10 was analyzed using a nonlinear least-squares estimation of parameters and their standard errors. For normal muscle, the [^{3}H]STX uptake curve consists of a linear and a single saturable component, with a maximum specific uptake, $M = 9.0$ fmol/mg wet, and $K_d = 0.49$ nM. For denervated muscle, the uptake curve consists of a linear component and two hyperbolic saturable components of uptake. Accurate determination of ligand binding parameters ordinarily requires 90%–95% saturation of the receptor sites.[25] Although the high-affinity saturable component in FIGURE 10B can be well characterized, the low-affinity

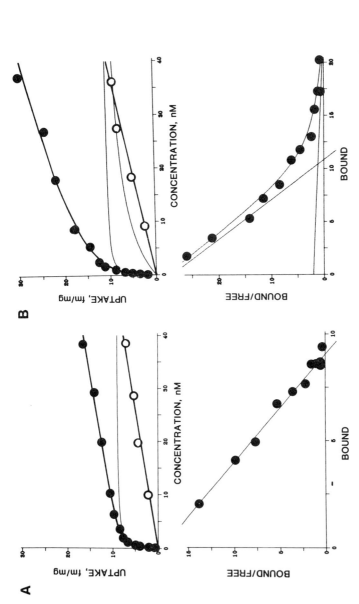

FIGURE 10. [³H]STX uptake to high- and low-affinity Na⁺ channels: normal and denervated muscle. The uptake of labeled saxitoxin ([³H]STX) by (**A**) normal and (**B**) denervated rat skeletal muscle, as a function of increasing [³H]STX concentration. Muscle homogenate samples (10–15 mg wet weight of tissue, homogenized with a Polytron homogenizer, centrifuged at 27,000 to 35,000 g for 20–30 minutes, and resuspended with a glass-glass homogenizer) were exposed to labeled [³H]STX ranging from 9 to 50 nM concentration in 1.5 ml of an isotonic assay solution containing 154 mM choline chloride, 0.8 mM CaCl₂, and 10 nM MOPS. Nonspecific [³H]STX uptake was measured in the presence of an excess of unlabeled STX (5 – 10 μM) and was the nondisplaceable linear portion of the total (●) and linear (○) uptake. Specific saturable [³H]STX binding, defined as the difference between the total and linear uptake components, is a *light solid* line shown as in **A**; two *light lines* show the low- and the high-affinity components of saturable uptake in **B**. *Below,* Scatchard plots are shown for specific [³H]STX uptake. The binding parameters were (**A**) $M = 9.3 \pm 9.3$ fmol/mg wet, $K_d = 0.56 \pm 0.09$ nM, and $B = 0.195 \pm 0.007$ fmol/mg wet; (**B**) $M_H = 11.2 \pm 0.9$ fmol/mg wet, $K_H = 0.45 \pm 0.03$ nM, $M_L = 10.8 \pm 1.9$, $K_L = 12.9 \pm 5.4$ nM, and $B = 0.17 \pm 0.006$ fmol/mg wet.

component reaches only about 70% saturation, leading to some uncertainty in the estimation of its binding parameters.

Detailed characterization of the low-STX-affinity component of [^{3}H]STX binding was achieved by studying the displacement of 2 nM and 20 nM labeled [^{3}H]STX by unlabeled STX over the concentration range of 0–300 nM. The displacement curves achieve saturation of the low-STX-affinity binding sites over a concentration range of 2–300 nM. At a concentration of 20 nM, [^{3}H]STX is bound to both high-STX-affinity and low-STX-affinity binding sites (line at 20 nM, FIG. 10B). The competition curve at 20 nM [^{3}H]STX (FIG. 11A) is therefore determined by four parameters (K_L and M_L for the low-STX-affinity component, and K_H and M_H for the high-STX-affinity component). For a similar competition curve at 2 nM [^{3}H]STX concentration (line at 2 nM, FIG. 11B), ligand is bound almost entirely to high-STX-affinity binding sites. Hence, the displacement curve in FIGURE 11B is approximately that of a single population of binding sites, with parameters M_H and K_H. With good estimates of M_H and K_H, FIGURE 11A can then be resolved into its high-STX-affinity and low-STX-affinity components. (M_L and K_L can be accurately estimated from the portion of [^{3}H]STX uptake found at 20 nM [^{3}H]STX, which is not accounted for by a high-affinity component with parameters M_H and K_H.) The data in FIGURE 11 were analyzed by simultaneously fitting the two competition curves at 2 nM and 20 nM [^{3}H]STX, using a weighted nonlinear least-squares method.

The uptake curve from FIGURE 10B was then simultaneously fitted with the competition curves in FIGURE 11, constraining all three sets of data to common K_H and K_L values. The low-STX-affinity specific uptake in FIGURES 10B and 11 was characterized by M_L = 11.4 fmol/mg wet, and K_L = 11.4 nM. Na$^+$ channels with low-affinity toxin binding sites therefore account for 50%–60% of the total channels for the muscle preparation 4 days after denervation.

FIGURE 12 shows two competition curves obtained using unlabeled TTX to displace [^{3}H]STX binding at 2 nM and 20 nM. FIGURE 12B is well approximated by a single population of high-STX-affinity [^{3}H]STX binding sites with parameters M_H(TTX) and K_H(TTX). Simultaneous analysis with the two population competition curves in FIGURE 12A allows determination of K_H(TTX), equaling 1.8 nM, and K_L(TTX), equaling 497 nM, for TTX binding to the high-STX-affinity and low-STX-affinity toxin binding sites, respectively.

Low-STX-Affinity Na$^+$ Channels in Mouse Cerebellum

While measuring the development of high-STX-affinity Na$^+$ channels in mouse cerebellum, we were surprised to find that in postnatal mice aged 6–14 days[26] we observed[27] a second population of Na$^+$ channels with low STX affinity. The time course over which we noted the appearance of the low-STX-affinity Na$^+$ channel corresponds to a period of neurogenesis and morphogenic activity. The low-STX-affinity receptor has a K_L of 12–16 nM, and a K_L of 300 nM for TTX. Thus, the low-STX-affinity receptor in young mouse cerebellum appears similar to the low-STX-affinity receptor found in newborn and denervated mammalian muscle and in mammalian heart, based upon its affinity for STX and TTX.

In these latter preparations, a TTX-insensitive action potential had previously been observed in electrophysiological studies. This is the first time that we have found a low-STX-affinity receptor in a preparation before physiological studies demonstrating a TTX-insensitive AP have been described. We believe that a population of TTX-insensitive Na$^+$ channels with a low-affinity STX and TTX receptor probably accounts

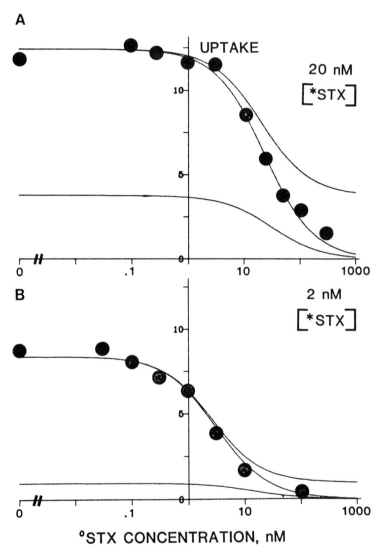

FIGURE 11. Inhibition of specific [³H]STX binding by unlabeled °STX. Displacement in rat denervated skeletal muscle of (A) 20 nM and (B) 2 nM [³H]STX by unlabeled STX ranging in concentration from 0 to 1000 nM. Specific uptake was that portion of the total uptake that was displaceable by 10 μM unlabeled STX. Points shown are the means of four samples. The *solid line* connecting the *filled circles* shows the curve describing total inhibition of specific [³H]STX uptake by unlabeled STX. This total inhibition curve is the sum of two components, the inhibition of [³H]STX binding by unlabeled STX to high-affinity and low-affinity receptors. These high-affinity and low-affinity inhibition curve components are shown as the upper and lower solid lines, respectively, for each inhibition curve. The binding parameters determined were $M_H = 8.8 \pm 0.5$ fmol/mg wet; $K_H(\text{STX}) = 0.40 \pm 0.08$ nM; $M_L = 5.9 \pm 0.9$ fmol/mg wet; $K_L = 11.4 \pm 4.4$ nM.

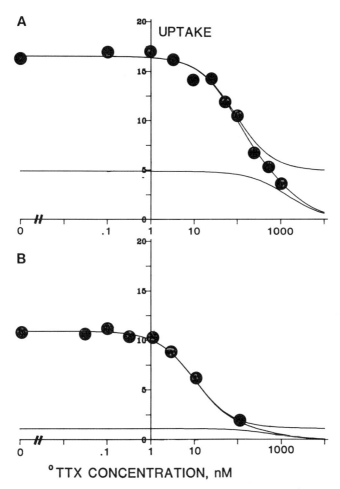

FIGURE 12. TTX competition: denervated rat muscle. Inhibition of specific [³H]STX binding to rat denervated skeletal muscle at (**A**) 2 nM and (**B**) 20 nM [³H]STX by unlabeled STX ranging in concentration from 0 to 1000 nM. Specific uptake was that portion of the total uptake which was displaceable by 10 μM unlabeled STX. Points shown are the means of four samples. The *solid line* shows the total specific uptake and the two calculated lines show the high- and low-affinity components of uptake. The binding parameters determined were: M_H = 9.3 ± 9.5 fmol/mg wet; K_H(STX) = 0.45 ± 0.03 nM; M_L = 5.6 ± 1.9 fmol/mg wet; K_L = 12.9 ± 5.3 nM.

for this observation, providing yet another example of this Na⁺ channel subtype in an immature, developing nerve membrane system. Although the toxin-insensitive AP has been described most frequently in muscle preparations lacking innervation, this low-STX-affinity Na⁺ channel found in the nervous system in mouse cerebellum is probably like that in muscle in that it is also present in postsynaptic uninnervated membrane.

DISCUSSION

Saxitoxin and tetrodotoxin have been used successfully and interchangeably to characterize many features of the Na^+ channel in nerve and skeletal muscle, to which they bind and block Na^+ currents with high affinity at nanomolar concentrations. For this high-STX-affinity Na^+ channel, electrophysiological and pharmacological studies with TTX and STX have been in good agreement in (1) inhibition of the Na^+ current at the same concentration range as saturable toxin binding (1–10 nM), (2) matching of cation permeability sequences for the Na^+ channel with cation inhibition of labeled toxin binding, (3) pH-dependent inhibition of Na^+ current size and of toxin binding, and (4) estimation of Na^+ channel density from toxin binding measurements and from gating current, noise, and patch-clamp measurements.

The studies presented here demonstrate that pharmacological studies with these toxins can also define many characteristics of a second type of low-STX-affinity Na^+ channel which we observe in cardiac and postsynaptic uninnervated membranes. When we began these studies, a toxin-insensitive AP had been observed in electrophysiological studies in a variety of cardiac uninnervated membranes,[3] but previous studies[4-12] had failed to detect a corresponding low-affinity STX and TTX binding site. The low-affinity [³H]STX binding site that we observe has properties that correspond to the physiologically described toxin-insensitive action potential. The interactions of STX and TTX at their low-affinity receptor sites, however, are not identical.

A new two-step ligand binding technique has been introduced[21] that substantially reduces nonspecific ligand uptake, and is essential for allowing us to study the low-STX-affinity receptor. The method facilitates studies in which elevated ligand concentrations are necessary to saturate low-affinity receptors, where other ligand binding techniques would result in a nonspecific ligand uptake that would obscure the specific ligand binding. The improved 20–40–fold reduction in nonspecific uptake of labeled saxitoxin achieved here was essential to detect the low-affinity [³H]STX binding sites. This method is generally applicable for other ligands binding to low-affinity receptors.

The ability to detect and quantitate the two Na^+ channel subtypes in unpurified membrane by direct ligand binding of a radiolabeled ligand provides the ability to perform the following characterizations. (1) The ratio of the two Na^+ channel subtypes can be determined in homogenate membrane, prior to any purification steps altering this ratio. (2) The purification of the two Na^+ channel subtypes can be quantitated during various steps, starting with that in unpurified membrane. (3) Expression and metabolism of the Na^+ channel subtypes can be followed in the unpurified membrane, eliminating any distortions created by membrane purification.

The Low-Affinity Mammalian Cardiac Na^+ Channel: Physiological Comparisons

Rat brain membrane has only a single population of Na^+ channels with high-affinity receptors for [³H]STX. Rat cardiac membrane, however, has two populations of Na^+ channels with high-affinity and low-affinity receptors for [³H]STX.[21,23] There are approximately four times as many low-affinity [³H]STX receptors as high-affinity receptors. Subsequent studies have demonstrated high-affinity and low-affinity receptors for a derivative of TTX in rat heart,[28] and for [³H]STX in purified sheep cardiac membrane.[29]

Correlation of pharmacological and physiological studies of membrane receptors is essential to optimize the information obtained from both studies. Comparison of the affinity of a labeled ligand with the ligand's physiological effect is required to validate identification of the binding sites. To make this comparison, the K_d values for [³H]STX binding obtained here must be corrected for the differing experimental temperatures, and for the differing cationic composition of the bathing solution used in physiological experiments. The values here can be extrapolated to the physiological conditions of a temperature of 37°C, using Q_{10} of 1.2–1.3, and a bathing solution (154 mM NaCl, 2 mM CaCl₂, and 0.8 mM MgCl₂) using inhibitory K_{ions} at the STX binding site of 40–100, 16, 22 mM respectively for Na⁺, Ca²⁺ and Mg²⁺ ions.[30] For the low-STX-affinity receptor in rat cardiac membrane, the affinities found were $K_L(STX)$ = 13.5 nM and $K_L(TTX)$ = 300 nM in choline-substituted Locke solution (free of Na⁺ and divalent cations) at a temperature of 2°–4°C. By extrapolating to the physiological conditions above, we obtain $K_L(STX)$ = 75 nM and $K_L(TTX)$ = 1.2 μM. These values correspond well with physiological estimates of $K_L(STX)$ = 100 nM for STX and K_L (TTX) = 1.2–4 μM, identifying the low-affinity [³H]STX receptor with the physiologically observed mammalian cardiac Na⁺ channel.

Although good correlation is found between the low-affinity [³H]STX receptors and physiological block of cardiac Na⁺ currents by STX and TTX, physiological studies in mammalian cardiac membrane have not observed a TTX-sensitive Na⁺ current that corresponds with the high-affinity [³H]STX receptor we observe. Several explanations may be considered for the function of the high-affinity [³H]STX receptor observed in rat cardiac membrane:

- The presence of four times as many low-affinity STX receptors as high-affinity receptors may obscure detection of TTX-sensitive Na⁺ currents in mammalian heart. Studies of TTX and STX on cardiac AP may have missed a high-affinity effect since decrease in AP size is extremely nonlinear with block of g_{Na}, requiring a high percentage of channels to be blocked before AP height is reduced by 50%. Studies of rate of rise of the AP and voltage-clamp studies of Na⁺ currents, however, have also failed to show the occurrence of block of channels by STX and TTX at low concentrations.

- High-affinity and low-affinity ³H-labeled STX and TTX receptors in mammalian cardiac membrane may be located in different regions of the membrane. For example, the low-affinity receptor might be located in the sarcolemma, and the high-affinity receptor may be localized in the T-tubule. Supporting this hypothesis for regional localization of different types of [³H]STX receptors, Frelin et al.[31] have observed Na⁺ channels in skeletal muscle sarcolemma and T-tubule with a 20-fold difference in affinity for [³H]TTX-en. Sodium currents observed electrophysiologically arise almost exclusively from the surface sarcolemma. Hence, TTX-sensitive Na⁺ currents from different membrane portions in cardiac membrane may correlate with high-affinity receptors for [³H]STX. Further fractionation and characterization of mammalian cardiac membrane will be necessary to test this hypothesis.

- High-STX-affinity Na⁺ channels in mammalian heart may represent a precursor pool, localized in internal membrane, for the functional low-STX-affinity Na⁺ channel in surface membrane which expresses functional properties.

- Catterall and Coopersmith[7] have hypothesized that high-affinity [³H]STX receptors in rat cardiac membrane were found in autonomic nerve terminal endings in heart tissue. Their study did not observe low-affinity [³H]STX receptors. Renaud et al.,[28] however, have found that rat cardiac muscle cells in tissue culture develop high-affinity receptors for [³H]TTX-en. They also observed the time course of development of high-affinity TTX-en receptors in embryonic rat cardiac tissue, and found that the high-affinity receptors developed before autonomic innervation of the heart occurred. Hence, it seems unlikely that high-affinity [³H]STX receptors simply arise from contaminating nerve tissue in rat cardiac membrane preparations.

● Renaud et al.[28] have hypothesized that the high-affinity [³H]TTX-en receptors in rat cardiac membrane are "latent" or "silent" channels that are not observed physiologically.

Further studies will be required to judge the accuracy of these hypotheses.

The Low-Affinity Mammalian Denervated Muscle Na⁺ Channel: Physiological Comparisons

The studies here identify two subtypes of high-STX-affinity and low-STX-affinity Na⁺ channels in mammalian muscle showing differences in affinity of 30-fold for STX and 250-fold for TTX. Both Na⁺ channel subtypes are found in denervated mammalian skeletal muscle, whereas normal muscle contains only the high-affinity Na⁺ channel subtype.

For comparison with physiological measurements, the K_d values for toxin binding obtained here must again be corrected for differing experimental temperatures (assuming a $Q_{10} = 1.2-1.3^{6,7}$), and for the differing cationic composition of the bathing solution used (assuming simple competition by cations with $K_{Na} = 40-100$ mM and $K_{Ca} = 16mM^{26}$). For 25°C and a bathing solution containing 154 mM Na⁺ and 2.2 mM Ca²⁺, a 3-5–fold correction results in estimated values of $K_L(STX) = 35-55$ nM and $K_L(TTX) = 1500-2500$ nM. Comparable functional estimates for STX and TTX binding affinity to the toxin-insensitive Na⁺ channel have been made in a number of studies. Harris and Thesleff[32] found that 40 nM STX and 600 nM TTX reduced the maximum rate of rise of the action potential, V_{max}, in denervated rat skeletal muscle by 50%, although the nonlinearity between V_{max} and Na⁺ conductance precludes a direct comparison of these values with toxin K_d values. Half-maximal inhibition of veratridine-stimulated Na⁺ fluxes occurred in primary cultures of mammalian skeletal muscle at 150–300 nM STX and at 500–1000 nM TTX,[33] and in cultured rat heart cells at 50 nM STX and 960 nM TTX.[34] In voltage-clamped denervated skeletal muscle, 75% of the Na⁺ conductance was blocked by TTX with $K_d = 5.1$ nM ("type I" Na⁺ channels) and 25% was blocked with $K_d = 1\mu M$ ("type II" Na⁺ channels).[35]

These relative conductances of 75% and 25% contributed by type I and type II channels are the only estimates presently available to compare to our finding of 40%–50% high-affinity and 50%–60% low-affinity channels in denervated muscle. The following factors may account for the differing ratio we observed: high-affinity and low-affinity channels may have a different single channel conductance; the younger rats (100 to 150 g) used in our study may respond differently to denervation than the older rats (400–800 g) used by Pappone[35]; or mixed hind limb muscle (our preparation) may respond differently to denervation than the extensor digitorum longus muscle (EDL) fibers that Pappone[35] selected.

The observation that V_{max} of the AP drops to ⅔ normal in denervated muscle has remained puzzling, because the added conductance from the large population of newly synthesized low-affinity Na⁺ channels would normally be expected to increase V_{max}. Hodgkin,[36] however, showed in squid giant axon that if additional Na⁺ channels were added to the membrane, the additional capacitance contributed by the gating currents of the added channels would actually slow the AP conduction velocity (proportional to V_{max}). At the Na⁺ channel density which optimizes conduction velocity, the capacitance contributed by gating currents is approximately equal to the membrane capacitance; at about twice this channel density, conduction velocity drops to about ⅔ of the peak velocity. The decrease in V_{max} in denervated mammalian muscle may therefore reflect the increase in gating current capacitance due to the added low-affinity Na^+ channels.

The Low-STX-Affinity Na^+ Channel in Chick Cardiac Membrane: Physiological Comparisons

Electrophysiological studies have previously demonstrated a TTX-insensitive AP only in mammalian preparations such as heart and denervated skeletal muscle, suggesting that the low-STX-affinity Na^+ channel was unique to mammal. TTX sensitivity in chick nerve, skeletal muscle, and heart has been found to have only a single high-affinity site of action with an IC_{50} of about 10 nM. Hence, the chick cardiac Na^+ channel has been considered to have a high-affinity toxin binding site, similar in properties to the channel found in chick nerve.

The studies we have described here have demonstrated high-STX-affinity and low-STX-affinity Na^+ channel subtypes in chick nerve and heart respectively. Previous inability to identify these two Na^+ channel subtypes resulted from the nonselective nature of TTX as compared to STX. It is important to demonstrate that values for the K_d of STX and TTX binding to the chick cardiac Na^+ channel reported here are comparable to the values determined electrophysiologically in the literature. The K_d values for toxin binding must again be corrected for the differing experimental conditions used in [^{3}H]STX binding experiments and physiological experiments including temperature (assuming a $Q_{10} = 2.5$) and differing cations in the physiological solution (assuming simple competition with $K_{Na} = 30$ mM and $K_{Ca} = 1.5$ mM).[37] For comparison with electrophysiologic studies carried out at 30°C in a bathing solution with 150 mM Na^+ and 2.2 mM Ca^{2+}, we estimate a 20-fold correction.

Hence, the estimated corrected value for the K_d for binding of TTX to the low-affinity chick cardiac Na^+ channel is 12 nM. This is quite similar to values obtained in several electrophysiological studies for chick heart, including: (1) in chick heart, 50% reduction of V_{max} occurred at about 10 nM [TTX][16,18]; and (2) in cultured chick embryonic heart cells, 50% inhibition of veratridine-stimulated Na^+ flux was found at 1.6 nM TTX.[38]

From the data in this study, we make the following conclusions. (1) Chick possesses two subtypes of Na^+ channels, with high-affinity and low-affinity toxin binding sites that are analogous to the channel subtypes in mammal. This conclusion differs from that of other workers, who demonstrated toxin affinities in chick heart in the <10 nM range, and concluded that the chick cardiac Na^+ channel is identical to that in chick nerve. Since toxin affinities in chick nerve and heart were not compared directly, they failed to demonstrate the differing affinities found here. (2) The two chick channel subtypes are better recognized by STX (20-fold selectivity) than by TTX (2.5-fold selectivity). Further, comparison of the high-affinity and low-affinity Na^+ channel subtypes found in mammal and chick demonstrate: (1) chick Na^+ channels are more sensitive than mammalian channels to both STX and TTX; and (2) in distinguishing between Na^+ channel subtypes in chick, STX is more selective than TTX in chick (STX > TTX, 20:2.5), whereas TTX is more selective than STX in mammal (TTX > STX, 1000:40).

These data indicate that even though the mechanism of action of STX and TTX in blocking Na^+ currents may be identical, the two toxins cannot be used interchangeably. TTX and STX show differences in specificity in identifying high-STX-affinity and low-STX-affinity Na^+ channel subtypes, and hence are not equivalent selective antagonists at receptor subtypes. We make the assumption that Na^+ channels exist as several subtypes. These subtypes are defined by differences in toxin affinity, similar to a line of reasoning used to identify hormone and neurotransmitter receptors.[45] Hence, the identification of Na^+ channel subtypes depends upon demonstrating selective agonists and antagonists for each subtype with differing affinities. We have shown here that TTX and STX differ as selective antagonists in chick and rat; in different species, other selective antagonists also frequently show differing abilities to distinguish receptor subtypes.[46]

Identification of High-STX-Affinity and Low-STX-Affinity Sodium Channel Subtypes

Based upon the quantitative difference in STX and TTX affinity for cardiac and brain Na^+ channels in chick and mammal, we have previously proposed[19] the identification of two separate Na^+ channel subtypes with high-STX-affinity and low-STX-affinity receptor sites. Catterall and co-workers[7,33,34] and Lazdunski and co-workers[12,28,31] have also suggested this identification of Na^+ channel subtypes from their comparison of radiolabeled toxin binding to high-STX-affinity Na^+ channels and toxin inhibition of Na^+ fluxes in low-STX-affinity Na^+ channels. Although voltage-activated ionic channels are unlike neurotransmitter and hormone receptors in that they are not normally activated by specific physiological agonists, it is reasonable that the same criteria established for identification of other receptor subtypes apply to Na^+ channel subtypes as well.

In addition to identifying groups of Na^+ channel subtypes based upon their affinity for STX and TTX, this classification of channel subtype groups may also help to clarify the interaction of other pharmacological agents with the Na^+ channel, much as identification of other receptor subtype groups has helped clarify their response to agonists and antagonists. For instance, the low-STX-affinity cardiac Na^+ channel subtype appears to be more sensitive to local anesthetic/antiarrhythmic agents than the nerve Na^+ channel subtype.[19]

The criteria for classification of well-characterized receptor subtypes include differences in affinity for selective agonists and antagonists and anatomical localization. Our finding of a 15-30–fold and 100-150–fold difference in [³H]STX affinity for chick and mammal cardiac and brain Na^+ channels, respectively, is comparable to the 10-50–fold difference in inhibition by selective antagonists such as practolol, metoprolol, and atenolol of α_1- and α_2-adrenergic receptors, which are among the more clearly defined receptor subtypes. Our data also demonstrate a clearcut difference in anatomical localization of the two Na^+ channel subtypes in heart and brain. This important characteristic of receptor subtypes allows selective agonists and antagonists to mediate different physiological responses in tissues with a given receptor subtype.

Toxin-insensitive, or toxin-resistant, Na^+ channels have been postulated to account for the corresponding TTX-insensitive AP in mammalian cardiac and denervated skeletal muscle. Both of these terms are somewhat misleading in that they suggest that TTX and STX lack any activity at this toxin-insensitive Na^+ channel, in which case receptor sites for these labeled toxins should not exist.

If the TTX-insensitive AP is postulated instead to arise from Na^+ channels which are "partially sensitive" to toxins, then corresponding low-affinity toxin receptor sites would exist, as we have demonstrated here. We favor identifying the following two channel subtype groups observed in the studies described here as (1) high-STX-affinity Na^+ channels, including nerve and skeletal muscle channels, and (2) low-STX-affinity Na^+ channels, including cardiac and postsynaptic uninnervated membrane channels.

We do not assume that the Na^+ channels within these subgroups are identical, either within the same animal or across species. Instead, we suggest the following hypothesis, requiring further experimental study for Na^+ channels in the two major subtype groups:

- Na^+ channel subtypes within low-STX-affinity and high-STX-affinity Na^+ channels (nerve and innervated skeletal muscle) may share certain properties in common.
- High-STX-affinity and low-STX-affinity Na^+ channel subtypes are not restricted to mammals, but may be present in other species as well, such as in chick, as demonstrated here. However, interspecies differences in absolute toxin affinities may be found, so that recognition of Na^+ channel subtype groups in other species requires direct comparison of affinities using several different toxins, if possible, in the two tissues where the channel subtypes are to be identified.
- Even within the two major high-STX-affinity and low-STX-affinity Na^+ channel subtype groups various channel members are not identical, but have differentiating properties. Despite many features they may share in common (as in the first item in this list), substantial evidence has already accumulated demonstrating that the subtype groups contain subpopulations of Na^+ channels with differentiating features. In frog skeletal muscle, the high-STX-affinity Na^+ channels in sarcolemma and T-tubule differ in their affinity for derivatives of TTX.[47] Sarcolemma channels are also affected by *Centruroides* toxin[48] and *Tityus serrulatus* toxin,[49] whereas T-tubule channels are not. In rat brain and skeletal muscle,[50] anti-rat skeletal muscle Na^+ channel antibodies distinguish these two high-STX-affinity Na^+ channels, reacting strongly with muscle Na^+ channels, but showing little cross-reactivity with brain Na^+ channels. Furthermore, in rat skeletal muscle,[51] monoclonal antibodies against rat skeletal muscle T-tubule Na^+ channels can distinguish three subpopulations of high-STX-affinity Na^+ channels in end-plate, T-tubule, and sarcolemma membrane.

Studies of Na^+ channel homology at the nucleic acid level have also revealed subpopulations of Na^+ channel subtype. In rat brain, three subpopulations of presumably high-STX-affinity Na^+ channels have been distinguished in hybridization studies with cDNA probes from the eel electroplaque Na^+ channel. Furthermore, Northern blot analysis using rat brain and eel electroplaque cDNA probes fail to detect hybridization with rat muscle mRNA and detects only faint hybridization with rat cardiac mRNA.[52]

We have presented here only the most simple classification of Na^+ channels in two major subtype groups based upon their affinity for STX and TTX. The details of classification of Na^+ channel subtypes and their subpopulations will require further study. Molecular biology studies will determine the extent of sequence homology among various types of Na^+ channels, and will eventually provide exact sequences. Physiological and pharmacological study will be required to interpret this structural information about Na^+ channels in the framework of a functional classification.

CONCLUSION

We have demonstrated a new ligand binding assay that provides the resolution to study two Na^+ channel subtypes with high-affinity and low-affinity receptors for [³H]STX. Using this assay, we have used a simple classification to distinguish two Na^+ channel subtype groups in (1) chick brain, mammalian brain, and mammalian skeletal muscle, and (2) denervated muscle, chick heart, mammalian heart, mammalian skeletal muscle, newborn mammalian skeletal muscle, and developing mammalian cerebellum.

Key questions for the future will be to (1) determine the differences in function, biochemical structure, and control mechanisms for expression of the two Na^+ channel subtypes and (2) further refine the classification of Na^+ channel subtype groups and subpopulations.

ACKNOWLEDGMENT

I would like to thank Ms. Diane L. Perrin for her excellent secretarial assistance in preparation of this manuscript.

REFERENCES

1. RITCHIE, J. M., R. B. ROGART & G. STRICHARTZ. 1976. A new method for labelling saxitoxin and its binding to non-myelinated fibers of the rabbit vagus nerve, lobster walking leg, and garfish olfactory nerve fibres. J. Physiol. **261:** 477–494.
2. RITCHIE, J. M. & R. B. ROGART. 1977. The binding of saxitoxin and tetrodotoxin to excitable tissue. Rev. Physiol. Biochem. Pharmacol. **79:** 1–50.
3. ROGART, R. B. 1980. Sodium channels in nerve and muscle membrane. Ann. Rev. Physiol. **43:** 711–725.
4. COLQUHOUN, D., J. P. RANG & J. M. RITCHIE. 1974. The binding of tetrodotoxin and {alpha}-bungarotoxin to normal and denervated mammalian muscle. J. Physiol. **240:** 199–226.
5. HANSEN-BAY, C. M. & G. R. STRICHARTZ. 1980. Saxitoxin binding to sodium channels of rat skeletal muscles. J. Physiol. **300:** 89–103.
6. BARCHI, R. L. & J. B. WIEGELE. 1979. Characteristics of saxitoxin binding to the sodium channel of sarcolemma isolated from rat skeletal muscle. J. Physiol. **295:** 383–396.
7. CATTERALL, W. A. & J. COOPERSMITH. 1981. High-affinity saxitoxin receptor sites in vertebrate heart—evidence for sites associated with autonomic nerve endings. Mol. Pharmacol. **20:** 526–532.
8. LOMBET, A., J. F. RENAUD, R. CHICHEPORTICHE & M. LAZDUNSKI. 1981. A cardiac tetrodotoxin binding component: Biochemical identification, characterization, and properties. Biochemistry **20:**1278–1285.
9. RITCHIE, J. M. & R. B. ROGART. 1977. The binding of labeled saxitoxin to the sodium channels in normal and denervated mammalian muscle and in amphibian muscle. J. Physiol. **269:** 341–354.
10. SHERMAN, S. J. & W. A. CATTERALL. 1982. Biphasic regulation of development of the high-affinity saxitoxin receptor by innervation in rat skeletal muscle. J. Gen. Physiol **80:** 753–768.
11. SHERMAN, S. J., J. C. LAWRENCE, D. J. MESSNER, K. JACOBY & W. A. CATTERALL. 1983. Tetrodotoxin-sensitive sodium channels in rat muscle cells developing in vitro. J. Biol. Chem. **258:** 2488–2495.
12. LOMBET, A., C. FRELIN, J. F. RENAUD & M. LAZDUNSKI. 1982. Na^+ channels with binding sites of high and low affinity for tetrodotoxin in different excitable and non-excitable cells. Eur. J. Biochem. **124:** 199–203.
13. REDFERN, P. & S. THESLEFF. 1971. Action potential generation in denervated rat skeletal muscle. II. The action of tetrodotoxin. Acta Physiol. Scand. **82:** 70–78.
14. AGNEW, W. S., S. R. LEVINSON, J. S. BRABSON & M. A. RAFTERY. 1978. Purification of the tetrodotoxin-binding component associated with the voltage-sensitive sodium channel from *Electrophorus electricus* electroplax membranes. Proc. Natl. Acad. Sci. U.S.A. **75:** 2606–2610.

15. BARCHI, R. L., S. COHEN & L. E. MURPHY. 1980. Purification from rat sarcolemma of the saxitoxin-binding component of the excitable membrane sodium channel. Proc. Natl. Acad. Sci. U.S.A. **77:** 1306–1310.

16. HARTSHORNE, R. P. & W. A. CATTERALL. 1981. Purification of the saxitoxin receptor of the sodium channel from rat brain. Proc. Natl. Acad. Sci. U.S.A. **78:** 4620–4624.

17. MARCUS, N. C. & H. FOZZARD. 1982. Tetrodotoxin sensitivity in the developing and adult chick heart. J. Mol. Cell. Cardiol. **13:** 335–340.

18. INOUE, D. & A. J. PAPPANO. 1984. Block of avian cardiac fast sodium channels by tetrodotoxin is enhanced by repetitive depolarization but not by steady depolarization. J. Mol. Cell. Cardiol. **16:** 943–952.

19. ROGART, R. B., J. B. GALPER, L. J. REGAN & L. DZIEKEN. 1982. Identification of two sodium channel subtypes in chick heart and brain. Proc. Natl. Acad. Sci. U.S.A. **80:** 1106–1110.

20. ROGART, R. B., J. M. SPIVAK & J. B. GALPER. 1986. Species-dependent recognition of saxitoxin and tetrodotoxin identifies differences in Na^+ channel structure. J. Biol. Chem. Submitted.

21. ROGART, R. B. & L. J. REGAN. 1986. Saxitoxin binding to low-affinity sites on cardiac sodium channel: Resolution by a new assay method. In preparation.

22. ROGART, R. B., L. REGAN & J. B. GALPER. 1982. Cardiac and nerve Na^+ channels differ at their saxitoxin binding sites. Biophys. J. **37:** 101a.

23. REGAN, L. J. & R. B. ROGART. 1982. Binding of labeled saxitoxin to the TTX-resistant cardiac Na^+ channel in rat. Circulation **66:** II-96.

24. ROGART, R. B. & L. J. REGAN. 1985. Two subtypes of sodium channel with tetrodotoxin-sensitivity and insensitivity detected in denervated mammalian skeletal muscle. Brain Res. **329:** 314–318.

25. NORBY, J. G., P. OTTOLENGHI & J. O. JENSEN. 1980. Scatchard plot: Common misinterpretation of binding experiments. Anal. Biochem. **102:** 313–320.

26. ROGART, R. B., M. WILLINGER & G. KUZMA. 1983. Expression of excitable sodium channels in developing mouse cerebellum. Neurosci. Abstr. **9:** 504.

27. ROGART, R. B., M. WILLINGER & R. L. SIDMAN. 1987. Two subtypes of sodium channel with tetrodotoxin sensitivity and insensitivity detected in mouse cerebellum cells. In preparation.

28. RENAUD, J. F., T. KAZAZOGLOU, A. LOMBET, R. CHICHEPORTICHE, E. JAIMOVICH, G. ROMEY & M. LAZDUNSKI. 1983. The Na^+ channel in mammalian cardiac cells: Two kinds of tetrodotoxin receptors in rat heart membranes. J. Biol. Chem. **258:** 8799–8805.

29. DOYLE, D. D., D. M. BRILL, J. A. WASSERSTROM, T. KARRISON & E. PAGE. 1985. Saxitoxin binding and "fast" Na^+ channel inhibition in sheep heart plasma membrane. Am. J. Physiol. **249:** H328–H336.

30. ROGART, R. B. & E. GELLER. 1986. Characterization of "high-" and "low STX-affinity" Na^+ channels in rat myocardium. In preparation.

31. FRELIN, C., P. VIGNE & M. LAZDUNSKI. 1983. Na^+ channels with high and low affinity tetrodotoxin binding sites in the mammalian skeletal muscle cell. J. Biol. Chem. **258:** 7256–7259.

32. HARRIS, J. B. & S. THESLEFF. 1971. Studies on tetrodotoxin resistant action potentials in denervated skeletal muscle. Acta Physiol. Scand. **83:** 382–388.

33. LAWRENCE, J. C. & W. A. CATTERALL. 1981. Tetrodotoxin-insensitive sodium channels-ion flux studies of neurotoxin action in a clonal rate muscle cell line. J. Biol. Chem. **256:** 6213–6222.

34. CATTERALL, W. A. & J. COOPERSMITH. 1981. Pharmacological properties of sodium channels in cultured rat heart cells. Mol. Pharmacol. **20:** 533–542.

35. PAPPONE, P. A. 1980. Voltage clamp experiments in normal and denervated mammalan skeletal muscle fibers. J. Physiol. **306:** 377–410.

36. HODGKIN, A. L. 1975. The optimum density of sodium channels in an unmyelinated nerve. Phil. Trans. R. Soc. London Ser. **270:** 297–300.

37. ROGART, R. B., J. M. SPIVAK & J. B. GALPER. 1986. Characterization of two Na^+ channel subtypes in chick heart and brain. In preparation.

38. LOMBET, A., J. F. RENAUD, R. CHICHEPORTICHE & M. LAZDUNSKI. 1981. A cardiac

tetrodotoxin binding component: Biochemical identification, characterization, and properties. Biochemistry **20:** 1279–1285.

39. MINNEMAN, K. P., R. N. PITTMAN & P. B. MOLINOFF. 1981. Annu. Rev. Neurosci. **4:** 419–461.
40. MINNEMAN, K. P. & P. B. MOLINOFF. 1980. Biochem. Pharmacol. **29:** 1317–1323.
41. JAIMOVICH, E., R. CHICHEPORTICHE, A. LOMBET, M. LAZDUNSKI, M. ILDEFONSE & O. ROUGIER. 1983. Differences in the properties of Na$^+$ channels in muscle surface and T-tubular membranes revealed by tetrodotoxin derivatives. Pfluegers Arch. **397:** 1–5.
42. JAIMOVICH, E., M. ILDEFONSE, J. BARHANIN, O. ROUGIER & M. LAZDUNSKI. 1982. Centruroides toxin, a selective blocker of surface channels in skeletal muscle: Voltage clamp analysis and biochemical characterization of the receptor. Proc. Natl. Acad. Sci. U.S.A. **79:** 3896–3900.
43. BARHANIN, J., M. ILDEFONSE, O. ROUGIER, S. V. SAMPAIO, J. R. GIGLIO & M. LAZDUNSKI. 1984. Tityus toxin, a high affinity effector of the Na$^+$ channel in muscle, with a selectivity for channels in the surface membrane. Pfluegers Arch. **400:** 22–27.
44. HAIMOVICH, B., E. BONILLA, J. CASADEI & R. BARCHI. 1984. Immunocytochemical localization of the mammalian voltage-dependent sodium channel using polyclonal antibodies against the purified protein. J. Neurosci. **4:** 2259–2268.
45. BARCHI, R. L. 1986. Biochemistry of sodium channels from mammalian muscles. This volume.
46. NUMA, S. & M. NODA. 1986. Molecular structure of the sodium channel. This volume.
47. JAIMOVICH, E., R. CHICHEPORTICHE, A. LOMBET, M. LAZDUNSKI, M. ILDEFONSE, & O. ROUGIER. 1983. Differences in the properties of Na$^+$ channels in muscle surface and T-tubular membranes revealed by tetrodotoxin derivatives. Pfluegers Arch **397:** 1–5.
48. JAIMOVICH, E., M. ILDEFONSE, J. BARHANIN, O. ROUGIER & M. LAZDUNSKI. 1982. Centruroides toxin, a selective blocker of surface channels in skeletal muscle: Voltage clamp analysis and biochemical characterization of the receptor. Proc. Natl. Acad. Sci. U.S.A. **79:** 3896–3900.
49. BARHANIN, J., M. ILDEFONSE, O. ROUGIER, S. V. SAMPAIO, J. R. GIGLIO & M. LAZDUNSKI. 1984. Tityus toxin, a high affinity effector of the Na$^+$ channel in muscle, with a selectivity for channels in the surface membrane. Pfluegers Arch. **400:** 22–27.
50. HAIMOVICH, B., E. BONILLA, J. CASADEI & R. BARCHI. 1984. Immunocytochemical localization of the mammalian voltage-dependent sodium channel using polyclonal antibodies against the purified protein. J. Neurosci. **4:** 2259–2268.

Properties of the Sodium Gating Current in the Squid Giant Axon

R. D. KEYNES

Physiological Laboratory
University of Cambridge
Cambridge CB2 3EG, United Kingdom

Somewhat paradoxically, one of the most important contributions of tetrodotoxin and saxitoxin to our knowledge of the molecular biology of the sodium channel arises from an effect that they do not exert. The original discovery of the sodium gating current[1,2] depended on the use of TTX to block the channels completely to the passage of ionic current without at the same time interfering with the operation of the voltage-gating mechanism, so enabling the very much smaller asymmetrical displacement current to be recorded. Yet although the statement that TTX has no marked effect on the kinetics of the gating current is reasonably secure, the point has not as far as I am aware been examined really rigorously. There is, unfortunately, a technical complication in making the necessary control measurements of the gating current in the absence of TTX, which arises because the sodium reversal potential for the normal rapidly inactivating channels differs by some 20 mV from that for the noninactivating channels that are always present when there is fluoride at the inside of the membrane.[3] This difficulty should not be insuperable, and more attention should clearly be paid to the whole question of the modification of the behavior of sodium channels by fluoride, instead of sweeping it under the carpet as I am afraid we so often tend to do.

Let me now turn to a description of the asymmetrical displacement current, the sodium gating current, that accompanies the opening and closing of the sodium channels in a squid giant axon treated with 1 μM TTX and dialyzed with CsF to block the potassium channels. As shown in FIGURE 1, the gating current is not homogeneous, but consists of two readily separable components, one of which is tightly linked with the process of inactivation, the other entirely independent of inactivation.[4]

The kinetics and steady-state behavior of the inactivating $(I_{g,i})$ and noninactivating $(I_{g,n})$ components differ in a number of ways. On application of a positive voltage-clamp step, $I_{g,n}$ is recorded as a pulse of outward current that rises very fast to its peak and relaxes with a single exponential time constant. At the conclusion of the clamp pulse, an equal charge moves inwards with a similar time course. Neither the amount of charge Q_n transferred for a given potential step, nor its kinetics, are measurably affected by the state of inactivation of the sodium system. $I_{g,i}$ behaves very differently, since as may be seen in FIGURES 1 and 2, the "on" response reaches its peak more slowly with a rise time constant of the order of 25 μs, and displays both a fast and a slow relaxation time constant. If the pulse duration is long enough for inactivation of the sodium conductance to be complete, the rapidly relaxing fraction of $I_{g,i}$ disappears, and the "off" response becomes a single slow relaxation with a time constant of several ms.

In order to obtain the steady-state charge transfer curves of the two components shown in FIGURE 3, the sodium system was inactivated by applying a prepulse taking the membrane to a potential in the neighborhood of 0 mV, so that records of Q_n by itself could be made. Subtraction of Q_n from the total unfractionated charge Q_t measured without a prepulse then yields the Q_v curve for the inactivating component Q_i. This

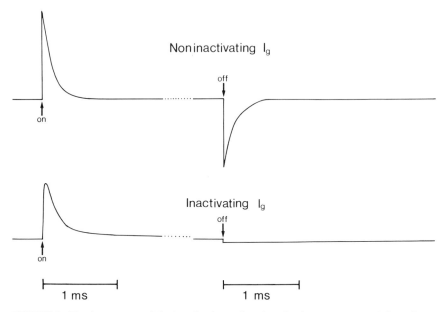

FIGURE 1. The time courses of the inactivating and noninactivating components of the sodium gating current for a pulse to $+20$ mV from a holding potential of -80 mV. T $= 5°$C.

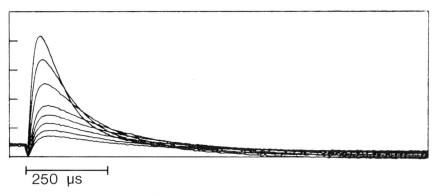

FIGURE 2. A low-noise family of records of $I_{g,i}$ for test pulses to -40, -30, -20, -10, 0, 20, 40, 60, and 80 mV. For each test pulse, $I_{g,n}$ was recorded 0.5 ms after the end of a 20 ms inactivating prepulse to 0 mV, and subtracted from a corresponding record of the total unfractionated gating current with no prepulse. Sixteen pairs of such traces were averaged. Holding potential $= -80$ mV. T $= 5°$C. The axon was bathed in artificial sea water containing 111 mM NaCl, 413 mM TrisCl (pH 7.3), 11 mM $CaCl_2$, 55 mM $MgCl_2$, and 1 μM TTX. The internal dialysis solution contained 330 mM CsF, 20 mM NaF, 400 mM sucrose and 10 mM HEPES buffer (pH 7.3). (From an unpublished experiment by N. G. Greeff, J. M. Bekkers, and R. D. Keynes.)

procedure demonstrates that the curve for Q_n has a slope at its midpoint corresponding to an effective valency of about 0.9, and an equilibrium potential V'_n falling at -50 mV. The curve for the fast fraction of Q_i, on the other hand, has twice as great a slope, with an effective valency of 1.9, and an equilibrium potential $V'_i = +3$ mV. It should be noted particularly that on the negative side of -50 mV, the whole of the charge transfer must be attributed to Q_n, and that there is no movement of inactivable gating charge in this potential region.

The two components of the gating charge may be distinguished not only by their very different kinetics and voltage dependences, but also by their contrasting sensitivities to various drugs. FIGURE 4 shows than low concentrations of local anaesthetics like benzocaine and QX-314 reduce Q_i by more than half, while leaving Q_n unchanged.[6] Other drugs as colchicine[7] and formamide[8] also appear to act in a similar way on the gating charge, strongly supporting the legitimacy of fractionating it into two components, and suggesting that Q_n and Q_i may not arise in the same part of the sodium channel.

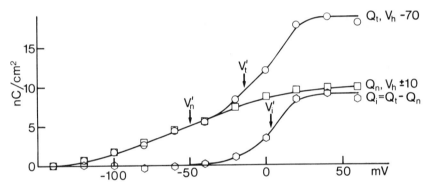

FIGURE 3. Steady-state charge transfer curves for the fast fractions of the total gating charge Q_t, the noninactivating charge Q_n, and the inactivating charge Q_i. Q_t was measured at a holding potential of -70 mV. Q_n is the average of measurements made with the sodium system inactivated by superimposed potential wells to -10 and $+10$ mV. $Q_i = Q_t - Q_n$. (From an unpublished experiment by R. D. Keynes, D. F. van Helden, and N. G. Greeff.[5])

One further experimental observation that needs to be described before I consider possible models of the sodium channel concerns the effect on the sodium system of making the starting potential more negative. It was first shown by Keynes and Rojas,[10] and later confirmed by others,[5,11,12] that the application of a negative prepulse preceeding the test pulse delays the rise of I_{Na} with very little alteration in its slope, in a manner very similar to the well known[9,13-15] and much larger effect on I_K. In the experiment illustrated in FIGURE 5, the extra delay in the rise of I_{Na} induced by lowering the starting potential from -50 mV to -180 mV was 65 μs at 5°C, and the peak of the gating current was delayed to exactly the same extent.[12] Employment of our standard pulse protocol for fractionation of the gating current showed that the rise of $I_{g,n}$ remained fast throughout, and that it was exclusively the rise of $I_{g,i}$ that was further slowed up.

In the light of our demonstration of the existence of two components of the sodium gating current with markedly different characteristics, I have previously put forward[9] what I termed the parallel activation model of the sodium channel shown in FIGURE 6, according to which the channel is gated in two places by more or less independent systems operating in parallel, one generating Q_n and the other generating Q_i. The model satisfies the requirement based on the findings of a single-channel studies[16] that direct access must exist from the resting to the inactivated state without necessarily passing through the open state, and accounts satisfactorily for the rapid closure of the channels when the membrane is repolarized while the sodium conductance is at its peak. It also possesses the merit of allowing the behavior of the sodium current to be calculated directly from that of the gating current without making any further assumptions, since it predicts that the fraction of channels in the open state is given by the product of the fraction of the noninactivating system in state A_n and of the fraction of the inactivating system in state A_i. Preliminary tests made by calculating the product of the running integrals of $I_{g,n}$ and $I_{g,i}$ from the experimental data gave quite

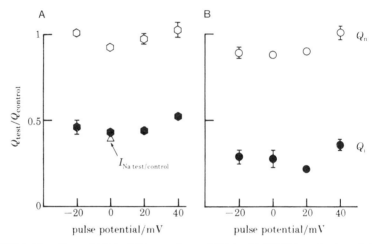

FIGURE 4. The effects of (A) 1 mM benzocaine, and (B) 1 mM QX-314, on the sizes of the two components of the gating charge. The points plotted are the mean values of $Q_{test}/Q_{control}$ for Q_n (*open symbols*) and for Q_i (*filled-in symbols*), with an indication of the standard error of the determinations where it was larger than the size of the symbol. (From Keynes.[9] Reprinted by permission from the Proceedings of the Royal Society of London, Series B.)

good agreement both with the steady-state behavior of g_{Na} and with its kinetics,[9] and later calculations have shown that the fit becomes better still when correction is made, as it needs to be, for the contribution to Q_i of charge movement arising from the slow final step leading to inactivation.

　　Despite the fact that the parallel activation model reconciles the data for the gating and ionic currents as accurately as one could wish, the original version shown in FIGURE 6 is defective in two respects. As depicted, it cannot account satisfactorily for the delaying effect of negative prepulses, for although the existence of a precursor step with an appropriate equilibrium potential could result in the observed sensitivity of the delay in the peak of $I_{g,i}$ and the opening of the channel to prepotentials out to -180 mV, transitions from R_i to R_i' would necessarily be accompanied by a corresponding flow of inactivable gating current, and as is clear from FIGURE 3, no such gating charge is actually recorded on the negative side of -60 mV.

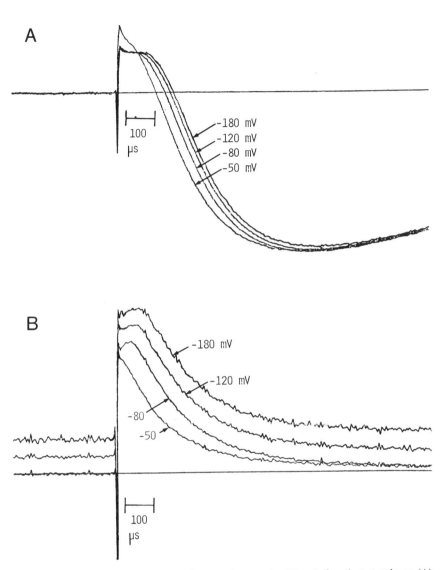

FIGURE 5. The effect of applying negative prepulses starting 20 ms before the test pulse on (**A**) the rise of I_{Na}, and (**B**) the total unfractionated gating current. (**A**) Records of gating current and sodium current in $\frac{1}{5}$ Na artificial sea water for a test pulse to $+20$ mV. The trace for the -50 mV prepulse was scaled up to make the peak of I_{Na} roughly equal in height in all four traces. (**B**) Records of gating current alone after adding 1 μM TTX to the bathing solution. The traces for the prepulses to -120 and -180 mV have been displaced upwards for the sake of clarity. There was an initial transient arising from a slight asymmetry in the voltage-clamp amplifier which distorted the first 10 μs of the traces. (From an unpublished experiment by J. M. Bekkers, R. D. Keynes, and B. Neumcke.)

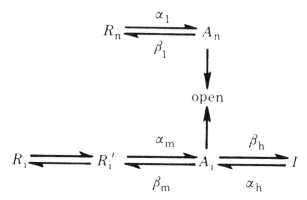

FIGURE 6. The parallel activation model of the sodium channel.[9] The fraction of channels in the open state equals $[A_n]/([R_n] + [A_n])$ multiplied by $[A_i]/([R_i] + [R'_i] + [A_i] + [I])$.

There is a second difficulty in that the model will only yield gating current with a slow rising phase, and at the same time produce the cube law inflection in the rise of I_{Na} that is an essential feature of the sodium system, if the activation step $R'_i \rightarrow A_i$ is assumed to obey unorthodox kinetics with a slow transition. Although the generation of gating current with a slow rising phase by a conventionally coupled sequence of individually fast transitions obeying Eyring-Boltzmann kinetics is certainly possible, it requires that the first transition in the sequence should be the slowest one.[5,17] Cube law kinetics for the achievement of the open state at all pulse potentials are, on the other hand, exhibited only by a sequence in which the first transition is the fastest one, and the forward rate constants decrease successively in a 3:2:1 fashion.[5] Hence there is no easy way to devise a conventional sequence that will correctly predict the delay both in the peak of the gating current and in the opening of the channel.

It is clear that the kinetics of activation cannot be fully explained without postulating the existence of more than one closed state preceding the open one, but serious difficulties are thus seen to arise if it has to be assumed that these closed states are sequentially coupled in the conventional way with transitions obeying Eyring-Boltzmann kinetics. In trying to think of a way out of this dilemma, it has recently occurred to me[5] that there is no conceptual reason why the conformational changes involved in activation should always be regarded as being sequentially coupled, and that it could equally well be supposed that there is an alternative mode of coupling that would result in one change being modulated by another in such a way that change A would affect the kinetics of change B, but not the reverse.

This hypothesis would immediately explain both the delaying effect of negative prepulses and the slow rise of $I_{g,i}$. One way of representing such a type of coupling is shown in FIGURE 7, which postulates that transition between states R_i and A_i of the activating system is blocked when the modulating system is in state R_b, and can proceed only after the transition to state A_b has taken place. An equivalent state diagram can be proposed in which there are parallel transitions of which certain ones are not permitted, but for an initial exploration of the properties of this kind of system, I find it easier to think in terms of a blocking and unblocking of one pathway by another.

According to the modified model of the sodium channel pictured in FIGURE 7, the noninactivated component of the gating charge Q_n would be generated partly by the parallel activating pathway $R_n \rightarrow A_n$ and partly by the modulating pathway $R_b \rightarrow A_b$. The relative sizes of Q_n and Q_i are compatible with there being two sources of charge movement with similar voltage dependences contributing to Q_n.[5] If the fraction of channels free to make the transition from R_i to A_i is determined by the rate of the transition from R_b to A_b, it is easy to calculate both the resulting time to peak of $I_{g,i}$, and the delay in the arrival at state A_i caused by a negative prepulse. From the experimental data for a test pulse to $+20$ mV at 5 °C (see FIG. 2) the observed value of the time to peak of $I_{g,i}$ is 60 μs; the value calculated from the characteristics of Q_n is 47 μs.[5] For the same test pulse with a holding potential of -50 mV, the observed value of the extra delay in the rise of I_{Na} following a prepulse to -180 mV is 65 μs (see FIG. 5), as compared with a calculated value of 83 μs.[5] Hence the modified model of FIGURE 7 passes a preliminary quantitative test well enough for the principle of cross-modulation to deserve examination in greater detail.

As to how the several conformational changes taking place within the sodium channel might interact to bring about this type of modulation of one by another, I can only speculate. A physically plausible possibility that has been suggested to me by Dr. Donald Edmonds is that the modulating pathway might be a four-state system incorporating a movement of charge in the electric field coupled energetically with a lateral movement of a blocking charge that would be electrically silent. A system of this kind would have the advantage of accounting readily for the observed discrepancy between the equilibrium potential of Q_n (V_n' in FIG. 3) and the potential at which the relaxation time constant of $I_{g,n}$ attains its peak value,[5] which is otherwise difficult to explain.

There is more than one way in which the laterally moving charge might then influence the kinetics of the activating pathway, however, and Dr. Edmonds and I are not yet in a position to put forward a detailed model operating on these lines. Nevertheless, it appears to me that the experimental evidence definitely requires that any valid model must incorporate some type of modulation mechanism in addition to a chain of sequentially coupled transitions. Moreover, there are very severe constraints imposed if the model is to predict at the same time both the cube law kinetics of the channel opening observed at all pulse potentials, and the properties of the closed states implied by the evidence on the two components of the gating current that I have assembled here. There is therefore good reason to hope that any model that sucessfully complies with all these constraints will provide a unique solution to the problem.

The main conclusion I would like to make is that studies of the sodium gating current in the squid giant axon, which remains the best preparation at present available to us for a critical analysis of its kinetic and steady-state properties, offer an excellent prospect of arriving at a molecular model of the channel that can be correlated with the outstandingly elegant evidence on the chemical structure of the channel that is presented in this volume.

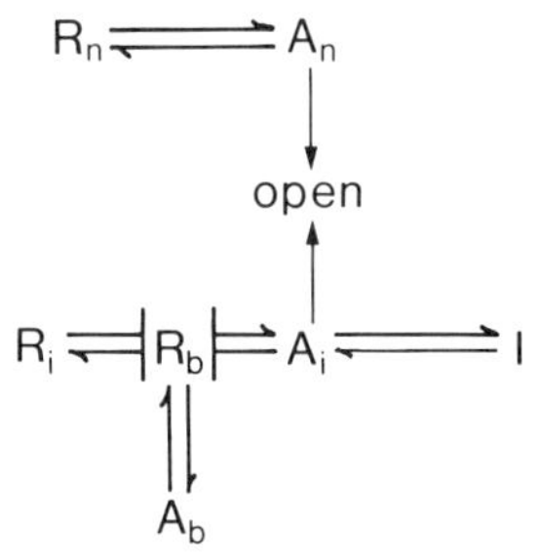

FIGURE 7. Modification of the parallel activation model to account for the slow rising phase of the inactivating component of the gating current.

REFERENCES

1. ARMSTRONG, C. M. & F. BEZANILLA. 1974. Charge movement associated with the opening and closing of the activation gates of the Na channels. J. Gen. Physiol. **63**: 533–552.

2. KEYNES, R. D. & E. ROJAS. 1974. Kinetics and steady-state properties of the charged system controlling sodium conductance in the squid giant axon. J. Physiol. (London) **239**: 393–434.

3. BEKKERS, J. M., N. G. GREEFF & R. D. KEYNES. 1986. The conductance and density of sodium channels in the cut-open squid giant axon. J. Physiol. (London) **377**: 463–486.

4. GREEFF, N. G., R. D. KEYNES & D. F. VAN HELDEN. 1982. Fractionation of the asymmetry current in the squid giant axon into inactivating and non-inactivating components. Proc. R. Soc. London, Ser. B. **215**: 375–389.

5. KEYNES, R. D. 1986. Modelling the sodium channel. *In* Ion Channels in Neural Membranes. J. M. Ritchie, R. D. Keynes & L. Bolis, Eds.: 85–101. Alan R. Liss. New York.

6. BEKKERS, J. M., N. G. GREEFF, R. D. KEYNES & B. NEUMCKE. 1984. The effect of local anaesthetics on the components of the asymmetry current in the squid giant axon. J. Physiol. (London) **352**: 653–668.

7. MATSUMOTO, G. & M. ICHIKAWA. 1985. Kinetics of sodium activation in giant axons of squid (*Doryteuthis bleekeri*). Neuroscience **14**: 327–334.

8. SCHAUF, C. L. & M. A. CHUMAN. 1986. Mechanisms of sodium channel gating revealed by solvent substitution. *In* Ion Channels in Neural Membranes. J. M. Ritchie, R. D. Keynes & L. Bolis, Eds. pp. 3–23. Alan R. Liss. New York.

9. KEYNES, R. D. 1983. Voltage-gated ion channels in the nerve membrane. Proc. R. Soc. London, Ser. B. **220**: 1–30.

10. KEYNES, R. D. & E. ROJAS. 1976. The temporal and steady-state relationships between activation of the sodium conductance and movement of the gating particles in the squid giant axon. J. Physiol. (London) **255**: 157–189.

11. KEYNES, R. D. & J. E. KIMURA. 1983. Kinetics of activation of the sodium conductance in the squid giant axon. J. Physiol. (London) **336**: 621–634.

12. TAYLOR, R. E. & F. BEZANILLA. 1983. Sodium and gating current time shifts resulting from changes in initial conditions. J. Gen. Physiol. **81**: 773–784.

13. COLE, K. S. & J. W. MOORE. 1960. Potassium ion current in the squid giant axon: Dynamic characteristic. Biophys. J. **1**: 161–202.

14. BEGENESICH, T. 1979. Conditioning hyperpolarization-induced delays in the potassium channels of myelinated nerve. Biophys. J. **27**: 257–266.

15. KEYNES, R. D. & J. E. KIMURA. 1980. The effect of starting potential on activation of the ionic conductances in the squid giant axon. J. Physiol. (London) **308**: 17P.

16. HORN, R. & C. A. VANDENBERG. 1984. Statistical properties of single sodium channels. J. Gen. Physiol. **84**: 505–534.

17. WHITE, M. M. & F. BENZANILLA. 1985. Activation of squid axon K^+ channels. J. Gen. Physiol. **85**: 539–554.

Future Directions in Sodium Channel Research

Moderator: S. R. LEVINSON
Panel Members: ARTHUR KARLIN, H. RON KABACK, RICHARD D. KEYNES, AND CHARLES F. STEVENS

[MODERATOR'S NOTE: A unique feature of this conference was a concluding panel discussion concerning the future of sodium channel research. The panel consisted of four eminent researchers who together represented a broad spectrum of experience in the study of transport mechanisms. These panelists were invited to observe the conference and then share their observations on what paths might most profitably be taken in the study of the molecular mechanisms of sodium channels. The discussion that ensued was remarkably lively, and the audience as well as the panel expressed a number of controversial views.]

A. KARLIN (*Columbia University, New York, N.Y.*): I'm going to deal with the question of the molecular mechanism of action of the sodium channel. What do we need in order to understand the function of the sodium channel in terms of its molecular structure? What we need is a detailed three-dimensional structure. Now, would that be enough? No, that would not be enough, because, in fact, the sodium channel operates only in a membrane. We need this three-dimensional structure in the membrane. Would that be enough? No. I'm afraid that would also not be enough, because we need to know where in this three-dimensional structure the functional sites are. Now, the sodium channel has a number of wonderful functional sites. For example, there are binding sites for different kinds of effectors, about which we've heard a lot in this conference. In addition, there is the channel, which may contain binding sites and which certainly contains regions involved in cation translocation. We need to locate all of these sites and regions in the structure.

All right, if we located the important functional sites in an exquisitely detailed three-dimensional structure would we then know the molecular mechanism? No, not yet. Because there are at least three major functional states—the resting, active, and inactive states. And we would need to know this exquisitely detailed three-dimensional structure in these three different states.

Now, these states, some of them, are transient and so it may be necessary, in fact, to do X-ray "movies" of this channel. I think this is in the realm of possibility, but it's not going to happen tomorrow.

What is actually accessible with present technology? I think we could use the information that has come from Professor Numa's elucidation of the primary sequence and locate the functional sites in the primary sequence. What is required are specific labels, with which we can covalently label the protein, cleave the labeled subunit, and separate and identify the labeled fragments. We must further identify by microsequencing where the fragment is in the primary sequence and identify which residues are labeled. Now, obviously, I'm a little biased because in my laboratory we have been taking this approach with the acetylcholine receptor. I'm not saying it's going to give us the molecular mechanism but we are going in the right direction.

Another important task is to figure out the folding of the sodium channel subunits in the membrane. The approach that should work is to use impermeant reagents which will label on one side or the other of the membrane. These should label loops of the subunits that are on the outside and loops that are on the inside. Once these sites of labeling are identified, we should be able to decide whether or not the inferences from the primary sequence were correct.

I think the next stage for us would be to get two-dimensional crystals in membranes and analyze these by electron microscopy. It should be possible to construct a crude, 10–20 Å resolution, three-dimensional structure, and, using some kind of electron-dense labels, locate the functional sites in this crude structure. Finally we want three-dimensional crystals and a good three-dimensional structure.

These are some of the directions that I think the sodium channel field will take.

H. R. KABACK (*Roche Institute of Molecular Biology, Nutley, N.J.*): I study the *lac* permease of *E. coli*, an integral membrane protein representative of many membrane proteins including the sodium channel. Thus the problems that we face are very similar to the problems you face with the sodium channel, except we're a little further ahead because it's an easily manipulated bacterial system. Without meaning to be either pessimistic or depressing, I think it's fair to say that in order to really understand any of these membrane proteins one has to do a lot of difficult work. Let me give you an example with *lac* permease which, as you'll see, is similar in many respects to much that has been presented at this meeting.

The *lac* permease is encoded by the *lac-Y* gene of *E. coli* and it catalyzes transport of the disaccharide lactose in symport (co-transport) with protons. In the late 1970s the *lac Y* gene was cloned into a recombinant plasmid so that the permease could be amplified, and in 1981 a purification technique was developed that allows purification of this protein to a high degree of homogeneity in a completely functional state. *Lac Y* encodes a single gene product, *lac* permease, and the purified protein does everything that the permease does in the native membrane. Furthermore, since the *lac-Y* gene has been sequenced, we are able to do site-directed mutagenesis or make site-directed antibodies and so forth. One can make mosaics, deletions, and do all sorts of manipulations. At the present time, however, there is no straightforward way to figure out how the permease works.

In my view, molecular genetics has provided techniques for examining a protein at the level of individual amino acid residues. However, what are lacking are the corresponding physical approaches. That is, physical techniques that divulge information about the *dynamics* of a membrane protein on the level of amino acid residues. One can, however, begin to use techniques like site-directed mutagenesis to complement physical approaches. For instance, one can put reactive amino acid residues into proteins in places where reporter groups can be attached in order to search for conformational changes that will yield information about mechanism. However, techniques that will resolve the problems in a straightforward manner don't exist at present.

J TALVENHEIMO (*University of Miami, Coral Gables, Fla.*): Any idea of the physical techniques that you would think are going to be more promising?

H. R. KABACK: I think that depends on the protein. With the *lac* permease, if it were possible to do proton NMR, that would be marvelous because the system moves protons. However, the possibility of doing protein NMR on the *lac* permease is very limited because we're about four orders of magnitude off the concentration required because of the solubility of the permease. There are problems at every level that look to be insurmountable at present, if you look at them all at the same time. However, the next generation of investigators will take individual portions of these problems and begin to resolve them. For example, a technology for doing hydrophobic HPLC on very hydrophobic proteins will be established! I don't think, however, there is any single technique that will yield the answer ultimately.

There is one physical technique that can yield lots of structural information, X-ray crystallography, but preparing crystals from something as hydrophobic as a membrane protein is not easy. This being the case, it is common practice these days to derive secondary structure models from DNA sequences, and some take these models as gospel, not as working models. This is not to say that this approach is not useful. Rather, it provides the investigator with a testable model. The difficulty is that there is no good way to test the model short of crystallization.

From DNA sequence data, the *lac* permease for instance yields models with 12–14 transmembrane helices which correlate reasonably well with data from circular dichroism and laser Raman spectroscopy. Based on such a model, we have synthesized every putatively exposed portion of the permease and made site-directed polyclonal antibodies. In principle, the approach seems reasonable. However, out of 16 or 20 of these antibodies, only 3 are useful, possibly because when the protein folds into its tertiary structure, not all of these loops are exposed. Alternatively, of course, the model could be wrong. The point is that a lot of time and effort is spent for minimal information. Perhaps the time would have been better spend trying to crystallize the permease.

I stress that I'm not pessimistic. To the contrary, I feel very enthusiastic about resolving these problems and I think they will be solved. However, I think it's going to take a lot of hard work from many directions. I don't think any single technique, site-directed mutagenesis included, is going to yield a complete solution. Site-directed mutagenesis is powerful, but it can't give all the answers in itself. One can determine what parts of a protein are interesting but not why unless one has more information.

R. D. KEYNES[a] (*University of Cambridge, Cambridge, United Kingdom*): I'd like to describe briefly a new model of the sodium channel gating mechanism which is based on observation of the sodium channel gating current (the asymmetrical displacement current) in the squid giant axon. First, the sodium gating current is not homogeneous but consists of two readily separable components with very different kinetics. One of these components has a fast rise, relaxes with a single time constant, and does not appear to be related to the state of inactivation of sodium conductance. The other component has a slower rise and double exponential relaxation, but appears to inactivate in a way that is closely linked to the inactivation of sodium conductance. These two components also display quite different sensitivities to drugs; for example, certain local anesthetics can dramatically reduce the inactivating component without affecting the noninactivating component of the gating current.

Several years ago I suggested that these components may arise in different parts of the membrane, and I proposed a "parallel activation model" in which the channel opens only when both components are in an open state. However, while this previous model can account very well for the observed properties of the sodium conductance, it leaves two features of the gating current unexplained. These features are the slow rise of the inactivating component and the increasing delay of this component at more negative starting potentials. In order to account for these observations I have made a modification of the parallel model by introducing a principle of "cross modulation." It is thus my suggestion that we ought to think harder about how two voltage-dependent conformational changes might modulate one another, as opposed to the sequential-coupling schemes that are in the literature at present. I also believe that modulation coupling may turn out to apply rather widely in channel gating.

C. F. STEVENS (*Yale University, New Haven, Conn.*): How can we find out the properties of the sodium channel, for example, the rate constant, the dependence of rate constant on voltage, how much charge moves from one conformational state to the

---

[a]For a further elaboration of these remarks, see Dr. Keynes's paper "Properties of the Sodium Gating Current in the Squid Giant Axon" in this volume.

next? Classically, what one does is start with a family of sodium currents and fit the Hodgkin-Huxley equations or some alternative theory to them. Then one extracts all the rate constants and tries to identify those rate constants with, say, the conformational change of a protein, for example moving a helix up one notch or something like that.

Now if one makes a list of the assumptions that one must have in order to make progress with those equations, it is quite a long list. For example, are channels identical and independent in their operation, or are they not? Assume that one is 90% sure that they are. Do channels have only one open state or do they have more than one open state? Say one is 90% sure that they have only one open state. Do they have more than one closed state or just one closed state? Let's say one can be 90% sure that they have more than one closed state. Anyway, by going through a list like this even with 90% certainty of each one of those assumptions that one has to make, when one multiplies 0.9 by 0.9 by 0.9 by 0.9—the number of times one has to for each assumption—the chances that the theory is going to be right is well less than 50–50. And I'm not even sure that I know 90% whether channels are identical and independent with 90% probability. So what I've been doing personally, then, is trying to get around this problem by getting functional information in a model-independent way.

What I really want to talk to you about are three areas I think are extremely important for sodium channel research that we need to focus on. The first one is structural information. We're not going to make any progress at all until at least we get low-resolution EM pictures of sodium channels, to put constraints on what they're going to be. It's been enormously helpful for the acetylcholine receptor channel and it's got to happen for the sodium channel.

Secondly, while I firmly believe that the clones we've seen so far are the sodium channel, until we can get expression of the RNA made from cDNA clones, we don't know what we have. For example, we don't know if they're missing subunits, or we don't know if we have potassium channels when we think they're sodium channels. Although we have the sequence, we've got to find out what the sequence corresponds to and if it's all there. That's a terribly important thing to be done before we can take the next step. Thirdly, some informed speculations.

Let me reiterate those three priorities. The first is structure, the second is finding out precisely what we have and how it relates to other things we know, and the third is guessing for the future what's going to be important. I think family relationships are going to be enormously important. I think it's going to be really revealing to see the sequence of sodium channels, calcium channels, various potassium channels, because I think that as soon as we can start defining relationships between families of channels, we'll be able get valuable clues about how individual channels work. I think that is going to be one of the most revealing things.

E. MOCZYDLOWSKI (*University of Cincinnati, Cincinnati, Ohio*): With the structure of channels that we've seen so far, it seems that we need to have an arrangement of subunits or homologous regions which are required to form a pore, which traverses the membrane. With carrier proteins and pumps, there must be some sort of hydrophilic pathway through the membrane for many of the polar molecules that get through. Is there any clue in the primary structure of the carriers that can allow us to relate carriers to channels?

H. R. KABACK: It is surprising to me that there is this kind of homology among different sodium channels, because with the three bacterial permeases that have been sequenced thus far, there is no homology at all. However, the hydropathic profiles are almost identical. Thus this could be either a good example of convergent evolution in which nature developed 30 different ways for proteins to snake through the membrane or of so many mutations since the primordial permease that the proteins no longer bear any resemblance.

J. YEH (*Northwestern University, Chicago, Ill.*): It is worth mentioning the use of interacting chemical probes to investigate channel mechanisms. For example, TTX blocks sodium current only when applied on the outside of the membrane, while the local anesthetic QX-314 only blocks current when it has access to the internal side of the channel. Neither of these agents produces a block in gating current when it is applied alone. However, when they are applied together a block of gating current results, in addition to the inhibition of sodium current. We have seen a similar effect with TTX and guanidine derivatives only when the guanidine is linked to a suitable long alkyl chain; shorter chains, for example propyl guanidine, block sodium current but do not block gating current in conjunction with TTX, whereas octyl guanidine does. We have evidence that this interaction is not based on length of the alkyl chain per se but rather on its hydrophobicity, suggesting that a hydrophobic domain of the channel is involved in this phenomenon. I suggest that these interactions could serve as a valuable approach for identifying structural domains involved in channel mechanism.

W. ALMERS (*University of Washington, Seattle, Washington*): This is sort of a more general point of an impression that I've gotten by listening to some of the talks here. Electrophysiologists can't measure very much. What they can measure they measure with tremendous accuracy. Consequently they are obsessed with details. Electrophysiologists have studied sodium channels in detail and they've found small differences between them. For instance, Pappone found that denervated sodium channels in muscle fibers that are TTX-insensitive are a little slower than the ones in squid axons; and you can go on like that. You can look for small differences and find them. Then electrophysiologists worry. What are those differences to mean in molecular terms? Do they mean anything at all? How much difference in the molecule do you need to produce these tiny differences that electrophysiologists see?

We've heard from people who've studied sodium channels biochemically, that they really are quite different. The brain channel, for instance, needs the β subunit that the eel channel does not need. The brain channel has a piece that the eel channel is missing altogether. Yet we have electrophysiological data for eel and brain; and they've been presented here and I've looked for differences and I've found none. So, where are we going to look to interpret differences that electrophysiologists see? We sort of get the feeling that the differences that we see are minor and perhaps irrelevant and yet there are large differences in the molecule that seem to not be at all reflected in the differences the electrophysiologists see.

O. ANDERSEN (*Cornell Medical College, New York, N.Y.*): Based upon low molecular-weight ion channels one can study in a planar bilayer, ion selectivity and voltage gating might only require a structure with a molecular weight of between 20,000 and 30,000 to be able to do anything the sodium channel is able to do. It seems unlikely that the tenfold larger molecule that represents the sodium channel is there just by random chance. A lot of that molecule might be there for reasons that we don't know.

I think the other question is that each time we want to take some of these extremely precise electrophysiological measurements and we'd like to interpret them in molecular terms, we first have to be quite certain that we actually are able to formulate the problem in such a way that the question is meaningful. Is it, for example, meaningful to talk about transition between discrete states? The more states that seem to come up in various gating states, the more you have to worry about whether that is no longer a fruitful way to look upon the problem. Very often I have a feeling that the problems we deal with may be that we have macroscopic intuitive notions of how the world should operate, but they are in no way relevant in trying to correlate detailed functional measurements in terms of molecular characteristics.

I would like to make two points regarding "group-specific modification" and "site-specific mutagenesis." First of all, even if one has detailed molecular resolution for a protein, how does one know after site-specific mutagenesis that the general structure is the same? That's important because in my own lab we found that the small peptide gramicidin channels actually can adopt a completely different conformation when simply modified.

Secondly, in terms of site-directed mutagenesis, one has to worry about the interpretation of the results. Is the site of altered function the point where one made the amino acid change? Is it in close or maybe not very close proximity to the point where one observed the functional perturbation? For example, one can have interactions over distances of at least 15 Å, which means that even though one modified amino acids and saw changes in gating or permeation, that may essentially just be a random finding which results from an ion dipole effect where two places in the molecule interact. Thus there is no critical functional basis for why this modulation occurs.

K. ANGELIDES (*University of Florida, Gainesville, Fla.*): I think we could probably learn a lot from previous examples of enzymes. We can look at enzymes which have the same functional groups and carry out the same organic chemistry yet have very different molecular shapes or structures. For example, simple enzymes like chymotrypsin and trypsin have the same functional groups and carry out the same catalysis, but have very different specific sites and their reactions are very different. So, I think what we should think of is a very restricted region where the catalysis is taken care of, but the extra baggage that this protein (or the channel) actually carries along with it confers the very subtle conformational flexibility necessary for function.

W. S. AGNEW (*Yale University, New Haven, Conn.*): One of the concerns I think we should have in thinking about site-specific mutagenesis is that especially for the elaborate proteins, these very large structures don't adopt the lowest thermodynamic conformation, the lowest energy conformation in the membrane. Rather the folding pattern that they're likely to adopt is going to be a product of the history of folding during biosynthesis, and thus modifying certain particularly conformationally important domains may produce a markedly altered structured in the final product. This consideration suggests that major controls have to be considered in designing a whole program of site-specific mutagenesis to avoid misinterpretation.

B. KRUEGER (*University of Maryland, Baltimore, Md.*): I wonder if it would be possible for one of the panelists to present to us a hypothetical, very simplified strategy by which site-directed mutagenesis could lead to some specific information about the structure of a particular site on the sodium channel. Frankly, it's not entirely clear to me how in a step-by step manner that process could really elucidate structure.

C. F. STEVENS: One has to start with some hypotheses. So, just hypothetically, suppose that one had two proposed structures for the sodium channel. What one might do then is find a bunch of amino acids that would provide negative charges around the mouth of the channel in either model, and one would then change those amino acids for other amino acids. Of course, one would have to think about what these substitutions might do to the whole structure, and one might have to do different kinds of controls. Next one would do voltage-current relationships.

Finally one would figure out what voltage-current relationships ought to occur if a certain number and concentration of charges where changed at the mouth of the channel. Thus, insofar as two different schemes would make different predictions about these changes, one is then testing each of those schemes by changing the amino acids. In summary, one has to make a specific hypothesis, test it in several different ways, and make alternative hypotheses.

B. KRUEGER: Where did the original model come from and how were the particular amino acids identified that would be altered?

C. F. STEVENS: One has to have some model for the structure. For example, for the acetylcholine receptor, we knew that the acetylcholine receptor binding site was near a cystine that you could identify (*i.e.*, Cys 192–193). Thus one knows that the amino acids that end up near that are going to be involved in acetylcholine binding. That's one way of identifying which amino acids one would be interested in.

Another way is to propose models for how the channel might be folded up, and one could test those models in various ways. For example, suppose that a certain folding scheme is proposed from hydropathic analysis and a certain reactive group is predicted that ought to get labeled on the outside. One could then do the labeling experiment with a group-specific reagent and then check and see if that specific group was labeled.

So one can obtain biochemical evidence for locating particular amino acids and a very low resolution kind of proposed structure can be inferred which predicts a number of membrane crossings. Then one might make use of molecular biology or other techniques to find out whether that model is correct. So it's just hard work, but the more information, the more chemical information, the more structural information one has, and the more other constraints one has in the models, the better the work one can do with them.

H. R. KABACK: One can always ask the question whether the functional effect of a site-directed modification is secondary to a local conformational alteration, especially when precise structural information is lacking. However, there are genetic approaches that can be used to approximate answers to such questions. One can start with a given site-directed mutant, select reversions to the wild-type phenotype, and then sequence the revertant genes. If the original mutation is retained and a secondary mutation cures the defect, it is apparent that the original mutated residue cannot be obligatorily involved in the mechanism. On the other hand, if all of the revertants are shown to be back mutations to wild-type in the mutated codon, one can conclude that the residue encoded is important in the mechanism. However, without further information, one cannot differentiate whether it is important for structural or mechanistic reasons.

T. NARAHASHI (*Northwestern University, Chicago, Ill.*): Just a brief comment on the environment of channels. We now know the amino acid sequence of the sodium channel, but this only gives a static picture. As a physiologist, I look at channels in dynamic equilibrium, embedded in a lipid environment. Nobody has been able to measure channel activity alone without this environment, and this environment could be very important, for example, in the differences we see in TTX sensitivity in different tissues and at different stages of development and so on and so forth. Thus these differences may not be due to the channel per se but may be the result of different environments. So we have to take a look at the effect of environment, because channel-gating kinetics obviously will be affected by what lipid surrounds the channel and what environment the channel is embedded in.

S. R. LEVINSON (*University of Colorado, Denver, Colorado*): That's a point we were trying to make too, namely that there might be lipids in very close association with the channel and that it might be hard to distinguish between channel mechanism due to protein and channel mechanism due to general membrane structure. This consideration adds a further complication to this whole business of how you go about elucidating mechanism.

Index of Contributors

447